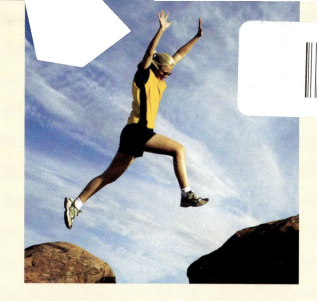

A Fit and Well Way of Life

GWEN ROBBINS / DEBBIE POWERS / SHARON BURGESS

Ball State University

Boston   Burr Ridge, IL   Dubuque, IA   New York   San Francisco   St. Louis
Bangkok   Bogotá   Caracas   Kuala Lumpur   Lisbon   London   Madrid   Mexico City
Milan   Montreal   New Delhi   Santiago   Seoul   Singapore   Sydney   Taipei   Toronto

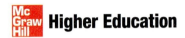

Higher Education

Published by McGraw-Hill, an imprint of The McGraw-Hill Companies, Inc., 1221 Avenue of the Americas, New York, NY 10020. Copyright © 2008 by The McGraw-Hill Companies. All rights reserved. No part of this publication may be reproduced or distributed in any form or by any means, or stored in a database or retrieval system, without the prior written consent of The McGraw-Hill Companies, Inc., including, but not limited to, in any network or other electronic storage or transmission, or broadcast for distance learning.

This book is printed on acid-free paper.

1 2 3 4 5 6 7 8 9 0 DOW/DOW 0 9 8 7

ISBN: 978-0-07-352365-1
MHID: 0-07-352365-8

Vice President and Editor-in-Chief: Emily Barrosse
Publisher: William R. Glass
Executive Editor: Christopher Johnson
Director of Development: Kathleen Engelberg
Developmental Editors: Sarah B. Hill and Carlotta Seely
Executive Marketing Manager: Nick Agnew
Media Project Manager: Michele Perez
Developmental Editor for Technology: Julia D. Akpan
Production Editor: Leslie LaDow
Designer: Cassandra Chu

Cover Designer: Joan Greenfield
Interior Designer: Susan Breitbard
Photo Research Coordinator: Natalia Peschiera
Art Editor: Emma Ghiselli
Production Supervisor: Randy Hurst
Composition: 10.5/12 Garamond by Carlisle Publishing Services
Printing: 45# Publishers Matte Plus by RR Donnelley & Sons

Cover image: © Brand X Pictures/Punchstock

Credits: The credits section for this book begins on page C-1 and is considered an extension of the copyright page.

Library of Congress Cataloging-in-Publication Data

Robbins, Gwen
    A fit and well way of life / Gwen Robbins, Debbie Powers, Sharon Burgess.–1st ed.
        p. cm.
    Includes bibliographical references and index.
    ISBN-13: 978-0-07-352365-1 (alk. paper)
    ISBN-10: 0-07-352365-8 (alk. paper)
        1. Health. I. Powers, Debbie. II. Burgess, Sharon. III. Title.

RA776.R63 2006
613–dc22

                                        2006044961

The Internet addresses listed in the text were accurate at the time of publication. The inclusion of a Web site does not indicate an endorsement by the authors or McGraw-Hill, and McGraw-Hill does not guarantee the accuracy of the information presented at these sites.

www.mhhe.com

Brief Contents

Preface xiii

1   **Understanding Wellness**   1

2   **Changing Behavior**   31

3   **Developing and Assessing Physical Fitness**   57

4   **Maximizing Cardiorespiratory Fitness**   107

5   **Developing Flexibility**   159

6   **Developing Muscular Fitness**   177

7   **Exploring Special Exercise Considerations**   225

8   **Preventing Common Injuries and Caring for the Lower Back**   251

9   **Maximizing Heart Health**   277

10   **Coping with Stress**   315

11   **Eating for Wellness**   363

12   **Achieving a Healthy Weight**   407

Appendixes A-1

Credits C-1

Glossary G-1

Index I-1

Contents

Preface   xiii

CHAPTER 1 Understanding Wellness   1

Healthy Life Expectancy and the Costs   3
  Determinants of Health and Longevity   4
    Heredity   4
    Social Circumstances   4
    Environmental Conditions   5
    Medical Care   5
    Lifestyle Behaviors   5
  The Power of Prevention   5
  Healthy People 2010   5
  Understanding Risks   6
High-Level Wellness   7
  The Dimensions of Wellness   9
    Physical Dimension   9
    Intellectual Dimension   9
    Emotional Dimension   10
    Social Dimension   10
    Spiritual Dimension   10
    Environmental Dimension   11
    Occupational Dimension   11
  Growth in Wellness   11
    Awareness   12
    Assessment   12
    Knowledge   12
    Self-Management Skills   13
    Motivation   13
    Support and Opportunity   13
    Self-Responsibility   13
Societal Norms   14
  Changing Times: Making Wellness the Norm   15
Frequently Asked Questions   16
Summary   17
Internet Resources   17
Lab Activity 1-1   Healthy Lifestyle: A Self-Assessment   21
Lab Activity 1-2   Assessing Your Wellness   25
Lab Activity 1-3   Societal Norms: The Unwritten Codes   29

CHAPTER 2 Changing Behavior   31

More Than Willpower   32
The Transtheoretical Model of Behavior Change   33
  The Processes of Change   35
Making a Plan   39
  Identifying Your Goal   39
  Listing Pros and Cons   41
Preventing Relapse   42
  Factors That Contribute to Relapses   43
Frequently Asked Questions   44
Summary   45
Internet Resources   45
Lab Activity 2-1   Identify Your Current Stage of Change   47
Lab Activity 2-2   Identify Your S.M.A.R.T. Goal   49
Lab Activity 2-3   Behavior-Change Contract (Using the Transtheoretical Model)   51
Lab Activity 2-4   Behavior-Change Log/Journal   53
Lab Activity 2-5   I've Had a Setback. . . . Now What?   55

CHAPTER 3 Developing and Assessing Physical Fitness   57

Importance of Exercise   58
Physical Activity and Health: A Report of the Surgeon General   59
  Moderate Physical Activity for Health Promotion   61
  The Activity Pyramid   62
What Is Physical Fitness?   63
Health-Related Components of Fitness   64
  Cardiorespiratory Endurance   64
  Muscular Strength   64
  Muscular Endurance   64
  Flexibility   64
  Body Composition   64

Physical Fitness and Wellness   64

Three-Part Workout   65
Warm-Up   65
Conditioning Bout   66
Cool-Down   66

Principles of Fitness Development   66
Progressive Overload   66
Specificity   66
Reversibility   66
Individual Differences   67

Cross Training   67

Assessing Physical Fitness   67

Guidelines for Medical Clearance   68

Cardiorespiratory Endurance Tests   68
Pretest Instructions   69
1.5-Mile Run Test   69
1-Mile Walk Test   70
3-Mile Bicycling Test   70
500-Yard Swim Test   70
500-Yard Water Run Test   70
3-Minute Step Test   71

Muscular Strength and Endurance Tests   72
Abdominal Curls   72
Push-Ups   72
Leg Press Strength Test   72
Bench Press Strength Test   75

Flexibility Tests   75
Quick Checks for Flexibility   75
Sit and Reach Test   75
Sit and Reach Wall Test   77

Body Composition Tests   77
Body Composition Assessment Using Skinfold Calipers   78
Body Girth Measures   79
Body Girth Measures of Body Fat   79
Waist-to-Hip Ratio and Waist Girth   81

Frequently Asked Questions   82

Summary   82

Internet Resources   83

Lab Activity 3-1   Student Precourse Health Assessment   87

Lab Activity 3-2   Physician-Approved Exercise Clearance Form   88

Lab Activity 3-3   Personal Fitness Profile   89

Lab Activity 3-4   Evaluating Your Cardiorespiratory Fitness: 1.5-Mile Run Test and 1.0-Mile Walk Test   91

Lab Activity 3-5   Evaluating Your Cardiorespiratory Fitness: 500-Yard Water Run Test and 500-Yard Swim Test   93

Lab Activity 3-6   Evaluating Your Cardiorespiratory Fitness: 3-Minute Step Test   95

Lab Activity 3-7   Evaluating Your Muscular Endurance: Abdominal Curls Test and Push-Ups Test   97

Lab Activity 3-8   Evaluating Your Muscular Strength: Leg Press Strength Test and Bench Press Strength Test   99

Lab Activity 3-9   Evaluating Your Flexibility: Sit and Reach and Flexibility Quick Checks   101

Lab Activity 3-10   Body Composition Assessment   103

Lab Activity 3-11   Fitness Goals   105

CHAPTER 4   *Maximizing Cardiorespiratory Fitness   107*

Cardiorespiratory Endurance and Maximal Oxygen Uptake   108
Benefits of Aerobic Exercise   108
Improved Mental Health   109
Improved Cognitive Function   110
Improved Sleep   110
Immune System Function   110
Improved Body Composition and Weight Management   110
Reduced Risk of Chronic Diseases   110

The FITT Prescription for Cardiorespiratory Fitness   111
"F" Equals Frequency   111
"I" Equals Intensity   111
Target Heart Rate: Karvonen Equation   112
Talk Test   113
Rate of Perceived Exertion (RPE)   113
Target Heart Rate: Percentage of Maximal Heart Rate   114
"T" Equals Time   114
"T" Equals Type   114
How Long Before Results Become Apparent?   115
Various Exercise Guidelines Lead to Confusion   115

Lifetime Exercise Activities   115

10,000 Steps: A Daily Lifestyle Goal   116

Aerobic Dance   118
Advantages/Disadvantages   118
What to Wear   119
Technique and Safety Tips   120
How to Begin and Progress   120
Variety   121
Step Aerobics   121
Indoor Cycling Classes (Spinning or Fit Ride)   121
Common Discomforts   122

Bicycling   122
Advantages/Disadvantages   122
What to Wear   122
Equipment   122
Technique and Safety Tips   123
How to Begin and Progress   124
Variety   125
Common Discomforts   125

Fitness Swimming   125
  Advantages/Disadvantages   125
  What to Wear   126
  Technique and Safety Tips   126
  How to Begin and Progress   126
  Variety   126
  Discomforts   127

Fitness Walking   127
  Advantages/Disadvantages   127
  What to Wear   128
  Technique and Safety Tips   128
  Tips for Increasing Walking Pace   129
  How to Begin and Progress   130
  Variety   131
  Common Discomforts   132

Indoor Exercise Equipment   133
  Advantages/Disadvantages   133
  What to Wear   133
  Equipment   133
  Stationary Bikes   134
  Advantages/Disadvantages   134
  How to Select   134
  Technique and Safety Tips   134
  Steppers   134
  Advantages/Disadvantages   134
  How to Select   134
  Technique and Safety Tips   134
  Treadmills   134
  Advantages/Disadvantages   134
  How to Select   135
  Technique and Safety Tips   135
  Ski Machines   135
  Advantages/Disadvantages   135
  How to Select   135
  Technique and Safety Tips   135
  Rowing Machines   135
  Advantages/Disadvantages   135
  How to Select   135
  Technique and Safety Tips   135
  Elliptical Trainers   136
  Advantages/Disadvantages   136
  How to Select   136
  Technique and Safety Tips   136
  How to Begin and Progress   136

In-Line Skating   137
  Advantages/Disadvantages   137
  What to Wear   138
  Necessary Gear   138
  Technique and Safety Tips   138
  Skate Maintenance   139
  How to Begin and Progress   139
  Variety   139
  Common Discomforts   139

Jogging   140
  Advantages/Disadvantages   140
  What to Wear   140

  Technique and Safety Tips   140
  How to Begin and Progress   141
  Variety   141
  Common Discomforts   142

Water Exercise/Aqua Aerobics   142
  Advantages/Disadvantages   142
  What to Wear   142
  Technique and Safety Tips   142
  How to Begin and Progress   143
  Variety   143
  Common Discomforts   144

Frequently Asked Questions   145

Summary   146

General Resources   147

Internet Resources   147

Lab Activity 4-1 Calculate Your Target Heart Rate (THR) Range   149

Lab Activity 4-2 Using a Pedometer: "How Many Steps Do I Take?"   151

Lab Activity 4-3 30-Minute Treadmill Workouts   155

Lab Activity 4-4 Cardiorespiratory Exercise Log Sheet   157

CHAPTER

5

Developing Flexibility   159

Flexibility   160
  Benefits of Flexibility   160
    Cautions   161
  Factors Affecting Flexibility   161
    Joint Structure   161
    Soft Tissues   161
    Inactivity   161
    Muscle Temperature   161
    Age   162
    Genetics   162
    Gender   162
    Obesity   162
    Injury and Scar Tissue   162
    Neural Factors   162
  Types of Flexibility   162
  Guidelines for Flexibility Development   163
  Principles of Flexibility Development   164
    Progressive Overload   164
    Specificity   164
    Reversibility   164
    Individual Differences   164
    Balance   164
  Flexibility Exercises for Basic Fitness   164
  PNF Partner-Assisted Stretches   165
  Other Programs for Enhancing Flexibility   166

Contraindicated Exercises   167

Frequently Asked Questions   **171**

Summary   **172**

Internet Resources   **172**

Lab Activity 5-1   Sample Flexibility Program   173

Lab Activity 5-2   Hatha Yoga Workout: Sun Salutation (or Salute to the Sun)   175

CHAPTER 6
Developing Muscular Fitness   177

Muscular Fitness   **178**

Resistance Training: Benefits and Cautions   178

Muscle Function   181

Determinants of Muscular Fitness Gains   181

Muscle Fiber Recruitment   *181*

Muscle Atrophy and Hypertrophy   *182*

Gender Differences   *182*

Types of Resistance Training Programs   182

Static (Isometric) Exercise   *182*

Dynamic (Isotonic) Exercise   *182*

Principles of Resistance Training   183

Progressive Overload   *183*

Specificity   *183*

Recovery   *183*

Guidelines for Developing Muscular Fitness   183

Sequence   *184*

Form   *184*

Rest Between Sets   *184*

Muscle Balance   *184*

Breathing   *185*

Speed of Movement   *185*

Resistance Training Programs   185

Weight Training   *185*

Equipment   *186*

Weight Room Etiquette   *186*

Program for Health Fitness   *187*

How to Begin and Progress   *191*

Establishing Your Workload   *191*

Increasing Your Workload   *192*

Variety   *192*

Common Discomforts and Training Errors   *193*

Performance Aids   *193*

How to Shape and Tone Without Weights   193

Abdominal and Core Strengthening Exercises   *194*

Hip and Thigh Exercises   *196*

Upper Body Exercises   *197*

Stability Balls   *198*

Pilates   *201*

Elastic Resistance   201

Partner Resistance Exercises   204

Frequently Asked Questions   **206**

Summary   **207**

Internet Resources   **208**

Lab Activity 6-1   Resistance Training Log   211

Lab Activity 6-2   Weight Training Experience   213

Lab Activity 6-3   Abdominal and Core Strengthening Workout   217

Lab Activity 6-4   Stability Ball Workout   219

Lab Activity 6-5   Elastic Band Workout   221

Lab Activity 6-6   Partner Resistance Workout   223

CHAPTER 7
Exploring Special Exercise Considerations   225

Similarities and Differences in Men's and Women's Exercise Performance   **226**

Females and Exercise   **226**

Menstruation   226

Female Athlete Triad   228

Pregnancy   229

Stress Incontinence   *230*

Kegel Exercise   *230*

Postpartum: Getting Back into Shape   *231*

Breast Support   *231*

Males and Exercise   **231**

Exercise Addiction   **232**

Exercise and Disease Resistance   **233**

Environmental Considerations   **233**

Exercising in the Cold   233

Exercising in the Heat   235

Heavy Sweating During Exercise   *235*

Electrolyte Replacement   *236*

Fluid Replacement: Water or Sports Drinks?   *237*

Water: Are Americans Dehydrated?   237

Aging and Physical Activity   **238**

Aging and Performance   239

Does Exercise Increase Life Span?   241

Exercise and Chronic Health Conditions   **242**

Arthritis   242

Asthma   242

Diabetes Mellitus   243

Hypertension   244

Osteoporosis   244

Frequently Asked Questions   **246**

Summary   **247**

Internet Resources   **247**

Lab Activity 7-1   Exploring Special Exercise Considerations Challenge   249

CHAPTER 8

Preventing Common Injuries and Caring for the Lower Back   251

Injury Prevention   252
Overuse   252
Footwear   254
Weakness and Inflexibility   254
Mechanics   255

P.R.I.C.E.   256
P = Protect   257
R = Rest   257
I = Ice   257
C = Compress   258
E = Elevate   258

Heat and Pain Relievers   258

Common Injuries   258
Ankle Sprain   258
Blisters   259
Bursitis   260
Chafing   260
Heel Spur   260
Iliotibial Band Syndrome   260
Muscle Cramp   260
Muscle Soreness   260
Muscle Strain   261
Patellofemoral Syndrome   261
Plantar Fasciitis   261
Shin Splint   262
Side Stitch   263
Stress Fracture   263
Tendinitis   263

When to Seek Medical Help   264

Getting Back into Action   265

Care of the Lower Back   265
Ways to Avoid Lower Back Pain   265
Back Tips for Sitting, Standing, and Driving   268
Lower Back Injuries   269
Core Exercises for Lower Back Health   269

Frequently Asked Questions   270

Summary   271

Internet Resources   271

Lab Activity 8-1   Phil A. Case Study   273

Lab Activity 8-2   Action Plan for the Back   275

CHAPTER 9

Maximizing Heart Health   277

Impact of Cardiovascular Disease   278
Coronary Heart Disease (CHD)   280
Atherosclerosis   280
Angina Pectoris   281
Myocardial Infarction (MI)   282
Stroke (Brain Attack)   282

Risk Factors   283
Primary Risk Factors   283
1. Inactivity   283
2. High Blood Pressure (Hypertension)   285
3. High Blood Lipid Profile (Cholesterol and Triglycerides)   286
4. Cigarette Smoking   291
5. Obesity   292
6. Diabetes Mellitus (Type 1 and Type 2)   293
Secondary Risk Factors   295
1. Stress   295
2. Emotional Behavior   296
3. Age   297
4. Male Gender   297
5. Race   297
6. Positive Family History   298
The Emerging Risk Factors   298
Metabolic Syndrome   298
Homocysteine   298
C-Reactive Protein (CRP)   299

Treatment for Blocked Coronary Arteries   299
Drug Therapy   300
Angioplasty (or Balloon Angioplasty)   300
Coronary Bypass Surgery   300

The Future . . . Focus on Lifestyle   300
Mind and Body Connection   301

Frequently Asked Questions   302

Summary   303

Internet Resources   304

Lab Activity 9-1   Are You at Risk for Heart Disease?   307

Lab Activity 9-2   Evaluation of "Are You at Risk for Heart Disease?"   309

Lab Activity 9-3   How to Mend a Broken Heart   311

Lab Activity 9-4   Are You at Risk for Diabetes?   313

CHAPTER 10

Coping with Stress   315

What Is Stress?   317

The Stress Response: A Three-Stage Process   317
Fight-or-Flight (Alarm Reaction)   318
Stage of Resistance   319
Stage of Exhaustion   320

Perception and Control   320

Harmful Effects of Stress   321

Measuring Your Stress   322

Daily Hassles and Uplifts   325

Type A, B, and D Personalities and Stress   326
The Hot Reactor   327

Angry/Hostile Behavior Modification   328

The Stress-Resistant Hardy Person   329

Building Skills for Stress Management   331

Strategy #1: Exercise   332

Strategy #2: Relaxation Techniques   332
  2a. Meditation   332
  2b. Autogenic Training and Imagery   333
  2c. Jacobson's Progressive Relaxation   334
  2d. Abdominal Breathing   334
  2e. Hatha Yoga   334
  2f. Massage   335
  2g. Biofeedback Training   335

Strategy #3: Lifestyle Change   335
  3a. The Impact of Diet   335
  3b. Time Management   336
  3c. Alcohol, Drugs, and Cigarettes   337
  3d. Get Plenty of Restful Sleep   337
  3e. Develop Satisfying Relationships   338
  3f. Learn When to Seek the Help and Support of
      Others   338
  3g. Schedule "Me Time" and Listen to Music   338

Strategy #4: Reframing   339

Strategy #5: Laughter and Humor   339

Strategy #6: Create a Memory Bank   339

Frequently Asked Questions   340

Summary   341

Internet Resources   342

Lab Activity 10-1   Evaluation of the Life Event Stress
                    Test   345

Lab Activity 10-2   How to Meditate and Experience the
                    Relaxation Response   347

Lab Activity 10-3   Becoming Stress-Resistant and
                    Hardy   349

Lab Activity 10-4   Relaxation   351

Lab Activity 10-5   Measuring Your Stress and Coping
                    Skills   353

Lab Activity 10-6   Time Management   357

Lab Activity 10-7   Changing Behavior Using the
                    Transtheoretical Model   361

CHAPTER 11 Eating for Wellness   363

Changing Times   364
  Dietary Guidelines for Americans   366

Nutrition Basics   367
  Carbohydrates   367
    Simple Carbohydrates (Sugars)   367
    Complex Carbohydrates (Starches)   367
    Whole Grains Versus Refined Flours   369
    Glycemic Index   369
  Proteins   370
  Fats   370
    Fish Oils   372
    Cholesterol   373
  Vitamins   373
  Minerals   373
    Calcium   374
    Iron   377
    Sodium   377
  Water   377

Phytochemicals and Antioxidants: Disease
  Fighters   378
  Nutritional Supplements   378

The Well-Balanced Diet   379
  USDA's MyPyramid   380
  DASH Eating Plan   382
  Making Positive Changes   383
  Nutrition Labeling   384

Eating Out   386

Special Nutritional Concerns   387
  Vegetarian Diet   387
  Pregnancy   387
  Aging   388
  Sports and Fitness   389

Frequently Asked Questions   390

Summary   391

Internet Resources   391

Lab Activity 11-1   Food Log   395

Lab Activity 11-2   Analyze Your Diet   397

Lab Activity 11-3   How Much Fat?   399

Lab Activity 11-4   Label Reading Assignment   401

Lab Activity 11-5   Changing Behavior Using the
                    Transtheoretical Model   403

Lab Activity 11-6   Can You Eat Healthy at a Fast-Food
                    Restaurant?   405

CHAPTER 12 Achieving a Healthy Weight   407

Understanding Body Composition   410
  Overweight Versus Obesity   410
  Risks Associated with Obesity   411
    Location of Fat   412

The Surgeon General Steps In   413

What Causes Obesity?   414
  The Energy Balance Equation   414
  Fat-Cell Theory   414
  Set-Point Theory   416
  Heredity   417
  Metabolism   417

What About "Dieting"?   418
  Weight Cycling   420
  Reliable Weight-Loss Programs   420

Lifetime Weight Management: Staying Lean in Fattening Times   420
  Food Management   421
    Recognizing Portion Distortion   421
    Avoiding Mindless Eating   422
    Understanding Our "Toxic" Environment   422
  Emotional Management   422
  Exercise Management   424

Gaining Weight: A Healthy Plan for Adding Pounds   427

Culture and Weight   428
  There She Is . . . Miss Unrealistic America   428
  Men Are Joining In   429

Eating Disorders   429
  Bulimia Nervosa   430
  Anorexia Nervosa   430
  Binge Eating Disorder   431
  Eating Disorders Not Otherwise Specified (EDNOS)   432
  What Can Be Done?   432

Frequently Asked Questions   433

Summary   434

Internet Resources   435

Lab Activity 12-1   Why Do You Eat? (A Food Journal)   439

Lab Activity 12-2   How Active Are You?   441

Lab Activity 12-3   Estimating Your Basal Metabolic Rate (BMR)   443

Lab Activity 12-4   Weight Management Plan   445

Lab Activity 12-5   Are You at Risk for an Eating Disorder?   447

Appendixes   A-1

Credits   C-1

Glossary   G-1

Index   I-1

Preface

This book is your guide for how to live life to your fullest potential. In the past, people delegated responsibility for their health and well-being to medical professionals. Today the tide is changing as evidence points to healthy behaviors as the key to lifelong vitality, wellness, and longevity. This means the lifestyle choices you make every day can dictate your present and future well-being. The purpose of *A Fit and Well Way of Life* is to help you pursue your wellness potential. Do you want straightforward explanations on how to live your best life? Do you want to know what really counts? This book is a road map for this exciting journey. The road map includes two essential components: (1) knowledge and (2) tools for action.

You may have heard the phrase "Knowledge is power." However, we believe that "Knowledge is *potential* power." It is vitally important to have accurate, up-to-date information about exercise, nutrition, stress, heart disease, weight management, and other health topics. So we have sorted through the array of confusing and sometimes contradictory health information to provide information in this book based on solid research. We have minimized technical jargon and have presented the material in consumer-friendly language. But knowledge alone is not enough to change behavior. If so, no one would smoke and everyone would wear seat belts. Many people know what to do but just don't do it! To make lifestyle changes, you need to take knowledge and move into *action*. *A Fit and Well Way of Life* sets the stage for this by providing many useful tools for action so you can apply the information to your everyday life. As you read each chapter, you'll find self-assessments, behavior-change strategies, and tips for making daily decisions that can lead to enhanced wellness. We hope that these practical suggestions will guide and motivate you. Assuming responsibility for your own well-being is a powerful step toward wellness. There is no better feeling than to know that you are empowered to take charge of your health—and resist cultural norms that challenge this way of thinking.

A Fit and Well Way of Life is designed to help you become an informed wellness consumer who acknowledges control of your own lifestyle decisions and embraces the opportunity to make positive choices for a lifetime. The result will be the joy of knowing that you are working toward your highest potential for well-being. And you will discover that this proactive, take-charge attitude becomes a normal way of thinking—truly a way of life! We have been successful in teaching and guiding thousands of college students and colleagues to embrace wellness as a positive way of living. We can help you, too. Are you ready? Let's go!

AUDIENCE

This text is designed to meet the needs of a course that goes beyond the basics of physical fitness to encompass the broader scope of wellness. The content—covering all aspects of fitness, heart health, stress management, nutrition, and weight management—easily accommodates a variety of fitness, wellness, and health courses. It is a flexible book that fits nicely into a lecture/fitness activity format.

WHY THE PROCHASKA TRANSTHEORETICAL MODEL OF BEHAVIOR CHANGE?

The Prochaska transtheoretical model of behavior change is included in this text because of its proven effectiveness in changing behavior. This easy-to-use model presents concrete strategies rather than vague resolutions to help people make permanent lifestyle changes. Psychologists James Prochaska, John Norcross, and Carlo DiClemente studied individuals who had successfully changed health-related behaviors on their own. What these researchers discovered during their years of studying behavior change is that individuals progress through distinct stages of change on their way to improved well-being. Their initial research was done on people who quit smoking but has expanded to cover other health behaviors. The stages of change are as follows:

1. *Precontemplation.* People at this stage see no problem with their behavior and have no intention of changing it.
2. *Contemplation.* In this stage, people come to understand their problem and its causes, and they start to think about taking action to solve it.
3. *Preparation.* In the preparation stage, people are planning to take action within the next month and are putting together a plan of action.
4. *Action.* A person in the action stage has taken the leap and is actively making behavior changes.
5. *Maintenance.* Even after action has been taken successfully, it must be maintained to prevent relapse.

Prochaska and his colleagues noted that certain behavioral change techniques work better than others in some stages of change. This model has received a great deal of attention in the popular press and among health educators. We hope this method assists you in your wellness journey.

SUCCESSFUL FEATURES

A Fit and Well Way of Life includes a number of features that make learning easy:

Chapter Objectives

Each chapter begins with a list of objectives, providing students with a starting point and a focus for the chapter.

Key Terms

Important terms are highlighted in boldface to capture students' attention, increase retention, and identify those terms found in the Glossary.

Top 10 Lists

Appearing in each chapter, the Top 10 boxes offer additional insight into chapter topics. Examples include ways to exercise if you have diabetes and tips for having a safer party.

Diversity Issues

This feature addresses fitness and wellness issues for various cultures and ethnic backgrounds. Sample topics include health disparities among Americans, the nutritional value of different ethnic foods, and weight differences in various ethnic groups.

Frequently Asked Questions

This popular feature highlights the questions about fitness and wellness that seem to be on everyone's mind. It addresses myths and offers practical approaches to fitness and wellness.

Chapter Summary

Each chapter includes a summary at the end that reinforces learning and helps students review for exams.

Internet Resources

This end-of-chapter list offers suggestions for further exploration of chapter-related topics.

Bibliography

The bibliography at the end of each chapter includes the sources used as references for the chapter content.

Lab Activities

Conveniently located at the end of each chapter, these labs help students apply their learning to their everyday lives.

Appendixes

The appendixes to *A Fit and Well Way of Life* include Outside Reading Assignment and Reaction Paper to Guest Speaker forms.

SUPPLEMENTS FOR INSTRUCTORS

Instructor's Media DVD-ROM (0-07-327780-0)

Organized by chapter, this instructor DVD-ROM includes all the resources you need to help teach your course: Course Integrator Guide, Test Bank, Computerized Test Bank, PowerPoint slides, and high-definition videos. The DVD-ROM works in both Windows and Macintosh environments and includes the following resources:

✔ **Course Integrator Guide.** This manual includes all the features of a useful instructor's manual, such as key concepts, lecture outlines, suggested activities, media resources, and Web links. It also integrates the text with all the related resources McGraw-Hill offers, such as the Online Learning Center, and the high-definition videos included on the DVD-ROM.
✔ **Test Bank.** The electronic Test Bank (Microsoft Word files) offers more than 1,800 questions,

including multiple choice, true-false, and short answer questions.

✔ **Computerized Test Bank.** The Test Bank is available with the EZ Test computerized testing software, which provides a powerful, easy-to-use way to create printed quizzes and exams. EZ Test runs on both Windows and Macintosh systems. For secure online testing, exams created in EZ Test can be exported to WebCT, Blackboard, PageOut, and EZ Test Online. EZ Test is packaged with a Quick Start Guide. Once the program is installed, you have access to the complete User's Manual, including Flash tutorials. Additional help is available at www.mhhe.com/eztest.

✔ **Classroom Performance System Test and Polling Questions.** These questions have been written for use with the Classroom Performance System and include objective test questions and subjective polling questions. Please see Other Resources for a full description of CPS.

✔ **PowerPoint Slides.** A comprehensive set of PowerPoint lecture slides, ready for use in your class, was prepared by a wellness professional. The slides correspond to the content in each chapter of *A Fit and Well Way of Life,* making it easier for you to teach and ensuring that your students will be able to follow your lectures point by point. You can modify the presentation as much as you like to meet your teaching needs.

✔ **High-Definition Videos.** These videos are correlated to *A Fit and Well Way of Life* and are designed to help you engage students in class discussions and promote critical thinking about fitness and wellness topics. The videos feature student interviews and historical health videos on body image, depression, and many other topics. Videos and images can be searched by chapter, topic, or media type. Once a video is located, it can be downloaded to a computer, saved to a playlist for later viewing, or simply viewed by double-clicking. For selected video clips, an Instructor's Guide is available to describe the objective of the clip, provide critical thinking questions to ask before the video is shown, and suggest follow-up discussion questions.

✔ **Image Bank.** This collection of illustrations from the text of *A Fit and Well Way of Life* can be used to highlight lecture points or be incorporated into PowerPoint slides.

Online Learning Center
www.mhhe.com/robbinsfitwell1e

The Online Learning Center to accompany *A Fit and Well Way of Life,* designed with different features for in-

structors and for students, offers a number of special resources for instructors:

✔ Downloadable PowerPoint presentations
✔ Course Integrator Guide
✔ Downloadable quizzes and polling questions (for use with Classroom Performance Systems)
✔ Lecture-launcher videos
✔ Links to professional resources
✔ Image Bank

Online Interactive Labs

Online interactive Lab Activities that enable students to assess their wellness and plan for a healthier lifestyle are available for instructors using Blackboard and WebCT course management systems. These labs can be assigned to and completed by students online and submitted to the instructor via the Blackboard or WebCT gradebook. The completed labs can also be printed.

SUPPLEMENTS FOR STUDENTS

Online Learning Center
www.mhhe.com/robbinsfitwell1e

The Online Learning Center contains many study tools, including the following:

✔ Self-scoring chapter quizzes
✔ Flashcards and concentration games
✔ Key terms
✔ Learning objectives
✔ HealthQuest activities
✔ Web links
✔ Extra Lab Activities
✔ Additional resources

Exercise Band (0-07-039473-3)

The elastic exercise band (Thera-Band™), packaged with the text of *A Fit and Well Way of Life,* is lightweight and portable and is used to add resistance when performing exercises. A comprehensive exercise program with instructions for using the exercise band is described and illustrated in Chapter 6. This program also appears conveniently on the inside and outside back cover of this text.

Health and Fitness Pedometer (0-07-320933-3)

An electronic digital pedometer (step counter) can be packaged with *A Fit and Well Way of Life.* This pedometer is useful in tracking walking steps, miles/kilometers, and kilocalories.

OTHER RESOURCES

Daily Fitness and Nutrition Journal (0-07-302988-2)

This logbook helps students track their diet and exercise programs. It can be packaged with any McGraw-Hill textbook for a small additional fee.

HealthQuest CD-ROM (0-07-295117-6)

This interactive CD helps students explore and change their wellness behavior. It includes tutorials, assessments, and behavior change guidelines in key areas such as nutrition, fitness, stress, cardiovascular disease, cancer, tobacco, and alcohol.

NutritionCalc Plus http://nutritioncalc.mhhe.com

✔ Online 2.0 (Package 0-07-321925-8; Standalone 0-07-321924-X)
✔ CD-ROM 2.0 (Package 0-07-319570-7; Standalone 0-07-319532-4)

NutritionCalc Plus 2.0 is a suite of powerful dietary self-assessment tools. Students can use it to analyze and monitor their personal diet and health goals. The program is based on the reliable ESHA database and has an easy-to-use interface.

Wellness Worksheets (0-07-297649-7)

This collection of 120 assessments is designed to evaluate health behaviors and knowledge. Categories of topics include General Wellness and Behavior Change, Stress Management, Psychological and Spiritual Wellness, Intimate Relationships and Communication, Sexuality, Addictive Behaviors and Drug Dependence, Nutrition, Physical Activity and Exercises, Weight Management, and Consumer Health.

PageOut: The Course Website Development Center www.pageout.net

PageOut, available free to instructors who use a McGraw-Hill textbook, is an online program that lets you create your own course website. PageOut offers the following features: a course home page, an instructor home page, a syllabus (interactive and customizable, including quizzing, instructor notes, and links to the text's Online Learning Center), Web links, discussions (multiple discussion areas per class), an online gradebook, and links to student Webpages. Contact your McGraw-Hill sales representative to obtain a password.

Course Management Systems www.mhhe.com/solutions

McGraw-Hill's Instructor Advantage program offers customers access to a complete online teaching website called the Knowledge Gateway, pre-paid toll-free phone support, and unlimited e-mail support directly from WebCT and Blackboard. Instructors who use 500 or more copies of a McGraw-Hill textbook can enroll in our Instructor Advantage Plus program, which provides on-campus, hands-on training from a certified platform specialist. Consult your McGraw-Hill sales representative to learn what other course management systems are easily used with McGraw-Hill online materials.

Classroom Performance System

Classroom Performance System (CPS) brings interactivity into the classroom or lecture hall. It is a wireless response system that gives instructors and students immediate feedback from the entire class. The wireless response pads are essentially remotes that are easy to use and engage students. CPS is available for both Microsoft Windows and Macintosh computers.

Primis Online www.mhhe.com/primis/online

Primis Online is a database-driven publishing system that allows instructors to create content-rich textbooks, lab manuals, or readers for their courses directly from the Primis website. The customized text can be delivered in print or electronic (eBook) form. A Primis eBook is a digital version of the customized text (sold directly to students as a file downloadable to their computers or accessed online with a password). *A Fit and Well Way of Life* is included in the database.

ACKNOWLEDGMENTS

We wish to express our gratitude to the following individuals for their assistance in the development of this book:

Sam Minor II, Department of Art, College of Fine Arts, Ball State University for artwork.

Edgar Self and John Huffer for photography.

Katherine Barnet, Margaret Phillips, Boung Jin Kang, Chris Powers, Melissa Smith, Kelley Jarvis, Erika Hogan, Karlyn Rent, Jamie Troxell, and Lowell Faison for modeling for photographs.

Brian Dietz, Program Advisor, Ball State University, for consultation on higher education alcohol programming.

Jesse Neal, Investigator and Director, Muncie and Delaware County Drug Task Force, for consultation on illegal drugs.

A very generous thank you goes to the dedicated Ball State University Physical Education Fitness/Wellness (PEFWL) faculty for their vigorous commitment to quality teaching.

Special recognition is extended to Dr. Mitchell Whaley, School of Physical Education, Sport, and Exercise Science, and Dr. Nancy Kingsbury, Dean of the College of Applied Sciences and Technology, and Dr. JoAnn M. Gora, President of Ball State University, for their continuing support of the fitness/wellness program at Ball State University. We are fortunate to have administrators who have the vision to recognize that participating in a fitness/wellness program will have a positive impact on students' lives now and in the future.

We dedicate this first edition to Carlotta Seely. This one's for you!

Gwen Robbins
Debbie Powers
Sharon Burgess

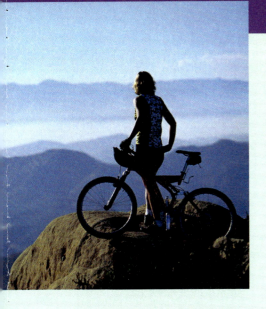

1

Understanding Wellness

Life is not merely to be alive, but to be well.
—Martial

Objectives

After reading this chapter, you will be able to:

1. Identify the top three causes of death in the United States.
2. Define *healthy life expectancy* and explain why it is low in the United States compared with other industrialized countries.
3. Discuss the impact of lifestyle choices on health and longevity.
4. Explain the focus of the publication *Healthy People 2010*.
5. List five lifestyle habits that can reduce the risk of chronic diseases.
6. Define *wellness*.
7. Identify the seven dimensions of wellness and give three examples within each dimension.
8. List and describe the six factors that influence growth in wellness.
9. Give four examples of ways society supports wellness and four examples of ways society detracts from wellness.

Terms

- chronic diseases
- emotional dimension
- environmental dimension
- health
- health promotion
- healthy life expectancy
- intellectual dimension
- locus of control
- occupational dimension
- physical dimension
- social dimension
- societal norm
- spiritual dimension
- wellness

A Fit and Well Way of Life Online Learning Center www.mhhe.com/robbinsfitwell1e
Go to the Online Learning Center for chapter quizzes, outlines, flashcards, and additional lab activities.

As Rob lay in the coronary care unit, his eyes surveyed the various tubes and wires connected to his tired body. The nightmare of the last 24 hours was over, but the pain and confusion lingered.

"How can this be? I'm only 49 years old. How could I have had a heart attack? What if I die? What about my wife? My son? My daughter? I've just become a grandpa. I was given a big promotion at work. Why now?" Rob's mind drifted.

"But I'm an athlete! Well, I *was* an athlete back in high school. Once I started college, there was no time for sports or exercise. Started smoking, too. Figured I'd stop when the deadlines subsided, but the stresses never ended. Drank too much, too; partied a lot. Still like a couple of drinks to end the day. I always thought I'd lose those extra 30 pounds—always next year, always a New Year's resolution. Diet? Too busy. Vending machines, hot dog stands, snacks in front of the TV, fast food. No time. Too much to do. Money to make. A lot of stress. Can't stop now. There'll be time later."

Rob's mind drifted back to his room. He could faintly hear his doctor's voice—"Stop smoking. Change in lifestyle. Low-fat diet. Start exercising. Cholesterol is 280. Break old habits." Rob thought, "How I wish I could turn back the clock!"

This scenario is too common in the United States. More than half of all deaths in this country are attributed to coronary heart disease and stroke. Although most heart attacks occur after middle age, many result from years of lifestyle abuse. Table 1-1 lists the leading causes of death in the United States. One hundred years ago the leading causes of death were infectious diseases such as tuberculosis, polio, diphtheria, pneumonia, and influenza and various diseases of infancy. Advances in medicine, the discovery of antibiotics, and improved sanitation diminished the incidence of these ravaging diseases and increased the average life span. Through scientific discovery, technology, industrial growth, and automation, the entire American lifestyle has changed. We use remote controls to change television channels and open garage doors. Appliances wash our clothes, dishes, and teeth. We ride vehicles to work, to school, and even while playing golf. "Surfing the 'Net" is much more popular than surfing the ocean. We allow ourselves to be bused and trucked, elevated and escalated, and then wonder why we get fat and are out of shape. This so-called good life has created sedentary living, changes in eating habits (fast foods, increased fats and sweets, processed foods), stress, alcohol and drug abuse, and obesity. Although social scientists predicted in the 1960s that technology would create a future of abundant leisure time, in actuality, most of us face an unrelenting pace of increased expectations and demands. Chronic hurrying

---

TABLE 1-1   *Leading Causes of Death in the United States (annual deaths in parentheses)*

Rank	All Ages	Ages 15–24	Ages 25–44	Ages 45–64
1	Heart disease (684,462)	Accidents	Accidents	Cancer
2	Cancer* (554,643)	Homicide	Cancer	Heart disease
3	Stroke (157,803)	Suicide	Heart disease	Accidents
4	Chronic respiratory diseases (126,128)	Cancer	Suicide	Diabetes mellitus
5	Accidents (105,695)	Heart disease	Homicide	Stroke
6	Diabetes mellitus (73,965)	Congenital abnormalities	HIV	Chronic respiratory diseases
7	Pneumonia and influenza (64,847)	Pneumonia and influenza	Chronic liver disease and cirrhosis	Chronic liver disease and cirrhosis
8	Alzheimer's disease (63,343)	Stroke	Stroke	Suicide
9	Kidney disease (42,536)	Chronic respiratory diseases	Diabetes mellitus	HIV
10	Systemic blood infections (34,243)	HIV	Pneumonia and influenza	Systemic blood infections

*AMONG PEOPLE UNDER AGE 85, CANCER IS THE LEADING CAUSE OF DEATH.

SOURCE: Centers for Disease Control and Prevention. National Center for Health Statistics. *National Vital Statistics Reports*, Vol. 53, No. 15, February 2005.

has created chronic stress. Life has gotten out of balance for many. As Mahatma Gandhi once said, "There is more to life than increasing its speed."

The harsh truth is that a high percentage of disease and disability affecting the American people is preventable, a consequence of unwise behavior and lifestyle choices. The decision to smoke, for instance, is responsible for one of every six deaths in the United States each year. With the rapidly increasing obesity rate, health officials predict that obesity will soon surpass tobacco as the leading contributor to premature death in the United States. Instead of infectious diseases, we now die of **chronic diseases**—diseases that develop over many years and are heavily influenced by lifestyle. Examples of chronic diseases are heart disease, cancer, stroke, type 2 diabetes, atherosclerosis, obesity, and osteoporosis.

If you are like most people, you underestimate your future risk of chronic diseases. Studies show that many young adults already possess several risk factors that can lead to these lifestyle diseases. Underestimation of your risk is of substantial concern because action should be an outcome of your health knowledge. After all, the truly educated individual understands cause and effect. Nevertheless, many young adults are much more interested in the present than the future. Good health often is taken for granted until it is lost. You make choices every day that either increase or decrease your risk for developing chronic diseases.

This chapter introduces you to the concept of high-level wellness. You will see that wellness living and healthy lifestyle interventions that begin early in life can shape your health destiny and lead to a vibrant life.

HEALTHY LIFE EXPECTANCY AND THE COSTS

Life expectancy in the United States is 77.6 years (74.8 years for men and 80.1 years for women). In 2000 the World Health Organization (WHO) began calculating **healthy life expectancy** in 191 countries. Healthy life expectancy is the number of years a person is expected to live in *good* health. This number is obtained by subtracting years spent in poor health from overall life expectancy. The United States ranks 29th in the world

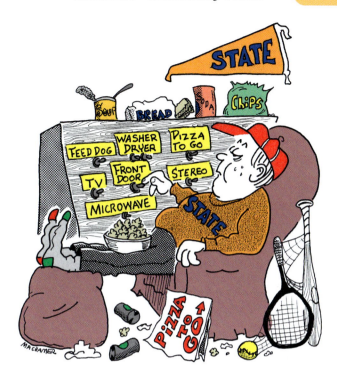

The "good life"?

using this measurement, with an average of 69.3 years of healthy life expectancy. Japan ranks number 1 with a healthy life expectancy of 75.0 years.

The ranking of the United States is surprisingly low in light of its status as a country with one of the best medical care systems in the world. The WHO report indicates that Americans die earlier and spend more time disabled than do people in most other advanced countries. Several factors are cited in the WHO report to explain why the United States ranks relatively low among wealthy nations:

1. Some groups, such as American Indians, rural African Americans, and the inner-city poor, have extremely poor health that is more characteristic of a poor developing country than of a rich industrialized one.
2. The HIV epidemic causes a higher proportion of death and disability in the United States than in other developed countries.
3. The United States is one of the leading countries for cancers because of the high incidence of tobacco use.
4. The United States has a high incidence of coronary heart disease.
5. The United States has a fairly high level of violence, especially homicides, compared with other industrialized countries.

In contrast, the United States spends more than twice as much for health care than any other nation. Yet,

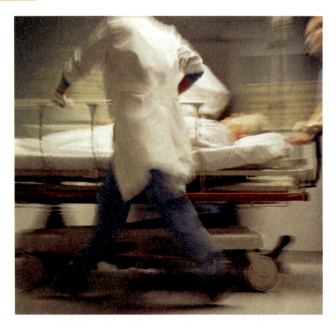

Cardiovascular diseases, the number one killer of both men and women, are considered "lifestyle" diseases.

we are among the sickest in the world! The national health-care expenditures in the United States exceed 1.5 trillion dollars and are rising every year. If current policies and conditions hold true, by the year 2011 this amount will jump to $2.8 trillion. Smoking alone costs our society over $150 billion annually in health-care costs and lost productivity (and causes 435,000 premature deaths). Cardiovascular diseases cost $351 billion annually, and the financial burden of obesity nearly rivals that of smoking. In fact, for the first time in history, experts predict a decline in life expectancy in the United States in the 21st century due to the rising prevalence of obesity. During the last few years expenditures for prescription drugs have grown at a faster rate than has any other type of health cost. Unfortunately, very few health-care expenditures go toward prevention. America is terrific at expensive, heroic care but very poor at low-cost preventive care!

This burden will continue to grow as the population ages. By 2011, if trends continue, health-care costs will double. According to government statistics, as much as two-thirds of disability and death up to age 65 would be preventable in total or in part if we applied what we know about the effects of lifestyle on premature illness and death. You may be thinking . . . "but we all have to die sometime!" Of course that is true. But we are born to last nearly 100 years, and not meant to suffer from chronic diseases in our 40s and 50s. Former U.S. Surgeon General C. Everett Koop states, "We are in an era of self-induced premature deaths."

Determinants of Health and Longevity

As a result of the curative focus of our health-care system, a majority of our health-care dollars are spent on procedures for patching people up after the damage has been done. Since billions of dollars are spent to treat the results of bad eating and drinking habits, sedentary living, stress, and smoking, our system probably should be renamed "sickness care" rather than "health care." Because of the medical procedures, drugs, and technologies currently available, many people have become complacent about their health habits. They think they can be "bailed out" by medical science.

A range of factors underlies one's susceptibility and predisposition to ill health. (See Figure 1-1.) Rather than working independently, all of these factors interact. It is important to understand how all of these factors work in combinations and affect each other. Nevertheless, the largest contributing factor is lifestyle behaviors.

Heredity

Predisposition to health or disease begins at conception. Each of us has cellular codes that dictate our size, shape, personality, and biological limits. However, our hereditary tendencies are strongly affected by other determinants like social circumstances and behavioral choices.

Social Circumstances

Powerful influences on our health are derived from circumstances such as education, income, housing, employment, poverty, crime, and other community forces.

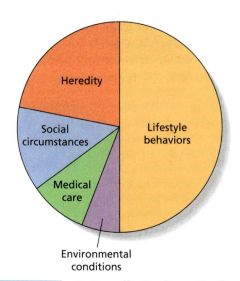

FIGURE 1-1 Factors affecting longevity. Our longevity is affected by a combination of factors. SOURCE: Adapted from J. M. McGinnis, *American Journal of Health Promotion* 18 (Nov./Dec. 2003): 146–150.

Environmental Conditions

Home, work, and community environments sometimes present us not only with barriers to active lifestyles but also with toxic hazards. Environmental pollutants, chemical contaminants, radon, occupational hazards, and tobacco smoke all have the potential for triggering cellular changes.

Medical Care

Despite the expensive and stunning feats of our medical care system, the contribution of medical treatment to overall gains in the function and quality of life has been limited in recent years. Whereas the introduction of antibiotics and improved sanitation in the early 1900s increased our life span by more than 60 percent, modern-day medical treatments and technologies have had far less dramatic impact.

Lifestyle Behaviors

In the United States, lifestyle behaviors represent the single most controllable influence over our health prospects. The daily choices we make with respect to diet, physical activity, stress management, tobacco and alcohol use, sexual practices, and safety issues are the most important determinants of well-being. It has been well documented that the top three lifestyle contributors to premature deaths in the United States are tobacco use, poor diet, and lack of exercise. Hopefully as people learn more about the effect of behavioral factors, they will accept the personal responsibility for making changes in their lifestyles and find joy in discovering how much power they truly have in determining their health destinies.

The Power of Prevention

Empowering individual responsibility involves aggressive health promotion. **Health promotion** is the science and art of helping people change their lifestyles to move toward a state of optimal health. Health promotion involves systematic efforts by organizations to create healthy policies and supportive environments as well as the reorienting of health services to include more than clinical and curative care. Lifestyle change is motivated not by knowledge alone but also by supportive social environments and the availability of facilitative services. Examples of health promotion programs are weight-loss workshops, smoking cessation clinics, and stress management seminars. Laws and policies such as those prohibiting drunk driving, those curtailing pollution, and those establishing smoke-free businesses and restaurants also assist in health promotion.

Because the preventive aspects of health have become more publicized, research studies involving diet

---

TOP **10** LIST

Lifestyle Practices That Enhance Wellness

1. Exercise aerobically at least four to five times per week.
2. Eliminate all tobacco products.
3. Limit animal fats, cholesterol, trans fats, and saturated fats in the diet.
4. Eat five to nine daily servings of fruits and vegetables and include other high-fiber foods and whole grains every day in the diet.
5. Assess personal stressors and practice stress management techniques, including maintaining a strong social support system.
6. Limit the consumption of alcohol to no more than one drink (women) or two drinks (men) per day.
7. Pursue and maintain a healthy weight.
8. Fasten seat belts.
9. Practice safe sex habits.
10. Balance work, social, and personal time, including getting 7 to 9 hours of sleep every night.

---

and exercise often become instant headlines (e.g., Which is better . . . butter or margarine? coffee or tea? protein or carbohydrate?). Sometimes the information is reported only partially, resulting in confusion, contradiction, and even sensationalism. Bewildered and wary, many Americans reject or ignore many legitimate health pronouncements such as *cutting saturated fat in their diets. Exercising aerobically 30 minutes five times per week. Eating five or more fruits and vegetables daily.* It is a challenge to recognize legitimate health pronouncements. Being educated about wellness will empower you to make informed decisions and distinguish between legitimate health pronouncements and fads and illegitimate assertions. Regardless of the messages, a majority of present-day Americans continue to be sedentary and overweight. Stress levels, blood cholesterol readings, and blood sugars continue to soar. Though the relationship between lifestyle and health is clear, adopting healthy lifestyle habits can be challenging in our environment where fast food is everywhere, we ride rather than walk, and we sit rather than play. But the good news is it can be done and it does make a difference in health, longevity, and vitality.

Healthy People 2010

Because of the concern for our nation's health and vitality, a vigorous national crusade for health promotion has been initiated. *Healthy People 2010: Understanding and Improving Health* is a publication facilitated by the

U.S. Department of Health and Human Services. *Healthy People 2010* is a statement of national opportunities and challenges communities to support health-promoting policies.

This document is a road map for improving the health of all people in the United States during the first decade of the 21st century. *Healthy People 2010* is committed to one overarching purpose: promoting health and preventing illness, disability, and premature death. The document identifies two broad goals as the means of bringing about fuller human potential:

1. Increase quality and years of healthy life
2. Eliminate health disparities

To achieve these goals, 467 objectives have been targeted for the year 2010 in areas such as environmental health, violence, cancer prevention, and obesity reduction, among others.

Table 1-2 lists a few of the objectives found in *Healthy People 2010* as well as estimates of our current status. Because of the diversity and varying needs of Americans, reaching these goals is a challenge. (See Diversity Issues.) Nevertheless, the federal government is playing a leadership role in cultivating a culture of healthier, life-enhancing habits for all Americans, regardless of income, race, sex, or other status. We must do our part to help.

A companion document to *Healthy People 2010* is *Healthy Campus 2010*, which establishes national health objectives for the nation's colleges and universities. The health indicators in this document are similar to *Healthy People 2010* in regard to physical activity, overweight and obesity, tobacco use, and other practices. The goal of both of these documents is to motivate people into personal action. Surveys have revealed that since 1990 young adults ages 18–24 from all racial and ethnic groups have shown a larger increase in several risk behaviors than all other age groups in the United States.

Those risk behaviors are increases in tobacco use (especially among women), obesity, inactivity, and low vegetable and fruit intake. This is a particular public health concern since this is the age when independent lifelong habits are established. Young adults, apparently believing they are immune from risk, are not too far from entering the ages of high chronic disease burden. Most of the proposals in these two government documents are linked to everyday practices, so it is up to each of us to develop strategies for incorporating healthy habits into our daily lives. Look at the Top 10 List "Lifestyle Practices That Enhance Wellness." How many of these habits do you practice?

There is nothing extreme or magical in this list. It shifts the main responsibility for health to the individual rather than relegating the individual to a position of passivity amid excessive surgeries, medications, and medical tests. One physician has summarized the issue by stating, "One of my frustrations in medicine was having people come to me expecting way too much of me and not expecting anything of themselves."

To evaluate your personal lifestyle habits, look to *Healthy Lifestyle: A Self-Assessment*, Lab Activity 1-1.

Understanding Risks

Often in this book we will talk about risks. In an effort to prevent disease and promote health, it is important to identify the factors that cause disease and injury. From this process, probabilities are determined as to the chances for occurrence. Like placing a bet at a racetrack, identifying risks is a way of quoting the odds. No one can promise you that doing something or refraining from doing it will keep you safe or that doing one thing will kill you. You must draw your own conclusions from the evidence. There is no such thing as absolute safety, and so you can choose only to widen or narrow your risk margins with your habits.

TABLE 1-2	*A Sample of Health Objectives from* **Healthy People 2010**		
Objective		**Goal (%)**	**Current Status (%)**
• Reduce cigarette smoking prevalence of adults age 18 and older		12	21
• Increase the use of sun protection measures among adults		75	59
• Increase the proportion of adults age 18 and older who engage in regular moderate physical activity		50	33
• Increase the prevalence of healthy weight among adults age 20 and older		60	33
• Increase the use of seat belts in motor vehicles		92	75
• Reduce overall colorectal cancer deaths per 100,000 people		13.9	19.1
• Increase the proportion of people age 2 and older who consume at least 2 servings of fruit daily		75	28
• Increase the proportion of people age 2 and older who consume at least 3 servings of vegetables daily		50	3
• Increase the proportion of people age 2 and older who consume at least 6 servings of grains daily (with at least 3 being whole grain)		50	7

SOURCE: Centers for Disease Control and Prevention. National Center for Health Statistics. *DATA2010 . . . the Healthy People Database*, January 2006. http://wonder.cdc.gov/data2010/

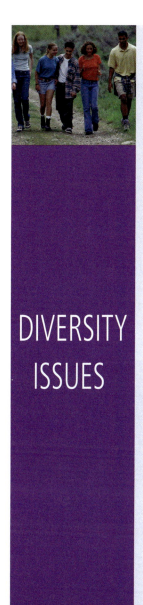

DIVERSITY ISSUES

Health Disparities Among Americans

Although the diversity of the American population may be one of our nation's greatest assets, diversity also presents a range of health improvement challenges. Causes for these disparities could be variances in education and income levels, accessibility to health care, health insurance coverage, cultural preferences and influences, and discrimination. A few examples of major disparities include:

- More than half of persons who die of heart disease each year are women.
- HIV/AIDS is the leading cause of death for African American men ages 25–44.
- American Indians suffer from type 2 diabetes at 3 times the average rate.
- Lung cancer kills twice as many men as women.
- African American women die from breast cancer 1.3 times more than white women, 2 times more than Hispanic women, and almost 3 times more than American Indians.
- Lower-income persons consume fewer fruits and vegetables than do those with higher income levels.
- Deaths from chronic liver disease and cirrhosis are 4 times more prevalent among American Indians than among the general U.S. population.
- African American men suffer from heart disease at twice the rate of other men.
- Whites die from lung cancer 2.5 times more than Hispanics.
- Whites suffer 1.5 times more coronary heart disease deaths than American Indians.

- Of white teens, 40 percent smoke, compared with 25 percent of white adults (over age 18).
- People from households with an annual income of at least $25,000 live an average of 3 to 7 years longer than people from households with annual incomes of less than $10,000.
- African American men die from prostate cancer at more than twice the rate of other men.
- The prevalence of diabetes is 70 percent higher among African Americans and nearly 100 percent higher among Hispanics than among whites.
- Among adolescent minorities, African Americans show the lowest prevalence of heavy drinking; Hispanic adolescents have the highest prevalence, followed by whites.
- Health screening rates in Hispanic communities are substantially lower than national rates.
- African Americans, American Indians, and Hispanics engage in less vigorous exercise than whites.
- Obesity prevalence is higher for African American women at every age compared with every other gender and racial or ethnic group.
- Hispanic children (ages 6–19) have twice the obesity rate of other children.

DATA FROM: U.S. Department of Health and Human Services. *Healthy People 2010: National Health Promotion and Disease Prevention Objectives.* DHHS. Publication #19-50212, 2000; Centers for Disease Control and Prevention, National Center for Chronic Disease Prevention and Health Promotion. "Chronic Disease Overview." National Center for Health Statistics; U.S. Department of Health and Human Services. *Health, United States, 2004. Reach 2010 Surveillance for Health Status in Minority Communities—United States, 2001–2002.*

One ongoing study has resulted in much of the information we have about the risk factors associated with several chronic diseases. The people of Framingham, Massachusetts, a community 18 miles west of Boston, have been studied and charted since 1950. The Framingham Study, as it has become known, has resulted in information about how heredity, environment, medical care, and lifestyle factors affect heart disease and well-being. A comprehensive longitudinal study such as this, in contrast to a short-term, isolated study involving only a few people, results in reputable data pertaining to risks. So although the risk of most chronic diseases can't be totally eliminated, it can be significantly reduced using information from studies such as this. We hope you are thinking beyond mere "risk avoidance" to a life full of enrichment, self-fulfillment, and satisfaction. This dramatic shift in emphasis toward self-responsibility and an expanded quality of life has evolved into a concept called *wellness.*

HIGH-LEVEL WELLNESS

In 1948 the World Health Organization defined **health** as "a state of complete physical, mental and social well-being and not merely the absence of disease or infirmity." In the late 1950s Dr. Halbert Dunn began writing about the upper limits of health—the *ultimate* in health.

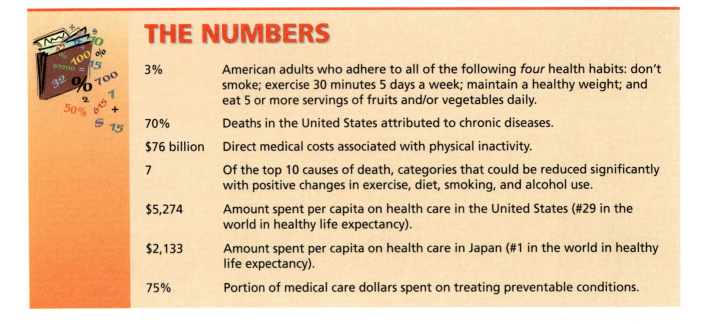

THE NUMBERS

3%	American adults who adhere to all of the following *four* health habits: don't smoke; exercise 30 minutes 5 days a week; maintain a healthy weight; and eat 5 or more servings of fruits and/or vegetables daily.
70%	Deaths in the United States attributed to chronic diseases.
$76 billion	Direct medical costs associated with physical inactivity.
7	Of the top 10 causes of death, categories that could be reduced significantly with positive changes in exercise, diet, smoking, and alcohol use.
$5,274	Amount spent per capita on health care in the United States (#29 in the world in healthy life expectancy).
$2,133	Amount spent per capita on health care in Japan (#1 in the world in healthy life expectancy).
75%	Portion of medical care dollars spent on treating preventable conditions.

He was the first to use the word *wellness* in his writings in reference to the pursuit of optimal well-being. Dunn viewed "health" as a relatively passive and neutral state of existence—in contrast to "wellness," which he described as an ever-changing process of growth toward an *elevated* state of superb well-being, and where one is actively working to reach it. Today, **wellness** is defined as *an integrated and dynamic level of functioning oriented toward maximizing potential, dependent on self-responsibility.* Wellness involves not only preventive health behaviors but also a shift in *thinking* and *attitude.* Wellness is a mind-set of lifelong growth and achievement in the emotional, spiritual, physical, occupational, intellectual, environmental, and social dimensions. It means a lifetime of striving toward ever higher levels of functioning where complacency and passivity are not tolerated.

High-level wellness is achievable by people of all ages, all socioeconomic groups, and all types. It involves working toward becoming the best you can be without accepting "traditional" limitations (i.e., age, race, gender, heredity). Wellness is a way of living in which growth and improvement are sought in all areas. It involves a lifestyle of deliberate choices and self-responsibility, requiring conscientious management and planning. Living a wellness lifestyle does not come about by accident or luck. It also involves much more than curing sickness, counting fat grams, jogging, and measuring body fat. It is a *mind-set* of personal empowerment. It means approaching life with optimism, confidence, and energy. Unlike sickness care, which involves treatment, wellness is a lifelong quest toward optimal functioning in which *you* take charge. Individuals who strive for wellness have an exceptional openness to experience. Rather than fearing new experiences and life's changes, they welcome them as a way to grow. They do not allow prejudices or

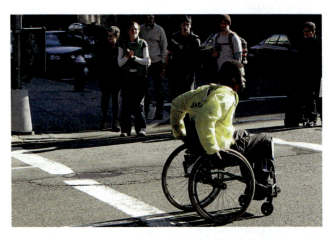

Wellness means striving to be the best you can be regardless of life's situations or circumstances.

stereotypes to distort their perceptions. They take control of life and face it with creativity and freshness. Living a wellness lifestyle has good potential for increasing longevity. However, this is not the sole purpose of wellness living. Wellness author and advocate Donald Ardell agrees. He states, "Wellness is not a goal to be attained but a process to be maintained." Simply put, wellness is the idea of being aware of and actively working toward better health. When you think of wellness, think of the phrase, "Make the *rest* of your life the *best* of your life." No matter where you are starting from or what you've done in the past, you have the capacity to take steps to improve your personal well-being.

Figure 1-2 shows a wellness continuum. You do not attain a "state of wellness" and then stop. Your personal choices dictate whether you are moving upward toward high-level wellness or downward away from your well-

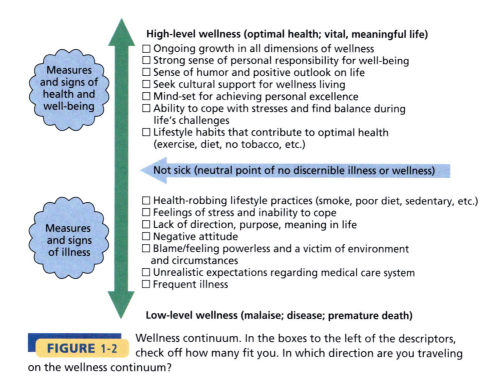

High-level wellness (optimal health; vital, meaningful life)
☐ Ongoing growth in all dimensions of wellness
☐ Strong sense of personal responsibility for well-being
☐ Sense of humor and positive outlook on life
☐ Seek cultural support for wellness living
☐ Mind-set for achieving personal excellence
☐ Ability to cope with stresses and find balance during
   life's challenges
☐ Lifestyle habits that contribute to optimal health
   (exercise, diet, no tobacco, etc.)

Not sick (neutral point of no discernible illness or wellness)

☐ Health-robbing lifestyle practices (smoke, poor diet, sedentary, etc.)
☐ Feelings of stress and inability to cope
☐ Lack of direction, purpose, meaning in life
☐ Negative attitude
☐ Blame/feeling powerless and a victim of environment
   and circumstances
☐ Unrealistic expectations regarding medical care system
☐ Frequent illness

Low-level wellness (malaise; disease; premature death)

Measures and signs of health and well-being

Measures and signs of illness

FIGURE 1-2 Wellness continuum. In the boxes to the left of the descriptors, check off how many fit you. In which direction are you traveling on the wellness continuum?

ness potential. In what direction are you traveling on the wellness continuum?

The Dimensions of Wellness

The wellness lifestyle is a coordinated and integrated living pattern that involves seven dimensions: physical, intellectual, emotional, social, spiritual, environmental, and occupational. There is a strong interconnection among these dimensions. For example, joining an exercise class in your community most notably enhances your physical well-being, but it can also be socially enriching and intellectually stimulating as you learn more about the functional capacity of the human body. It can also help relieve emotional stress. Attending the class with coworkers after work may improve your occupational wellness. In each dimension there is opportunity for personal growth, and due to the dimensions' interrelationships, growth in one area often sparks interest in another. *Balancing* these dimensions, however, is important in pursuing wellness. For example, being an avid reader yet not being able to get along with anyone is not an example of balanced wellness.

Physical Dimension

The **physical dimension** deals with the functional operation of the body. It involves the health-related components of physical fitness—muscular strength, muscular endurance, cardiorespiratory endurance, flexibility, and body composition. Dietary habits have a significant ef-

fect on physical well-being. Your sexual, drinking, and drug behaviors also play a role in physical health. Do you smoke? Do you get enough sleep? Are you overweight? Do you catch many colds? These questions deal with your physical dimension.

The physical dimension also includes medical self-care—regular self-tests, medical and dental checkups, proper use of medications, taking necessary steps when you are ill, and appropriate use of the medical system. Managing your environment also affects physical well-being. For example, do you try to minimize your exposure to tobacco smoke and harmful pollutants? Since your body is the vehicle in which you travel throughout life, treat it like the precious entity it is.

Intellectual Dimension

The **intellectual dimension** involves the use of your mind. Maintaining an active mind contributes to total well-being. Intellectual growth is not restricted to formal education—that is, school learning. It involves a continuous acquisition of knowledge throughout life, engaging your mind in creative and stimulating mental activities, and opening your mind to new ideas. Curiosity and learning should never stop. Reading, writing, and keeping abreast of current events are intellectual pursuits. Being able to think critically and analyze, evaluate, and apply knowledge also are associated with this dimension. Do you visit museums or attend cultural events? Do you watch educational programs on television? The link between intellectual stimulation and healthy living is undeniable.

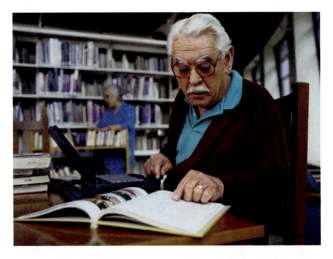

Having a strong desire to continue learning throughout life shows strength in the intellectual dimension of wellness.

Emotional Dimension

The abilities to laugh, enjoy life, adjust to change, cope with stress, and maintain intimate relationships are examples of the **emotional dimension** of wellness. Emotional wellness includes three areas: awareness, acceptance, and management. Emotional awareness involves recognizing your feelings as well as the feelings of others. Emotional acceptance means understanding the normality of human emotion in addition to assessing your personal abilities and limitations realistically. Emotional management is the ability to control or cope with personal feelings and knowing how to seek support when necessary. It involves having adequate stress-coping mechanisms. The ability to maintain emotional stability at some mid-range between the highs and the lows is essential.

Research shows that optimistic people live longer. They become masters of their own fate not just because they *believe* good things will happen but also because they believe they can *make* good things happen. Having a positive mental state is directly linked to wellness.

Social Dimension

Everyone must interact with people. The **social dimension** of wellness involves the ability to get along with others and appreciate the uniqueness of others. It means exhibiting concern for the welfare of your community and fairness and justice toward others. Social wellness also involves concern for humanity as a whole. You have achieved social wellness when you feel a genuine sense of belonging to a large social unit. Good friends, close family ties, volunteerism, community involvement, and trusting relationships go hand in hand with high-level wellness. Whereas feelings of isolation and loneliness are linked to ill health, feeling "connected" to a person, group, cause, or even pet is a health strengthener.

Spiritual Dimension

The **spiritual dimension** involves the personal search for meaning and direction in life. For many people spiritual wellness means identifying a creator, a god, or a specific religion. However, the spiritual dimension is not always synonymous with religion. In its purest sense, spiritual wellness involves cultivating beliefs, principles, and values that provide guidance and strength throughout all of life's experiences. Why am I here? What path will lead to fulfillment in my life? What is life about? What are my values? These questions are most often answered within the context of a larger reality beyond the physical and material aspects of existence. Selflessness; compassion; honesty; joy for living; forgiveness; charity; and the development of a clear, comfortable sense of right and wrong are components of spiritual wellness. The Top 10 List "Components of Spirituality" will help you gain an understanding of the components of a spiritual life.

TOP 10 LIST

Components of Spirituality

Spirituality and religion are related but not always synonymous. However, the practice of religion may deepen spirituality for some. One cannot discount the importance of organized religion to the spirituality of millions. Nevertheless, it is inappropriate to suggest that one must practice a specific religion to develop spiritual wellness. This list includes components that are typically seen in a spiritual life. Those who develop spiritual wellness see spirituality as a journey or process, not a destination. How many of these 10 components do you possess?

1. Belief in a higher power, being, or energy force greater than oneself that provides strength in coping with the demands and challenges of life
2. Feelings of hope about the future
3. Feelings of purpose, meaning, and direction in life
4. Feelings of optimism; ability to see the best side of a situation
5. Regular worship, prayer, meditation, or spiritual study/reflection
6. Universal love and devotion to the welfare of others
7. Possession of moral and ethical principles that reflect one's spiritual beliefs
8. Possession of a clear set of values and ability to live according to those values
9. Ability to share spiritual values with others and tolerance of others whose beliefs are different from yours
10. Feeling a sense of unity with nature and the universe; inner peace

There is a strong connection between spirituality and self-esteem because of the internal feelings of self-worth that occur when a sense of hope, purpose, and morality is developed. Attempts to achieve long-term self-esteem through external constructs of power, socioeconomic status, or physical appearance fail. Like all dimensions of wellness, spirituality does not "happen." It is a process of growth requiring time and attention. Medicine has begun to recognize the strong influence of spirituality on health and illness. Studies at UCLA of cancer patients have shown that those who continuously pursue goals related to living a meaningful life boost the natural killer cell activity in their immune systems.

Environmental Dimension

The **environmental dimension** of wellness deals with the preservation of natural resources as well as the protection of plant and animal wildlife. We have basic biological needs that include safe air, water, and food. Our dependence on the automobile and the general industrialization of our world have created worldwide pollution and changes in the atmosphere. Habits such as recycling, limiting the use of pesticides, carpooling, and conserving electricity show positive involvement in the environmental dimension of wellness. Demonstrating a commitment to the protection of wildlife and plants is also a component of environmental wellness. We must *all* take part in sustaining and improving the quality of the environment for current and future generations.

Occupational Dimension

The **occupational dimension** involves deriving personal satisfaction from your vocation. Much of your life will be spent at work. Therefore, it is important that your chosen career provide the internal and external rewards you value. Do you want a job that allows for creativity, interaction with others, daily challenge, or autonomy? Do you prefer opportunities for advancement, personal entrepreneurship, leadership, or helping others? How do you feel about mobility? Is salary your major motivation? Answering these questions may help you with career selection. Occupational wellness also involves maintaining a satisfying balance between work time and leisure time. It involves a work environment that minimizes stress and exposure to physical health hazards. A majority of your college life is spent analyzing your skills and interests and integrating them with career choices. It is vital that your vocational choice be personally enriching and stimulating. If you are not happy with your occupation, you will find that your entire well-being suffers.

Wellness is a combination of all seven dimensions. It means striving for growth in each dimension and appreciating the interconnectedness between all of them. Is there one dimension in which you are strongest? Which dimension is your weakest? Neglecting any di-

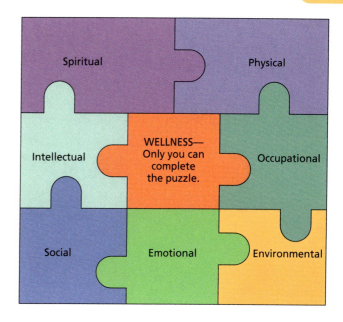

mension destroys the balance critical to high-level wellness. Certain dimensions may take on a greater importance at different times throughout your life. Nevertheless, striving for balance contributes to your wholeness. To evaluate your wellness in the seven dimensions, you are encouraged to do Lab Activity 1-2, *Assessing Your Wellness.* Doing this assessment will also help you understand the broad array of choices within each dimension.

Growth in Wellness

We have described wellness as a dynamic course of action based on self-responsibility. The goal is to assume greater responsibility for your quality of life by making positive lifestyle decisions. How do you begin making positive lifestyle choices? How do you know the options

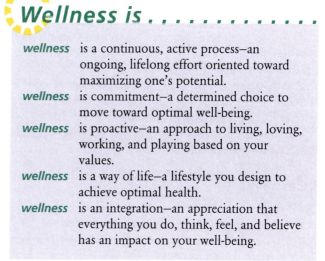

Wellness is . . . .

wellness   is a continuous, active process—an ongoing, lifelong effort oriented toward maximizing one's potential.

wellness   is commitment—a determined choice to move toward optimal well-being.

wellness   is proactive—an approach to living, loving, working, and playing based on your values.

wellness   is a way of life—a lifestyle you design to achieve optimal health.

wellness   is an integration—an appreciation that everything you do, think, feel, and believe has an impact on your well-being.

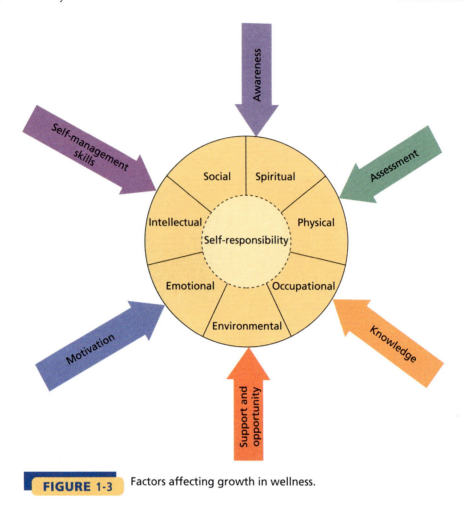

FIGURE 1-3   Factors affecting growth in wellness.

available to you? How do you grow in wellness? As Figure 1-3 shows, growth in wellness is influenced by many factors. Wellness living is an *active* process, and so understanding how each of the factors contributes to your growth in each dimension is important.

Awareness

Before you can grow in wellness, you must have an awareness of wellness options. You are now aware that your health, happiness, and quality of life are strongly affected by your willingness to make wellness choices. Your well-being is not solely the responsibility of the medical care system. You have choices. The increasing general interest in wellness has made it easier for an individual to adopt a wellness lifestyle, because wellness choices now are not only available but valued.

Assessment

Once you are aware of the wellness option, you should assess your lifestyle. Assessment allows you to see how you are conducting your life and identify where changes should occur. An assessment can be anything from med-

ical tests (cholesterol profile, blood pressure, bone density, etc.) to physical fitness tests. They can be stress inventories, health-risk appraisals, dietary logs, or even attitude questionnaires. Personality assessments can help you understand your social and professional relationships. Assessment offers an opportunity to begin the process of self-observation as you confront a wellness issue. You will find a wide variety of assessments throughout this book.

Knowledge

Having knowledge in the lifestyle areas helps you make decisions. For example, suppose from an assessment you learn your blood cholesterol level. What level constitutes high blood cholesterol? How do you go about reducing your cholesterol? What dietary changes can make an impact? Will exercise help? Having accurate knowledge about nutrition, fitness, stress, and other areas of health can help you understand your risks and become a foundation for you to build upon. However, knowledge is not enough. You must have self-management skills and motivation to put that knowledge to good use.

Self-Management Skills

Self-management skills help you try some of the options. Skills in goal setting, behavior modification, and personal strategy building enable you to make the necessary lifestyle changes. How do I go about managing stress? Eating nutritiously in the residence hall or on a tight budget? Fitting regular exercise into my busy schedule? Self-management skills help you incorporate strategies of self-change into your life so that daily lifestyle choices are habitually "wellness choices." Realize that it takes time and practice to develop these skills into lifetime habits.

Motivation

Motivation is the desire to do something—a stimulus to action. Motivation gets you started and keeps you going as you strive for continued wellness growth. It is also very personal and complex. It changes throughout life and is specific to each person. For example, a 19-year-old may be motivated to lose weight to look better. A 55-year-old may want to lose weight to help reduce high blood pressure.

Motivation is strongly influenced by locus of control. **Locus of control** is an individual's belief about how much power he or she has in regard to what happens to him or her. If you believe that personal actions can make a difference in your life, you have an internal locus of control. If you feel, however, that factors beyond your control—environment, heredity, chance, friends, luck—play a greater role, you have an external locus of control. Since those with an external locus of control do not relate their personal behavior to outcomes, they are less likely to be motivated to take charge of their lives. Having an internal locus of control makes it easier to be motivated and committed to a wellness lifestyle. Whether the goal is to lose weight, manage stress, or get along better with a roommate, a variety of complex factors affect a person's ability to change the behavior and sustain motivation. More detailed information relating to behavior change techniques and motivation is given in Chapter 2.

Support and Opportunity

Maintaining positive lifestyle choices is best achieved when there is support and encouragement from the organizations and environments surrounding you. For example, suppose you join a smoking cessation class. You are starting your climb toward permanent behavior change. If you face returning every day to a roommate who smokes or to a workplace where coworkers smoke, your chances of maintaining your new behavior are considerably lower. Your family, friends, and group affiliations have a strong influence on your behavior. It has been found that there are significant correlations among self-esteem, social support, and a healthy lifestyle.

Choices are not made in a vacuum, and so the aim should be to establish a health-promoting environment in which persons like you can easily make health-significant decisions. Choosing a living or working environment where others strive for wellness can assist you in wellness growth. That is why it is important for schools, communities, and government agencies to provide wellness support to cultivate lifestyle changes. When people have an opportunity to practice healthy behaviors, they are more likely to do them. Making healthy choices is easier when one has access to healthy foods, safe and inviting places to exercise, and stress-reducing activities. Having a supportive environment may be the most powerful factor of all. Do you feel your roommates, friends, and family are supportive of wellness? How about your campus? Why or why not?

Self-Responsibility

At the center of wellness growth is self-responsibility. The goal is to assume greater responsibility for your quality of life by making positive lifestyle decisions. Understandably, for every decision to be made there are alternatives and consequences. Your challenge is to make thoughtful decisions that direct you toward high-level wellness. You know what you can and cannot control. Some circumstances are beyond your control. Part of self-responsibility is recognizing this and adjusting to strive continuously toward full potential. Heredity is an example of something you cannot control. You had no voice in selecting your genetic tendencies. A physical disability is another uncontrollable life situation. Self-responsibility in wellness is making the best of the "hand you are dealt" regardless of your stage in life or circumstances.

Self-responsibility in wellness also means active involvement. Having realistic expectations, a sense of personal accountability, and a sense of humor will help you see wellness living as a joyful experience. Self-responsibility involves self-control as opposed to going along with the crowd or merely reacting to what seems to happen. Because everyone else is eating a triple order of french fries, that does not mean you must. When everyone else is grumbling about the weather, why not find something positive about it? Wellness is about personal empowerment—having a sense of ownership and control of the decision-making process. With that in mind, how do you make lifestyle changes? To make any permanent behavior change, you need a distinct, systematic plan of action.

As you travel this wellness path, you will probably become more aware of how society can help and hinder your trip. Societal or environmental support has the most powerful influence on promoting and maintaining a wellness lifestyle. A challenge we all face in attempting to pursue a wellness lifestyle is societal norms.

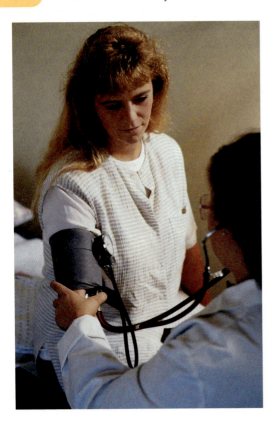

Having your blood pressure checked is an example of a wellness assessment.

SOCIETAL NORMS

We are influenced by what we encounter every day. We are constantly bombarded by subtle yet extremely powerful messages that are sometimes obstacles to wellness. Our behavioral choices are strongly affected by unwritten codes that permeate our daily lives and can contradict and sabotage a wellness lifestyle. **Societal norms** are behaviors or practices that are expected in a culture and that are accepted and supported by its members. Our society often makes it easy to do things we know are not good for us.

These unwritten rules are carried on from generation to generation. Table 1-3 lists circumstances and norms you have probably grown up with. As you look at them, consider the messages they give. Do they promote wellness as you know it? You can probably think of more examples.

Many of our norms encourage a sedentary lifestyle. Somehow we've absorbed the notion that minimal exertion is better. Heaven forbid if, when operating your car, you have to roll down your own windows, walk around the car to unlock the doors, or keep constant pressure on the accelerator while driving on the interstate. We push buttons to open garage doors, change television channels, and order food delivery. You can go to

TABLE 1-3	*Societal Norms That Promote "Unwellness"*

- The idea that everyone must be extremely thin (especially women)
- The assumption that alcohol abuse is an acceptable rite of passage into college
- The media's portrayal of sex as being glamorous, without commitment or consequences
- Social events, parties, celebrations where alcohol and food abuse is expected (New Year's Eve, wedding receptions, Super Bowl parties, etc.)
- The number of high-sugar and high-fat gifts associated with holidays such as Valentine's Day, Easter, Halloween, and Christmas
- The habit of driving a car to go short distances
- Equating tanned skin with beauty, wealth, power, and sex appeal (thus, the emergence of thousands of tanning salons)
- Vending machines at offices and schools loaded with candy bars, chips, cookies, and doughnuts
- Fast-food restaurants that offer burgers and fries (with few healthy alternatives)
- Miles and miles of roads built *without* sidewalks or bike lanes
- The elimination of daily physical education in the schools coupled with the parental push for private sports lessons and competitive Little League football, baseball, soccer, etc. (often serving only the best athletes and emphasizing "winning" rather than lifetime participation)
- Access to television 24 hours a day, with a choice of 100 cable stations—all changed by remote control
- Meals built around a red meat entree
- The notion that as you grow older it is okay to be inactive and fat
- Consistently driving 5–15 mph over the speed limit
- Extra large portions or an "all you can eat" emphasis at restaurants

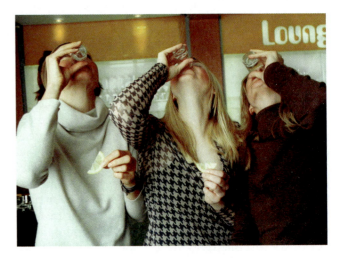

The notion that alcohol is a rite of passage into college is an example of a societal norm that is unhealthy.

the bank, a fast-food restaurant, a dry cleaner, and a drug store without ever leaving the comfort of your car. What kind of message is this sending?

The advertising industry is especially effective at influencing us with messages. We see former star athletes guzzling beer that is "less filling." Every Saturday morning high-sugar snacks are displayed on television. If thin, attractive movie stars enjoy smoking, perhaps you will, too. Lab Activity 1-3 allows you to explore the norms in your community or campus.

In traveling the road to optimum well-being, be aware of these pitfalls and obstacles in our society. Remember, it is you who will make the daily choices as to how to live your life. You are the one who must assess the traps that may impede your pursuit of wellness. Self-responsibility is the key.

Changing Times: Making Wellness the Norm

Now that the wellness concept has begun to invade the health-care profession and society as a whole, we can see some norms changing. Twenty years ago the only people jogging were athletes in training or fitness "nuts." Now no one takes a second look even at senior citizens fitness walking along roads. Businesspeople pack their workout gear next to their business reports. Hotels hand out jogging maps to guests. Stress management, parenting, addictive behavior management, smoking cessation, and a multitude of other wellness topics are offered in community classes and workshops. As wellness permeates our society, there are more resources that support this lifestyle. There are positive choices available in grocery stores—more whole-wheat breads and cereals, low-sugar and low-salt products, low-fat dairy items, even take-out salad and fruit bars. Restaurants are also responding to consumer demand for more nutritious food selections.

These are a few of the positive changes that reflect wellness awareness. Only by drawing together all available resources (individual, community, media, school, corporate, government) will we fix current health problems. This multilevel approach is necessary to bring about changes in societal norms.

For example, a study by the RAND Corporation found that as communities become more spread out and less walkable, chronic disease rates go up. Therefore, suburban design may be an important new avenue for health promotion. Our choices are shaped by our surroundings. If you live in a subdivision or work in an office park where you can't buy a stamp without getting on the interstate, you are going to rely on a car more than your own legs. Health messages and advice only go so far. The real secret to wellness is making the healthy choice the *easy* choice! City planners are now looking at ways to improve people's options. Bike lanes, walking paths, neighborhoods with sidewalks, shops, healthy restaurants, and office structures connected by walking bridges, etc., encourage more activity. This is a positive change from past cultural norms that engineered physical activity out of our daily lives.

Beyond the physical, health-related factors of wellness, it is important to change people's attitudes. It should not be considered bizarre for people to arrive at

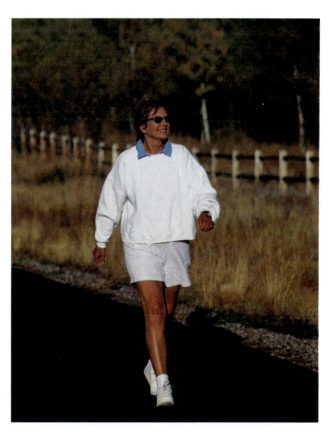

Many communities are converting old railroad tracks to paved exercise trails—an example of a commitment to wellness.

℞ₓ ## Prescription For Action

Date *Do one or more today*

✔ Schedule into your planner an exercise "appointment" with yourself.

✔ Read the entire front page of a major newspaper.

✔ Write down three positive wellness behaviors you can do today. Then do them!

✔ Do two anonymous good deeds for someone.

✔ Get 7 to 9 hours of sleep tonight.

Prescribed by *YOU*

Many success coaches and business consultants use the acronym S.M.A.R.T. to explain goal setting. S.M.A.R.T. refers to **S**pecific, **M**easurable, **A**chievable, **R**eward, and **T**ime-defined.

S = Specific

Goals need to be specific, not vague. *Not* "study history" *but* "read pages 15–35 in the history text, write notes in the margins, and answer the study questions." *Not* "lose weight" *but* "lose 5 pounds." *Not* "save some money" *but* "set aside $50 per paycheck."

M = Measurable

Goals should have concrete criteria for measuring progress (How much? How many? How will I know when it is accomplished?). *Not* "start exercising" *but* "go to the gym M, W, F, S at 5:30 P.M." *Not* "eat better" *but* "eat three pieces of fresh fruit every day." *Not* "handle stress better" *but* "get up 15 minutes earlier in the morning to meditate."

A = Achievable

Goals should be challenging but also within your capabilities—something you know you can achieve! *Not* "win Wimbledon" *but* "learn to play tennis at an intermediate level." *Not* "make straight A's all 4 years" *but* "maintain a 3.5 GPA." *Not* "run a marathon next month" *but* "run a 5K race next month."

R = Reward

You need to reward yourself along the way as you reach certain milestones (new shoes, a pedometer, a massage, a new CD, concert tickets, etc.).

T = Time-defined

Establish some time frames for your goal—either when you'll do it or when you'll accomplish it. ("I'll study between 8 and 10 P.M. Sundays through Thursdays." "I'll lose 8 pounds by summer break." "I'll cycle the Hilly Hundred by October 15.")

Get started today by establishing your S.M.A.R.T. goal (see Lab Activity 2-2).

Listing Pros and Cons

The decision to move from one stage to the next is based largely on the weight given to the pros and cons of changing behavior. The pros represent positive aspects or benefits of changing. The cons represent negative aspects of changing behavior and may be thought of as barriers to change. It's helpful to make a list of the pros and cons as

---

TOP 10 LIST

Keys for Success in Changing Behavior

1. Self-monitor your behavior by keeping a log or record of your habit. This increases self-awareness of cues, triggers, consequences, and challenges.
2. Focus on one habit at a time; don't try to change everything at once.
3. Set reasonable expectations; be realistic but also challenge yourself!
4. Divide large tasks into a number of small steps.
5. Find someone or a group of people who will support you actively.
6. Each day make a list of three things you *can* and *will* do to reach your goal.
7. Spend time with people who already do what you are trying to do. ("It's hard to soar like an eagle if you hang around with the turkeys.")
8. Practice stress management strategies daily and use positive attitudes and affirmations. Emotional distress is a primary factor in lapses and relapses.
9. Expect occasional setbacks; they are part of change. Plan what you'll do if things don't work out as expected or if you face a high-risk situation.
10. Don't let the change be an obsession; try to maintain a sense of humor and don't take yourself too seriously.

---

you contemplate a change. Seriously ask yourself how your life will be affected by your changed behavior. Realize that changing behavior brings consequences to yourself and, most likely, others. (By quitting drinking I will have better health and less likelihood of suffering from an alcohol-related accident. However, I will lose some social friends and my "mood medication.")

In the precontemplation stage of the transtheoretical model, the cons of changing outweigh the pros. In the contemplation stage, the pros may begin to match the cons. However, because they are so close to being equal, the resulting indecision and lack of commitment cause many individuals to become stuck in the contemplation stage. These individuals substitute *thinking* for *action* while continually weighing the costs and benefits of changing. As individuals move into preparation and through the final two stages, the positive aspects (pros) of changing progressively outweigh the negative aspects (cons).

Honestly assessing the costs of changing will help you face yourself and your true motivations. This will help you anticipate the obstacles ahead of you. To increase your motivation, you might talk to acquaintances who have successfully made the change you are attempting.

Check out the Top 10 List "Keys for Success in Changing Behavior." Keep these in mind as you use the behavior strategies that correspond with your stage of change.

PREVENTING RELAPSE

In the first line of his best-selling book *The Road Less Traveled*, Dr. M. Scott Peck writes, "Life is difficult." He further adds that "life is always difficult and is full of pain as well as joy." Changing a habit takes *effort*, but the joy in the growth and self-empowerment is the wellness journey. In our society we have become accustomed to the quick fix: instant cash at the ATM machine, fast food, credit cards, 24-hour Internet shopping, fax machines. Changing a behavior takes *time*, and setbacks are not uncommon. Instead of giving up forever, try to learn from your experiences. Since new behaviors are fragile, maintaining your plan will require flexibility, particularly if the plan is not working properly, if unexpected obstacles arise, or if a support system is failing. Reevaluation is a necessary component in making a permanent lifestyle change. A lapse or setback should be viewed as a mere "bump in the road" where learning and growth can occur. One problem many people have is believing that a setback is a *failure* rather than a temporary obstacle. How you respond to a temporary lapse determines what you will do after it occurs. Often the first line of defense against relapse is *planning*. If chocolate chip cookies are your downfall, don't buy any. (They'll keep calling your name from the cupboard.) If you've tried and can't get up 45 minutes earlier in the mornings to exercise, what about using your lunch hour to exercise? Take your walking shoes to work with you and invite a colleague to exercise with you. If you are trying to con-

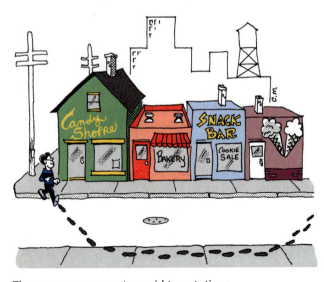

There are many ways to avoid temptations.

trol your weight, you'll likely do better ordering from a menu than choosing the all-you-can-eat buffet. Plan so you'll *succeed*. It is important to recognize "high-risk" situations and have specific coping skills for those situations. If successfully managed, high-risk situations can lead to increased feelings of self-efficacy. This means you've increased your behavior-changing skills, which in turn leads to decreased chances of relapse.

As you become the *cause* rather than the *effect* of actions, your confidence and self-esteem are enhanced. Emphasize the positive. Value your successes and your worth as a human being. Most of us do not realize that the majority of our supportive messages come from our internal thought processes rather than from external sources. We carry on a continuous dialogue with ourselves each day. Called *self-talk*, our inner voice can be a positive source of motivation. Mental health experts recognize self-talk as a powerful force for changing the way we think and behave. "We have a choice about how we think," states Martin Seligman, author of *Learned Optimism*. Self-talk that encourages us and reminds us of our achievements helps increase our self-esteem. Self-talk can also be negative and, as a result, a source of discouragement. For example, when confronted with tempting desserts at a holiday party, a positive self-talk statement would be: "I'll have just a small amount because I am looking forward to wearing my new clothes." A negative self-talk statement would be: "I'm already overweight, so it doesn't matter if I eat a lot." Remem-

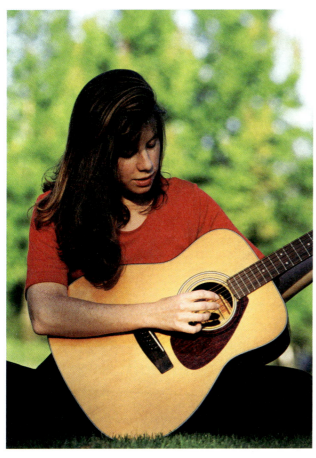

By playing the guitar to distract herself from the urge to smoke, this young woman is utilizing the *countering* process of change.

ber . . . you control your thoughts, and they can be very powerful.

Factors That Contribute to Relapses

Several factors can cause a relapse. The top contributors are (1) stress, (2) social situations, and (3) cravings.

- Stress has a tendency to drain our energy and blur our focus. For example, suppose you have been exercising every Monday, Wednesday, and Thursday evening at the recreation center. Then you suffer a breakup with your girlfriend. Feeling stressed, you suddenly find yourself skipping workouts and immersing yourself in television. These are times when it is important to have healthy stress-coping strategies. We all face life's stresses at times, and it is important not to give up during these times. See Chapter 10 for information on stress management techniques.
- Social situations often present a challenge when trying to change a behavior. Other people may be ambivalent about your change, and can consciously or unconsciously tempt you to revert to old habits. For example, suppose you have been cutting back on eating candy, limiting yourself to one small treat a week. Then, at a campus party, you find yourself eating handfuls of chocolate peanuts from a big bowl. A remedy for social situations is to plan ahead for such high-risk situations—chew gum, position yourself away from the candy bowl, eat before the party, and so on.
- Cravings are intense urges that involve emotional and physiological wants and needs. For example, suppose you haven't smoked a cigarette for 3 weeks. Then you attend your high school reunion and find yourself smoking again with old classmates. By using positive self-talk, mental imagery, and countering strategies, cravings can be controlled.

Regardless of the cause, if a relapse does occur, analyze what happened. Learn what you could do better in the next similar situation. Check out Table 2-2 for more specific tips.

Remember that changing a behavior is a process involving growth. It is a process of assessing and reassessing goals, monitoring behavior, reviewing strategies, learning from setbacks, and acknowledging the joy in the effort to be the best you can be. Successful behavior change requires time, attention, and effort. But you'll find it is well worth it!

Paul J. Meyer, an international self-empowerment author, acknowledges such effort by saying, "Ninety percent of all those who fail are not actually defeated. They simply quit."

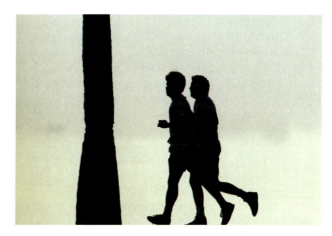

It is much easier to stick with a program when you have someone doing it with you. This is a strategy in the *helping relationships* process of change.

TABLE 2-2 *Tips for Getting Back on Track After a Setback*

1. Cut yourself some slack.

   Accept that you are human and that no one is perfect. If you slipped today, tomorrow is another day. More importantly, what have you learned from this setback? Remember that success does not hinge on 1 or 2 bad days. Therefore, praise yourself for the successes you *have* experienced. In this way you shift your focus from failures to successes. ("I did this successfully for 5 days; what made it work?")

2. Review your goal and plan.

   Make sure it is realistic and achievable. Don't set yourself up for failure. If you have never been an early riser, perhaps a 6:00 A.M. workout is not the best time for you. November, just before the holidays, may not be the best time to start a new weight-loss program. Readjust your plan: e.g., exercise at 3:00 P.M., set a goal to *not gain* extra weight over the holidays.

3. Review your pros for changing.

   You must have had strong reasons for wanting to change. Was it to fit into that new swimsuit? Was it to lower your blood pressure? Was it to develop muscle definition? Go over your motivations again. Write them down and post them in a prominent place.

4. Anticipate obstacles.

   Try to anticipate roadblocks and find ways around them, or at least prepare for them. For example, your exercise routine may run afoul amidst holidays, travel, vacations, or bad weather. Look for hotels with fitness centers; pack a jump rope and exercise band; investigate indoor facilities during bad weather; ask the concierge about jogging routes, facilities, etc.; organize a family walk after Thanksgiving dinner.

5. Look for role models.

   Do you know people who have reached the goal you are striving for? If you do, chat with them about how they overcame obstacles and setbacks. Gain strength from their experiences. Even reading stories about strangers or celebrities who have succeeded can provide inspiration and hope. Tell yourself, "If they can do it, so can I!"

6. For cravings, use the 3 D'S.

   Delay at least 10 minutes so that your actions are conscious, not impulsive.

   Distract yourself by engaging in an activity that requires concentration (e.g., play the piano, surf the Internet, do a crossword puzzle).

   Distance yourself from the temptation (e.g., stand away from the buffet table; don't walk past the donut shop; sit in the non-smoking area).

   Substitute (e.g., a fun-size candy bar for a king-size, a low-fat fudgesicle for a super premium turtle sundae, a mint rather than a cigarette, or chew on a toothpick rather than fingernails).

Frequently Asked Questions

Q. One of the processes of change in the transtheoretical model is called "countering." What are some of the specific strategies of this process?

A. Countering behaviors replace the problem behavior. This strategy is useful when one faces a craving or a social pressure. Try reading a magazine article; abdominal breathing; calling a friend; surfing the Internet; playing a musical instrument; putting on a CD and dancing or singing; going for a walk; watching a television program; playing a game of solitaire; practicing positive self-talk; doing sit-ups/push-ups; cross-stitching; watching a movie; reading scriptures; chewing gum; closing your eyes and practicing imagery; shooting baskets; practicing a new skill; drinking a diet soda; e-mailing a friend/family member. There are many more. The intention is to divert your attention for 10 to 15 minutes while you refocus on your goals.

Q. My behavior-change needs involve time management—specifically, making myself go to the library 4 nights per week from 7:00 to 10:00 P.M. to do homework. I wrote a contract and did well for 4 weeks; then I missed several nights. Now I feel like a failure and am having a hard time getting back on track. Help!

A. The problem of relapse is an important challenge in changing behavior. When individuals experience a *lapse* (a few days of not complying with a new behavior), they need to avoid the feeling that they are doomed. For dieters, it is the belief that one cookie terminates a diet. For exercisers, it is the belief that one missed exercise class means they are no longer "exercisers." Remember that a lapse is a slip, a *relapse* is a string of lapses, and a *collapse* is when the person gives up and returns to past behaviors. Everyone has lapses. Analyze what influenced your lapse. Did you have some other commitments? An invitation to go shopping? A birthday party to attend? Maybe you'd be better off scheduling your 3 hours at the library from 2:00 to 5:00 P.M. Readjust, refocus, recommit, and don't let a mere lapse turn into a major relapse or collapse.

Q. Is there a way to increase my self-efficacy?

A. Yes. Since self-efficacy deals with your perception of your ability to perform a task or engage in a behavior, you can improve your confidence by using four methods: (1) hands-on practice (give it a try!), (2) observing others like you who are doing it successfully (modeling), (3) internalizing the benefits you'll be getting (positive expectations), and (4) beginning to feel or see results (positive feedback/reinforcement).

Q. My best friend is very inactive, even though I am an avid exerciser. She even makes fun of me sometimes! Even though she is trim, I worry about her future health. I have begged her to go to the gym with me, but she just laughs and says she doesn't need to exercise since she is slim. What can I do to change her mind?

A. Like millions of others, your friend is in the precontemplation stage. She doesn't see the need for exercise or is in denial about the benefits of exercise

for her. The three processes that will have the most impact on her are consciousness-raising, social liberation, and emotional arousal. Therefore, find opportunities to casually bring up the benefits of exercise. Verbalize how good you feel after your workout and how it reduces your stress. Talk about how nice the campus recreation center is, or how you've met some great new friends there. Mention the awesome aerobics class that you are taking, or how excited you are about the bike club trip next weekend. Making comments like these in a nonthreatening manner raises your friend's awareness. Letting her know about available campus resources may also help. As time goes by, she may consider giving it a try—or at least move on to the contemplation stage.

Summary

Following a great musician's performance, an admirer said to him, "I'd give my life to play like that." The brilliant performer hesitated for a moment and then replied, "I did." We often view a performance by an athlete or artist with envy. Accomplishment is often deceptive, because we don't see the perseverance that produces it. We don't see the good times and bad, the setbacks and the obstacles. Changing behavior also involves a certain amount of perseverance and discipline. Many desire the benefits of a healthy lifestyle but fail to commit to its precepts.

It takes more than willpower to change a behavior. Permanent behavior change involves passing through five distinct transitional stages while using the corresponding problem-solving processes and strategies within each stage. Just as special tools are needed in building a house, having skills in the various processes of change will help you

"build your new self." Making a plan, S.M.A.R.T. goal setting, listing pros and cons, and understanding relapses are important skills. Writing a contract helps you construct a plan in its entirety, and keeping a behavior-change log helps you monitor daily activity. Though setbacks may occur, a mind-set of commitment and self-empowerment can help you continue the journey.

Think about a business that places a sign in its window: "UNDER NEW MANAGEMENT." Imagine that your body/life is your "business" and you're the new manager who's been brought in to turn this business around. It's going to be challenging, and you're going to have to make some tough decisions. It'll take effort and commitment, but it is your job! And think of the benefits! So declare it now: "MY LIFE IS UNDER NEW MANAGEMENT!"

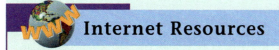

Internet Resources

American Academy of Health Behavior
www.ajhb.org
Offers current and archived abstracts of articles from the *American Journal of Health Behavior* with an emphasis on health behavior research.

Health Behavior News Service
www.hbns.org
Has recent scientific research and news stories pertaining to how people can change their behavior to improve and manage existing illnesses.

Home of the Transtheoretical Model
www.uri.edu/research/cprc
Offers detailed information about the transtheoretical model of behavior change. Included are assessment inventories for various behaviors and habits.

Psychology Today
www.psychologytoday.com
Accesses thousands of articles related to a variety of psychological topics: anxiety, behavior, depression, family, personality, relationships, stress, and addictions.

Small Steps
www.smallstep.gov
From the U.S. Department of Health and Human Services, gives helpful hints in making lifestyle changes, particularly related to weight loss.

Bibliography

Barry, T. R., and B. L. Howe. "The Effects of Exercise Advertising on Self-Efficacy and Decisional Balance." *American Journal of Health Behavior* 29 (March/April 2005): 117–126.

Bedford, P. "Watch Old Habits Disappear." *IDEA Health & Fitness Source* (May 2004): 46–50.

Brown, S. "Measuring Perceived Benefits and Perceived Barriers for Physical Activity." *American Journal of Health Behavior* 29 (March/April 2005): 107–116.

Chapman, M. A. "Bad Choices: Why We Make Them, How to Stop." *Psychology Today* 32 (September/October 1999): 36–39, 71.

Gallagher, K. I., and J. M. Jakicic. "Overcoming Barriers to Effective Exercise Programming." *ACSM's Health & Fitness Journal* 6 (November/December 2002): 6–12.

Goldberg, S. "The 10 Rules of Change." *Psychology Today* 35 (September/October 2002): 38–44.

"How to Banish a Bad Habit." *Consumer Reports on Health* (March 2003): 8–9.

Jakicic, J. M., and A. D. Otto. "Motivating Change: Modifying Eating and Exercise Behaviors for Weight Management." *ACSM's Health & Fitness Journal* 9 (January/February 2005): 6–12.

King, A. C., J. E. Martin, and C. Castro. "Behavioral Strategies to Enhance Physical Activity Participation." In Kaminsky, L. A. (ed.). *ACSM's Resource Manual for Guidelines for Exercise Testing and Participation*. Philadelphia: Lippincott Williams & Wilkins, 2006.

Kottler, J. A. *Making Changes Last*. Philadelphia: Brunner-Routledge, 2001.

Marano, H. E. "Reinvention: How to Be Perfect." *Psychology Today*, February 3, 2004. www.psychologytoday.com

Mellin, L. *The Pathway*. New York: Regan Books, 2003.

Napolitano, M. A., et al. "Principles of Health Behavior Change." In Kaminsky, L. A., ed. *ACSM's Resource Manual for Guidelines for Exercise Testing and Participation*. Philadelphia: Lippincott Williams & Wilkins, 2006.

Prochaska, J. O., J. C. Norcross, and C. C. DiClemente. *Changing for Good*. New York: William Morrow, 1994.

Prochaska, J. O., and W. F. Velicer. "The Transtheoretical Model of Health Behavior Change." *American Journal of Health Promotion* 12 (September/October 1997): 38–44.

Seligman, M. E. P. *Authentic Happiness*. New York: Free Press, 2002.

Seligman, M. E. P. *Learned Optimism*. New York: Simon & Schuster, 1998.

Shilts, M. K., M. Horowitz, and M. S. Townsend. "Goal Setting as a Strategy for Dietary and Physical Activity Behavior Change: A Review of the Literature." *American Journal of Health Promotion* 19 (November/December 2004): 81–93.

Wallace, L. S., and J. Buckworth. "Application of the Transtheoretical Model to Exercise Behavior Among Nontraditional College Students." *American Journal of Health Education* 32 (January/February 2001): 39–47.

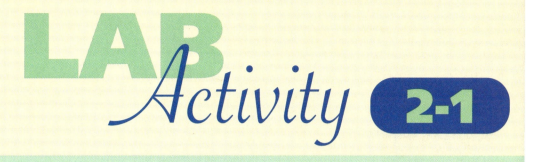

Name _____ **Class/Activity Section** _____ **Date** _____

Identify Your Current Stage of Change

On the line, write a lifestyle question (see Figure 2-1). Then, using a highlighter, trace a path on the algorithm as you answer each question. Highlight your stage of change. On the back of this sheet, write another lifestyle question and highlight your stage of change for that particular habit.

Do you _____?

Yes   No

Have you done this consistently over the last 6 months?   Do you plan to adopt this practice within the next 6 months?

Yes   No   Yes   No

Within the next month?

Yes   No

| Maintenance | Action | Preparation | Contemplation | Precontemplation |

Do you _____?

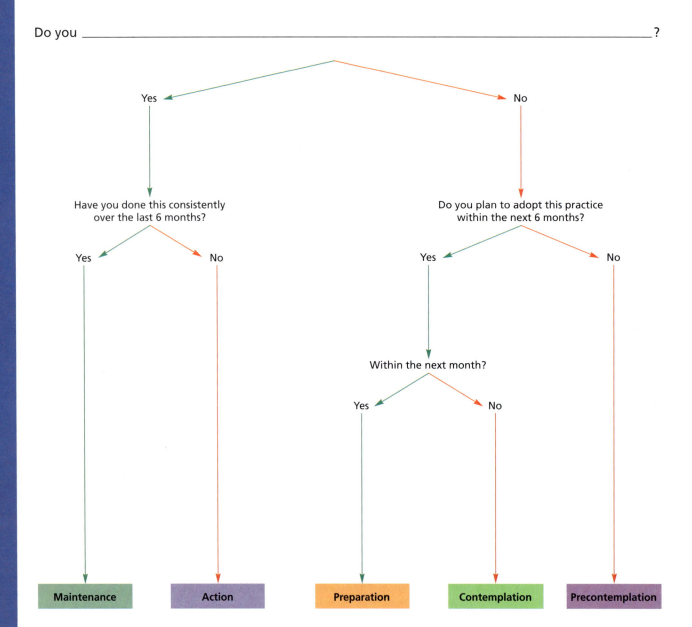

Yes   No

Have you done this consistently   Do you plan to adopt this practice
over the last 6 months?   within the next 6 months?

Yes   No   Yes   No

                                    Within the next month?

                                    Yes   No

| Maintenance | Action | Preparation | Contemplation | Precontemplation |

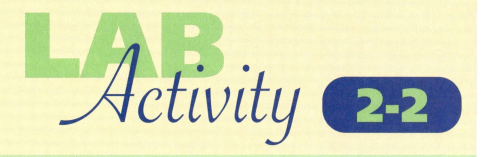

Identify Your S.M.A.R.T. Goal

By using the information in this chapter on goal setting, identify your **S.M.A.R.T.** goal.

S (Specific):

M (Measurable):

A (Achievable):

R (Reward):

T (Time-defined):

(continue on the back)

Anticipated obstacles, barriers, or high-risk situations:

Strategies for overcoming obstacles, barriers, or high-risk situations:

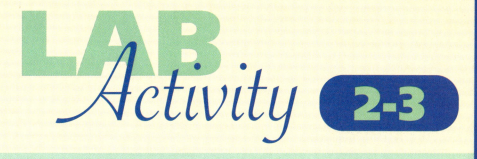

LAB *Activity* 2-3

Behavior-Change Contract
(Using the Transtheoretical Model)

Writing a contract makes you think through your plan in its entirety. It specifies the *details* for carrying out your plan. See Figure 2-3 for a sample contract.

Goal (specific and measurable):

Pros/benefits:

Cons/barriers:

Identify stage of change currently in:

_____ Precontemplation   _____ Preparation   _____ Maintenance

_____ Contemplation   _____ Action

PROCESSES

Identify and circle the *processes* that correspond to the stage of change you are in (refer to Figure 2-2). Then list three specific behavioral strategies you will use for each process. (See Table 2-1 and Figure 2-3 for examples of behavioral strategies.)

1. Consciousness-raising

   a.

   b.

   c.

2. Social liberation

   a.

   b.

   c.

3. Emotional arousal

    a.

    b.

    c.

4. Self-reevaluation

    a.

    b.

    c.

5. Self-liberation

    a.

    b.

    c.

6. Reward

    a.

    b.

    c.

7. Countering

    a.

    b.

    c.

8. Environmental control

    a.

    b.

    c.

9. Helping relationships

    a.

    b.

    c.

Witness (optional): _____

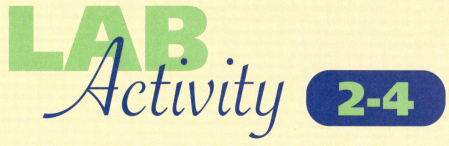

LAB Activity 2-4

Behavior-Change Log/Journal

Rather than writing a formal contract, you may find it easier to simply keep a log or journal of your behavior. In this way you can monitor your behavior, track your progress, identify stumbling blocks, incorporate coping behavior strategies, and readjust your plan as circumstances dictate. (Make copies as needed.)

Goal (specific and measurable):

Potential obstacles/challenges:

Behavioral/coping strategies to overcome obstacles:

Day/date	Today's challenges/obstacles	Today's behavioral/ coping strategies	Comments (personal and/or instructor)

Day/date	Today's challenges/obstacles	Today's behavioral/ coping strategies	Comments (personal and/or instructor)

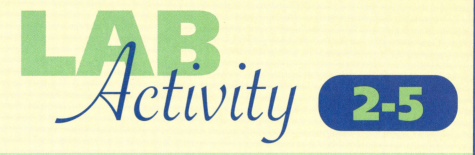

I've Had a Setback. . . . Now What?

Setbacks (or relapses) are not uncommon when undergoing a behavior change. Many factors can contribute to a setback: stress, social situations, cravings, illnesses, holidays, vacations, family issues, and so on. It is important to be able to recover from a setback and get back on track. Use this activity to help you rebound from a setback. See Table 2-2 for additional tips.

1. Describe your setback:
   (Examples: "I'd been exercising regularly for 6 weeks, then caught a cold and never started up again after I got well." "I'd been cutting back on fatty foods, then went to a party and ate a whole bag of potato chips.")

2. What do you feel triggered this setback?

3. What have you learned about yourself from this setback?

4. List three strategies you can use to get back on track and prevent this from happening again.

Name _____   **Class/Activity Section** _____   **Date** _____

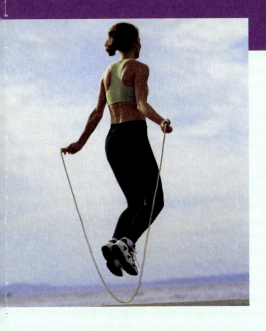

Developing and Assessing Physical Fitness

Our medicines are no further away than the shelves of the grocery and the sidewalks that we can use for a brisk walk.
—Tommy Thompson, former Secretary of Health and Human Services

Objectives

After reading this chapter, you will be able to:

1. Identify the five health-related fitness components.
2. Describe the purpose, content, and time of the three parts of a workout.
3. Identify one or more tests for each component of health-related fitness.
4. Complete the personal fitness assessment at the end of this chapter.
5. Use textbook norms to identify fitness levels in health-related fitness components, based on the results of fitness assessments.
6. Determine an appropriate fitness program by using workout charts for specific aerobic activities in Chapter 4 and the results of a cardiorespiratory fitness assessment.

Terms

- ballistic stretching
- body composition
- cardiorespiratory endurance (CRE)
- conditioning bout
- cool-down
- cross training
- exercise tolerance test
- fat-free tissue
- flexibility
- hypokinetic disease
- lean body mass
- muscular endurance
- muscular strength
- physical fitness
- principle of individual differences
- principle of reversibility
- principle of specificity
- progressive overload
- skinfold calipers
- static stretching
- subcutaneous fat
- task-specific activity
- warm-up

A Fit and Well Way of Life Online Learning Center www.mhhe.com/robbinsfitwell1e
Go to the Online Learning Center for chapter quizzes, outlines, flashcards, and additional lab activities.

*I*f there was a magic potion that you could take to increase your energy and help you manage weight, decrease stress, feel better, and decrease the risk of heart disease, cancer, and diabetes, would you be interested? The benefits of regular physical activity include these and many more. It is perhaps our cheapest preventive medicine. To live a wellness lifestyle, you must be physically active. While moderate levels of activity produce improvements in health, physical fitness requires higher-intensity activity and produces greater benefits. Physical fitness is an important component of wellness, because what affects the body ultimately affects the mind. Physical fitness enables you to function at the peak of your capacity physically and mentally—to enjoy life more fully—to be all that you can be.

You want to become more physically fit. How do you begin? This chapter discusses the benefits of physical activity and how much activity is needed to maintain health. It reviews basic principles of developing physical fitness, gives a prescription for physical fitness, and details methods of assessing the health-related physical fitness components. This enables you to measure your current fitness levels, set goals, and develop a plan for working toward those goals. It will provide you with the information you need to begin a fitness program so that you can reap the benefits for life!

IMPORTANCE OF EXERCISE

The natural peak of fitness occurs at physiological maturity, in the late teens to early twenties. After this, life becomes a slide down the aging curve for sedentary individuals, who gradually lose 1 to 3 percent per year of their cardiorespiratory endurance, muscle mass, flexibility, and so on. If you have observed friends who are older, you have seen that many of them are beginning to show physical deterioration due to lack of exercise: decreasing energy levels, increasing body fat, loss of muscle tone. Our bodies were designed for physical activity, but few occupations provide enough to maintain health or fitness. The homemaker, office worker, attorney, and student have busy, stressful lives and may feel tired at the end of the day, but they often lack the physical activity vital to tone muscles, stimulate the heart and lungs, or produce a training effect. This has resulted in

an epidemic of **hypokinetic diseases** related to an inactive lifestyle such as obesity, coronary heart disease, cancer, osteoporosis, and diabetes. Older adults are sometimes erroneously told to "slow down" and "take it easy," resulting in increasing weakness and accelerated physical decline. Unfortunately, too many people feel that they don't have time for exercise and are satisfied with minimal exertion in their lives. Approximately 250,000 premature deaths per year in the United States can be attributed to lack of exercise. According to Dr. Steven Blair, epidemiologist for the Cooper Institute for Aerobics Research, a sedentary lifestyle is as much a risk factor for disease as are smoking, obesity, and high blood pressure, but inactivity is more prevalent.

Inactivity also contributes to the problem of obesity in our country. Over 60 percent of American adults are overweight, and nearly a third are obese. In the last 10 years, adults have shown an average weight gain of nearly 8 pounds per person. Our nation's children are fatter, too, and about half are not physically active enough for aerobic benefit; this increases their risk of heart disease. Too many calories consumed and not enough exercise are to blame. The problem is compounded by the abundance of labor-saving devices, in other words, remote controls, computers, and riding lawn mowers. Children's playtime often consists of watching television; surfing the Internet; or sports lessons where sitting, standing, or watching consumes a major portion of the time. To make matters worse, although childhood is the best time to develop a lifelong habit of physical activity, many physical education programs face elimination because they are considered a frill when educational budgets are crunched. In a world filled with labor-saving devices, it is more important than ever to build exercise into our lives for optimal health and well-being.

For young people, levels of physical activity decline sharply through adolescence. Many college stu-

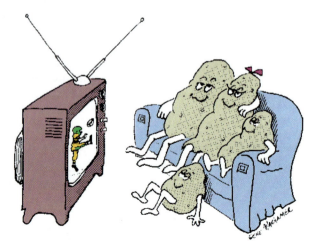

We have become a nation of spectators.

dents show early signs of hypokinetic disease. If you are concerned about slowly gaining weight from pizza, shakes, and fries, a good fitness program can reverse the trend. If normal daily activities leave you feeling worn out, you can boost your energy with regular exercise 3 to 5 days a week. Because routine activities such as sitting in class, watching TV, and walking across campus seldom require the physical effort needed to develop fitness, we must plan for daily vigorous exercise. The old saying "Use it or lose it" has never been more true.

PHYSICAL ACTIVITY AND HEALTH: A REPORT OF THE SURGEON GENERAL

We know that many people can improve their health and the quality of their lives with lifelong physical activity, yet about 60 percent of Americans are not regularly active and, worse, 29 percent are not active at all. Nearly 90 percent need more physical activity to improve their health. Almost half of our young people are not vigorously active. To encourage Americans to get moving and reverse the increasing toll of health-care costs related to chronic diseases, Surgeon General Audrey F. Manley produced a report, *Physical Activity and Health*. This report summarized the literature on the role of physical activity in preventing disease and came to these conclusions:

1. People of all ages can benefit from regular physical activity.
2. People can gain significant health benefits by including a moderate amount of physical activity on most, if not all, days of the week. This is equal to physical activity that uses 150 calories of energy per day, about 1,000 calories per week. It may include such activities as washing the car, dancing, and gardening (see Figure 3-1). With this modest level of physical activity, Americans can improve their health and quality of life.
3. Because amount of activity is related to frequency, intensity, and duration, the same caloric expenditure can be obtained in longer sessions of moderately intense activities (such as brisk walking) and shorter sessions of more vigorous activities (such as running). See Table 12-8 for the

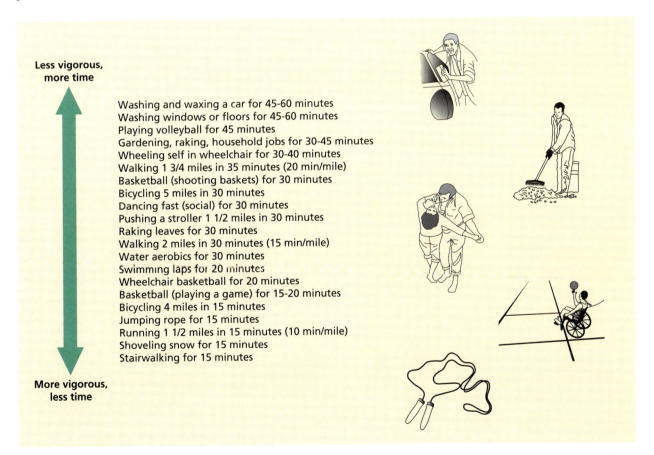

Less vigorous, more time

Washing and waxing a car for 45-60 minutes
Washing windows or floors for 45-60 minutes
Playing volleyball for 45 minutes
Gardening, raking, household jobs for 30-45 minutes
Wheeling self in wheelchair for 30-40 minutes
Walking 1 3/4 miles in 35 minutes (20 min/mile)
Basketball (shooting baskets) for 30 minutes
Bicycling 5 miles in 30 minutes
Dancing fast (social) for 30 minutes
Pushing a stroller 1 1/2 miles in 30 minutes
Raking leaves for 30 minutes
Walking 2 miles in 30 minutes (15 min/mile)
Water aerobics for 30 minutes
Swimming laps for 20 minutes
Wheelchair basketball for 20 minutes
Basketball (playing a game) for 15-20 minutes
Bicycling 4 miles in 15 minutes
Jumping rope for 15 minutes
Running 1 1/2 miles in 15 minutes (10 min/mile)
Shoveling snow for 15 minutes
Stairwalking for 15 minutes

More vigorous, less time

FIGURE 3-1   Moderate amounts of physical activity. SOURCE: U.S. Department of Health and Human Services Centers for Disease Control and Prevention, National Center for Chronic Disease Prevention and Health Promotion. *Physical Activity and Health: A Report of the Surgeon General*. Atlanta: USDHHS (1996).

caloric expenditure per minute for various activities.

4. Cardiorespiratory endurance activity should be supplemented with strength-developing exercises at least twice per week.

5. Greater amounts of physical activity (longer duration or greater intensity) can provide additional health benefits. The American College of Sports Medicine (ACSM) recommends that as fitness increases, individuals should move toward 300 to 400 calories of energy expenditure per day for high-level fitness.

6. Physical activity provides the following benefits:

- Reduces risk of premature death.
- Reduces risk of dying from coronary heart disease, and developing high blood pressure, cancer, and diabetes (see Figures 3-2 and 3-3).
- Helps reduce body fat and control weight. The ACSM recommends at least 60 minutes of moderately intense activity daily to lose weight and at least 90 minutes to manage body weight and fat.
- Helps reduce blood pressure in some people who already have high blood pressure.
- Helps build and maintain healthy bones, muscles, and joints.
- Reduces the risk of developing metabolic syndrome, a deadly combination of three or more of abdominal obesity, insulin resistance, elevated triglycerides, low HDL, and elevated blood pressure.
- Prevents cognitive decline in older individuals and may improve cognitive performance.
- Reduces anxiety and depression and improves mood.
- Promotes psychological well-being.

A landmark study conducted at the Institute for Aerobics Research in Dallas by Steven Blair et al. provides evidence that physical fitness is associated with longevity (Figure 3-3). In this 8-year study, physical fitness was quantified by using an exercise tolerance test on a treadmill. The subjects were categorized into five levels of physical fitness based on the treadmill test. The greatest reduction in risk of death occurred between the two lowest levels of fitness. Therefore, a modest improvement in fitness among the most unfit can bring about substantial health benefits.

Healthy People 2010 (see Chapter 1) also contains exercise objectives, which include the following:

✔ To reduce to 20 percent the proportion of adults who engage in no leisure-time physical activity.

✔ To increase to 30 percent the proportion of adults who engage regularly in moderate physical activity for at least 30 minutes or more.

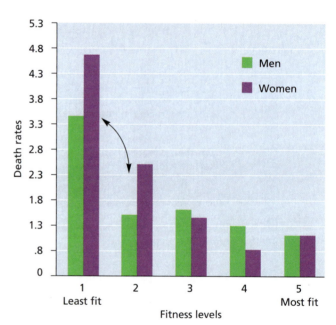

FIGURE 3-3 Comparison of fitness levels and risk of death. The death rates for the least fit men (level 1) were 3.4 times higher than those for the most fit men (level 5). Death rates for the least fit women (level 1) were 4.6 times higher than those for the most fit women (level 5). **The most dramatic drop in risk of death occurs between levels 1 and 2** (from 3.4 to 1.4 for men, from 4.6 to 2.4 for women). SOURCE: Steven Blair et al. "Physical Fitness and All-Cause Mortality: A Prospective Study of Healthy Men and Women." *Journal of the American Medical Association* 262 (November 3, 1989): 2395–2401.

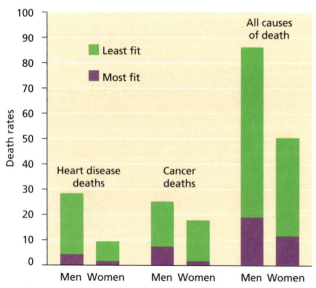

FIGURE 3-2 Exercise and health. An 8-year study of 13,344 people (10,224 men, 3,120 women) shows that physical activity reduces the risk of death from most causes. Charts compare death rates. SOURCE: Institute for Aerobics Research, "Physical Fitness and All-Cause Mortality." *Journal of the American Medical Association* 262, no. 17 (November 3, 1989).

Accomplishing these objectives would greatly reduce mortality rates. Then, perhaps, these individuals will enjoy a new active lifestyle and begin to see and feel the benefits of exercise. Eventually, they may invest additional time and energy, increasing the potential to acquire greater benefits from increased levels of activity.

Moderate Physical Activity for Health Promotion

There are differences in the intensity and duration of physical activity needed for health, for physical fitness, and for performance, such as in athletics. What is involved in adopting a moderately active lifestyle?

First, realize that physical activity does not have to be punishing to be beneficial. The emphasis should be on activity of *moderate* intensity. This would be equivalent to walking approximately 2 miles at a pace of 15 minutes per mile. You don't have to be soaked with sweat for improvements in health to occur.

Second, exercise does not have to be done all at one time. We know that 20 to 30 minutes or more of vigorous exercise is recommended for high-level fitness (full cardiorespiratory benefit), but all activity is beneficial to our health. Something is better than nothing. Incorporate bits of activity every day whenever and wherever you can. For example: Ride your bike to mail a letter; play racquetball, walk, swim, or run at noon; take a walk after dinner; walk to the grocery when you need only a few items. *Look* for opportunities to add daily activity—get up earlier, use TV commercial time, when working out a problem, when visiting a friend, and so on.

How much exercise is needed for health—30, 60, 90 minutes? The amount of daily physical activity recommended depends on your goal. To lower the risk of chronic diseases, 30 minutes of moderate activity is recommended on most, if not all, days of the week. This is important for reducing risk of coronary heart disease, diabetes, and cancer. Walking 2 miles in 30 minutes, or mowing the lawn with a push mower for 30 minutes, would meet the goal. However, this may not be enough to prevent weight gain. People can get greater health

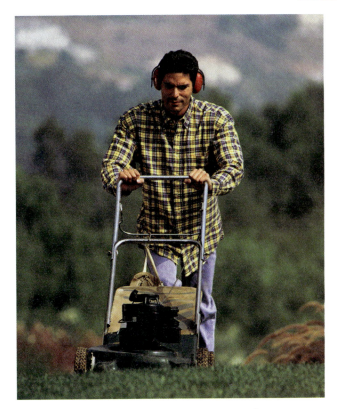

Just 30 minutes of moderate activity can provide many health benefits.

and fitness benefits from more vigorous activity or longer duration. Studies of people who have lost weight and kept it off for several years show that 60 minutes of moderate intensity activity, or lesser amounts of vigorous activity, are needed to lose weight. For those who have lost weight and are trying to keep it off, 60 to 90 minutes of physical activity are recommended to prevent gaining it back.

Most people declare lack of time as a reason for not exercising, but out of the nearly 40 hours a week of discretionary time available to the average person, 15 to 20 hours are spent watching television. For the time-crunched, Figure 3-1 has some suggestions for working exercise into your day.

THE NUMBERS

250,000	Premature deaths per year in the United States attributable to lack of exercise.
89%	Adults who need more physical activity to improve their health.
60%	Adults who are not regularly active.
29%	Adults who are not active at all.
30	Minutes of daily moderate activity needed to gain health benefits.

The Activity Pyramid

The Activity Pyramid (Figure 3-4), like the Food Guide Pyramid (see Chapter 11), is a guide to help you choose activities to improve your health and fitness level. The activities at the base of the pyramid, such as walking the dog and using the stairs more often, can be built into your everyday life. If you are currently sedentary, this is the place to start. If you are already moderately active, begin a formal exercise program (the second level of the pyramid) at least three times per week. Aerobic exercise is the most beneficial in promoting health benefits and cardiorespiratory fitness. Vigorous recreational sports also promote cardiorespiratory fitness. Extra healthful benefits can be achieved at the third level, which recommends strength exercises at least twice per week to build balanced fitness, especially if you already do aerobic exercise regularly. The fourth level adds flexibility and leisure activities two or three times per week. The top of the pyramid suggests what to do *least*, including sitting and watching TV.

You are faced with a tremendous challenge. Because you are our nation's future homemakers, parents, and leaders, the responsibility for the health and well-being of the next generation rests in your hands. You can make an enormous impact on the activity patterns of your children, family, friends, and neighbors by setting a good example. So go to it: Get up off the sofa, turn off the TV, and accept the challenge to enjoy exercise daily.

Encourage your friends and neighbors to get out and work in the garden, walk around the block, mow the

Prescription for Action

Date: *Do one or more today*

✔ Write down three reasons your last exercise program did not work and a solution for each.

✔ Schedule exercise on your calendar for a specific time 3 to 5 days this week.

✔ Take a 15-minute study break and go for a walk.

✔ Get to your job 30 minutes earlier and walk before starting work.

✔ Pack a sack lunch and take a 30-minute walk on your lunch break.

✔ Call a friend and make a date to bicycle or play tennis.

✔ Jump rope or use a stationary cycle while watching the news.

Prescribed by: _____*YOU*_____

TOP 10 LIST

Ways to Exercise on the Go

When you travel for business or pleasure, fitting in exercise presents a special challenge. As much as possible, plan ahead when/where you will fit in exercise during your trip. Pack your exercise clothes and a small towel so that you will be ready to go. Here are some suggestions for incorporating exercise into your travel plans.

1. Pack an exercise band and instructions (see the back cover of this book). Exercise bands are lightweight and take very little space in the suitcase. They are inexpensive and allow a wide variety of exercises for different muscle groups.

2. Lace up your shoes and walk for both sightseeing and exercise. You can often get route directions and maps from hotel personnel or a city guidebook. Walk wherever and whenever possible, avoiding cars and cabs. If the weather is extreme and you would rather walk inside, combine a trip to a mall with a 30-minute walk. Try to go early when the mall is least crowded.

3. Before you leave home, check the Internet for a list of gyms close to your destination and call or check online for classes (yoga, spinning, kickboxing) that you would like to try.

4. Use the Internet or a guidebook to check out local activities that you can incorporate into your trip like kayaking, climbing, swimming, and horseback riding.

5. With a laptop or portable DVD player, you can work out with an exercise DVD. A morning exercise program on TV may also be an option.

6. Pack two large empty plastic water bottles. When at your destination, fill the bottles with water to use as hand weights for upper body exercises.

7. An inexpensive exercise mat is easy to pack and can be used for stretching and calisthenics as shown in Chapters 5 and 6.

8. If you have a few hours between flights, use them to walk the airport, stretch, or do a few exercises with your exercise band. Some airports have a fitness facility that you can use for a small fee. You can also stretch and use the exercise band for sitting exercises while on the plane.

9. If you would rather exercise inside, take a jump rope. It can provide an aerobic workout in a small area.

10. If you are spending time on the beach, take a Frisbee and plan to be active rather than lying in the sand all day.

lawn, walk the dog, participate in recreational sports (bowling, tennis, golf, softball), and go dancing. Anyone can begin the journey toward wellness with a single step and begin reaping health benefits immediately.

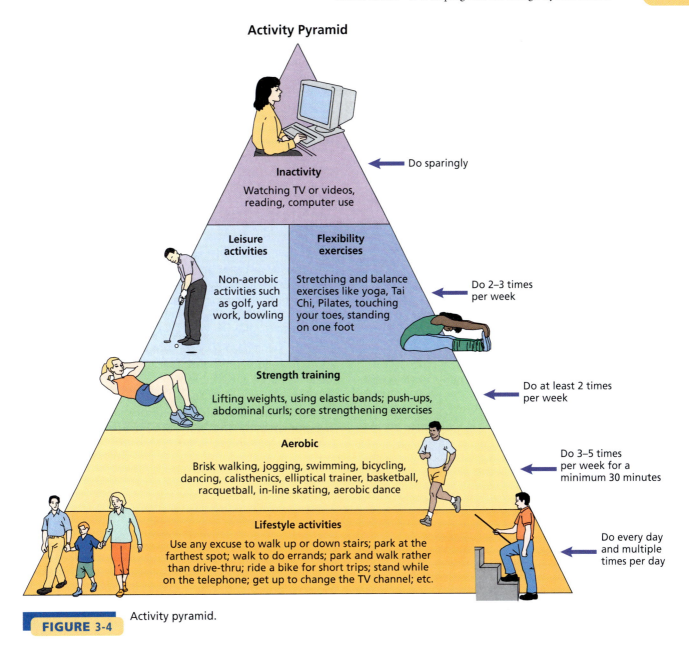

FIGURE 3-4   Activity pyramid.

While moderate activity can improve health, physical fitness requires more vigorous exercise to cause long-term beneficial physiological changes. Specific activity examples are given in Figure 3-1. Next, we will look at the components of physical fitness and basic principles of fitness development.

WHAT IS PHYSICAL FITNESS?

Physical fitness is the ability of the body to function at optimal efficiency. The fit individual is able to complete the normal routine for the day and still have ample reserve energy to meet the other demands of daily life—recreational sports and other leisure activities—and to handle life's emergency situations. Physical fitness involves skill-related and health-related components. The *skill-related* components of fitness are important to athletic success and are not crucial for health. The five *health-related components* of fitness are important for health and performance of daily functional activities. The skill-related and health-related components of fitness are:

Skill-Related
✔ Speed
✔ Power
✔ Agility
✔ Balance
✔ Reaction time
✔ Coordination

Health-Related
✔ Cardiorespiratory endurance
✔ Muscular strength
✔ Muscular endurance
✔ Flexibility
✔ Body composition

HEALTH-RELATED COMPONENTS OF FITNESS

Cardiorespiratory Endurance

Probably the most important fitness component is **cardiorespiratory endurance (CRE)**, the ability of the heart, blood vessels, and lungs to deliver oxygen and essential nutrients to the working muscles and remove waste products during vigorous physical activity. Your life depends on the efficient functioning of your cardiorespiratory system. Research shows that vigorous exercise is needed to keep your heart healthy and prevent heart disease. Good CRE is also needed if you want to enjoy running, swimming, cycling, and other vigorous activities to live at the peak of health and enjoy a full life. For more information on CRE, see Chapter 4.

Muscular Strength

Muscular strength is the ability of a muscle to exert one maximal force against resistance. Short-duration, high-intensity efforts such as moving furniture, lifting a heavy suitcase, and lifting a 100-pound weight one time are examples. Strength is important in sports whether you are hitting a tennis ball, running, jumping, or throwing. Weight training (see Chapter 6) is the best way to enhance strength and provides health benefits needed across the life span.

Muscular Endurance

Muscular endurance is the ability of a muscle to exert repeated force against resistance or to sustain muscular contraction. It is characterized by activities of long duration but low intensity, such as doing repetitions of push-ups or sit-ups. Muscular endurance is essential in everyday activities such as housework, yard work, and recreational sports. Muscular strength and endurance tend to decline with age along with activity levels, making it difficult to perform daily activities such as getting in and out of a car and standing up from the floor. This loss can be delayed and muscular fitness can be maintained by participating in a resistance training program.

Flexibility

Flexibility is movement of a joint through a full range of motion. Flexibility is essential to smooth, efficient movement and may help prevent muscle strains. It is specific to each joint; you may have flexible shoulders but tight hip flexors or vice versa. Can you sit and touch your toes without bending your knees? This requires hamstring flexibility. You need arm and shoulder flexibility to scratch your back. Women usually have more joint flexibility than men because men have bulkier skeletal muscles. Older adults may have trouble performing routine tasks such as turning to watch traffic while driving and fastening clothes at the back when dressing because flexibility diminishes with age. This loss can be countered if stretching is part of your lifetime exercise program. Chapter 5 has more information about flexibility.

Body Composition

Body composition is the amount of body fat in proportion to fat-free weight. The ratio between body fat and fat-free weight is a better gauge of fatness than is body weight alone. There are various ways to measure body composition, and all are superior to the height/weight chart method. For instance, a height/weight chart may label a 6-foot, 210-pound football player as overweight, when in reality he has only 10 percent body fat, as measured with skinfold calipers. On the other hand, a sedentary person may look okay, but when body composition is analyzed, it is calculated to be 30 percent body fat. Have your body composition analyzed by a professional. Obesity is unhealthy, is uncomfortable, and is associated with increased risk for heart disease, diabetes, high blood pressure, cancer, and joint and lower back problems.

PHYSICAL FITNESS AND WELLNESS

Becoming physically fit is a positive health habit that has a major impact on all dimensions of wellness (Table 3-1). It is one area where you can assume control of your lifestyle.

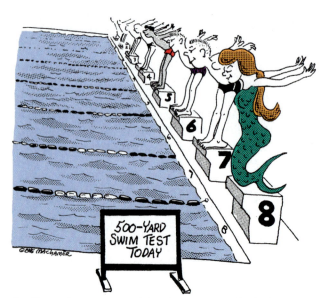

Cardiorespiratory potential varies among individuals.

TABLE 3-1	*Benefits of Physical Fitness on Wellness Dimensions*
Physical	Slows the aging process; increases energy; improves posture and physical appearance; helps control weight; improves flexibility; improves muscular strength and endurance; strengthens bones and reduces osteoporosis; reduces risk for coronary heart disease
Emotional	Relieves tension; aids in stress management; improves self-image; evens emotional swings; provides time for adult play; promotes psychological well-being
Social	Enhances relationships with family and friends; increases opportunity for social contacts
Intellectual	Develops concepts of mind and body oneness; increases alertness; enhances concentration; motivates toward improved personal habits (smoking cessation, reducing drug and alcohol use, better nutrition); stimulates creative thoughts
Occupational	Decreases absenteeism; increases productivity; decreases disability days; lowers medical care costs; lowers job turnover rate; increases networking possibilities
Spiritual	Develops appreciation of body-mind connection; enhances appreciation for healthy environment; builds compassion for those less able
Environmental	Develops appreciation for healthy air and water; increases concern for recycling and preservation of natural resources; increases interest in eliminating toxins and chemicals from food chain

THREE-PART WORKOUT

An exercise session includes three parts: a warm-up, a conditioning bout, and a cool-down.

Warm-Up

The **warm-up** is an important beginning to an exercise session. Two important physiological changes occur during the warm-up. The internal temperature of the muscles increases, enhancing their elasticity. Heart rate and respiration increase, thus providing greater blood flow to the exercising muscles. The warm-up prepares the body physically and mentally for the conditioning bout and may reduce the chance of injury while exercising.

There is no set length of time for the warm-up, although 5 to 15 minutes is adequate. On cold days or when you feel sluggish, the warm-up may take longer. When you're feeling energetic or when the temperature is warm, the warm-up period may be shorter. A good method of gauging whether you have had an adequate warm-up is to pay attention to how you feel. Do you feel ready to exercise vigorously? If you still feel stiff and sluggish, you need a longer warm-up. A slight sweat, reflecting an increase in deep muscle temperature, is a good indication of an adequate warm-up.

Three activities may be included in the warm-up: calisthenics (such as jumping jacks), mild stretching exercises, and a short period of task-specific activity. Stretching during a warm-up is mainly preparation for the activity, not for flexibility. Gentle **static stretching**, in which a stretch is held for 10 to 30 seconds, is best. **Ballistic stretching**, with jerking and bouncing movements, should not be used because it can strain cold muscles. See Figures 5-1 and 5-2 for more information on types of stretching and specific exercises. Most experts agree that the best time to stretch for flexibility is during the cool-down phase because the muscles are warmer and more elastic.

The **task-specific activity** is an exercise using the same muscles that will be used in the conditioning bout but at a lowered intensity level (lower heart rate). For example, joggers should include a short period of walking or slow jogging before increasing to normal intensity.

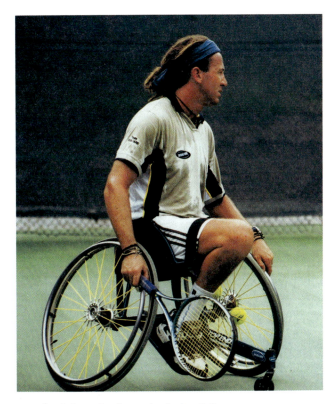

Everybody benefits from physical activity.

Conditioning Bout

The **conditioning bout** is the main part of the workout: 20 to 30 minutes or more. It may include a variety of activities for building cardiorespiratory endurance, muscular strength and endurance, or flexibility, depending on your goals. Gradually increase the frequency, time, and intensity of your exercise sessions until you reach a maintenance level. Progress slowly and listen to your body. If the exercise is at an appropriate level, you should recover within an hour. If you are too tired afterward or if the fatigue lingers until the next day, ease back on the workout time, intensity, or frequency to find an appropriate level. Your goal is a lifetime of exercise. Select an activity you will enjoy. Depending on your age, current fitness level, and physical abilities, enjoy walking, cycling, weight training, or any other vigorous activity you prefer.

Cool-Down

The **cool-down** is the final segment of the exercise session. The purpose of the cool-down is to ease your body back to its resting state. It will usually take 5 to 15 minutes to reduce the intensity of exercise. It should begin with the same activity performed in the conditioning bout, but at a lowered intensity. For example, if you jog, reduce the pace and end with a period of walking. Failure to cool down may allow the muscles to tighten further, potentially causing soreness and stiffness. Another problem with an inadequate cool-down is the possibility of venous blood pooling in the lower extremities, resulting in faintness and dizziness. The cool-down should continue until the heart rate is approximately 100 to 110 beats per minute or less. In the cool-down, spend a few minutes stretching while the muscles are thoroughly warm and elastic. Use the stretching exercises illustrated in Figures 5-1 and 5-2. Greater flexibility is achieved when stretching occurs in the cool-down segment of the workout.

PRINCIPLES OF FITNESS DEVELOPMENT

When a person begins an exercise program, over time the body adapts to the demands placed on it. The beneficial long-term changes that occur with regular exercise depend on several factors. To put together an effective exercise program, it is important to understand several principles of fitness development, including overload, specificity, reversibility, and individual differences.

Progressive Overload

Progressive overload is a gradual increase in physical activity, working a muscle group or body system beyond accustomed levels. Overload is perhaps the most important factor in developing physical fitness. When the amount of exercise is gradually increased, the muscle group or system, such as the cardiorespiratory system, gradually adapts, resulting in improved physiological functioning. In addition, a decrease in the severity and a delay in the onset of fatigue occur. If there is insufficient overload, there is no fitness improvement, but too much overload can cause injury. The key to gradual overload is to increase slowly.

To progress in cardiorespiratory exercise, gradually increase the frequency of workouts, starting with three and progressing to five workouts per week, adding one workout each week. Second, increase time. Start with workouts of 20 minutes (or less, if your fitness is very low) and lengthen the workouts by no more than 10 percent per week. For example, if the conditioning bout is 20 minutes, the next week's workout can be 22 minutes. Third, increase the workout intensity by no more than 10 percent per week. See Chapter 4 for further information on developing cardiorespiratory fitness.

The old saying "No pain, no gain!" is inappropriate advice for fitness exercisers. To increase your level of fitness and minimize the risk of overuse injury, follow the prescription factors in the correct order and listen to your body. Don't rush to get into shape in a few weeks. Exercise is for a lifetime.

Specificity

The **principle of specificity** means that only the muscles or body systems being exercised will show beneficial changes. To improve the cardiorespiratory system, exercise the heart and lungs through aerobic activities; to improve flexibility, do stretching exercises; and to improve muscular strength, lift weights. You cannot strengthen the muscles of the arms by jogging or increase cardiorespiratory fitness by doing yoga. This principle also helps explain why you are "wiped out" after swimming 10 minutes even though you can run for 30 minutes.

Reversibility

The **principle of reversibility** states that changes occurring with exercise are reversible and that if a person stops exercising, the body will decondition and adapt to the decreased activity level. Rate of fitness loss varies, but if a person stops exercising, a gradual loss of fitness begins within 48 hours. All fitness improvements can be lost within 2 to 4 months. If a person must decrease activity, the greatest benefits can be retained by maintaining intensity while decreasing the frequency or time of exercise. For example, if a person is traveling for 2 weeks and doesn't have time for the regular 30-minute run, 5 days a week, dropping to 20 minutes or 3 days a week at the usual target heart rate (THR) will help maintain training effect benefits.

Individual Differences

The **principle of individual differences** states that people vary in their ability to develop fitness components. Some people find that it is relatively easy to build strength, but they have to work hard to maintain their desired body composition. Others find that it is easier to increase their cardiorespiratory endurance than their flexibility. We differ in our genetic endowment, and there are limits on our ability to improve any particular fitness component. Some have estimated that maximal oxygen uptake can be improved by only about 15 to 30 percent with aerobic exercise. Even that amount of increase can make a tremendous difference in a person's quality of life. Within our genetic endowment, we have potential for improvement. You don't have to be an Olympic athlete to gain the health benefits of physical activity.

CROSS TRAINING

Cross training involves participating in two or more types of exercise in one session or in alternate sessions for balanced fitness. An easy way to start is to vary activities; for example, you could add one swimming session and two weight training days to a three-times-per-week jogging program and stretch daily. Or within one exercise bout you may spend a few minutes warming up on a treadmill, lift weights, do stationary cycling for 20 minutes, and finish with stretching. See Table 3-2 for cross-training activities. Cross training provides several advantages:

✔ It adds variety to your exercise sessions, preventing boredom and making it easier to stick to an exercise program.

✔ It provides a greater variety of fitness benefits than does any single activity alone. For example, weight training improves muscular strength and endurance but does little for cardiorespiratory endurance or flexibility. Running increases cardiorespiratory endurance but does little for upper body strength. It can be used to develop all five fitness components.

✔ It reduces the risk of injury because the bones, joints, and muscles are not subjected to the same repetitive stresses of one activity, which leads to overuse injuries (e.g., shin splints from excessive impact).

✔ Changing activities utilizes muscles differently, promoting muscle symmetry, a balance of strength, and flexibility in opposing muscle groups. Using only one activity tends to cause some muscles to grow strong and their opposing muscles to grow disproportionately weak.

✔ You may continue to train while allowing an injury to heal by using activities that do not stress the injured area.

TABLE 3-2	Activities for Cross Training
Exercise Goal	**Activity**
Cardiorespiratory endurance	Running, fitness walking, aerobic dance, bench and stair stepping, rope jumping, cross-country skiing, swimming, cycling, water exercise, in-line skating, ice skating, full-court basketball, ultimate Frisbee, soccer
Flexibility	Stretching, yoga, Tai Chi, Pilates
Muscular strength	Resistance training with weight machines, free weights, elastic bands, gymnastics
Muscular endurance	Calisthenics (push-ups, pull-ups, abdominal curls), weight training with light weights and high repetitions
Body composition	Cardiorespiratory endurance exercises burn calories at the highest rate per minute. Resistance training builds muscle, which increases metabolic rate for a greater calorie burn 24 hours a day.

✔ It develops high levels of fitness, because peak performance in any activity usually requires more than one fitness component. For example, a distance runner may benefit from greater strength and anaerobic fitness to run uphill or sprint to the finish line.

ASSESSING PHYSICAL FITNESS

Physical fitness tests are often divided into two categories: health-related and skill-related. Skill-related tests, such as a vertical jump or shuttle run, are performance-based and are related to athletic ability. Health-related tests are related to functional well-being in the areas of cardiorespiratory endurance, muscular strength and endurance, flexibility, and body composition. These areas of physiological functioning can be improved or maintained through regular exercise and offer protection against the negative effects of a sedentary lifestyle.

Do you know how fit you are? We seem to have a natural curiosity about how we compare to others. The purpose of fitness testing is to help you identify your current fitness levels in several health-related categories. Such an evaluation should tell you whether your current lifestyle is effective in developing and maintaining a level of fitness conducive to optimal wellness. Your results can be used as a basis for setting personal fitness goals; for developing an appropriate individualized exercise prescription; and finally, for measuring the effectiveness of your fitness program in reaching your goals.

The remainder of this chapter gives norms that enable you to compare your fitness levels with those of other students. Norms reflect achievements of thousands of people who have completed a 12- to 15-week fitness course. When evaluating your fitness and setting goals, keep in mind that scoring in the "low" category does not reflect negatively on you. While "superior" is an attainable goal for some, relatively few people achieve this level in one or more areas of fitness. Bodies are different. Your current fitness level does not indicate your potential. Physical capacity to achieve any particular level of fitness is partially genetically determined. You may find that you gain strength easily but must constantly work on flexibility or vice versa. Health-related fitness benefits can be experienced at the "average" fitness level. Also keep in mind that all tests are subject to some measurement variability. Results of tests of aerobic capacity and muscular fitness are influenced by a person's level of motivation. If you don't try hard, your fitness will be underestimated. Use these norms as guidelines. Finally, testing should not dominate your program but help you measure its effectiveness. You may wish to measure at the beginning of your program and remeasure 8 to 12 weeks into the program to see how you are progressing.

A *Personal Fitness Profile* is located in Lab Activity 3-3. When completed, it will indicate areas of fitness you can maintain and areas needing improvement. It will help you decide where to begin in your fitness program.

GUIDELINES FOR MEDICAL CLEARANCE

According to American College of Sports Medicine guidelines, it is generally safe to begin a vigorous exercise program if you are under 40 years of age for men and under 50 for women, are healthy, and have had a satisfactory medical checkup in the last 2 years. Also, if you have been exercising regularly, it is probably safe to continue progressing gradually from your current activity level. Prior to participation, you should complete the *Student Precourse Health Assessment* form found in Lab Activity 3-1 to identify any potential health concerns.

If you are over these age guidelines or if, regardless of age, you have noted health concerns on the *Student Precourse Health Assessment* form, it is important to check with your physician before taking a cardiorespiratory fitness test or participating in vigorous exercise. The *Physician-Approved Exercise Clearance Form* in Lab Activity 3-2 is designed for individuals with special health

concerns to assist your instructor in individualizing your fitness program according to your physician's recommendations. You may need to have a medical checkup and a diagnostic exercise test. If you smoke cigarettes, have been sedentary over the last several months, are pregnant, have diabetes, are 20 or more pounds overweight, or have family members who have positive risk factors for heart disease, it is particularly important that you see your physician and ask him or her to fill out the *Physician-Approved Exercise Clearance Form*. Also, check with your physician if you are unsure or have concerns about your health.

CARDIORESPIRATORY ENDURANCE TESTS

High-level wellness is inextricably tied to a physically active lifestyle. If you want to be an active participant in life—not just a spectator—cardiorespiratory fitness is essential. A person with a high level of cardiorespiratory fitness can do more work with less fatigue than can a person with low cardiorespiratory fitness. Increased cardiorespiratory fitness can enhance quality of life by increasing the rate of energy production during physical activity. Low levels of cardiorespiratory fitness may result in a limited lifestyle due to low energy reserves, quick exhaustion after moderate exertion, and resulting inability to participate in vigorous, oxygen-demanding activities. The ability of your heart and lungs to supply oxygen during activity is one of the best indicators of overall physical fitness. There are several ways to measure your body's ability to use oxygen. The most accurate method is an **exercise tolerance test** on a treadmill or on a bicycle ergometer in a laboratory (see Figure 3-5). In an exercise tolerance test, a person exercises strenuously while heart rate and oxygen consumption are measured. This, however, is complex, expensive, and time-consuming and requires elaborate equipment and trained personnel. It is impractical for testing large numbers of people.

Cardiorespiratory fitness can also be measured in field tests conducted out of the laboratory setting. What they lose in accuracy these tests make up in the practicality of self-testing or testing many people at the same time. Field tests of cardiorespiratory endurance are generally based on physiological performance (distance or time tests) or a parameter such as pulse rate (step test).

A field test used to estimate oxygen consumption measures the time it takes you to jog 1.5 miles. Studies have shown that time on the 1.5-mile run correlates well with your maximal ability to utilize oxygen. The faster you cover the distance, the more efficient your heart and lungs are at their job of supplying oxygenated blood and nutrients to the working muscles. Field tests make it easy

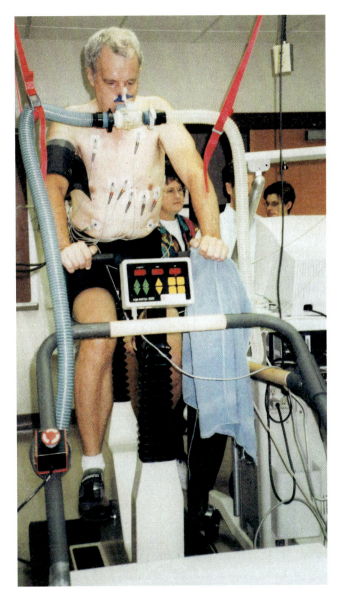

FIGURE 3-5 Exercise tolerance test on a bicycle ergometer.

for you to measure your fitness and detect progress as you train. Keep in mind that if you retest within a few weeks, early improvements may be due to a "learning effect" rather than true cardiovascular changes. That is, you will learn to pace yourself better throughout the distance. It will take 8 to 12 weeks for significant cardiovascular improvement to occur. You should take the *1.5-Mile Run Test* only if you are conditioned for it. It is best if you have been building up to the distance gradually for several weeks prior to taking the test. Other field tests that measure cardiorespiratory endurance are the *1-Mile Walk Test*, the *3-Mile Bicycling Test*, the *500-Yard Swim Test*, the *500-Yard Water Run Test*, and the *3-Minute Step Test*. You can choose the test most appropriate for your chosen physical conditioning activity.

Pretest Instructions

For any of the cardiorespiratory endurance tests, you will need comfortable clothes appropriate for the activity and a stopwatch or a watch with a second hand.

> ✔ If possible, avoid taking the test under conditions of extreme heat or cold, particularly if you are not accustomed to exercising under those conditions.
> ✔ Do not eat a heavy meal, consume alcohol, take caffeine, or smoke for up to 3 hours prior to the test.
> ✔ Drink plenty of fluids the day before testing.
> ✔ Rest from vigorous exercise at least 1 day prior to taking the test.
> ✔ Get adequate sleep (7 to 9 hours) the night before testing.
> ✔ Warm up and stretch before taking the test and then cool down and restretch afterward.
> ✔ If at any point during the test you begin to feel ill, dizzy, faint, or extremely short of breath, stop! Your body is telling you that you are not ready for this level of exertion.

Do not be ashamed of stopping before completing the test, especially if you are unfit. Test performance may be limited by local muscular endurance or by aerobic capacity. You may record the amount of time in the test you were able to complete and work toward a fitness level that will enable you to complete the test.

1.5-Mile Run Test

The *1.5-Mile Run Test* requires six laps around a standard quarter-mile track, or it can be done on a measured section of road. Consider taking this test only if you have been exercising previously. The *1-Mile Walk Test* may be more appropriate for you if you are over 35 years of age or 20 or more pounds overweight or if you have been out of shape for some time but are otherwise in good health.

Goal: To run 1.5 miles as quickly as you can.

Directions:
1. Locate a standard quarter-mile track or measure a section of road that has few stoplights.
2. Have a stopwatch or a watch with a second hand.
3. Before taking the test, warm up with walking, stretching, and a slow jog.
4. This is a test of your maximum capacity, so do the best you can. Push yourself to cover the distance as fast as possible without overdoing it. Try to maintain a continuous, even pace. Run as long as you can and then walk when necessary. In a group of runners, it is helpful for runners to be given the

right-of-way on the inner lanes and for people who need to walk to move to the outer lanes.

5. When you complete the 1.5-mile distance, record your time and exercise pulse and then cool down with walking and stretching.
6. Check Table 3-4 for your fitness level.

1-Mile Walk Test

For those who are starting a walking program or for whom the *1.5 Mile Run Test* may be too vigorous, the *1-Mile Walk Test* is an option. You will need a 1-mile measured course (four laps of a quarter-mile track), your walking shoes, and a watch with a second hand.

Goal: To walk 1 mile as quickly as you can.
Directions:

1. Warm up and stretch before beginning.
2. Walk 1 mile as quickly as you can.
3. Record your time to the nearest second. Record your exercise pulse.
4. Cool down and stretch.
5. Locate your fitness level in Table 3-4.

3-Mile Bicycling Test

If your main fitness activity is bicycling, you can test your cardiorespiratory fitness with a timed 3-mile bicycle ride. This test can be done on a bike track or on a measured section of road with few stoplights or stop signs.

Goal: To bicycle 3 miles as quickly as possible.
Directions:

1. Warm up by riding for a few minutes and stretching.
2. Cycle 3 miles as quickly as you can. If you are doing this on the road, be careful to obey traffic rules.
3. Try to pace evenly. Time the ride with a stopwatch or a watch with a second hand. Record the time. Record your exercise pulse.
4. Cool down and stretch.
5. Check your results in Table 3-4.

500-Yard Swim Test

If your fitness program primarily involves swimming, you will find a swimming endurance test useful. A regulation 25-yard pool is recommended, and you will need a friend to time you. You may swim any stroke, although best results will be obtained with the front crawl.

Goal: To swim 500 yards as quickly as you can.

Directions:

1. Warm up.
2. Have a friend time you and count lengths. In a 25-yard pool, 500 yards is 20 lengths.
3. Record your time and your exercise pulse, cool down, and stretch.
4. Check Table 3-4 for your fitness level.

500-Yard Water Run Test

The *500-Yard Water Run Test* (Figure 3-6) was designed for those involved in aerobic water exercise programs in which swimming skills are not required. It can be done lengthwise in a pool of constant depth or widthwise across the shallow end of a pool of variable depth. It helps to work in pairs, with one partner on deck counting completed laps for the other. For the most accurate results, runners should carve their own paths through the water and avoid drafting in the wake of other runners. Runners should use their arms to pull as they run but must maintain a vertical body position. No swimming is allowed.

Goal: To run 500 yards in the water as quickly as possible.

Directions:

1. Measure pool width and calculate the number of lengths required to cover 500 yards.
2. Have a partner on the deck count laps and keep the time.

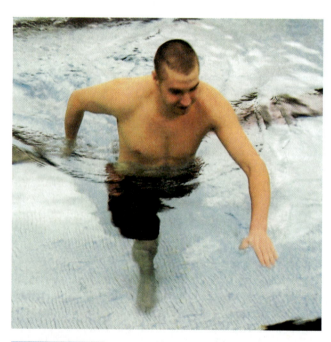

FIGURE 3-6 500-yard water run test. This is a valid field test for nonswimmers. (Note: The water level should be midpoint between navel and nipple.)

3. Warm up with a couple minutes of easy jogging in the water.
4. To give runners of different heights a similar level of water resistance in a variable depth pool, select a starting point along the pool wall where the water level is at a midpoint between the runner's navel and nipple. Shorter runners will start in shallower water, taller runners in deeper water.
5. Take a position in the water, note your starting time, and run the necessary number of widths. Record your time to the nearest second. Record your exercise pulse.
6. Cool down and stretch.
7. Check Table 3-4 for your fitness level.

3-Minute Step Test

A variety of step tests are useful for testing cardiorespiratory fitness indoors. They involve stepping on and off a bench for a 3- to 5-minute period and measuring the heart rate recovery. The step test is based on the fact that the heart rate of a person who is physically fit is lower at any work load and recovers faster than does the heart

rate of a person who is unfit. Although it is not the best measure of cardiorespiratory fitness, it is a quick and simple way to evaluate the heart's response to exercise. It is easy to administer to an individual or to large groups, requires no special skill to perform, and requires little equipment (Figure 3-7).

Goal: To step on and off a bench for 3 minutes.

Directions:

1. Locate a 15-inch bench or a 16-inch roll-out bleacher step.
2. Warm up.
3. Work with a partner. While your partner is stepping on and off the bench, stand in front of him or her to prevent falling. Then switch.
4. You will need to step up and down at 96 counts per minute. A metronome or recorded music at a tempo of 96 beats per minute will help you keep cadence, or your instructor will call the cadence: "Up-up-down-down." At the signal "Begin," step up with your right foot and then your left foot and then step down with your right and then your left. Continue for 3 minutes. Straighten your knees as you step up on the bench. To prevent leg soreness, you may want to switch lead legs about halfway through the test.
5. Stop at the end of 3 minutes and sit down. Five seconds after completing the test, the tester should count the partner's pulse for 15 seconds. The tester can check the partner's carotid pulse by lightly pressing against the neck under the jawbone. The partner being tested can double-check his or her own pulse at the radial artery, located on the thumb side of the wrist. The partners' pulse counts should not vary more than one or two beats if counting is accurate.
6. Record the pulse.
7. Cool down and stretch.
8. Compare your pulse with the norms given in Table 3-3 to assess your cardiorespiratory fitness. If you are unable to keep the cadence for the full 3 minutes, consider yourself to have low cardiorespiratory endurance.

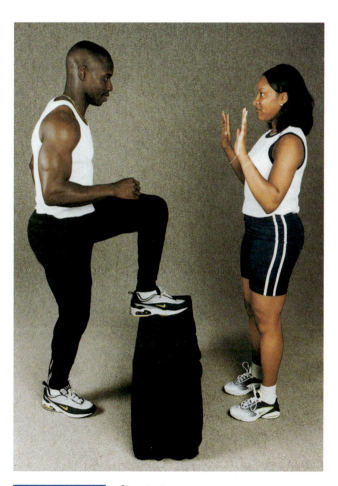

FIGURE 3-7   Step test.

TABLE 3-3	3-Minute Step Test Norms	
	Men	**Women**
Superior	<31	<37
Good	31–37	37–41
Average	38–41	42–44
Fair	42–45	45–49
Low	>45	>49

SOURCE: F. W. Kasch and J. L. Boyer. *Adult Fitness: Principles and Practices.* Mountain View, CA: Mayfield, 1968. Used by permission.

MUSCULAR STRENGTH AND ENDURANCE TESTS

Muscular strength and endurance are assets in the ability to perform daily activities—lifting, carrying, pushing, pulling—without strain or undue fatigue. Strength and endurance of the abdominal muscles are particularly important for good posture and lower back health. Muscular fitness activities add shape and firmness to muscles, resulting in a trim, well-toned appearance.

Muscular strength and muscular endurance tests have been used as a measure of physical fitness for years. Physical conditioning activities require and can develop both components. Strength is best developed by weight training and is often measured by one maximal lift with weights. Muscular endurance can be measured without special equipment by using the tests provided here. Abdominal curls are perhaps the best way to assess the endurance of the abdominal muscles. The traditional bent-knee sit-up test requires use of the thighs and hip flexors as well as abdominals and may put the back at risk. Abdominal curls isolate and test only abdominal muscles, decreasing risk to the lower back. Directions and norms for abdominal curls are given. To test the muscular endurance of the arms and upper body muscles, norms are also given for push-ups.

Muscular strength and muscular endurance are measured by different tests. You can assess the strength of major muscle groups by taking the *Leg Press Strength Test* and the *Bench Press Strength Test* using the guidelines provided.

Abdominal Curls

Goal: To complete as many abdominal curls as possible in 1 minute.

Directions:

1. Tape a 3-inch-wide strip on the floor and lie on your back on the floor with your fingertips at the edge of the strip (Figure 3-8). Bend your knees, and bring your heels as close as possible to your buttocks.
2. Curl forward until your fingertips have moved forward across the 3-inch strip and then curl back until your shoulder blades touch the floor. Your shoulders should lift from the floor with each curl, but the lower back should stay on the ground. If you are working with a partner who is counting your curls, your partner should not hold your feet down, nor should your feet lift off the ground—if they do, you are curling too high.
3. Complete as many curls as possible in 1 minute; then check the results in Table 3-4.

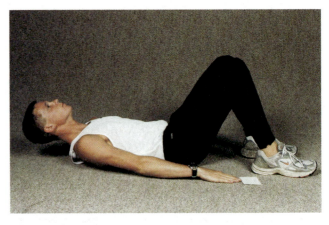

FIGURE 3-8   Abdominal curls (fingertips move forward 3 inches).

Push-Ups

Goal: To complete as many push-ups as possible in 1 minute.

Directions:

1. Start in an "up" position with your weight on your toes (men) or knees (women) and hands (Figures 3-9 and 3-10).
2. Lower yourself until your elbows form a right angle and your upper arm is parallel to the floor.
3. Complete as many full push-ups as you can in 1 minute. Be sure to keep your abdominals tight, your hips slightly piked, and your back straight to protect your lower back. Record and check your score in Table 3-4.

Leg Press Strength Test

The best measure of strength is one single maximal lift (one-rep max). This should be attempted only after several sessions of weight training, emphasizing proper lifting form for safety, as the risk of injury is high for an inexperienced lifter. If you have knee, ankle, or lower back problems, check with your physician before attempting a maximal lift. As there is no industry standard for resistance levels on weight machines, "70 pounds" will give a slightly different resistance level on a Universal, Cybex, or Nautilus. Strength testing using a machine is encouraged as it is safer than using free weights. You will need a leg press machine and a weight scale.

Goal: To find the heaviest weight you can press one time using the leg press.

Directions:

1. Warm up with several light lifts and stretching.
2. Set the machine for a weight lighter than you think you can press one time. Press to full extension. If you can press the weight to

TABLE 3-4 — Fitness Test Norms*

1.5-Mile Run

Age	18–29 F	18–29 M	30–39 F	30–39 M	40–49 F	40–49 M	50–59 F	50–59 M
Superior	<12:34	<8:26	<13:34	<9:10	<14:34	<9:55	<15:34	<10:40
Good	12:34–13:40	8:26–10:24	13:34–14:40	9:10–11:10	14:34–15:40	9:55–12:00	15:34–16:40	10:40–12:50
Average	13:41–14:45	10:25–12:31	14:41–15:45	11:11–13:45	15:41–16:45	12:01–14:55	16:41–17:45	12:51–16:05
Fair	14:46–16:00	12:32–14:49	15:46–17:00	13:46–16:00	16:46–18:00	14:56–17:15	17:46–19:00	16:06–18:30
Low	>16:00	>14:49	>17:00	>16:00	>18:00	>17:15	>19:00	>18:30

1-Mile Walk

Age	18–29 F	18–29 M	30–39 F	30–39 M	40–49 F	40–49 M	50–59 F	50–59 M
Superior	<12:34	<11:39	<13:34	<12:40	<14:34	<13:40	<15:34	<14:10
Good	12:34–13:40	11:39–12:59	13:34–14:40	12:40–14:00	14:34–15:40	13:40–14:40	15:34–16:40	14:10–15:20
Average	13:41–14:45	13:00–14:21	14:41–15:45	14:01–15:20	15:41–16:45	14:41–15:55	16:41–17:45	15:21–16:25
Fair	14:46–16:00	14:22–15:43	15:46–17:00	15:21–16:15	16:46–18:00	15:56–16:45	17:46–19:00	16:26–17:25
Low	>16:00	>15:43	>17:00	>16:15	>18:00	>16:45	>19:00	>17:25

3.0-Mile Bicycle Ride

Age	18–29 F	18–29 M	30–39 F	30–39 M	40–49 F	40–49 M	50–59 F	50–59 M
Superior	<9:18	<8:24	<9:54	<9:00	<10:30	<9:36	<11:06	<10:12
Good	9:18–10:06	8:24–9:12	9:54–10:42	9:00–9:42	10:30–11:06	9:36–10:12	11:06–11:36	10:12–10:42
Average	10:07–11:06	9:13–10:12	10:43–11:42	9:43–10:48	11:07–12:18	10:13–11:24	11:37–12:54	10:43–12:00
Fair	11:07–12:00	10:13–11:06	11:43–12:30	10:49–11:35	12:19–13:00	11:25–12:06	12:55–13:30	12:01–12:48
Low	>12:00	>11:06	>12:30	>11:35	>13:00	>12:06	>13:30	>12:48

500-Yard Swim

Age	18–29 F	18–29 M	30–39 F	30–39 M	40–49 F	40–49 M	50–59 F	50–59 M
Superior	<7:05	<6:12	<7:35	<6:30	<8:05	<7:00	<8:35	<7:30
Good	7:05–8:49	6:12–7:44	7:35–9:19	6:30–8:14	8:05–9:49	7:00–8:44	8:35–10:19	7:30–9:14
Average	8:50–10:34	7:45–9:19	9:20–11:04	8:15–9:49	9:50–11:34	8:45–10:19	10:20–12:04	9:15–10:49
Fair	10:35–12:19	9:20–10:51	11:05–12:49	9:50–11:22	11:35–13:19	10:20–11:52	12:05–13:49	10:50–11:22
Low	>12:19	>10:52	>12:49	>11:22	>13:19	>11:52	>13:49	>11:22

500-Yard Water Run

Age	18–29 F	18–29 M	30–39 F	30–39 M	40–49 F	40–49 M	50–59 F	50–59 M
Superior	<7:59	<6:53	<8:30	<7:20	<9:00	<7:50	<9:30	<8:20
Good	7:59–8:38	6:53–7:44	8:30–9:08	7:20–8:15	9:00–9:38	7:50–8:45	9:30–10:08	8:20–9:15
Average	8:39–9:18	7:45–8:38	9:09–9:48	8:16–9:05	9:39–10:18	8:46–9:35	10:09–10:48	9:16–10:05
Fair	9:19–9:58	8:39–9:32	9:49–10:28	9:06–10:00	10:19–10:58	9:36–10:30	10:49–11:28	10:06–11:00
Low	>9:58	>9:32	>10:28	>10:00	>10:58	>10:30	>11:28	>11:00

*Norms reflect the achievements of thousands of people who have completed a 12- to 15-week fitness course. Norms are revised yearly.

(continued)

TABLE 3-4 *Fitness Test Norms* (continued)

1-Minute Abdominal Curls

Age	18–29 F	18–29 M	30–39 F	30–39 M	40–49 F	40–49 M	50–59 F	50–59 M
Superior	>88	>93	>70	>78	>56	>65	>45	>49
Good	75–88	79–93	60–70	62–78	48–56	53–65	38–45	42–49
Average	60–74	64–78	47–59	51–61	37–47	42–52	29–37	35–41
Fair	45–59	50–63	35–46	40–50	27–36	36–41	21–28	28–34
Low	<45	<50	<35	<40	<27	<36	<21	<28

1-Minute Push-Ups

Age	18–29 F	18–29 M	30–39 F	30–39 M	40–49 F	40–49 M	50–59 F	50–59 M
Superior	>54	>64	>43	>54	>33	>43	>23	>33
Good	44–54	51–64	32–43	41–54	26–33	32–43	18–23	26–33
Average	32–43	37–50	22–31	27–40	17–25	22–31	11–17	17–25
Fair	20–31	23–36	13–21	18–26	8–16	13–21	6–10	8–16
Low	<20	<23	<13	<18	<8	<13	<6	<8

Sit and Reach (inches)

Age	18–29 F	18–29 M	30–39 F	30–39 M	40–49 F	40–49 M	50–59 F	50–59 M
Superior	>8.5	>7.0	>8	>6	>7	>5	>6	>4
Good	6.5–8.5	4.0–7.0	5–8	3–6	4–7	2–5	3–6	1–4
Average	4.0–6.4	1.0–3.9	3–4.9	0–2.9	2–3.9	–1–1.9	1–2.9	–3–0
Fair	1.0–3.9	–2.0–0.9	0–2.9	–3--0.1	–1–1.9	–4---1.1	–2–0.9	–5--3.1
Low	<1.0	<–2.0	<0	<–3	<–1	<–4	<–2	<–5

Leg Press (max/body weight)

Age	18–29 F	18–29 M	30–39 F	30–39 M	40–49 F	40–49 M	50–59 F	50–59 M
Superior	>1.97	>2.39	>1.67	>2.19	>1.56	>2.01	>1.42	>1.89
Good	1.68–1.97	2.13–2.39	1.47–1.67	1.93–2.19	1.37–1.56	1.82–2.01	1.25–1.42	1.71–1.89
Average	1.50–1.67	1.97–2.12	1.33–1.46	1.77–1.92	1.23–1.36	1.68–1.81	1.10–1.24	1.58–1.70
Fair	1.37–1.49	1.83–1.96	1.21–1.32	1.65–1.76	1.13–1.22	1.57–1.67	.99–1.09	1.46–1.57
Low	<1.37	<1.83	<1.21	<1.65	<1.13	<1.57	<0.99	<1.46

Bench Press (max/body weight)

Age	18–29 F	18–29 M	30–39 F	30–39 M	40–49 F	40–49 M	50–59 F	50–59 M
Superior	>1.00	>1.62	>.79	>1.34	>.76	>1.19	>.67	>1.04
Good	.80–1.00	1.32–1.62	.70–.79	1.12–1.34	.62–.76	1.00–1.19	.55–.67	.90–1.04
Average	.70–.79	1.14–1.31	.60–.69	.98–1.11	.54–.61	.88–.99	.48–.54	.79–.89
Fair	.59–.69	.99–1.13	.53–.59	.88–.97	.50–.53	.80–.87	.44–.47	.71–.78
Low	<.59	<.99	<.53	<.88	<.50	<.80	<.44	<.71

SOURCE: For norms in 1.5-mile run, 1.0-mile walk, 3.0-mile bicycle ride, 500-yard swim, 500-yard water run, 1-minute abdominal curls, 1-minute push-ups, and sit and reach: E. Keener et al. "Undergraduate Student Physical Fitness Assessment." Muncie, IN: Ball State University (originally published Spring 1989; latest compiled data shown here). For norms in leg press and bench press: based on norms from the Cooper Institute for Aerobics Research, Dallas, TX, revised 2000, used with permission.

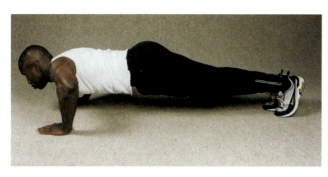

FIGURE 3-9 Push-up—standard position. (Note the 90-degree elbow angle.)

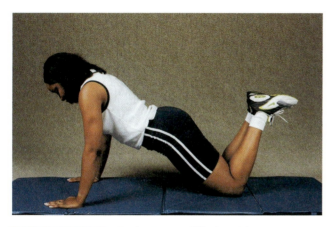

FIGURE 3-10 Push-up—modified position.

extension, add more weight and try again. Rest a few minutes between attempts. It probably will take several attempts to find your maximum. Stop when you reach a weight that you cannot move through a full range of motion. The heaviest weight that you could move through a full range of motion is your max. Divide your max by your body weight. Record.

3. Check Table 3-4 for your fitness level.

Bench Press Strength Test

If you have shoulder problems, check with your physician before attempting a maximal lift. While free weights may be used, strength testing using a machine is encouraged because it is safer than using free weights. You will need a bench press machine and a weight scale.

Goal: To find the heaviest weight you can press one time using the bench press.

Directions:
1. Warm up with several light lifts and stretching.
2. Set the machine for a weight lighter than you think you can press one time. Press to full extension. If you can press the weight to

extension, add more weight and try again. Rest a few minutes between attempts. It probably will take several attempts to find your maximum. Stop when you reach a weight that you cannot move through a full range of motion. The heaviest weight that you could move through a full range of motion is your max. Divide your max by your body weight. Record.

3. Check Table 3-4 for your fitness level.

FLEXIBILITY TESTS

Flexibility is a valuable asset in daily activities or in any type of vigorous exercise program. The ability to move joints through a full range of motion without stiffness or tightness makes exercise more comfortable and may decrease the risk of injury. The tests included in this section will indicate whether you have a normal range of motion in the lower back and other important areas.

Quick Checks for Flexibility

The quick checks for flexibility shown in Figures 3-11 to 3-15 are easy ways of measuring the flexibility of major muscle groups often shortened and tightened in daily activities. Each quick check is also a stretch, so if your range of motion is limited or if you feel excessive tightness in a joint or muscle group, use the same position to improve flexibility in that area (see Chapter 5 for basic fitness flexibility guidelines). Note that the hamstring flexibility test (Figure 3-14) eliminates the problem of arm-leg length discrepancy found in the traditional sit and reach test.

Sit and Reach Test

The *Sit and Reach Test*, which measures back and hamstring flexibility, can be done with a flex box. If you do not have a flex box, the test can be performed with a ruler on a bench or on the ground with feet flexed (Figure 3-16). Norms are given using the soles of the feet as the 0-inch mark.

Goal: To measure flexibility of the back and hamstrings.

Directions:
1. Warm up.
2. Sit with your feet flat against the flex box about 5 inches apart. Keep your legs straight.
3. Place your hands together. Without bending your knees, reach as far forward as possible, extending fingertips along the box. Hold the position for 3 seconds.
4. Find your flexibility in Table 3-4.

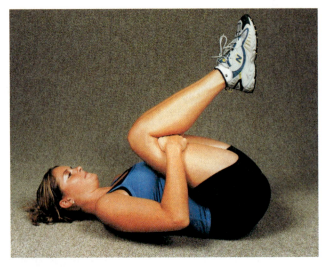

FIGURE 3-11   Low back flexibility test.
Muscle: Erector spinae (lower back)
Test: Lying on your back, pull thighs to chest.
Passing: Thighs should touch chest.

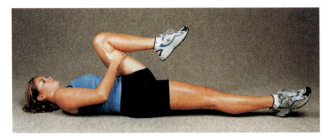

FIGURE 3-12   Hip flexor flexibility test.
Muscle: Iliopsoas (hip flexor)
Test: Lying on your back, pull one knee to chest, keeping other leg fully extended on the floor.
Passing: Calf of extended leg must remain on the floor; knee must not bend.

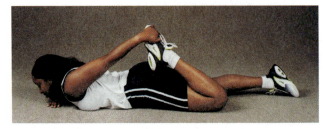

FIGURE 3-13   Quadriceps flexibility test. Caution: Avoid if you have or experience knee problems.
Muscle: Quadriceps (front of thigh)
Test: Lying face down with knees together, pull heel toward buttocks.
Passing: Heel should comfortably touch buttocks.

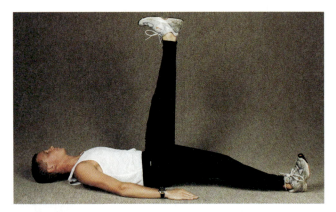

FIGURE 3-14   Hamstring flexibility test.
Muscle: Hamstring (back of thigh)
Test: Lying on your back, lift one leg, keeping other leg straight on the floor without bending either knee.
Passing: The raised leg must be vertical (90 degrees).

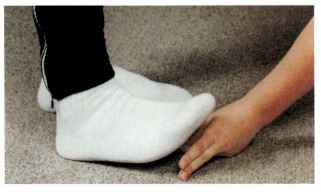

FIGURE 3-15   Calf flexibility test.
Muscle: Gastrocnemius (calf)
Test: Standing without shoes, raise one forefoot off floor, keeping knees relaxed and heels down.
Passing: Ball of foot should clear floor by height equal to width of two fingers.

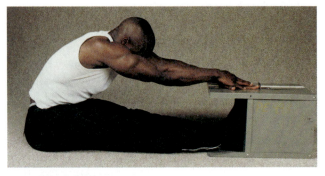

FIGURE 3-16   Sit and reach test.

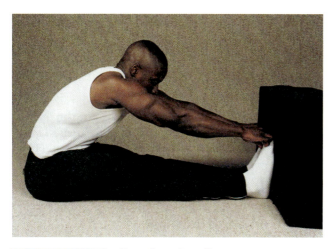

FIGURE 3-17   Sit and reach wall test.

Sit and Reach Wall Test

The *Sit and Reach Wall Test* is a self-check for flexibility and can quickly be performed by a large number of people. All you need is a wall (Figure 3-17).

Goal: To measure flexibility of the hamstrings.

Directions:

1. Warm up by walking and static stretching.
2. Remove shoes, sit facing a wall, and keep your feet flat against the wall and your knees straight.
3. Reach forward as far as possible to touch your fingertips, knuckles, or palms to the wall and hold the position for 3 seconds.
4. Check your flexibility evaluation in Table 3-5.

BODY COMPOSITION TESTS

A certain amount of body fat is essential to good health. Fat acts as an insulator, conserving body heat. It pads bones and cushions internal organs, and it stores and supplies energy for later use.

In a diet-obsessed society in which both obesity and eating disorders abound, few people realize that excessive leanness can be as unhealthy as excessive fatness. For young adults, an average range of body fat for women is 21 to 24 percent, and for men it is 14 to 17 percent (Table 3-6). Keep in mind that each of us has inherited a certain body build and fat distribution; it is natural for some bodies to carry more fat than others do. It is also natural to increase body fat slightly as we age.

While weight scales can tell you how much you weigh, they cannot tell you how much of your body is composed of fat or lean tissue. A sedentary individual may maintain a normal weight for height but increase fat

TABLE 3-5	*Sit and Reach Wall Test Scores*
Result	**Flexibility**
Cannot touch wall	Low
Fingertips touch wall	Average
Knuckles touch wall	Good
Palms touch wall	Superior

and lose **lean body mass** (muscle tissue) over time. A body builder may be "overweight" according to height-weight charts, but this is due to the development of muscle and bone rather than fat. Being overweight due to having a substantial amount of lean muscle tissue is not the same as being overweight due to excess fat tissue. A person who has a muscular build may think she is too heavy when the weight is mainly lean tissue. She could jeopardize her health trying to lose weight unnecessarily. On the other hand, a sedentary person who is satisfied with her weight may be shocked to discover that her body fat percentage is over 30 percent, high enough to pose a health risk. In the early stages of a fitness program, excess fat will often be lost and lean muscle weight will increase as fitness improves. Even if no significant weight change occurs, the exerciser is leaner and appears trimmer because a pound of muscle is denser than a pound of fat.

Body fat is measured by using several different techniques. Laboratory tests include DEXA and hydrostatic weighing. Nonlaboratory tests that use indirect techniques to estimate body composition include bioelectrical impedance, skinfold assessment, and measurements of circumference.

Dual energy X-ray Absorptiometry (DEXA) is a laboratory test that uses very low dose X-ray energy to measure body fat, muscle, and bone mineral. It is considered to be more accurate and valid than underwater weighing. When having the scan done, a person lies still on the DEXA table for about 12 minutes as the computer produces an estimate of body fat, muscle, and bone mineral. Two drawbacks are that this is an expensive test and that it is not readily available to fitness participants.

Underwater (hydrostatic) weighing is based on Archimedes' principle, which states that when a body is submerged in water, there is a buoyant counterforce equal to the weight of the water that is displaced. A person's weight on land and weight in water are compared. Because bone and muscle are denser than water, a person with a larger percentage of **fat-free tissue** is heavier in the water and records a lower percentage of body fat. However, fat floats, and so a large amount of fat mass will weigh less in the water. This technique reports an accuracy of ±2 percent and has been used by research laboratories to assess body composition for decades. The drawbacks are that it requires elaborate equipment, trained personnel, and about 30 minutes to test each person. Also, emptying the lungs of air (since air makes the body float) and repeatedly submerging underwater may be difficult for some individuals.

Bioelectrical impedance analysis (BIA) is based on the principle that an electrical current travels through fat-free tissue (all parts of the body except fat) with its high water and electrolyte content more readily than it does through fat. By measuring resistance to the current (which is too mild to be felt), the machine estimates body fat. Machines are inexpensive, are easy to use, and include handheld devices and weight scales with built-in electrodes (see Figure 3-18). However, the results vary with differences in hydration, placement of electrodes, and type of machine. BIA tends to overestimate lean individuals and underestimate those who are obese. Hydration plays an important role in BIA and can cause inaccurate results. Dehydration, which can be caused by exercising before testing, not drinking enough fluids, diuretics, illness, and drinking alcohol or caffeine, will cause overestimation of fat percentage. If these variables are controlled, BIA gives a fairly good estimate of body fat.

Another technique for measuring body composition involves the use of **skinfold calipers**. A caliper is a device that compresses the skin at a pressure determined by a spring. Skinfold measurements can be used to assess your proportion of fat to lean tissue because about 50 percent of your fat is **subcutaneous fat**—located directly under the skin between the skin and the underlying muscle. The amount of subcutaneous fat you have correlates highly with total body fat. An experienced measurer can assess body fat with skinfold calipers to within a range of plus or minus 2 to 5 percent. An inexperienced tester

may be less accurate. Two or more body sites may be measured, and accuracy increases with the number of sites sampled. Accuracy diminishes at the ends of the scale—for the very obese and the very lean—but for the average individual, skinfolds are reliable.

A self-test of body composition, though considerably less accurate than skinfold caliper measurements, involves body girth measures of body fat. Keep in mind that greater fitness is not guaranteed by low body fat, and what constitutes a healthy fat percentage is an individual matter.

Body Composition Assessment Using Skinfold Calipers

Goal: To measure subcutaneous body fat accurately.

Directions: Have a person trained in the use of skinfold calipers perform the following steps.

1. Measure skinfolds on the right side of the body by using a skinfold caliper.
2. Grasp a fold of skin between thumb and forefinger, pulling it away from the underlying muscle.
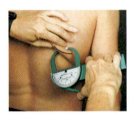
Skinfold measuring technique.
3. Apply the calipers about 0.25 inch below the fingers holding the skinfold.
4. For men, take triceps and thigh measurements on a vertical skinfold. For women, take subscapular and suprailiac measures on a slight lateral slant along the natural fold of the skin.
5. Measure twice. Take readings to the nearest 0.5 millimeter. If the readings do not match, take a third measurement and average the closest two measurements.
6. Skinfold sites for women are the following:
   a. Triceps. Measure a vertical skinfold on the back of the arm midway between the shoulder and the elbow.
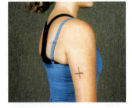
Triceps.
   b. Suprailiac. Measure a slightly lateral fold at the middle of the side of the body just above the hip bone (iliac crest).
7. Skinfold sites for men are the following:
   a. Subscapular. Measure a diagonal fold just under the right shoulder blade (scapula).
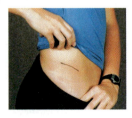
Suprailiac.

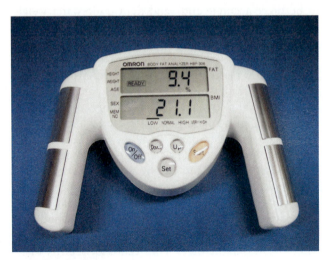
FIGURE 3-18 Bioelectrical impedance devices estimate body fat percentage.

b. Thigh. Measure a vertical fold on the front of the thigh midway between the inguinal fold (where the hip bends in front) and the top of the patella (knee cap).

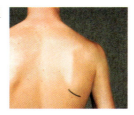

Subscapular.

8. Mark your two skinfold measurements on the *Percent Body Fat Nomogram* (Figure 3-20) and connect the marks with a straight line. Read your percent of fat on the center scale. See Table 3-6 for your body composition evaluation. If your body fat is not on the nomogram, use the following formula (Sloan-Weir):

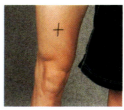

Thigh.

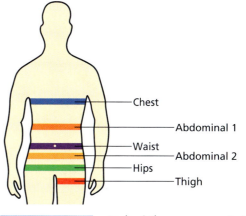

FIGURE 3-19   Body girth measurement sites.

Female (percent body fat formula)

% Body fat = [(4.57 ÷ (1.0764 − (0.00081 × suprailiac skinfold, mm) − (0.00088 3 triceps skinfold, mm))) 2 4.142] × 100

Male (percent body fat formula)

Percent body fat = [(4.57 ÷ (1.1043 − (0.00133 3 thigh skinfold, mm) − (0.00131 × subscapular skinfold, mm))) − 4.142] × 100

Example: A male with thigh skinfold = **10 mm** and subscapular skinfold = **10 mm**

Percent body fat = [(4.57 ÷ (1.1043 − (0.00133 × 10 mm) − (0.00131 × 10 mm))) − 4.142] × 100
= [(4.57 ÷ (1.1043 − 0.0133 − 0.0131)) − 4.142] × 100
= [(4.57 ÷ 1.0779) − 4.142] × 100
= .0977 × 100
= 9.77% body fat

Body Girth Measures

One reason many people begin a fitness program is that they are concerned about their physical appearance. Basic body build is an inherited characteristic, and less than 5 percent of the population can aspire to the current cultural "ideal" of model-like proportions. Take a look at your parents and grandparents to get an idea of your genetic endowment and what is realistic for you. While your basic structure cannot be altered, as fitness improves, fat may be lost from deposit areas and muscles will become firmer, enhancing body contours. You may notice a loss of unwanted inches from the waist, hips, or

thighs or a desirable reshaping of body contours before noticing any weight change. Body girth measures will help you set goals to work for a trim, healthy body shape.

Goal: To measure body girths.

Directions: Recruit a partner to measure you. You will need a measuring tape. For each measurement, pull the tape snugly but do not indent the flesh. Take the measurements at the following sites (Figure 3-19):

- *Chest:* across the nipple line at the midpoint of a normal breath
- *Abdominal 1:* across the floating ribs, halfway between the chest and waist, at the midpoint of a normal breath
- *Waist:* the narrowest point, across the navel
- *Abdominal 2:* across the iliac crest (hip bones), midway between waist and hips
- *Hips:* with feet together, across the pubic bone in front and across the widest part in back
- *Thigh:* right side, widest part, 1 inch below the crotch

Body Girth Measures of Body Fat

Body girth measures of fatness have greater variability than do other measures of body fat, such as skinfolds. However, their advantage is that they do not require special equipment or training and can be done with a measuring tape at home.

Directions:

1. Men should measure waist girth at the navel, and women should measure hips at the widest point. Pull the tape so it is snug but does not indent the skin.
2. Remove shoes. Men should measure their weight without clothing. Women should measure their height.

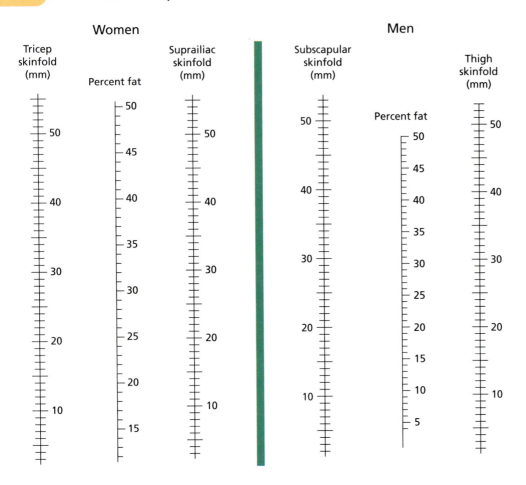

FIGURE 3-20   Percent body fat nomogram. Source: A. W. Sloan and J. Weir, "Nomograms for Prediction of Body Density and Total Body Fat from Skinfold Measurements." *Journal of Applied Physiology* 28:2 (1970): 221–222. Reprinted by permission of the American Physiological Society.

TABLE 3-6   *Body Fat Norm Percentages*

Ages	18–29		30–39		40–49		50+	
	F	M	F	M	F	M	F	M
Very low fat	<17	<10	<18	<11	<19	<13	<20	<15
Low fat (trim)	17–20	10–13	18–20	11–16	19–21	13–18	20–22	15–19
Average	21–24	14–17	21–24	17–19	22–24	19–21	23–25	20–22
Above average (fat)	25–27	18–20	25–27	20–22	25–27	22–23	26–28	23–24
High fat	28–30	21–25	28–30	23–25	28–30	24–25	29–31	25–26
Obese	>30	>25	>30	>25	>30	>25	>31	>26

Source: E. Keener et al. "Undergraduate Student Physical Fitness Assessment." Muncie, IN: Ball State University (originally published Spring 1997; latest compiled data shown here).

TABLE 3-7   *Waist-to-Hip Ratio, Waist Girth, and Health Risk**

Waist-to-Hip Ratio	High Risk	Waist Circumference	High Risk
Men	.95 or greater	Men	over 40 inches
Women	.80 or greater	Women	over 35 inches

*Risk of cardiovascular disease, hypertension, and type 2 diabetes

3. Mark the measurements on the appropriate circumference chart and connect them with a straight line (Figure 3-21).

Waist-to-Hip Ratio and Waist Girth

Investigations have begun pointing to the location of excess fat as a risk factor for heart disease and certain cancers. Fat distributed in the abdominal area is linked to increased health risks; hip/thigh fat is not as risky. As a result, the waist-to-hip ratio has become a common assessment for health-risk identification. To compute this ratio, divide the waist measurement by the hip measurement.

$$\frac{29 \text{ in. waist}}{38 \text{ in. hip}} = 0.76 \qquad \frac{42 \text{ in. waist}}{36 \text{ in. hip}} = 1.17$$

Studies indicate that health problems are increased for women whose ratio is 0.80 or higher and for men whose ratio is 0.95 or higher. You may also use waist girth alone. Health risks are higher for women with a waist measurement over 35 inches, and for men with one over 40 inches. (See Chapter 12 for more information on waist-to-hip ratio as a health-risk factor.)

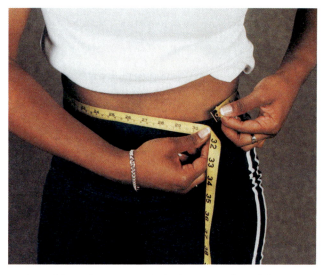

Waist-to-hip ratio or waist girth alone can identify health risk.

Circumference chart for women

Hip girth (inches)	% fat	Height (inches)
32	10	72
	14	70
34	18	
36	22	68
38	26	66
	30	
40	34	64
42	38	62
44	42	60

Circumference chart for men

Body weight (pounds)

% fat

Body weight (pounds)	% fat	Waist girth (inches)
120	40	45
140	30	
160	25 / 20	40
180	15	35
200	10	
220	5	30
240		
260		25

FIGURE 3-21 Circumference charts. Source: Nomograms developed by Jack Wilmore, University of Texas. Used by permission.

Frequently Asked Questions

Q. I want to exercise, but after a full day of work and classes I feel too tired, plus exercise makes me more tired. What should I do?

A. Schedule a time that works for you. Some people have more energy in the morning and get up a half hour early for a brisk walk. Others take time during their lunch hour. Still others schedule a class (like aerobics or spinning) at the end of the day. Whatever time you choose, schedule it in like an appointment. Some days you will start with more energy, and other days less, but generally, if the intensity is appropriate, you will find yourself invigorated rather than exhausted at the end of the workout. Use the "talk test" to judge if you are exercising at the correct intensity. It may also help if you exercise with a friend; that way it will seem more like fun and less like work. Review the Top 10 "Ways to Stick with Exercise" in Chapter 4 for more tips on maintaining your exercise program.

Q. How many calories do I burn while walking or jogging a mile?

A. Caloric expenditure is based on body weight. You burn about 62 calories per 100 pounds per mile whether walking or jogging. It's a principle of physics. It takes a certain amount of energy to move weight a certain distance. If you weigh 150 pounds, you burn $62 \times 1.50 = 93$ calories per mile.

Q. I want to lose weight. Is it better to exercise for a longer time at a lower intensity or for a shorter time at a higher intensity?

A. If your main goal is weight control, the most important factor, besides a low-fat, nutritious diet, is to be consistent about working aerobic exercise—of any length and intensity—into your daily schedule. Work out at least 5 days per week. Total of calories expended is more important than intensity of activity in maximizing weight loss. One or two weight-training sessions per week also lead to weight control. Moderate-intensity exercise is recommended because it allows you to exercise longer, accumulate more total work, and thus burn more calories, and it is less likely to cause discomfort or injury. Moderate-intensity activity can also help you keep off lost weight. If your goal is high-level fitness, exercise at a higher intensity is necessary.

Q. I swim/cycle regularly and feel like I'm in pretty good shape. Why did I score only "average" on the 1.5-mile walk/run?

A. It's the rule of specificity. Your aerobic fitness will show best if you use the test specific to your activity. Swimmers should use the 500-yard swim and cyclists the 3-mile ride for results, which are a better reflection of their aerobic fitness level. Likewise, someone who usually runs for exercise would find a cycling or swimming test more difficult.

Q. I had my body fat tested by skinfold calipers and bioelectrical impedance. They gave different results. Which is more accurate?

A. Both are reasonably accurate when used by an experienced tester, with average errors of 2 to 5 percent. Skinfold calipers are more accurate if multiple sites are measured to get a better picture of total fat distribution. Bioelectrical impedance can overestimate fat percentage if you are dehydrated, and results vary depending on where the electrodes are placed and the type of machine used.

Summary

The sedentary lifestyle of most Americans is seriously undermining the health and welfare of our nation. We are fast becoming overfat and underfit, resulting in reduced levels of well-being. From the information you have acquired in this chapter, you now have the necessary tools to develop a personalized physical fitness program based on sound scientific principles and using your age, resting heart rate, interests, and abilities. You also have gained a better understanding of the health benefits that can be achieved by incorporating moderate levels of physical activity into your daily life. By applying the concept of a three-segment workout and finding ways to increase daily activity, you can be on your way to a lifetime of improved health, fitness, and wellness.

Assessment is a critical tool in developing any dimension of wellness. It helps you understand your strengths and weaknesses and decide whether your current levels of cardiorespiratory endurance, muscular endurance, flexibility, and body fat are conducive to optimal wellness. With this knowledge, you can set reasonable fitness goals, establish a starting point for a fitness program, and develop a plan of action. Specific workout programs for different aerobic activities can be found in Chapter 4. A *Student Precourse Health Assessment* form and a *Personal Fitness Profile* are also available in the Lab Activities section of this chapter.

As you progress in your fitness program, it may be useful to retest occasionally. While testing should not dominate your program, it will allow you to monitor your progress and can give you additional motivation to continue regular exercise.

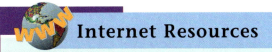

Internet Resources

American Academy of Family Physicians

www.familydoctor.org

Promotes healthy behaviors with fact sheets on many health topics, including exercise and fitness.

American College of Sports Medicine

www.acsm.org/sportsmed

Information on sports research, health and fitness, and aerobic exercise guidelines, along with a quarterly fitness newsletter. "Current Comments" gives information on a variety of exercise topics of recent interest.

American Council on Exercise

www.acefitness.org/fitfacts/

Features 100 fitness fact sheets, free e-newsletters, and a variety of different fitness activities from bicycling to swimming.

American Heart Association

www.americanheart.org

Health tools include an exercise diary and body mass calculator. Information includes exercise and fitness promotion for women, children, seniors; information on how exercise affects heart health; exercise tips; and a healthy heart workout quiz.

Centers for Disease Control and Prevention

www.cdc.gov/nccdphp/dnpa/

Information on getting started in physical activity, exercise tips, links to other fitness resources, and health promotion for increasing physical activity in your school or community.

Medline Plus

www.nlm.nih.gov/medlineplus

Consumer site with comprehensive information on many health topics, including physical fitness benefits, health, weight management, and fitness at any age.

National Center for Chronic Disease Prevention and Health Promotion

www.cdc.gov/nccdphp

Information on nutrition, physical fitness, and preventing chronic diseases such as diabetes and cancer.

National Institutes of Health

www.nhlbisupport.com/bmi

Calculate your body mass index, assess your risk, and find information and recipes for weight control.

President's Council on Physical Fitness and Sports

www.fitness.gov

Information on fitness and health, weight control, exercise for kids and seniors, videos, and sports and fitness awards, along with fact sheets on fitness and health.

Shape Up America!

www.shapeup.org

Information and guidance on weight management, plus a body fat lab.

Bibliography

American College of Sports Medicine. "ACSM Guidelines." October 2005. www.acsm.org

Avila-Funes, J. A., and E. J. Garcia-Mayo. "The Benefits of Doing Exercise in the Elderly." *Gaceta Medica de Mexico* 140 (July–August 2004): 431–436.

Barlow, C. E., et al. "Cardiorespiratory Fitness as a Predictor of Incident Metabolic Syndrome: Aerobics Center Longitudinal Study." *Medicine and Science in Sports and Fitness* 36 (May 2004): S7.

Bauman, A. E. "Updating the Evidence That Physical Activity Is Good for Health: An Epidemiological Review 2000–2003." *Journal of Science and Medicine in Sports* 7 (April 2004): 1 Suppl. 6–19.

Bigaard, J., et al. "Waist Circumference and Body Composition in Relation to All-Cause Mortality in Middle-Aged Men and Women." *International Journal of Obesity and Related Metabolic Disorders* 29 (July 2005): 778–784.

Blair, S. N., et al. "Influences of Cardiorespiratory Fitness and Other Precursors on Cardiovascular Disease and All Cause Mortality in Men and Women." *JAMA* 276, no. 3 (July 17, 1996): 205–210.

Blair, S. N., et al. "Physical Fitness and All-Cause Mortality: A Prospective Study of Healthy Men and Women." *JAMA* 262, no. 17 (November 3, 1989): 2395–2401.

Blair, S. N., Y. Cheng, and J. S. Holder. "Is Physical Activity or Physical Fitness More Important in Defining Health Benefits?" *Medicine and Science in Sports and Exercise* 33 (6Suppl) (June 2001): S379–399.

Blair, S. N., and A. S. Jackson. "Physical Fitness and Activity as Separate Heart Disease Risk Factors: A Meta-Analysis." *Medicine and Science in Sports and Exercise* 33 (May 2001): 762–764.

Borg, G. "Psychophysical Bases of Physical Exertion." *Medicine and Science in Sports and Exercise* 14 (1982): 707.

Casanova, R. M., et al. "Body Composition Analysis Using Bioelectrical and Anthropometric Parameters." *Annals of Pediatrics* 61 (July 2004): 23–31.

Castillo, G., P. Ortega, and R. Ruiz. "Improvement of Physical Fitness as Anti-Aging Intervention." *Medicina Clinica* 124 (February 2005): 146–155.

Chan, D. C., et al. "Waist Circumference, Waist-to-Hip Ratio and Body Mass Index as Predictors of Adipose Tissue Compartments in Men." *QJM* 96 (June 2003): 441–447.

Church, T. S., et al. "Usefulness of Cardiorespiratory Fitness as a Predictor of All-Cause and Cardiovascular Disease Mortality in Men with Systemic Hypertension." *American Journal of Cardiology* 88 (September 2001): 651–656.

Colcombe, S., et al. "Aerobic Fitness Reduces Brain Tissue Loss in Aging Humans." *Journal of Gerontology Psychological Science* 58 (February 2003): 176–180.

Colcombe, S. J., et al. "Cardiovascular Fitness, Cortical Plasticity, and Aging." *Proceedings of the National Academy of Science, USA* 101 (March 2004): 3316–3321.

Colcombe, S. J., et al. "Neurocognitive Aging and Cardiovascular Fitness: Recent Findings and Future Directions." *Journal of Molecular Neuroscience* 24 (January 2004): 9–14.

Cooper, K. H. "A Means of Assessing Maximal Oxygen Intake: Correlation between Field and Treadmill Testing." *Journal of the American Medical Association* 203 (January 1968): 201–204.

DuBose, K. D., et al. "Leisure-Time Physical Activity and the Metabolic Syndrome: An Examination of NHANES III." *Medicine and Science in Sports and Exercise* 36 (May 2004): S7.

Duncan, G. E., et al. "Effects of Exercise on Emerging and Traditional Cardiovascular Risk Factors." *Preventive Medicine* 39 (November 2004): 894–902.

Ekelund, U., et al. "Physical Activity Energy Expenditure Predicts Progression Toward the Metabolic Syndrome Independently of Aerobic Fitness in Middle-Aged Healthy Caucasians: The Medical Research Council Ely Study." *Diabetes Care* 28 (May 2005): 195–200.

Farrell, S. W., et al. "The Relation of Body Mass Index, Cardiorespiratory Fitness, and All-Cause Mortality in Women." *Obesity Research* 10 (June 2002): 417–423.

Garcia, A. L., et al. "Improved Prediction of Body Fat by Measuring Skinfold Thickness, Circumferences, and Bone Breadths." *Obesity Research* 13 (March 2005): 626–634.

Hagberg, J. M. "Exercise Your Way to Lower Blood Pressure." The American College of Sports Medicine, October 2005. www.acsm.org

Hawkins, S., and R. Wiswell. "Rate and Mechanism of Maximal Oxygen Consumption Decline with Aging: Implications for Exercise Training." *Sports Medicine* 33 (December 2003): 877–888.

Heyward, V. H., and D. R. Wagner. *Applied Body Composition Assessment*, 2nd ed. Champaign, IL: Human Kinetics, 2004.

Hu, F. B., et al. "Television Watching and Other Sedentary Behaviors in Relation to Risk of Obesity and Type 2 Diabetes Mellitus in Women." *New England Journal of Medicine* 348 (April 2003): 1625–1638.

Hwu, C. M., et al. "Waist Circumference Predicts Metabolic Cardiovascular Risk in Postmenopausal Chinese Women." *Menopause* 10 (January–February 2003): 73–80.

Jurca, R., et al. "Continuous Metabolic Syndrome Score as a Predictor of Mortality in Men with Metabolic Syndrome." *Medicine and Science in Sports and Exercise* 36 (May 2004): S7–S8.

Kaminsky, L., and G. Dwyer. "Body Composition." In Kaminsky, L. A., et al., eds., *ACSM's Resource Manual for Guidelines for Exercise Testing and Prescription,* 5th ed. Philadelphia: Lippincott Williams & Wilkins, 2006.

Kaminsky, L. A., et al. "Evaluation of a Shallow Water Running Test for the Estimation of Peak Aerobic Power." *Medicine and Science in Sport and Exercise* 25 (November 1993): 1287–1292.

Keener, E., et al. "Undergraduate Student Physical Fitness Assessment." Muncie, IN: Ball State University, Spring 1989.

Kemmler, W., et al. "Benefits of 2 Years of Intense Exercise on Bone Density, Physical Fitness, and Blood Lipids in Early Postmenopausal Osteopenic Women: Results of the Erlangen Fitness Osteoporosis Prevention Study." *Archives of Internal Medicine* 164 (May 2004): 1084–1091.

Kohl, H. W., et al. "Changes in Physical Fitness and All-Cause Mortality: A Prospective Study of Healthy and Unhealthy Men." *JAMA* 273, no. 14 (April 12, 1995): 1093–1098.

Lee, C. D., S. N. Blair, and A. S. Jackson. "Cardiorespiratory Fitness, Body Composition, and All-Cause and Cardiovascular Disease Mortality in Men." *American Journal of Clinical Nutrition* 69 (March 1999): 373–380.

Lee, I. M., C. Hsieh, and R. S. Paffenbarger. "Exercise Intensity and Longevity in Men: The Harvard Alumni Health Study." *JAMA* 273, no. 15 (April 19, 1995): 1179–1184.

Lee, I. M., H. D. Sesso, Y. Oguma, and R. S. Paffenbarger. "Relative Intensity of Physical Activity and Risk of Coronary Heart Disease." *Circulation* 107 (March 4, 2003): 1110–1115.

Lee, S., et al. "Cardiorespiratory Fitness Attenuates Metabolic Risk Independent of Abdominal Subcutaneous and Visceral Fat in Men." *Diabetes Care* 28 (April 2005): 895–901.

McAuley, E., A. F. Kramer, and S. J. Colcombe. "Cardiovascular Fitness and Neurocognitive Function in Older Adults: A Brief Review." *Brain and Behavior Immunology* 18 (May 2004): 214–220.

National Center for Chronic Disease Prevention and Health Promotion. "Physical Activity and Good Nutrition: Essential Elements to Prevent Chronic Diseases and Obesity." May 2003. www.cdc.gov/nccdphp/dnpa

Saris, W. H., et al. "How Much Physical Activity Is Enough to Prevent Unhealthy Weight Gain?" *Outcome of the IASO 1st Stock Conference and Consensus Statement. Obesity Review* 4 (May 2003): 101–114.

Sinaki, M., et al. "Site Specificity of Regular Health Club Exercise on Muscle Strength, Fitness, and Bone Density in Women Aged 29 to 45 Years." *Mayo Clinic Proceedings* 79 (May 2004): 639–644.

Sloan, A. W., and J. Weir. "Nomograms for Prediction of Bone Density and Total Body Fat from Skinfold Measurements." *Journal of Applied Physiology* 28 (1970): 221–222.

Stear, S. "Health and Fitness Series: 1. The Importance of Physical Activity for Health." *Journal of Family Health Care* 13 (January 2003): 10–13.

Stewart, K. J., et al. "Effect of Exercise on Blood Pressure in Older Persons: A Randomized Controlled Trial." *Archives of Internal Medicine* 165 (April 2005): 756–762.

Stewart, K. J., et al. "Exercise and Risk Factors Associated with Metabolic Syndrome in Older Adults." *American Journal of Preventive Medicine* 28 (January 2005): 9–18

U.S. Department of Health and Human Services. *Healthy People 2010.* Atlanta: U.S. Department of Health and Human Services, Centers for Disease Control and Prevention, 2000.

U.S. Department of Health and Human Services. *Physical Activity among Adults: United States, 2000.* Atlanta: U.S. Department of Health and Human Services, Centers for Disease Control and Prevention, May 2003.

U.S. Department of Health and Human Services. *Physical Activity and Health: A Report of the Surgeon General.* Atlanta: U.S. Department of Health and Human Services, Centers for Disease Control and Prevention, 2000.

Whaley, M., ed. *ACSM's Guidelines for Exercise Testing and Prescription,* 7th ed. Philadelphia: Lippincott Williams & Wilkins, 2006.

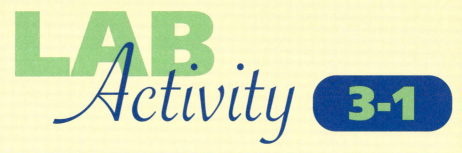

LAB Activity 3-1

Student Precourse Health Assessment

Student ID# _____ Age_____ Date of last medical checkup_____

Please answer all of the questions completely and honestly. This document is confidential between the student, instructor, and administration. This form is used to help you stay safe in courses that have physical activities. If at any time you do not feel well or experience an injury, please tell your instructor immediately. If you must leave the activity area to get water or use the restroom, take a classmate with you. While your participation in this course may enhance your health and well-being, you are advised that participation in some activities may be extremely vigorous and have potential risks. Some sports have inherent risks associated with them. If you have any questions about the course or activities, please talk to your instructor. If you are over age 40 (for men) or 50 (for women), it is highly recommended that you see your personal physician before you begin this class. The presence of some of the following conditions may affect your performance. Please check any conditions listed that pertain to you.

___ Cardiac/respiratory problems ___ Asthma (any) ___ High blood pressure (140/90 or above)

___ Chest pain or discomfort ___ Epilepsy (seizures/grand mal, 3+ min.) ___ Pregnancy

___ Severe allergic reactions ___ Diabetes ___ Severe headaches

___ Fainting spells/sudden unconsciousness ___ Family history of heart disease

___ Other life-threatening conditions (please list): _____

___ Knee injuries ___ Shoulder injuries ___ Ankle injuries

___ Back injuries ___ Neck/spinal injuries ___ Foot injuries

___ Scoliosis ___ Smoker ___ Allergies

___ Epilepsy (seizures/petit mal) ___ Other, please list below

Please list any other medical conditions or information you think should be brought to the attention of your instructor.

_____

_____

Please list all medications that you take regularly.

_____

_____

If during this class/course your physical health changes in regard to any of the listed or other conditions, please notify your instructor immediately. If you have concerns about your health, are sedentary, diabetic, pregnant, 20 or more pounds overweight, smoke, or have a family history of heart disease, it is important that you complete the *Physician-Approved Exercise Clearance Form*.

By signing this form, I accept responsibility for staying safe in this course and informing my instructor that I am not withholding any information regarding my health status. (Please sign, date, and return this form to your instructor.)

Student signature _____ Date _____

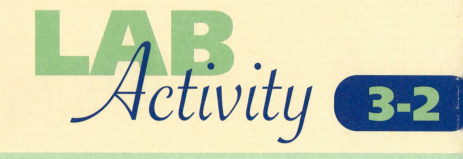

LAB *Activity* 3-2

Name _____   Class/Activity Section _____   Date _____

Physician-Approved Exercise Clearance Form

Student ID#_____ Age_____ Date of last medical checkup_____

This form is designed for individuals with special health concerns to assist your instructor in individualizing your fitness program according to your physician's recommendations. This form must be taken to your personal physician or the health center for review and a signature.

To be completed by the Lab Instructor:

(Name of student)_____ is presently enrolled in (name of course)_____
and he/she has identified the following health problems that may affect participation in the activities of this course:

_____

_____

This class/course will include the following activities:

_____

The above information was provided by **(instructor's name)**_____ Date _____

To be completed by the Physician:

NOTE TO PHYSICIAN: **PLEASE REVIEW THE REVERSE SIDE OF THIS DOCUMENT FOR HEALTH CONCERNS.**

After examining (student)_____, I recommend the following level of participation in the course described below:

_____ Full participation   _____ No participation*   _____ Modified participation as indicated:

_____

_____

*If the student may not participate in this class, list the activities in which the student may participate:

_____

_____

_____   _____   _____
Signature of physician   **Date**   **Physician's printed name**

                                                          _____
                                                          Physician's phone number

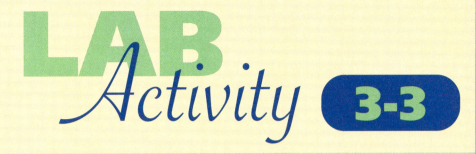

LAB Activity 3-3

Personal Fitness Profile

	Pretest Date: _____	Posttest Date: _____
1. **Resting heart rate**	_____	_____
2. **Cardiorespiratory endurance**		
1.5-mile run	_____	_____
1.0-mile walk	_____	_____
500-yard swim	_____	_____
Other_____	_____	_____
Exercise pulse	_____	_____
3. **Muscular endurance**		
Abdominal curls	_____	_____
Push-ups	_____	_____
4. **Muscular strength**		
Leg press	_____	_____
Bench press	_____	_____
5. **Body girth measurements**		
Hips–biggest part	_____	_____
Thigh–1 inch below crotch	_____	_____
Chest–nipple line	_____	_____
Waist–smallest part	_____	_____
Abdominal 1–halfway between chest and navel	_____	_____
Abdominal 2–halfway between navel and pubic bone	_____	_____
6. **Body composition**		
Female *Male*		
Triceps Subscapula	_____	_____
Iliac Thigh	_____	_____
Percent body fat (see nomogram in Figure 3-20)		
7. **Weight**	_____	_____
8. **Height**	_____	_____
9. **Waist-to-hip ratio**	_____	_____
10. **Flexibility**	_____	_____
Sit and reach		
Quick checks (pass or fail) (Figures 3-11 to 3-15)	P/F	P/F
a. Erector spinae	_____	_____
b. Iliopsoas	_____	_____
c. Quadriceps	_____	_____
d. Hamstrings	_____	_____
e. Gastrocnemius	_____	_____

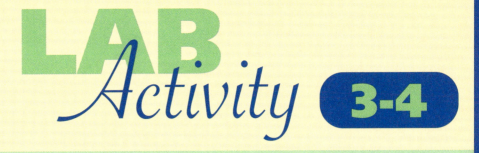

LAB Activity 3-4

Evaluating Your Cardiorespiratory Fitness: 1.5-Mile Run Test and 1-Mile Walk Test

1.5-MILE RUN TEST

Equipment Needed:

A track or premeasured course of 1.5 miles
Stopwatch

Procedure

1. Before taking the test, warm up with walking, stretching, and a slow jog.
2. This is a test of maximum capacity, so push yourself to cover the distance as quickly as possible without overdoing it. Try to maintain a continuous, even pace. Run as long as you can and then walk if necessary. When you complete the 1.5-mile distance, record your time.

   Running time: _____

3. Cool down by walking slowly for several minutes and stretching.

4. Check the table below for your fitness rating.

   Cardiorespiratory fitness rating: _____

1.5-Mile Run

Age	18–29		30–39		40–49		50–59	
	F	M	F	M	F	M	F	M
Superior	<12:34	<8:26	<13:34	<9:10	<14:34	<9:55	<15:34	<10:40
Good	12:34–13:40	8:26–10:24	13:34–14:40	9:10–11:10	14:34–15:40	9:55–12:00	15:34–16:40	10:40–12:50
Average	13:41–14:45	10:25–12:31	14:41–15:45	11:11–13:45	15:41–16:45	12:01–14:55	16:41–17:45	12:51–16:05
Fair	14:46–16:00	12:32–14:49	15:46–17:00	13:46–16:00	16:46–18:00	14:56–17:15	17:46–19:00	16:06–18:30
Low	>16:00	>14:49	>17:00	>16:00	>18:00	>17:15	>19:00	>18:30

1-MILE WALK TEST

Equipment Needed:

A track or premeasured course of 1.0 miles
Stopwatch

Procedure

1. Before taking the test, warm up with walking and stretching.
2. This is a test of maximum capacity, so push yourself to walk the mile as quickly as possible without overdoing it. Try to maintain a continuous, even pace. When you complete the 1-mile distance, record your time.

   Walking time: _____

3. Cool down by walking slowly for several minutes and stretching.

4. Check the table below for your fitness rating.

   Cardiorespiratory fitness rating: _____

1-Mile Walk

Age	18–29		30–39		40–49		50–59	
	F	M	F	M	F	M	F	M
Superior	<12:34	<11:39	<13:34	<12:40	<14:34	<13:40	<15:34	<14:10
Good	12:34–13:40	11:39–12:59	13:34–14:40	12:40–14:00	14:34–15:40	13:40–14:40	15:34–16:40	14:10–15:20
Average	13:41–14:45	13:00–14:21	14:41–15:45	14:01–15:20	15:41–16:45	14:41–15:55	16:41–17:45	15:21–16:25
Fair	14:46–16:00	14:22–15:43	15:46–17:00	15:21–16:15	16:46–18:00	15:56–16:45	17:46–19:00	16:26–17:25
Low	>16:00	>15:43	>17:00	>16:15	>18:00	>16:45	>19:00	>17:25

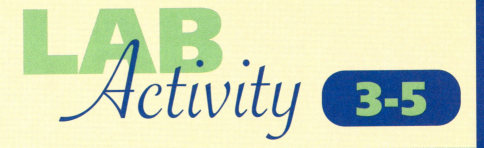

Name _____   **Class/Activity Section** _____   **Date** _____

Evaluating Your Cardiorespiratory Fitness: 500-Yard Water Run Test and 500-Yard Swim Test

500-YARD WATER RUN TEST

Equipment Needed:

A regulation 25-yard pool
Stopwatch
Partner to time you
Measuring tape to measure width of pool

Procedure

1. Measure pool width and calculate the number of widths required to cover 500 yards.
2. Have a partner on the deck to count laps and keep the time.
3. Before taking the test, warm up with a couple minutes of easy jogging in the water.
4. Select a starting point along the wall where the water level is at a midpoint between the runner's navel and nipple. Shorter runners will start in shallower water, taller runners in deeper water.
5. This is a test of maximum capacity, so push yourself to cover the distance as quickly as possible without overdoing it. Try to maintain a continuous, even pace. Run the necessary number of widths and record your time to the nearest second.

    500-yard water run time: _____

6. Cool down by walking in the water for several minutes and stretching.

7. Check the table for your fitness rating.

    Cardiorespiratory fitness rating: _____

500-Yard Water Run

Age	18–29		30–39		40–49		50–59	
	F	M	F	M	F	M	F	M
Superior	<7:59	<6:53	<8:30	<7:20	<9:00	<7:50	<9:30	<8:20
Good	7:59–8:38	6:53–7:44	8:30–9:08	7:20–8:15	9:00–9:38	7:50–8:45	9:30–10:08	8:20–9:15
Average	8:39–9:18	7:45–8:38	9:09–9:48	8:16–9:05	9:39–10:18	8:46–9:35	10:09–10:48	9:16–10:05
Fair	9:19–9:58	8:39–9:32	9:49–10:28	9:06–10:00	10:19–10:58	9:36–10:30	10:49–11:28	10:06–11:00
Low	>9:58	>9:32	>10:28	>10:00	>10:58	>10:30	>11:28	>11:00

500-YARD SWIM TEST

Equipment Needed:

A regulation 25-yard pool
Stopwatch
Partner to time you

Procedure

1. Have a partner on the deck to count laps and keep the time. In a 25-yard pool, 500 yards is 20 lengths.
2. Before taking the test, warm up with a couple of easy laps.
3. This is a test of maximum capacity, so push yourself to cover the distance as quickly as possible without overdoing it. Try to maintain a continuous, even pace. Record your time to the nearest second.

   500-yard swim time: _____

4. Cool down and stretch.

5. Check the table for your fitness rating.

   Cardiorespiratory fitness rating: _____

500-Yard Swim

Age	18–29		30–39		40–49		50–59	
	F	M	F	M	F	M	F	M
Superior	<7:05	<6:12	<7:35	<6:30	<8:05	<7:00	<8:35	<7:30
Good	7:05–8:49	6:12–7:44	7:35–9:19	6:30–8:14	8:05–9:49	7:00–8:44	8:35–10:19	7:30–9:14
Average	8:50–10:34	7:45–9:19	9:20–11:04	8:15–9:49	9:50–11:34	8:45–10:19	10:20–12:04	9:15–10:49
Fair	10:35–12:19	9:20–10:51	11:05–12:49	9:50–11:22	11:35–13:19	10:20–11:52	12:05–13:49	10:50–11:22
Low	>12:19	>10:52	>12:49	>11:22	>13:19	>11:52	>13:49	>11:22

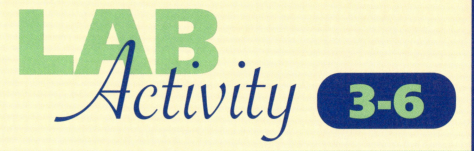

Evaluating Your Cardiorespiratory Fitness:
3-Minute Step Test

Equipment Needed:

A 15-inch bench or 16-inch roll-out bleacher step
Stopwatch
Metronome or recorded music at a tempo of 96 beats per minute

Procedure

1. Before taking the test, warm up with easy stepping and stretching.
2. You will need to step up and down at a tempo of 96 counts per minute. Step up with your right foot and then your left foot, and then step down with your right and then your left. Continue for 3 minutes. Straighten your knees as you step up on the bench. To prevent leg soreness, you may want to switch lead legs about halfway through the test.

   Pulse rate: _____

3. Stop at the end of 3 minutes and sit down. Five seconds after completing the test, the tester should count the partner's pulse for 15 seconds. The tester can check the partners' carotid pulse by lightly pressing against the neck under the jawbone. The partner being tested can double-check his or her own pulse at the radial artery, located on the thumb side of the wrist. The partner's pulse counts should not vary more than one or two beats if counting is accurate.

4. Record the pulse.

5. Cool down by walking slowly for several minutes and stretching.

6. Check the table below for your fitness rating.

   Cardiorespiratory fitness rating: _____

3-Minute Step Test Norms

	Men	Women
Superior	<31	<37
Good	31–37	37–41
Average	38–41	42–44
Fair	42–45	45–49
Low	>45	>49

SOURCE: F. W. Kasch and J. L. Boyer. *Adult Fitness: Principles and Practices*. Mountain View, CA: Mayfield, 1968. Used by permission.

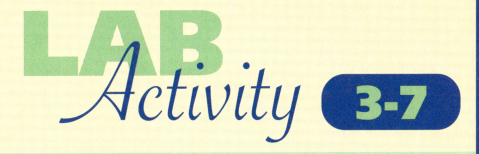

LAB *Activity* 3-7

Evaluating Your Muscular Endurance: Abdominal Curls Test and Push-Ups Test

ABDOMINAL CURLS TEST

Equipment Needed:

Ruler
Adhesive tape
Mat
Stopwatch or watch with a second hand

Procedure

1. Tape a 3-inch-wide strip on a mat or the floor and lie on your back with your fingertips at the edge of the strip. Bend your knees and bring your heels as close as possible to your buttocks.
2. Curl forward until your fingertips have moved forward across the 3-inch strip and then curl back until your shoulder blades touch the floor. Your shoulders should lift from the floor with each curl, but the lower back should stay on the ground.
3. Complete as many curls as possible in 1 minute, then check the results in the table below.

Number of abdominal curls: _____

Muscular endurance rating: _____

1-Minute Abdominal Curls

Age	18–29		30–39		40–49		50–59	
	F	M	F	M	F	M	F	M
Superior	>88	>93	>70	>78	>56	>65	>45	>49
Good	75–88	79–93	60–70	62–78	48–56	53–65	38–45	42–49
Average	60–74	64–78	47–59	51–61	37–47	42–52	29–37	35–41
Fair	45–59	50–63	35–46	40–50	27–36	36–41	21–28	28–34
Low	<45	<50	<35	<40	<27	<36	<21	<28

PUSH-UPS TEST

Equipment Needed:

Mat
Stopwatch or watch with a second hand

Procedure

1. Start in an "up" position with your weight on your hands and toes (men) or knees (women).
2. Lower yourself until your elbows form a right angle and your upper arm is parallel to the floor. Be sure to keep your abdominals tight, your hips slightly piked, and your back straight to protect your lower back.
3. Complete as many push-ups as possible in 1 minute; record, then check the results in the table below.

Number of push-ups: _____

Muscular endurance rating: _____

1-Minute Push-Ups

Age	18–29		30–39		40–49		50–59	
	F	M	F	M	F	M	F	M
Superior	>54	>64	>43	>54	>33	>43	>23	>33
Good	44–54	51–64	32–43	41–54	26–33	32–43	18–23	26–33
Average	32–43	37–50	22–31	27–40	17–25	22–31	11–17	17–25
Fair	20–31	23–36	13–21	18–26	8–16	13–21	6–10	8–16
Low	<20	<23	<13	<18	<8	<13	<6	<8

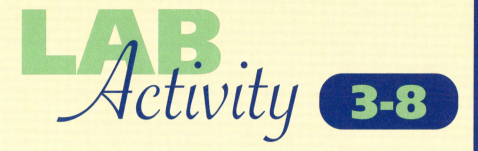

Name _____ **Class/Activity Section** _____ **Date** _____

Evaluating Your Muscular Strength: Leg Press Strength Test and Bench Press Strength Test

LEG PRESS STRENGTH TEST

Equipment Needed:

Leg press machine If free weights are used, the following equipment is needed:
Weight scale

Weight scale   Barbell
Squat rack   Assorted weight plates
One or two spotters

Procedure

1. If you have had a history of ankle, knee, hip, or lower back injuries, check with your physician before doing this test.
2. Before taking the test, warm up with several light lifts and stretching.
3. Set the leg press machine for a weight that is lighter than the amount you think you can press one time. Press to full extension. If you can press the weight to extension, add more weight and try again. Rest a few minutes between attempts. It may take several attempts to find your maximum lift.
4. Stop when you reach a weight that you cannot move through a full range of motion. The heaviest weight that you can move through a full range of motion is your max.
5. Divide your max by your body weight.
   Max: _____ Body weight: _____
   Max / Body weight = _____

   Check the table below for your fitness rating.
   Muscular strength rating: _____

	Leg Press (max/body weight)							
Age	**18–29**		**30–39**		**40–49**		**50–59**	
	F	M	F	M	F	M	F	M
Superior	>1.97	>2.39	>1.67	>2.19	>1.56	>2.01	>1.42	>1.89
Good	1.68–1.97	2.13–2.39	1.47–1.67	1.93–2.19	1.37–1.56	1.82–2.01	1.25–1.42	1.71–1.89
Average	1.50–1.67	1.97–2.12	1.33–1.46	1.77–1.92	1.23–1.36	1.68–1.81	1.10–1.24	1.58–1.70
Fair	1.37–1.49	1.83–1.96	1.21–1.32	1.65–1.76	1.13–1.22	1.57–1.67	0.99–1.09	1.46–1.57
Low	<1.37	<1.83	<1.21	<1.65	<1.13	<1.57	<0.99	<1.46

SOURCE: Based on norms from the Cooper Institute for Aerobics Research, Dallas, Texas, revised 2000. Used with permission.

BENCH PRESS STRENGTH TEST

Equipment Needed:

Bench press machine   If free weights are used, the following equipment is needed:
Weight scale   Weight scale   Barbell
                       Flat bench   Assorted weight plates
                       One or two spotters Weight scale

Procedure

1. If you have had a history of shoulder, wrist, or lower back injuries, check with your physician before doing this test.
2. Before taking the test, warm up with several light lifts and stretching.
3. Set the bench press machine for a weight that is lighter than the amount you think you can press one time. Press to full extension. If you can press the weight to extension, add more weight and try again. Rest a few minutes between attempts. It may take several attempts to find your maximum lift.
4. Stop when you reach a weight that you cannot move through a full range of motion. The heaviest weight that you can move through a full range of motion is your max.
5. Divide your max by your body weight.
   Max: _____ Body weight: _____
   Max / Body weight = _____

   Check the table below for your fitness rating.
   Muscular strength rating: _____

Bench Press (max/body weight)

Age	20–29		30–39		40–49		50–59	
	F	M	F	M	F	M	F	M
Superior	>1.00	>1.62	>.79	>1.34	>.76	>1.19	>.67	>1.04
Good	.80–1.00	1.32–1.62	.70–.79	1.12–1.34	.62–.76	1.00–1.19	.55–.67	.90–1.04
Average	.70–.79	1.14–1.31	.60–.69	.98–1.11	.54–.61	.88–.99	.48–.54	.79–.89
Fair	.59–.69	.99–1.13	.53–.59	.88–.97	.50–.53	.80–.87	.44–.47	.71–.78
Low	<.59	<.99	<.53	<.88	<.50	<.80	<.44	<.71

SOURCE: Based on norms from the Cooper Institute for Aerobics Research, Dallas, Texas, revised 2000. Used with permission.

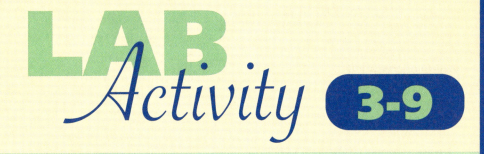

Name _____ **Class/Activity Section** _____ **Date** _____

Evaluating Your Flexibility: Sit and Reach and Flexibility Quick Checks

SIT AND REACH

Equipment Needed:

Flex box
Mat

Procedure

1. Warm up with walking or light calisthenics.
2. Sit with your feet flat against the flex box about 5 inches apart.
3. Place your hands together. Without bending your knees, reach as far forward as possible, extending fingertips along the box. Hold the position for 3 seconds.

   Sit and reach score: _____ inches

4. Check the table below for your flexibility rating.

   Flexibility rating: _____

Sit and Reach (inches)

Age	18–29		30–39		40–49		50–59	
	F	M	F	M	F	M	F	M
Superior	>8.5	>7.0	>8	>6	>7	>5	>6	>4
Good	6.5–8.5	4.0–7.0	5–8	3–6	4–7	2–5	3–6	1–4
Average	4.0–6.4	1.0–3.9	3–4.9	0–2.9	2–3.9	−1–1.9	1–2.9	−3–0
Fair	1.0–3.9	−2.0–0.9	0–2.9	−3−−0.1	−1–1.9	−4−−1.1	−2–0.9	−5−−3.1
Low	<1.0	<−2.0	<0	<−3	<−1	<−4	<−2	<−5

FLEXIBILITY QUICK CHECKS

Equipment Needed:

Mat

Procedure

1. Warm up with walking or light calisthenics.
2. Complete the flexibility quick checks shown in Figures 3-11 through 3-15. Record the results (*pass* or *fail*).

	Pass	Fail
Low back flexibility test	_____	_____
Hip flexor flexibility test	_____	_____
Quadriceps flexibility test	_____	_____
Hamstring flexibility test	_____	_____
Calf flexibility test	_____	_____

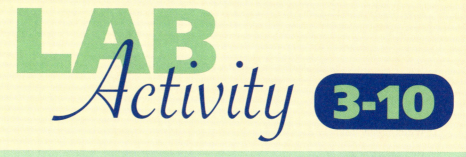

Name _____ **Class/Activity Section** _____ **Date** _____

Body Composition Assessment

Equipment Needed:

Measuring tape
Skinfold calipers
Height/weight scales

WAIST-TO-HIP RATIO

1. Measure your waist at the smallest circumference and hips at the greatest circumference. Record the results.

   Hips: _____ inches   Waist: _____ inches

2. Divide your waist measurement by your hip measurement and check your rating.

   Waist/Hip = _____   Rating: _____

Waist-to-Hip Ratio	High Risk
Men	.95 or higher
Women	.80 or higher

WAIST GIRTH

Measure your waist at the smallest circumference and record the results.

Waist: _____ inches   Rating: _____

Waist Circumference	High Risk
Men	over 40 inches
Women	over 35 inches

BODY MASS INDEX

1. Measure your height and weight and record the results.

   Height: _____ feet _____ inches   Weight: _____ pounds

2. Check your BMI using Table 12.1 on page 411.

   BMI: _____   Rating: _____

BODY FAT PERCENTAGE

1. Measure skinfolds on the right side of the body using a skinfold caliper and record the results.
2. Check the results on the nomogram in Figure 3-20 and Table 3-6.

   Female: Triceps   _____
                  Suprailiac   _____
                  Percent body fat   _____

   Male: Subscapular   _____
                  Thigh   _____
                  Percent body fat   _____

DESIRABLE WEIGHT

1. Percent body fat × weight (lbs) = Fat weight (lbs)

   _____ × _____ = _____ lbs

2. Weight (lbs) − fat weight = lean body weight (lbs)

   _____ − _____ = _____ lbs

3. Desirable weight for females (at 18%):
   lean body weight /.82 = desirable weight
   _____/.82 = _____ lbs

4. Desirable weight for males (at 12%):
   lean body weight /.88 = desirable weight
   _____/.88 = _____ lbs

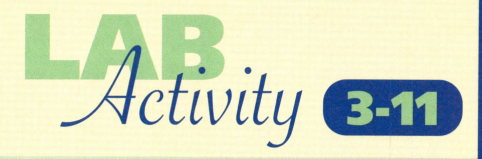

LAB Activity 3-11

Fitness Goals

Looking at the results of your fitness tests, evaluate yourself and set some realistic, personal goals.

	Test score time/number	Date of test	Fitness rating	Goal time/number	Fitness rating	By what date?
Cardiorespiratory Tests						
1-mile walk	_____	_____	_____	_____	_____	_____
1.5-mile run	_____	_____	_____	_____	_____	_____
500-yard swim	_____	_____	_____	_____	_____	_____
Other _____	_____	_____	_____	_____	_____	_____
Muscular Fitness Tests						
1-minute abdominal curls	_____	_____	_____	_____	_____	_____
1-minute push-ups	_____	_____	_____	_____	_____	_____
Sit and reach	_____	_____	_____	_____	_____	_____
Leg press	_____	_____	_____	_____	_____	_____
Bench press	_____	_____	_____	_____	_____	_____
Other Tests						
_____	_____	_____	_____	_____	_____	_____
_____	_____	_____	_____	_____	_____	_____
_____	_____	_____	_____	_____	_____	_____

Comments (e.g., Was this your best effort? Is this a realistic assessment of your abilities? Any surprises?) _____

_____

_____

_____

LAB Activity ■ **CHAPTER 3**

105

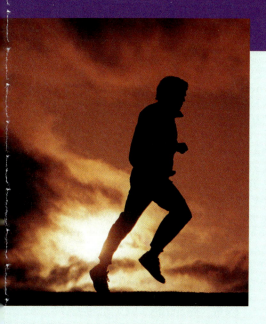

Maximizing Cardiorespiratory Fitness

A journey of a thousand miles starts with a single step.
—Lao Tse

Objectives

After reading this chapter, you will be able to:

1. Identify benefits of cardiorespiratory fitness.
2. Define and apply the FITT prescription factors for developing physical fitness.
3. Calculate training heart rate by using the Karvonen formula.
4. Explain how to use the Rate of Perceived Exertion Scale to measure workout intensity.
5. Describe how to apply the progressive overload principle to a cardiorespiratory exercise program.
6. Discuss the differences in the goals for the 30-minute, the 60- to 90-minute, and the FITT exercise guidelines.
7. Have a greater understanding of the eight aerobic exercise activities found in this chapter. You will discover each to be an excellent method for developing cardiorespiratory endurance (CRE). The eight activities include aerobic dance, bicycling, fitness swimming, fitness walking, indoor exercise equipment, in-line skating, jogging, and water exercise/aqua aerobics.
8. Describe and initiate the 10,000 steps per day wellness goal.
9. Pursue a lifetime of aerobic activity by selecting one of the eight exercise activities and following the guidelines established for that activity.

Terms

- aerobic
- anaerobic
- aerobic capacity
- cardiac output
- FITT factors
- heart rate reserve (HRR)
- Karvonen equation
- maximal heart rate (HR$_{max}$)
- maximal oxygen uptake (VO$_{2max}$)
- rate of perceived exertion (RPE)
- talk test
- target heart rate (THR)
- training effect

A Fit and Well Way of Life Online Learning Center www.mhhe.com/robbinsfitwell1e
Go to the Online Learning Center for chapter quizzes, outlines, flashcards, and additional lab activities.

The number one reason people begin exercising is to improve their physical appearance—to decrease body fat and develop firm, well-toned muscles. They find that these benefits are only the beginning. Cardiorespiratory endurance plays an important role in developing physical fitness and wellness. As was explained in Chapter 3, even modest levels of physical activity provide many health benefits and reduce health risks from several chronic diseases. There are a number of physiological (cardiorespiratory, body composition, and metabolic) and psychological (mental and emotional) health benefits that are yours in return for a small investment of time and effort.

A variety of exercise programs and recreational activities can enhance health and fitness. Nearly everyone can find one or two activities that are satisfying and enjoyable. This chapter focuses on the many benefits that can be gained from cardiorespiratory endurance, the prescription factors for fitness, and information about a variety of lifetime exercise activities to get you started on the path to a richly enjoyable life span.

CARDIORESPIRATORY ENDURANCE AND MAXIMAL OXYGEN UPTAKE

Cardiorespiratory endurance often is expressed in terms of your **maximal oxygen uptake** (VO_{2max} or **aerobic capacity**), the greatest amount of oxygen that can be taken in and used by the body during high-intensity exercise. You can go several days without water, several weeks without food, but only minutes without oxygen. Most fitness experts agree that VO_{2max} is the best measure of cardiorespiratory fitness. Energy for physical activity and body processes is produced by burning fuel in the presence of oxygen. For muscles to use oxygen, the lungs must take in air and transfer it to the blood. The blood must then be pumped to the muscles. Finally, the muscles must take the oxygen from the blood and use it. During exercise, the ability of the body to utilize oxygen and remove waste products depends on the efficient functioning of the cardiorespiratory system, which includes the heart, blood vessels, lungs, and muscles. When a person exercises, the working muscles demand more oxygen and nutrients and the heart must work harder to keep up with the demand. The demand for oxygen increases in direct proportion to the intensity of exercise.

VO_{2max} is determined partly by genetics and partly by training. As fitness improves, many factors contribute to greater VO_{2max}. The heart is a muscle and, like any muscle, grows stronger with training. A fit, trained heart can pump more oxygenated blood to exercising muscles than an unfit heart can. Cardiorespiratory training increases both stroke volume, the volume of blood pumped per heartbeat, and **cardiac output**, the volume of blood pumped per minute. Similarly, trained skeletal muscles can utilize oxygen and nutrients delivered by the blood to produce energy more efficiently than untrained muscles can. Ventilation and blood flow to the lungs improve. Blood flow of the muscles improves. Muscle cells become more efficient at extracting oxygen and producing energy for muscular contraction. Waste products are removed more efficiently. VO_{2max} determines how intensely and how long you can perform aerobic exercise and is considered one of the best overall indicators of physiological well-being.

While natural cardiorespiratory endowment may vary among individuals, with training, maximal oxygen uptake can improve 20 to 30 percent, depending on pretraining status and the frequency, intensity, and duration of training. Beneficial physiological changes persist as long as aerobic training continues, but inactivity produces physical decline. If training stops, VO_{2max} returns to pretraining levels within a few months. With aging, aerobic capacity decreases about 1 percent per year after age 25. This decline is related closely to decreasing levels of activity rather than to simply growing older. Declines in VO_{2max} may be slowed dramatically by those who exercise across the lifetime. See the section on aging in Chapter 7 for more information on the effects of exercise on aging.

The ability to utilize oxygen during exercise can be measured in a laboratory on a treadmill or in a field test. Several tests in Chapter 3 can be used to assess your cardiorespiratory endurance. They include the 1.5-mile run, the 1-mile walk, the 500-yard water run, the 500-yard swim, the 3-mile bicycling test, and the 3-minute step test. *Norms were developed by testing thousands of participants at the end of 12 to 15 weeks of aerobic fitness classes*, and so you can compare your results with the standards for your selected activity.

Benefits of Aerobic Exercise

Exercise has both short- and long-term effects. The immediate effects of vigorous exercise, regardless of fitness level, are an increase in the respiration rate, an increase in the heart rate, and an increase in body temperature. After a few weeks of regular, vigorous exercise, the body begins to adapt to meeting the demands. These physiological adaptations to exercise (the total beneficial changes) are called the **training effect** and are detailed in the following lists. The benefits of flexibility and muscular fitness will be discussed in Chapter 5 and Chapter 6.

Cardiorespiratory Benefits

1. Lower resting heart rate
2. Increased stroke volume (the amount of blood pumped out of the heart with each beat), improving heart efficiency
3. Increased rest for the heart between beats due to slower resting heart rate and increased stroke volume
4. Increased oxygen-carrying capacity of the blood due to the greater supply of red blood cells and hemoglobin; greater endurance in exercising muscles due to increased energy and improved elimination of waste products
5. Improved exercise performance on timed tests due to more efficient use of oxygen
6. Possible reduction in blood pressure
7. Improved blood lipid profile by increasing the number of protective high-density lipoproteins (HDLs)
8. Quicker recovery to resting heart rate after vigorous exercise due to improved cardiac efficiency
9. Possible regression of atherosclerosis
10. Fewer illnesses and deaths due to coronary heart disease

Body Composition/Physical Appearance Benefits

1. Reduced body fat percentage
2. Increased lean body mass
3. Firmer, more toned muscles
4. More positive body image

Psychological, Mental, and Emotional Benefits

1. Enhanced sense of well-being and self-esteem, resulting in increased energy, alertness, and vitality
2. Increased sense of self-discipline due to the determination needed to stick to an exercise program
3. Reduced state of anxiety and mental tension, thereby increasing stress coping ability
4. Improved quality of sleep; sleep soundly and wake up refreshed
5. Decreased level of mild to moderate depression
6. Improved mental acuity, learning, and memory
7. Feeling of relaxation

The psychological benefits are very rewarding and are often the main reason people keep exercising. More detail on these and other benefits of cardiorespiratory fitness follows.

Improved Mental Health

People who exercise regularly report improved mood, higher self-confidence and self-esteem, and less stress compared with nonexercisers. Research indicates that aerobic exercise also can enhance psychological well-being by reducing depression and anxiety. The best results were obtained after several weeks of regular exercise, with more vigorous exercise, and in those who were high in anxiety or depression to begin with. While it may not work for everyone and we can't say exactly how much exercise is needed, for many individuals being able to say "exercise makes me feel better" is a significant benefit.

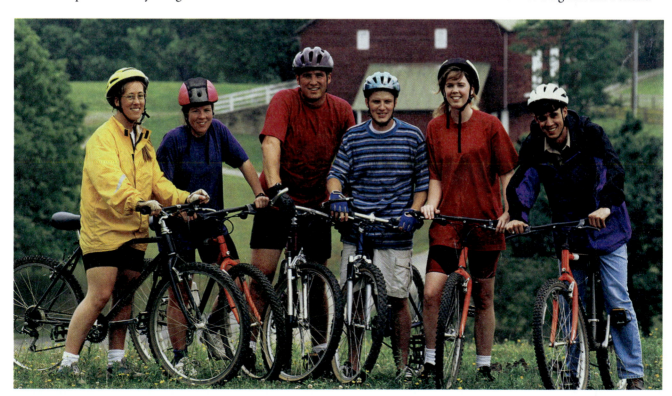

It's more fun to be a participant than a spectator.

Improved Cognitive Function

The human brain gradually loses tissue from age 30 onward, and this is reflected in gradual declines in cognitive function. Cardiorespiratory fitness has been associated with preservation of cognitive function in healthy adults. One study that followed subjects for 10 years indicated that middle-aged aerobic exercisers compared with sedentary individuals have a significantly slower rate of memory decline and better memory performance. In subjects over 55, the positive effect of exercise was greatest on the "executive control" functions of judgment, planning, and the coordination of actions to achieve a goal. In elderly subjects age 60 to 76, 2 months of aerobic training significantly improved cognitive test scores, and the effect was equal to 2 months of mental training. While we do not know exactly how this occurs, exercise does increase blood flow to the brain, which in turn can promote brain cell growth. Studies from the Institute for Brain Aging and Dementia suggest that exercise can increase levels of brain growth factors, stimulate neuron growth, and maintain brain function and plasticity, thus improving learning and mental performance.

Improved Sleep

Many studies support the positive effects of exercise on sleep. In studies of individuals who exercised aerobically, exercisers went to sleep more quickly, slept longer, and had a more restful sleep than did those who did not exercise.

Immune System Function

Those who participate in regular moderate exercise enjoy enhanced levels of well-being, including fewer colds and minor respiratory infections compared with sedentary peers. Avoid overtraining, however, as exercising to exhaustion can weaken immune system function.

Improved Body Composition and Weight Management

Regular endurance exercise burns excess calories and can help maintain muscle mass and reduce excess body fat. Increasing levels of overweight and obesity in the United States at all age levels may be due as much to decreased physical activity as to increased caloric intake. For this reason, at least 60 minutes of vigorous physical activity daily is recommended for weight management. Even if exercise does not reduce body fat significantly, research indicates that those who exercise regularly significantly reduce the risk of chronic diseases compared with sedentary individuals.

Reduced Risk of Chronic Diseases

Cardiorespiratory fitness can reduce the risk of developing several chronic diseases. For those who already have one of these diseases, a carefully monitored aerobic program is often recommended as a part of treatment to improve health and physiological resilience.

Cardiovascular Disease   Cardiorespiratory exercise reduces the risk of having cardiovascular disease and the risk of dying from it. Cardiovascular disease does not develop suddenly in middle age. It begins much earlier, in the teens and twenties, and continues to progress silently for many years. Young adults can reduce the risk of cardiovascular disease by developing a habit of regular exercise and managing the other risk factors described in Chapter 9.

High Blood Pressure   Exercise prevents or delays the development of high blood pressure. High blood pressure is associated with the risk of stroke, kidney failure, and coronary heart disease. If a person has high blood pressure, improving cardiorespiratory fitness can reduce it, particularly if that person loses weight as a result of exercise.

Type 2 Diabetes   Regular aerobic exercise is associated with a lower risk of developing type 2 diabetes. Type 2 diabetes is associated with the risk of several chronic diseases that can make one's life miserable and shorten one's life span. Exercise helps prevent obesity, which is related to the onset of diabetes. It burns excess blood sugar and increases cells' sensitivity to insulin, which helps regulate blood sugar. For those with diabetes, exercise is an important adjunct to other treatments. Additionally, regular exercise dramatically reduces the risk of metabolic syndrome, a dangerous group of risk factors that have been shown to raise the risk of diabetes and heart disease. See Chapter 9.

Cancer   Exercise is associated with a lower risk of certain types of cancer, including colon cancer. This may be due to increased intestinal motility, which decreases contact time between potential carcinogens and the intestinal wall. It also may be due in part to improved immune system function.

Osteoarthritis   Regular exercise may prevent or delay osteoarthritis. Osteoarthritis is most common at weight-bearing joints such as the hips, knees, and ankles and is exacerbated by increased weight on those joints. Exercise maintains the strength of the muscles that surround and support the joints and helps maintain normal joint function. For those who have osteoarthritis, regular exercise such as walking is recommended for maintenance of normal joint function and reduction of excess body fat.

Osteoporosis   Osteoporosis is another disease that has its beginning in the teens and twenties with inadequate exercise and eating habits. Weight-bearing exercise such as running, walking, and aerobics can decrease the risk of osteoporosis by building optimal bone mass in young adults and in slowing its loss with age.

The benefits of aerobic fitness can enhance health and well-being across the life span. They can be gained by following the FITT prescription for cardiorespiratory fitness.

THE FITT PRESCRIPTION FOR CARDIORESPIRATORY FITNESS

Cardiorespiratory fitness development involves four **FITT factors: F**requency, **I**ntensity, **T**ime, and **T**ype of exercise. The prescription for cardiorespiratory fitness for healthy adults is given in Figure 4-1. The prescription may be adjusted for older and sedentary individuals, who can begin with shorter times and lower intensity. While athletes may use this prescription to maintain fitness in the off-season, a greater investment of time and effort may be needed for in-season training.

"F" Equals Frequency

How often should you exercise? Exercise three to five times per week with no more than 48 hours between workouts. After 48 hours, the body starts to decondition and lose some of the benefits gained in the last workout. It is not necessary to exercise every day to develop fitness, although 5-day-a-week programs produce greater improvements than do 3-day-a-week programs. Working out three times per week is the *minimum* and approriate only for beginners or those recovering from an injury or illness. If your goal is to lose weight or reduce stress, at least 5 days of exercise a week is recommended. However, time for recovery is important, especially if you are just beginning a fitness program. The body needs time to adapt, so start slowly, working out every other day, gradually increasing the frequency as your fitness improves.

"I" Equals Intensity

How hard should you exercise? In athletics, a coach may ask you to give 100 percent effort, but this level of intensity is not needed to develop health-related fitness. Depending on the initial fitness level, about half to over three-quarters effort allows adequate stimulation of the cardiorespiratory system to produce training effect benefits. The American College of Sports Medicine (ACSM) recommends a workout intensity of 60 to 80 percent of your heart rate reserve for healthy, active in-

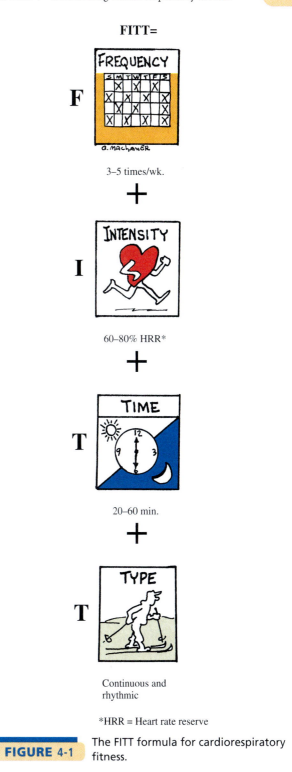

FITT=

FREQUENCY

3–5 times/wk.

+

INTENSITY

60–80% HRR*

+

TIME

20–60 min.

+

TYPE

Continuous and rhythmic

*HRR = Heart rate reserve

FIGURE 4-1 The FITT formula for cardiorespiratory fitness.

dividuals. For low fit, deconditioned, or older adults, intensities as low as 40 to 50 percent may be adequate for cardiorespiratory improvement. While this intensity will not produce excellent cardiorespiratory fitness, it does provide health benefits and reduces the risk for chronic diseases. Intensity of effort is directly reflected by exercise pulse rate and is perhaps the most important factor in gaining training effect benefits from your exercise program. You must put in enough effort to force the body to adapt and produce fitness improvements. If intensity is too low, there will still be health benefits but no increase in physical fitness. There are three ways to judge intensity: target heart rate, rate of perceived exertion, and the talk test.

Target Heart Rate: Karvonen Equation

To determine your **target heart rate (THR)** range for cardiorespiratory exercise, we will use the **Karvonen equation**, which takes into account your age and resting heart rate (RHR). Karvonen, a Finnish researcher, discovered that the heart rate during exercise must be raised by at least 60 percent of the difference between resting and maximal heart rates (called the **heart rate reserve, HRR**) to gain cardiorespiratory fitness. An adequate upper intensity is 80 percent of HRR.

It is necessary to know your **maximal heart rate (HR_{max})** to calculate your target heart rate range. The HR_{max} is your highest possible heart rate. It can be di-rectly determined during a treadmill exercise tolerance test in a laboratory or can be predicted based on your age. The maximal heart rate ranges from 180 to 200 beats per minute (bpm) in young people and decreases with age. Most people can estimate their HR_{max} by subtracting their age from 220. For example, if you are 23 years old, your estimated HR_{max} is $220 - 23 = 197$.

Next, you will need to know your RHR for 1 minute. Check it by using a stopwatch or a watch with a second hand. The best time to check it is in the morning before you get out of bed. You also may check it after you have been sitting quietly for 20 minutes or more. Ideally, you should check it several times over a few days. You can find the pulse with your fingertips (not the thumb) at the carotid artery in the neck or on the thumb side of the wrist (Figures 4-2 and 4-3). Be careful not to apply too much pressure at the carotid artery site because the body's natural response is to suppress the heart rate when this occurs. Count the number of beats for 30 seconds and multiply by two to calculate your 1-minute pulse. By using your age and your RHR, you can calculate your target heart rate range (Table 4-1). There is also a target heart rate worksheet in Lab Activity 4-1.

TABLE 4-1	***Calculating Target Heart Rate Range Using the Karvonen Formula***

This example shows a 23-year-old with a resting heart rate (HR_{rest}) of 72 bpm:

- Estimation of $HR_{max} = 220 - 23 = 197$
- HR_{rest} = pulse at complete rest for 1 minute
- Intensity = range of 60% to 80%

THR = (HR_{max} − HR_{rest}) × intensity + HR_{rest}

a. $\quad$ 220 $\quad$ − $\quad$ 23 $\quad$ = $\quad$ 197
$\quad$ (HR_{max}) $\quad$ (age) $\quad$ (estimated maximal heart rate [MHR])

b. $\quad$ 197 $\quad$ − $\quad$ 72 $\quad$ = $\quad$ 125
$\quad$ (MHR) $\quad$ (resting HR) $\quad$ (heart rate reserve)

c. $\quad$ 125 $\quad$ × $\quad$ .60 $\quad$ = 75 + $\quad$ 72 $\quad$ = $\quad$ 147
$\quad$ (HR reserve) $\quad$ (lower intensity) $\quad$ (resting HR) $\quad$ (lower target heart rate)

d. $\quad$ 125 $\quad$ × $\quad$ .80 $\quad$ = 100 + $\quad$ 72 $\quad$ = $\quad$ 172
$\quad$ (HR reserve) $\quad$ (higher intensity) $\quad$ (resting HR) $\quad$ (higher target heart rate)

Target heart rate is **147** to **172** beats per minute.

HR_{max} — 197
80% — 172
60% — 147
Target heart rate range
Heart rate reserve
HR_{rest} — 72

SOURCE: Adapted from M. Karvonen, K. Kentala, and O. Mustala. "The Effects of Training on Heart Rate: A Longitudinal Study." *Annals of Medicine and Experimental Biology* 35 (1957): 307–315.

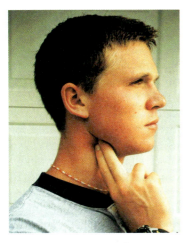

FIGURE 4-2   Pulse at carotid artery.

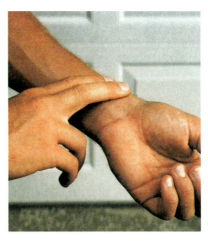

FIGURE 4-3   Pulse at the thumb side of wrist.

Now that you know your target heart rate range, you will be able to measure the intensity of every exercise session. Count your pulse during exercise and immediately after a conditioning bout. Because your pulse drops rapidly when you stop exercising, rather than counting your pulse for a full minute, you may find it easier to count for 6 seconds (e.g., if you count 15 beats in 6 seconds, your pulse is 150). It will take some practice, but in time you will become accurate at checking your heart rate.

Exercise heart rates differ by age (Figure 4-4). For most young adults, a THR is in the range of 140 to 170 beats per minute, but for older adults, a rate of 120 to 140 beats per minute may be adequate. Exercising at a heart rate above your THR is not necessary for fitness, does not increase health benefits, but may increase the risk of injury. Keep in mind that because the maximal heart rate is estimated, any error in that estimate is carried over into the THR calculation. Actual THR can vary plus or minus 10 beats. A general rule is to apply the **talk test** and/or the rate of perceived exertion (RPE).

Talk Test

The **talk test** is another way to gauge the intensity of exercise. You should be able to carry on a conversation with a companion while exercising. If you are too breathless to talk, you are exercising too hard. Research has confirmed that at the point where speech is just becoming difficult, the exercise intensity is almost exactly equivalent to the target heart rate. When speech is not comfortable, exercise intensity is consistently above target heart rate. Listen to your body and adjust exercise intensity accordingly.

Rate of Perceived Exertion (RPE)

Many people do not check their heart rate during exercise and judge intensity of exercise by **rate of perceived exertion (RPE)**, sensing how hard or easy a workout feels.

This method uses a scale developed by Gunnar Borg (see Table 4-2). Borg discovered that exercisers are able to "sense" their exercise intensity levels. He found that the RPE scale correlated with heart rate. Borg found that the descriptive words in the right column closely paralleled the heart rate of the exerciser, which is illustrated by the numbers in the left column. To develop fitness, exercisers should feel the effort is "Somewhat hard" to "Hard," or 12 to 16 on the Borg Scale. It is helpful to cross-check your heart rate with your perceived rating when you first begin to use this method. Experienced exercisers can use RPE to determine if they are in their target HR zone and adjust the exercise intensity accordingly. This is a safe and accurate way to monitor exercise intensity anywhere, anytime, without using a stopwatch.

THR During Non-Weight-Bearing Activities   When you swim, bike, or water run, an adequate target pulse rate is lower than it is when you are running. Weight-bearing activities, such as running and walking, use more oxygen and make your heart beat faster than it does when you exercise by cycling or swimming—at the same perceived level of effort. As a general rule, reduce cycling

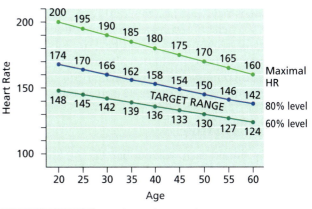

FIGURE 4-4   Estimated target heart rate range (based on RHR of 70 bpm).

TABLE 4-2	Borg's Rate of Perceived Exertion (RPE)	
(RPE) Chart		
6		
7	Very, very light	Warm-up/cool-down zone
8		
9	Very light	
10		
11	Fairly light	
12		
13	Somewhat hard	Target zone
14		
15	Hard	
16		
17	Very hard	
18		Working too hard zone
19	Very, very hard	
20		

SOURCE: G. Borg. "Psychophysical Bases of Physical Exertion–Perceived Rate of Exertion." *Medicine and Science in Sports & Exercise*, 1982: 14, 344–386. © by The American College of Sports Medicine.

THR by 5 percent and swimming THR by 10 percent. In any case, you should be able to pass the talk test. For example, if your THR for running/walking is 150–170 bpm, your swimming THR will be:

1. $150 \times .10 = 15$; $170 \times .10 = 17$
2. $150 - 15 = 135$; $170 - 17 = 153$
3. THR $= 135 - 153$ bpm

Also remember to set different goals for cross training. A good way to achieve an effective workout is to monitor your rate of perceived exertion (RPE).

Target Heart Rate: Percentage of Maximal Heart Rate

An old method of determining the target heart rate used a straight percentage of the maximal heart rate. The ACSM recommends using 70 to 90 percent of an individual's maximal heart rate to set exercise intensity. For example, if a person's estimated maximal pulse was 200, the target heart rate range would be 140 ($200 \times .7$) to 180 ($200 \times .90$) beats per minute. Its advantage is that it is simple to compute. The drawback of this method is that it does not take resting pulse into account.

"T" Equals Time

How long should each workout be? The ACSM recommends a conditioning bout of 20 to 60 minutes at an intensity of 60 to 80 percent, not including warm-up and cool-down. The 20 to 60 minutes does not have to be completed in one workout. It is acceptable to accumulate the time in 10-minute bouts of exercise throughout the day. For example: 10 minutes in the morning, 10 more minutes at lunch time, and 10 minutes (or more) after work or school.

Duration is inversely related to the intensity of the activity. A similar exercise volume may be obtained at a low intensity and a longer time (60 percent intensity, 30 to 60 minutes) or a higher intensity and a shorter time (80 percent intensity, 20 minutes). See Figure 3-1 for a comparison of exercise intensities and times. However, risk of injury does increase at higher intensities. Because many traditional-aged college students (18 to 24 years) have difficulty reaching their THR during some fitness activities (such as fitness walking), or find it is always at the low end of the THR range, they may wish to extend the time of the workout to 60 minutes or more. If time permits and the exercise session is enjoyable, if weight management is a goal, or if you are training for a long-distance event (e.g., mini-marathon), exercising for longer than 60 minutes is fine, but it is not necessary for cardiorespiratory fitness benefits. A typical exercise session would be as follows:

Warm-up 5 – 15 min.	+	Conditioning bout 20 – 60 min. or more	+	Cool-down 5 – 15 min.

When beginning a fitness program, it is best to limit your conditioning periods to 20 minutes or less (e.g., four 5-minute bouts with a rest in between if needed), then progress slowly until you can comfortably work out for 20 to 60 minutes or more in your target heart rate range. If you wish to progress beyond a basic level, the progressive overload principle discussed in Chapter 3 should be applied.

While many people feel that they don't have time to exercise, if you do the minimum 20 minutes, 3 days per week, it takes 1 hour out of 168 hours in your week–a small investment that pays big dividends.

"T" Equals Type

What type of exercise promotes aerobic fitness? The term **aerobic** means "with oxygen." Aerobic activities are activities that demand large amounts of oxygen and improve cardiorespiratory endurance. They are vigorous, continuous, and rhythmic. Aerobic dancing, swimming, cycling, and jogging are all good, as are other vigorous activities that sustain a target heart rate. However, riding a bike a short distance across campus is not adequate in intensity or time to develop fitness. Ask, "Did I keep my heart rate in the target heart range for 20 to 60 minutes or more?" In contrast, rope jumping or even stair climbing can be an aerobic activity as long as the FITT prescription factors are met. Bowling, golf, and softball, although enjoyable recreational activities, are not aerobic. What other activities meet the FITT prescription?

The term **anaerobic** means "without oxygen." Anaerobic activities are of high intensity and short duration, such as sprinting. This type of activity demands more oxygen than the body can supply while exercising, causing an oxygen debt. Anaerobic exercise causes waste products (lactic acid) to accumulate in muscles, which, along with the depletion of stored energy, leads to exhaustion. Many activities—tennis, volleyball, and weight training—are anaerobic. They aid in the development of agility, eye-hand coordination, and muscular strength and endurance, as well as flexibility, but they are not aerobic and are not an efficient way to increase cardiorespiratory fitness unless they follow the FITT formula.

How Long Before Results Become Apparent?

This varies with the individual. Within the first few exercise sessions, many people report that they feel better. Measurable differences such as decreased heart rate and improved aerobic fitness can occur within 8 to 12 weeks. The key is staying with the exercise program. Studies indicate that over 50 percent of adults who start an exercise program quit within the first 3 to 6 months. Regular exercisers focus on the positive benefits of exercise, reminding themselves how good they feel after exercise, and pat themselves on the back for making progress. So how do you stay with an exercise program long enough to experience the benefits of the training effect? See the Top 10 List "Ways to Stick with Exercise" for examples of ways to keep a commitment to a healthy lifestyle.

Various Exercise Guidelines Lead to Confusion

You have learned that to develop aerobic fitness you should follow the FITT prescription. Does this conflict with the U.S. Surgeon General's recommendation or the U.S. Government's recommendation that accompanies the new dietary food pyramid? No and no! While this may seem confusing at first, it is clear that the two recommendations have very different goals, and they both differ from the FITT goal.

For example, the 1998 U.S. Surgeon General's recommendation was to add 30 minutes of moderate-intensity activity each day. It was a warning that regardless of our age, we are not active enough. It was a health recommendation. It was designed to improve health by warding off chronic diseases (diabetes, heart disease, etc.) and is backed by solid scientific evidence.

The government's new dietary guidelines for the first time ever included physical activity recommendations. These new guidelines released in 2005 urged people to get 60 to 90 minutes of physical activity every day for weight management purposes. Their research found that 30 minutes of exercise was not enough to aid in

weight loss or to maintain weight loss in previously overweight people. Almost 65 percent of adults are either overweight or obese.

The differing recommendations confused many Americans. Which is it? Is 30 minutes enough? Do we need 60 to 90 minutes? What about the FITT guidelines? The answer is that it depends on your goals. The goal of the 30-minute recommendation is for health, to reduce risk of chronic diseases; the goal of the 60- to 90-minute recommendation is for weight management; and the FITT goal is for aerobic fitness. Although the goals are related, they are quite different. In the box below, notice that the exercise intensity differs for the FITT guidelines.

LIFETIME EXERCISE ACTIVITIES

Physical activity is touted as the single most effective lifestyle behavior for promoting better health. It has been identified as a major health indicator in *Healthy People 2010*, with specific objectives to increase the number of adults engaging in regular, preferably daily, moderate-intensity physical activity for at least 30 minutes. Only 25 percent of Americans achieve this. See "The Numbers" for the number of Americans who don't engage in sufficient exercise. What impact does this have on our nation's health?

You can do your part to help improve the health of our nation by selecting and participating in one of the eight exercise activities in this chapter. Select the activity you wish to pursue to reach your fitness goals and then

FITT Prescription	
For fitness aerobic benefits	• 20 to 60 minutes (Minimum of 20 to 30 minutes) • Moderate to vigorous intensity: 60%–80% HRR (Example: walking = 4.0 to 4.5 mph, jogging = 5 mph, biking = 10 mph) • 3–5 days per week
For health benefits	• 30 minutes (To ward off chronic disease) • Moderate intensity: 40%–60% HRR (Example: walking 3.5 mph) • Most days of the week
For weight loss or to prevent weight gain	• 60 minutes • Moderate intensity: 40%–60% HRR • Most days of the week
For weight loss maintenance (in previously overweight individuals)	• 60 to 90 minutes • Moderate intensity: 40%–60% HRR • Most days of the week

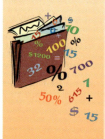

THE NUMBERS

3 in 4	Adults do not engage in sufficent exercise despite the common knowledge that inactivity is related to specific chronic diseases (e.g., heart disease, certain types of cancer, diabetes, obesity, and osteoporosis), leaving only 25% of Americans who do get the recommended amount.
18,000	Average number of steps that men in an Old Order Amish community in Ontario, Canada, took per day. On average, women in the same community took 14,000 steps per day. (Data from a University of Tennesee study.)
2,000–4,000	Number of steps the average American takes per day.
30,000	Number of steps per day that ancient people took just to survive and hunt for food.
3.4 times	Increased risk of early death attributed to the least fit men compared to the most fit men (according to studies conducted at The Aerobics Center, Dallas, Texas).
4.6 times	Increased risk of early death attributed to the least fit women compared to the most fit women (according the same studies noted above).
11.5	Calories per minute burned in deep-water running, about the same rate as a 9-minute-per-mile road run. (Data from University of New Mexico researchers.)
125	Number of steps per minute that meet the ACSM's fitness guidelines.
88%	Reduction in risk of brain injury associated with wearing a helmet while bicycling.
18%	Number of cyclists who wear a helmet all or most of the time while bicycling.

follow the FITT prescription factors. Next, thoroughly read the activity unit of your choice. This will provide you with the helpful guidelines necessary to assist you in reaching these goals.

As you begin your exercise program, let the thoughtful words of the Reverend Jesse Jackson inspire you: "Both tears and sweat are salty, but they render a different result. Tears will get you sympathy, sweat will get you change."

10,000 STEPS: A DAILY LIFESTYLE GOAL

Many fitness experts believe that we could manage weight control and enhance fitness if we would accumulate 10,000 steps in our activities each day. The goal of this new recommendation is to increase the activity levels of the American public by encouraging more people to move about at least 10,000 steps per day. Ten thousand steps is equivalent to about 5 miles. A mile can be anywhere from 1,800 to 2,000 steps, depending on

stride length and pace. Sedentary individuals typically move about (or walk) only about 2,000 to 4,000 steps in a day, moderately active people take 5,000 to 7,000 steps per day, and active people take at least 10,000 steps per day. The goal of 10,000 steps per day is applicable regardless of how much a person weighs or what his or her cardiorespiratory endurance fitness level is. A young person could accumulate steps through jogging, playing basketball, or other activities, while an older person could meet the recommendation by walking.

How do you measure the number of steps taken per day? A basic pedometer, which detects vertical movement of the hips, is an inexpensive and simple way to monitor the total volume of physical activity performed on a daily basis. See the Internet Resources section for information on pedometers. Pedometers are motivational, fitness experts contend. By keeping track of how many steps have been taken, one can check quickly to see how many more steps must be taken to reach the goal of 10,000 steps that day. You probably will discover that it is nearly impossible to get in 10,000 steps in a day without intentionally adding some type of fitness workout such as a jog, walk, or game of tennis or basketball, etc.

TOP 10 LIST

Ways to Stick with Exercise

1. *Pick an activity you enjoy.* Exercise should be fun, not merely work. Try different activities until you find one or two you like.

2. *Make exercise social.* Exercising with a partner or a group of friends is more fun than working out alone. Friends rely on each other for moral support and help each other stay committed to the fitness program. An "exercise date" once or twice a week can keep you going.

3. *Take lessons.* Join an aerobic dance class or a health club. Start slowly and progress gradually to avoid injuries. If exercise is too difficult or too intense, you are not likely to want to stay on the program.

4. *Make it convenient.* Develop a home gym or purchase a couple of exercise videos. Keep your exercise gear available so that you can squeeze in a quick workout.

5. *Treat exercise like an appointment.* Schedule a time that works best for you, whether morning, noon, or evening.

6. *Keep a chart to monitor your progress.* It's rewarding to see how much you have progressed.

7. *Add variety.* To keep your program fresh, walk or jog different routes or exercise in a park or around a golf course. Alternate swimming, walking, and bicycling. While pedaling a stationary bike, read, listen to music, or watch TV. (But don't wear headphones when exercising outside near traffic.)

8. *Have a backup plan in case of bad weather or conflicts.*

9. *Be patient with yourself.* Expect ups and downs. Some days you will be more energetic, some days less. If you're not feeling like a workout, tell yourself you will do a little, and you may find that you perk up after a few minutes. If you have been doing too much, a rest may do you more good than another workout.

10. *Finally, don't stop!* It's difficult to get going again. Remember to plan for changes in your schedule (for example, pack your exercise equipment when you travel). However, don't feel guilty if you miss an exercise session. Taking a few days off due to illness or injury isn't a disaster. Consider this a lifetime commitment and resume exercising as soon as possible.

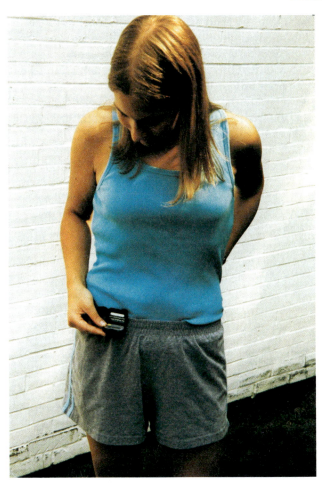

Use a pedometer to motivate you to get more activity every day. How many steps are you getting each day?

Pedometers accurately measure any form of physical activity that involves vertical movement at the hip, such as walking, jogging, tennis, basketball, some cardio machines, and even climbing stairs, shoveling, gardening, and raking. It is important to note that there are some activities and factors in which the pedometer will not accurately register movement counts at the hip. These include:

- ✔ cross-country skiing
- ✔ activities on wheels (e.g., bicycling, skateboarding, and in-line skating)
- ✔ swimming activity (most pedometers are not waterproof)
- ✔ moving slowly (less than 2.5 miles per hour)
- ✔ walking with an uneven gait or scuffing the feet
- ✔ walking on thick carpet
- ✔ wearing the pedometer on a flimsy waistband (this forces it out of the vertical position)

A good pedometer need not be expensive or have multiple functions in order to be reliable and valid. Pedometers requiring the calculation of the step-stride distance are not necessary either. Keep it simple but do get one with a safety strap. This protects against loss or damage if it should fall off the waistband.

Guidelines for using pedometers correctly include:

- ✔ Pedometers can be worn on either the right or the left side of the body.

✔ Place the pedometer on the waistband (or belt) in line with the midpoint of the thigh and kneecap. Reset it to zero. The pedometer will only register counts if the lid is closed (if the brand you have has a lid).

✔ Perform the 20-Step Accuracy Check before use to ensure the pedometer is in the correct spot on the waistband.

  • Begin walking at a normal cadence while counting the number of steps taken. Stop immediately when 20 steps are reached. Check the pedometer's step count reading. If the step count reads 19–21, the placement is accurate.

  • If the step count is not accurate, move the pedometer slightly to the right or left. Reset, take 20 steps, and recheck for accuracy as previously described. Continue with the 20-Step Accuracy Check until proper placement is reached.

✔ Attach a safety strap to clip the pedometer to your waistband, or simply use a safety pin to keep it from falling off.

✔ Pedometers *must remain in the upright vertical position to measure steps accurately*. Undercounting errors may occur for individuals who are overweight because the pedometer may be turned away from the vertical plane and moved toward the horizontal plane by the excess body fat around the waist. Loose-fitting clothing may also affect the accuracy of the pedometer because it absorbs slight vertical force that occurs with each step. In these cases, placement at waist level behind the hip on the back is often advised. Check the accuracy as described previously.

The 10,000-step goal may be too high for some people at first. Follow the five steps outlined in Table 4-3 for guidelines to safely reach your 10,000-step goal and for tips on how to incorporate more physical activity, fun, and variety into your daily life.

Use the *1-Mile Equivalent Chart* in Lab Activity 4-6 on the book's website for additional ideas on how to add more steps to your lifestyle. How many steps are you getting on most days of the week? Check "The Numbers" to see how modern society compares to ancient people and to the Amish lifestyle.

AEROBIC DANCE

(Including Step Aerobics and Spinning)
Advantages/Disadvantages

Aerobic dancing is a popular fitness activity. Usually performed under the leadership of an instructor, it combines the cardiovascular benefits of jogging with the joy

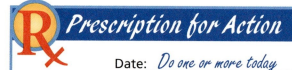

Prescription for Action

Date: *Do one or more today*

Select one of the following:

✔ Walk an extra 2,000 steps. Wear a pedometer all day today. (Hints: Pace around as you talk on the phone; take a walk as you return phone calls; take a marching-in-place minute once an hour; meet with a friend for a walk instead of a soda or coffee; walk around [even in place] during TV commercials.)

✔ Try a new cardio machine in the fitness gym.

✔ Enroll in a fitness class.

✔ Add hand weights to your walking workout.

Prescribed by: *YOU*

of dancing. The variety of movements not only strengthens the cardiorespiratory system but also increases flexibility, tones muscles, and enhances body composition. It is a total body workout. The upbeat music tempo creates an atmosphere of excitement; exercising in a group is fun and emotionally stimulating. The popular music and group camaraderie help prevent boredom and can keep you motivated. Aerobic dancing can be so much fun, you often forget you are exercising. Because the participants focus on the instructor, aerobic dance classes are good for the beginning or self-conscious exerciser. Aerobic dance allows for individualization of a workout. The same movement sequence or exercise can be done by a well-conditioned participant and a beginning exerciser with variation in the intensity or the number of repetitions. Because aerobic dance is done indoors, the environment provides security and comfort.

Aerobic dance has excellent potential for developing all components of physical fitness, but it can have some drawbacks. Although participants are urged by instructors to work at their own pace, some exercisers overdo it. These exercisers try to keep up with the group or work as hard as the instructor even though they may not be ready for this intensity. Many times the result is excessive soreness or fatigue. Performing aerobic dance on a hard, unyielding surface (such as cement) or while wearing inappropriate shoes also increases the risk of injury. Some overzealous aerobics participants attend classes one or more times a day, leading to overuse. Excessive impact may cause leg and foot problems. Also, not all aerobic dance instructors have had training in ex-

TABLE 4-3   *Five Steps to Reach 10,000 Steps a Day*

To avoid injury, you need to work up to 10,000 steps slowly. If you have any concerns about your joints (ankles, knees, hips), discuss your exercise plans with your physician. Check with your physician if you experience any pain or discomfort that concerns you. The goal is to be active for the rest of your life. Don't go overboard at the beginning and develop an injury that will prevent you from having an active lifestyle.

Step Conversion

1 step	=	2.64 feet
1 mile	=	2,000 steps
5 miles	=	10,000 steps
10 miles	=	20,000 steps
25 miles	=	50,000 steps

1. Week 1: Start by wearing the pedometer for one full "normal" or typical week. Record the number of steps taken each day. Use the log sheet in Lab Activity 4-4 Calculate a daily average for one week. This is your Baseline Activity Level and a reference point for setting a personal, realistic, and progressive goal.
2. Weeks 2 and 3: Establish your personal goal by taking the Baseline Activity Level and adding 10 percent more steps to that level.

   For example: If your baseline is 6,000 steps per day, your personal goal would be 6,000 steps plus 600 (10 percent) more steps for a total of 6,600 steps. This will be your personal goal for the next two weeks. If the goal is reached for a majority of days during this period, another 10 percent (600 steps) is added to the baseline and the process is repeated each two-week period thereafter until you reach the goal of 10,000 steps a day. (Example: Weeks 4–5 your goal will be 7,200 steps; weeks 6–7 your goal will be 7,800 steps, and so on.)

   Alternate Method: After the baseline is determined, establish progressive step goals based on the premise that approximately 100 steps are taken every minute. If you wish to increase your activity level by 5 minutes a day, then 500 steps should be added as a goal. One thousand steps should be added for an additional 10 minutes, and so on. Continue adding 500 steps per day (or 1,000 steps per day) to your daily goal until you reach the 10,000-step goal. (Example: If your Baseline Activity Level is 6,000 steps per day, your step goal for weeks 2–3 will be 6,500

steps; for weeks 4–5 your step goal will be 7,000 steps per day; and for weeks 6–7 your step goal will be 7,500 steps per day, and so on.)
3. Decrease your goal or stay at the same goal for longer if you wish or if you are not ready to increase.
4. Pedometers are accurate for walking, running, tennis, and so on, but not for bicycling, swimming, activities on wheels, and some cardio equipment in the fitness center. Use the *1-Mile Equivalent Chart* in Lab Activity 4-6 on the book's website to estimate your steps if you enjoy those activities. They can count toward the 10,000-step goal.
5. Use "Exercise Across the U.S.A." to have fun adding activity to your daily life. Pick a state and exercise/walk across it (see Lab Activity 4-6 on the book's website). At 10,000 steps per day, how many days would it take you to travel the length of the Mississippi River, the Grand Canyon, the circumference of the Earth, go to the Moon, or cross the state of Illinois? Or use the "Activity Step Equivalents" below if you enjoy these activities.

Activity Step Equivalents

Activity	Steps per Minute
Aerobic dance	150–200
Basketball	200–220
Bicycling (6 mph)	70–100
Bicycling (10 mph)	130–140
Gardening	100–130
Housework	80–100
Jumping rope	230–250
In-line skating	135–200
Rowing machine	170–200
Snow shoveling	140–180
Stair climbing	200–230
Swimming	200–300
Tennis (doubles)	100–150
Tennis (singles)	160–200
Weight training	100–130
Yoga	70–100

Example: A 30-minute aerobic dance workout would equate to 4,500–6,000 steps (or between 2.25 miles and 3 miles).

---

ercise instruction and safety and may teach improper technique. Unless good body mechanics and reasonable progressions are emphasized in a class, the result can be discomfort rather than exhilaration and a desire to continue exercising. Having to join or travel to a fitness facility to take an aerobics class may be viewed as a disadvantage by some exercisers. Others find it motivating to have a set time, to have made a financial investment, and to have a group of friends to exercise with. Aerobic dance videotapes are available for the home exerciser. They allow exercising in private but lack the

spontaneity, instruction, and enthusiasm available in a live class.

What to Wear

Although some aerobic dancers have color-coordinated leotards and fancy exercise apparel, any loose-fitting and comfortable clothing will do. A T-shirt and shorts are fine. More important than the clothing are supportive shoes. Shoes specially designed for the impact and movement of aerobic dance are recommended. A good aerobic shoe has a well-cushioned, resilient midsole to aid in shock dispersion and a sturdy heel counter to hold the foot in place. The shoe should allow for lateral movement and, as a result, not have the wide heel flare that is often seen in a jogging shoe. Like the jogger, the aerobic participant should replace old shoes when their cushioning ability has decreased.

Technique and Safety Tips

Many injuries and much discomfort can be avoided in aerobic dance with proper shoes, gradual progression, and exercising on a resilient surface. Chapter 8 gives several general suggestions for preventing injury in fitness activities. In aerobic dance, careful attention to technique and body mechanics further eliminates chance for injury and heightens the enjoyment of the activity.

1. *Always warm up with low-intensity, whole-body movements.* Your warm-up should include slow, full-range-of-motion joint movements. Static stretching should also be included in the warm-up.
2. *Keep abdominals pulled in and buttocks tucked under.*
3. *Avoid twisting the spinal column excessively* (windmill toe touches, elbow-to-knee lunges, etc.).
4. *Limit the hopping on one foot* to a maximum of four consecutive times.
5. *Soften your jumps and bounces by maintaining a slightly bent-knee landing position.*
6. *Try to make your heels go all the way to the floor when landing from jumps.*
7. *Never fling or throw your arms or legs.* Maintain control of limbs throughout movements.
8. *Avoid hyperextending your elbows, knees, or lower back.*
9. *Listen to your body.* If a stretch, exercise, or position causes pain or a burning sensation, do not do it.

The amount of concern for technique and safety in the class depends on your instructor. A wise wellness consumer chooses a knowledgeable, trained instructor. The popularity of aerobic dance has skyrocketed, and the number of qualified instructors has not kept pace. While standards and certification programs have been established, it is up to you to select a class. Do not be shy. Check the instructor's qualifications. Is she or he:

✔ Certified by a national fitness organization?
✔ Knowledgeable in anatomy, exercise physiology, kinesiology, and first aid?
✔ Currently certified in CPR (cardiopulmonary resuscitation)?
✔ Doing some health screening or fitness assessment of students?
✔ Supervising the class effectively?
✔ Monitoring the intensity of the workout with periodic heart-rate checks?
✔ Beginning with a good warm-up and ending with a cool-down period?
✔ Giving corrective cues and technique suggestions throughout the workout?

✔ Considering the variances in fitness levels in the class by showing how to modify the intensity of the workout?
✔ Easy to follow?
✔ Educating the participants on injury prevention and signs of fatigue?

Looking good in a leotard and being a fluid dancer are not requirements for being a quality aerobic dance instructor. Most important is the ability to conduct a safe yet invigorating workout from which all participants can benefit.

How to Begin and Progress

As with any other fitness activity, begin slowly. Attend no more than three classes per week for several weeks. Start with 5 to 10 minutes of the aerobic phase and progress gradually. If the aerobic portion of the class is 30 minutes, do low-impact moves or walk in place while the experienced exercisers continue. Monitor your pulse and stay within your target heart-rate range. You should be able to talk or sing with the music throughout the en-

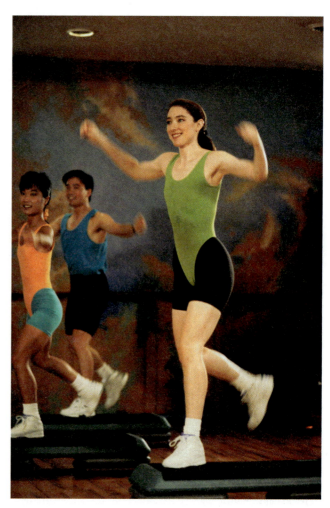

Working out in a class setting is social and fun.

tire workout. Gradually add a few minutes weekly to the aerobic phase until you can exercise aerobically for 20 to 60 minutes.

Some exercisers prefer low-impact aerobics to high-impact aerobics. Low-impact aerobics reduces the strain on knees and ankles by minimizing jumping and bouncing movements. In low-impact aerobics, one foot is in contact with the ground at all times. *Low impact* does not necessarily mean *low intensity*. To maintain a training heart rate, move your arms vigorously and travel along the floor by wide-stride walking, sliding, and sidestepping. Beginners and well-trained exercisers with joint problems can benefit from low-impact aerobics. You may want to combine low-impact and high-impact moves. Most jumps and steps can be modified to become low-impact steps.

Most aerobic dance classes incorporate in the workout a body toning segment. Once again, use common sense. Do not try to do as many repetitions as the teacher unless you are equally fit. Stop and stretch if you feel pain or a burning sensation in the muscle. Aerobic dance participants often tend to compare themselves or compete with others in the class. Avoid falling into this trap. Work to be the best you can be without shame or guilt.

Variety

It is easy to add variety to aerobic dance. Vary the music. Use pop, jazz, country, or classical music. Try some holiday or theme music when appropriate. Vary the routines or steps. Aerobics can be taught by using set routines (repetitive movements in a programmed format) or in a freestyle format (participants mimic the instructor and change accordingly). Varying between learned routines and a freestyle approach helps keep interest high. Try circuit aerobic dance. Set up exercise stations around the room. Do different aerobic movements for 1 to 2 minutes per station and then jog to the next station to sustain your training heart rate. There are many other ways to add variety to aerobic dance. Use 1- to 2-pound hand weights during aerobic routines to increase upper body endurance and maintain a training heart rate. Heavier hand weights are often used during stationary power moves to tone arms and legs. To prevent knee injuries, do not wear ankle weights while doing aerobic dance steps. Weights are, however, an effective way to add resistance while doing floor toning. Thick rubber bands and elastic tubing can also be used to increase the efficiency of body toning exercises.

Step Aerobics

Also known as *bench/step training*, step aerobics is an innovative activity that involves stepping up and down on a 4- to 12-inch platform. Combining a variety of stepping patterns with kicks, turns, and upper body move-

ments results in a brisk workout. Step aerobics appeals to a wide range of exercisers for several reasons: It can be a high-intensity workout with low-impact force; it is adaptable to different fitness levels by adjusting the bench height, adding jumps, varying arm gestures, and adding light hand weights; and it is easy to do. Step aerobics has become especially popular with men, who may be put off by "dancelike" aerobics classes. As with all aerobic exercise activities, proper form and technique are necessary to prevent injury.

To prevent injury while stepping:

1. *As much as possible, keep your shoulders aligned over your hips.*
2. *Step up lightly, making sure the whole foot lands on the platform.*
3. *Keep your knees aligned over your feet when they're pulling your body weight onto the platform.*
4. *At the top, straighten your legs but don't lock your knees.*
5. *Do not pivot a bent, supporting knee.*
6. *As you step down, stay close to the platform.*

If you are a beginner at step aerobics, start with the lowest bench and keep your eyes on the bench until you adjust to the activity. Once you learn the stepping patterns, you can add arm movements and light hand weights or challenge yourself by raising the height of the bench. (However, never use a height that flexes your knees to an angle less than 90 degrees.)

Step aerobics is a great workout for the lower body and, when combined with a variety of arm movements, an exciting variation in aerobic exercise.

Indoor Cycling Classes (Spinning or Fit Ride)

Indoor cycling class is a stationary cycling workout that uses motivational techniques. The instructor leads a group of riders on a scenic stationary trail ride by using visualization techniques, motivational strategies, and videotapes and music. The instructor prompts you on when to crank up or loosen the tension and when to pedal faster. The indoor cycling class allows people of all ages and fitness levels to take a stationary bike and transform it into a powerful workout. Participants vary the workout by making changes in the speed and resistance of the bike. Indoor cycling classes allow participants to experience road cycling without the associated dangers. The program is also a great choice for the cyclist who wants to take his or her outdoor program inside during inclement weather.

A drawback to this excellent aerobic exercise program is the necessity to join a class that provides the certified trained instructor and appropriate bikes. Access to a health/fitness club or university fitness class is usually required for this activity.

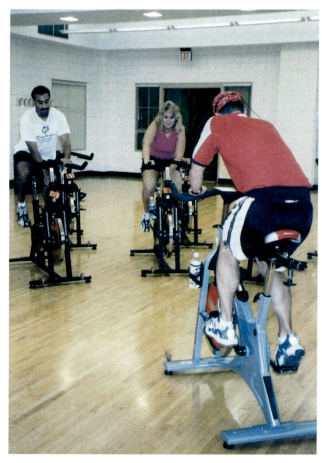

Indoor cycling class is a popular indoor fitness activity and can be quite challenging. The optimal pace is 60 to 80 rpm. A racer's pace is 80 to 100 rpm or more.

For added comfort and enjoyment, follow these guidelines:

1. Adjust the seat high enough so that the leg fully extends at the bottom of each pedal stroke with a slight bend in the knee.
2. If possible, move the seat forward or back so that the bent knee, at the top of the stroke, rests just above midfoot.
3. Attach toe clips to help prevent foot fatigue.
4. Tilt the seat slightly downward to avoid crotch numbness.
5. For added comfort, buy a cover to pad the seat (or a gel cover) and invest in cycling shorts.
6. Adjust handlebar height to reduce hand/wrist pressure.
7. Add resistance when pedals (instead of your thigh muscles) are propelling your foot or the instructor advises you to do so.
8. Always warm up and cool down properly. Don't try to compete with class members; ride at your fitness level. Use your THR or PRE as a guide.
9. Listen to your body and stop before you feel fatigued.

Common Discomforts

As in most fitness activities, mild soreness can be anticipated by the beginning exerciser. Some discomfort may be avoided by emphasizing stretching and toning the first 3 to 4 weeks to condition muscles and connective tissue for the stress of impact and the new movements. Veteran exercisers can suffer pain or injury by increasing frequency, time, or intensity too rapidly. Most aerobic dance discomfort is found in the legs, so be sure to warm up and stretch this area. Exercise fatigue can also occur due to dehydration or lack of sleep/rest. Refer to Chapter 8 for further information about prevention and treatment of injuries. If you use hand weights, elbow and shoulder strain can be avoided by not flinging the weights. Always move the weights with control. Having a towel or exercise mat with you provides additional comfort and padding for floor exercises.

BICYCLING

Advantages/Disadvantages

Cycling is a popular choice for people of all ages. You can fit in a cycling workout while running errands, while going to work, or at home in front of the TV (on rollers or a stationary bike). You can cycle alone, with family, or with friends. If you have a small child, you can take him or her along in a bike seat instead of having to hire a sitter while you get a workout. It is nonimpact exercise, minimizing stress to the back, shins, and ankles.

There are a few drawbacks, though. You must have a bicycle, keep it in good working condition, and store it securely to prevent theft. Cycling in traffic requires alertness and the use of defensive driving skills to prevent accidents. Cycling in rain, snow, or icy conditions is uncomfortable and hazardous. Also, bicycles are so efficient that they can do most of the work for you. Cycling to class or for short distances is fine for transportation, but if you want to get in shape, you will need to put in more effort. Nevertheless, cycling produces cardiorespiratory benefits without impact, making it the third most popular activity in the United States. It can be enjoyed throughout a lifetime.

What to Wear

To be clearly visible to vehicles, wear bright-colored clothing during the day and light-colored clothing at night. Fancy bicycling gear is not necessary, although if you really get into cycling, you might find that a pair of bicycling shorts makes long rides more comfortable. Hard-soled, athletic, or bicycling shoes are fine.

Equipment

There are plenty of bike-pedestrian and bike-car accidents, and usually it is the bicyclist who is at fault. Al-

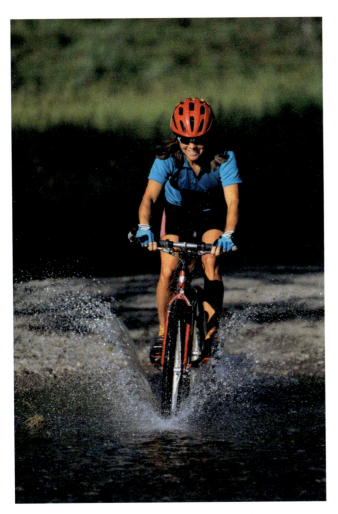

Bicycling is a great fitness activity across the life span. Always wear a helmet.

ways wear a helmet even if you're going only a short distance. The sidewalk is a hard surface. You may lose some skin in a slide or break some bones, but they will heal. Your brain won't. Head injuries account for over 75 percent of deaths and permanent disabilities in cycling crashes. If you hit something and go flying head first, wearing a good helmet is the best way to prevent serious injury.

When you are choosing a helmet, make sure that it has the following characteristics:

- ✔ Outer shell or cover that is brightly colored (e.g., yellow, white, or red) so that you are easily visible to drivers
- ✔ Hard shell lined with polystyrene or polystyrene alone
- ✔ Secure chin strap
- ✔ Label indicating that the helmet is ANSI or SNELL approved

Helmets are single-use devices designed to crush and absorb shock upon impact. You should replace a helmet that has been in a significant crash.

A water bottle is essential for workouts, particularly in the heat. Because sweat evaporates so quickly while you are riding, you may not realize how quickly water is lost. Dehydration, leading to heat illness, can easily occur. Drinking regularly from a water bottle to maintain an adequate level of hydration during a workout is a necessity, not a luxury.

Recumbent bicycles have recently become popular, especially for riders with back problems. Because they are low to the ground, they are not as visible to motorists. Be sure to use a warning flag on the bike.

It doesn't matter what type of bike you ride, but it does matter that it be kept in good working order. If you are not mechanically inclined, your local bicycle shop can help. Most people ride with the bike seat too low, which is inefficient and can make the knees hurt. The bike seat should be high enough that when you sit centered on the seat with your heel on the pedal at its lowest point, your knee is only slightly bent. That way, when you move the ball of your foot to its proper position on the pedal, your knee will be almost fully extended at the bottom of the stroke. If the seat is too high, you'll tend to rock from side to side with each footstroke and may develop a sore crotch. A sore crotch also can be caused by improper seat tilt. Start with the nose of the seat level. If it bothers you, tilt it down slightly. Pedals, wheels, and steering should turn or spin freely with no binding, catch, or click. The derailleur should shift smoothly. Brakes should close and release easily. Brake shoes should be ⅛ inch or less from and level with the rim of the bike. If they are badly worn, replace them. The air in the tires usually needs to be topped off weekly to keep them hard and rolling smoothly, but use caution when filling them. The air pumps at service stations are designed for cars, and it's easy to explode a bicycle tire by overfilling it. If a bike wheel is badly out of true and wobbles, it may hit the brake shoe with each revolution. A bike shop can true a wheel; lubricate sticky brake cables; adjust the derailleur; and show you how to keep your machine running smoothly, which makes riding safe and enjoyable.

Technique and Safety Tips

Shifting On multispeeds, the gears overlap slightly and you have to shift by feel. To shift, continue pedaling but ease up on the pedal pressure. Shifting without pedaling can cause a bent or broken chain or gear teeth. As you shift, you should not hear a loud clunk or a constant rubbing sound if you are shifting smoothly and getting it into gear correctly.

Most beginners gear too high and pedal too slowly. They feel like they're not getting any exercise unless they're pushing against resistance. This is inefficient and can increase fatigue and cause knees to ache. It is better to pedal quickly against light resistance. An optimal pedal rate is 60 to 80 rpm, with a range of 80 to 100 rpm. Racers and experienced tourists often cycle at 90 to 110 rpm.

If your bike has several gears, practice using them. Gearing is a matter of maintaining an even cadence regardless of terrain, weather, or wind conditions. If you're going uphill, shift before you have to slow your cadence so that you can go up smoothly. Also practice downshifting before stop signs so that you don't have to stand on the pedals to get going again.

Pedaling   Ride with the ball of your foot on the pedal. If you have toe clips, you can try ankling—pulling up as well as pushing down on the pedal with each stroke—which doubles your efficiency.

Braking   Look ahead, signal, slow down, and learn to anticipate problems instead of simply reacting to them. Be careful not to jam on the brakes too suddenly or you can pitch headfirst over the handlebars. The front brake is the most powerful because as you decelerate, your weight shifts forward, lessening the weight over the back tire. For the most efficient stop, keep the body weight back, gradually increase pressure on the front brake, and hold pressure on the back brake just below the point where the wheel will skid. In wet conditions, brakes lose up to 90 percent of their braking ability. It is good to frequently apply the brakes lightly to wipe water off the rims and allow extra stopping distance. When going downhill, pump the brakes to avoid overheating the wheel rims or brake shoes. When in doubt, favor the rear brake.

Bumps   When you come up to bumps, holes, and railroad tracks, shift your weight to pedals and handlebars to absorb the shock. It's better for you and for your bike.

Safety Tips

1. Wear brightly colored clothing, wear a helmet, and carry water.
2. Keep to the right side of the road and ride in a straight line. Always ride in single file with traffic.
3. Do not make sudden turns or swerves. Signal turns and stops.
4. Stay alert. Look out for cars pulling out into traffic or turning. Listen constantly for traffic approaching out of your line of vision.
5. Observe traffic regulations as if you were driving a car—red and green lights, one-way streets, stop signs. Slow down at all street intersections and look right and left before crossing.
6. Be sure the brakes are operating efficiently and keep your bicycle in perfect running condition. Keep your hands on or near the brakes at all times.
7. Keep speed under control, especially on long downhill runs. Speed should be low enough that you can stop quickly.
8. In rainy weather, allow much more distance for stopping and don't take corners too fast.
9. Watch for doors opening suddenly on parked cars. Ride at least 3 feet away from them.
10. Avoid sewer grates that parallel your direction.
11. If railroad tracks are rough, walk your bike across them (to prevent a blowout or other damage to the bicycle). If you choose to ride over the tracks, cross them at a 90-degree angle.
12. Make sure you are at least 3 feet off the traveled portion of the road when you stop or park.
13. Hug the right-hand shoulder of the road on all curves.
14. Give pedestrians the right-of-way. Avoid sidewalks.
15. Watch out for child cyclists. Children on bicycles usually weave from side to side and turn unpredictably without signaling and can run into you when you are passing them.
16. Dogs are potential adversaries. If a dog is far enough away, you can probably outrun it. Water from your bottle or a bike pump may scare the dog off. If you stop, keep the bike between you and the dog. Walk slowly away. Usually a dog will leave you alone, but watch the dog carefully before you get under way again. You can also buy a small can of "dog repellent," which will shoot a thin stream of chemical about 10 feet. Although the effects are potent, no permanent damage is done to the animal. Don't try to run down or kick at a dog—this can cause a crash. If you are scared, you can yell "Out" at the dog, mimicking a noise made by mother dogs when disciplining their puppies. This will usually startle a dog enough to give you a chance to escape.
17. Don't wear headphones—they block out street sounds that enable you to anticipate traffic.
18. Don't wear a heavy backpack. It can throw off your balance. Carry packages in baskets or bags attached to the cycle.
19. Learn to shift gears while keeping your eyes on the road.
20. If you use toe clips, practice getting in and out of them in a safe area.
21. Tuck in your shoelaces.

How to Begin and Progress

First, measure your fitness level by using the 3-mile timed ride test in Chapter 3. Remember that your *current* fitness level does not indicate your potential. Allow yourself several weeks to show significant improvement. Begin at the step indicated by your current fitness level. If you cannot complete the test, begin at level 1. Exercise 3 to 5 days a week at your training pulse. (An appropriate pulse for bicycling appears to be about 5 percent lower than that for other exercise, so subtract 5 percent to adjust for this difference.) It is also appropriate to use the RPE. You may work at one level until you can comfortably handle the recommended distance and intensity, then move to the next step. To develop balanced fitness, add 25 to 30 push-ups, a minute of abdominal curls, and 5 to 15 minutes of stretching to each workout.

Bicycling Program

Fitness Category	Starting Level
Low	1 or 2
Fair	3
Average	4
Good	5
Superior	6

Level	Cycling	Total Distance
1	20–30 min. (8–10 mph)	3–5 miles
2	20–30 min. (10–12 mph)	4–6 miles
3	30–45 min. (10–12 mph)	4–8 miles
4	30–60 min. (10–15 mph)	7–15 miles
5	40–75 min. (10–15 mph)	10–18 miles
6	40–90 min. (10–15 mph)	10–22 miles

Variety

Part of the appeal of bicycling is being able to explore an area and see things you normally wouldn't notice as you whiz past in a car. Try cycling to a park, a lake, or a scenic spot or just go exploring on a bicycle. Plan an outing with a picnic or refreshment break halfway. Ride to a nearby small town and back. Plan a bike rally, similar to a car rally with checkpoints, or a bike scavenger hunt in which you gather bits of information from locations (e.g., what is the name of the store at 21 Oak Street?). If you are interested in more alternatives, consult your local bicycle shop for bicycling organizations in your area and find out what rides and tours are planned.

Common Discomforts

Bicyclists beginning a conditioning program often experience a sore crotch the first week or two. As you and your saddle adjust to each other, the syndrome should disappear. Check to see that the seat is not too high. An overly high seat causes you to rock from side to side with each pedal stroke, and the constant rubbing will prolong soreness. It may help to tilt the nose of the saddle down a bit (not so much that you slide off!), to try a different saddle, one with padding under the "sit bones," or to consider padded cycling shorts. See the section "Males and Exercise" in Chapter 7.

Sore knees? A seat that is too low so that your knees are excessively bent throughout the pedal stroke is one cause. Riding with excessive resistance at too low a cadence increases pressure on the knees and is another easily remedied cause. A relatively high cadence against light resistance reduces the frequency of overuse injuries.

If your fingers feel numb after cycling, you need to change hand position more frequently and ride with the elbows slightly bent, not locked. The ulnar nerve runs across the palm, and constant pressure on the hands can temporarily cut off sensation to the area. Wearing padded cycling gloves or cushioning your handlebars with foam grips may also help.

Neck or back soreness usually disappears in a week or so once you grow accustomed to riding. If it does not, try changing hand positions frequently, riding with the elbows slightly bent, moving the seat forward a little, or perhaps switching to upright handlebars.

Do your toes tend to go numb on long rides? If you are using toe clips, it may be that pedaling tends to push your foot forward into your shoes until your toes touch the end, reducing blood flow to the area. Try lacing your shoes snugly enough so that they hold your foot back in the heel of the shoe but not so tightly that circulation is hindered. Also, try loosening your toe clips.

FITNESS SWIMMING

Advantages/Disadvantages

Swimming is a superb form of exercise. It is a total body workout that uses the major muscle groups of both the upper and lower body. Other forms of aerobic exercise, jogging, for example, use mainly large muscles of the lower body. In addition, water exercise is a natural form of strength training. Resistance of the water against the body's movements enhances muscle strength. Swimmers are also subject to fewer injuries than are participants in many other activities. Joint and muscle injuries are not common among swimmers because of water buoyancy.

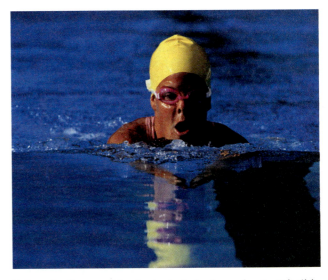

Swimming is one of the best whole-body workouts. It builds heart and lung capacity, tones all major muscles (arms, shoulders, waist, hips, and legs), improves flexibility, and reduces stress.

Water supports the body, alleviating the jarring effects of weight-bearing exercise such as aerobics or jogging. Swimming is ideal for the overweight, the arthritic, the injured, the elderly, and those prone to joint problems.

Another advantage of swimming is the rare occurrence of heat exhaustion and heat stroke. This can be a concern when exercising in hot, humid weather. If you don't like to sweat, you probably will prefer to exercise in water.

Swimming does have drawbacks. You must have some swimming ability and have access to a pool at a time convenient for you. That first plunge into the water may be difficult for some, but after a brief warm-up period, the cool water temperature will be invigorating. Warm water quickly becomes uncomfortable during a vigorous workout.

Although the injury rate is low, you may experience some minor annoyances as you train in water. Eye irritations and "swimmer's ear" are the most common.

The inconvenience of having to redo makeup and hair is minor when you measure the positive outcomes of aquatic exercise. After the workout, an efficient hair and makeup routine develops quickly.

What to Wear

Swimming is an inexpensive sport because the only equipment needed is a comfortable swimming suit. Many swimmers wear goggles to protect their eyes, and for added comfort, you may wish to use ear plugs and a swim cap. Swimmers can exercise indoors or outside, making this a year-round sport.

Technique and Safety Tips

Learn to swim the following five basic strokes efficiently: sidestroke, elementary backstroke, breaststroke, back crawl, and front crawl. Incorporate stroke mechanics sessions on these strokes into each workout. The butterfly stroke is too strenuous for most fitness swimmers.

Learn and practice the front crawl and back crawl turns. These will make lap swimming more enjoyable. Construct your daily training program to include a water warm-up, conditioning bout, and water cool-down. Monitor your heart rate (or use the RPE) and do not allow it to exceed your swimming target zone. Use hand paddles, kickboards, pull buoys, and swim fins to increase muscular strength and stroke efficiency. Hyperextension of the lower back (arching) is natural in water exercise. It is important to strengthen the abdominal muscles and always stretch the lower back area to counteract this tendency.

Here are other safety tips:

1. *Never swim alone.* A lifeguard should be present. Safety equipment, such as a ring buoy and a reaching pole, should also be available.
2. *Do not dive into the pool at the shallow end.* The risk is too great. Even experienced swimmers have misjudged the depth of the water and hit the bottom, resulting in serious injuries.
3. *Stay to the right of the lane and make your turns counterclockwise.*
4. *If resting at the pool edge, keep to one side of the lane to allow other swimmers to turn easily.*
5. *Be careful with electrical equipment around the pool* (radios, pace clocks, etc.). Make sure electrical outlets are grounded.
6. *Keep telephone and emergency rescue numbers in the pool area.*
7. *Keep all doors going into the pool area locked unless there is a lifeguard on duty.*

How to Begin and Progress

Assess your aerobic swimming fitness on the 500-yard swim test as described in Chapter 3. Based on your fitness category, begin at the appropriate starting S.W.I.M. level. Progress through each level, one step at a time. Do not skip steps and stay on each one as long as necessary to adapt to that workload. Remember to monitor your pulse and do not exceed your swimming target heart rate range. When you have completed level M, you may want to swim continuously for distance or time or continue with the routine of four lengths and a brief rest for the measured distance or time. Keep in mind the THR. for swimming is 10 percent less than for weight-bearing activities. You may also use the RPE.

In this program, swim the number of lengths suggested, but if the workout feels too hard, rest a few seconds by climbing out of the pool and walking back to the starting point or rest at the end of the pool for a few seconds before continuing the workout. Swim the front crawl, if possible, or any stroke that allows you to reach the prescribed swimming target heart rate. Consult the pool distance table.

Variety

To add variety to your swimming workouts, practice stroke mechanics on the five basic strokes. This will allow you to use a variety of strokes in your workouts instead of being limited to one or two. Swim for time instead of distance for a change or vice versa. Use equipment: a kick board is good for practicing kicks and for strengthening your legs; swim fins help you develop leg and abdominal muscles and increase ankle flexibility; hand paddles give your shoulders, chest, arms, and back an extra workout. Webbed gloves or a tethering system add interest to your workouts and improve strength and stroke efficiency. Use a waterproof CD player or digital music player if you find swimming monotonous. For a complete change of pace, try an aquacircuiting or water running session in shallow water or a deep water jogging workout using some type of flotation device. See the section on water exercise/aqua aerobics later in this chapter.

Pool Distance

Most standard pools are 25 yards in length
One length = 25 yards
One lap = two lengths (50 yards)

18 lengths = 1/4 mile	(approx. 450 yds.)
35 lengths = 1/2 mile	(approx. 875 yds.)
53 lengths = 3/4 mile	(approx. 1325 yds.)
70 lengths = 1 mile	(approx. 1750 yds.)

25 Meter Pools

16 lengths = 1/4 mile (approx. 402.25 m)
32 lengths = 1/2 mile (approx. 804.50 m)
48 lengths = 3/4 mile (approx. 1206.75 m)
64 lengths = 1 mile (approx. 1609 m)

FITNESS S.W.I.M. PROGRAM

Fitness Category	Starting Level
Low	S
Fair	S
Average	W
Good	I
Superior	M

S.W.I.M. Program

Level S			Level W		
Lengths	Repeats	Distance	Lengths	Repeats	Distance
1	× 4	= 100 yds./m	2	× 4	= 200 yds./m
1	× 6	= 150 yds./m	2	× 5	= 250 yds./m
1	× 8	= 200 yds./m	2	× 6	= 300 yds./m
1	× 10	= 250 yds./m	2	× 7	= 350 yds./m
			2	× 8	= 400 yds./m
			2	× 9	= 450 yds./m
			2	× 10	= 500 yds./m
			2	× 11	= 550 yds./m

Level I			Level M		
Lengths	Repeats	Distance	Lengths	Repeats	Distance
3	× 7	= 525 yds./m	4	× 7	= 700 yds./m
3	× 8	= 600 yds./m	4	× 8	= 800 yds./m
3	× 9	= 675 yds./m	4	× 9	= 900 yds./m
3	× 10	= 750 yds./m	4	× 10	= 1000 yds./m
3	× 11	= 825 yds./m	4	× 11	= 1100 yds./m
3	× 12	= 900 yds./m	4	× 12	= 1200 yds./m
3	× 13	= 975 yds./m			
3	× 14	= 1050 yds./m			

Discomforts

While swimmers are less susceptible to injuries, they may experience a few minor discomforts. Eye irritations are caused by an imbalance in the pH (balance of acidity and alkalinity) of the water or excessive amounts of chlorine. Wear goggles and you will have no problem. Swimmer's ear refers to a rashlike inflammation of the ear canal that is caused by frequent exposure to moisture. Dry your ears thoroughly with a towel to prevent this nuisance. If you have frequent ear infections, it would be wise to purchase a pair of ear plugs. See a specialist to get a good fit; those purchased over the counter do not fit well enough to keep water out of the ear canal. A few swimmers complain of sore shoulders. A certain amount of soreness is normal during the first weeks of training. But if pain persists, you may be developing tendinitis. Shoulder tendinitis may be caused by an inherent structural shoulder problem, the use of hand paddles, or improper stroke mechanics. See an orthopedic specialist if shoulder pain persists and use strokes with an underwater recovery (i.e., breaststroke, sidestroke, and elementary backstroke). Some swimmers experience knee pain, especially along the inner borders of the knees, when swimming the breaststroke and elementary backstroke. This is caused by the kick used in these strokes. Do not swim the breaststroke or elementary backstroke until the pain subsides or avoid them altogether. It is a common myth that you are more susceptible to colds if you participate in aquatic activities, especially during the winter. Colds and respiratory infections are caused by viruses and are spread by contact with infected individuals. You are more likely to catch a cold in a warm, dry, crowded room than in a swimming pool. Another myth is that swimming during menstruation is prohibited. Minor discomfort during this time may be alleviated by exercise. If cramps are severe, use your judgment.

FITNESS WALKING

Advantages/Disadvantages

Walking is simple, enjoyable, and probably the safest form of aerobic exercise known. It is inexpensive and can be done by almost anyone, any place, any time. There is no need to join a club or find partners or opponents. It is a wise exercise choice for the overweight, the older adult, the very out of shape, the postsurgical patient, and the individual in a cardiac rehabilitation program. Appropriate shoes and comfortable clothes are the only equipment you need. Walking is excellent for weight control. You use as many calories walking a mile as you would jogging the same distance. The difference is that walking takes longer. Even though the injury rate is low, some walkers who try to increase distance and pace too quickly may experience sore muscles and knees or other types of discomfort. Another disadvantage to walking is that the already physically fit may not be able to elevate the heart rate into the target zone. In this case, try one of the advanced forms of fitness walking, such as power walking (with hand weights or walking poles) or race walking. Dogs and inclement weather present other problems to the walker. Many shopping malls have opened their doors for early morning walking and also to provide a safe, weather-controlled environment year-round.

TOP 10 LIST

Reasons to Pursue Lifetime Exercise

In addition to helping maintain healthy weight, reducing unhealthy abdominal fat, and increasing energy, lifetime exercise:

1. Improves heart health by reducing heart disease
2. Lowers blood pressure and risk of stroke
3. Reduces risk of diabetes
4. Increases bone density, reducing osteoporosis
5. Lowers risk of some cancers, especially of the colon and breast
6. Improves sleep
7. Reduces joint pain in people with arthritis
8. Reduces likelihood of gallstone surgery
9. Reduces stress, anxiety, and depression
10. Increases HDL ("good") cholesterol and lowers triglycerides

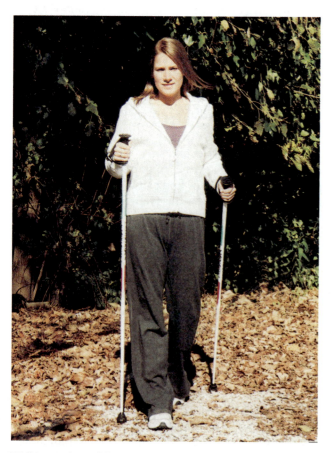

Walking poles safely increase the intensity of a fitness walking workout.

What to Wear

You don't have to buy special clothes; anything loose and comfortable will do. It is a good idea to have a pocket for carrying identification, keys, and a handkerchief. For suggestions on dealing with weather, read the tips for hot and cold weather dressing provided in the section on jogging.

Studies show that walking generates a downward force of about one and one-half times your body weight, so wearing appropriate shoes is important in helping you progress smoothly and injury-free. You may save a few dollars on inexpensive shoes, but a good pair of shoes will help protect your feet, legs, and back. When purchasing new shoes, go to a reputable store and ask for a trained salesperson. Look for shoes with a cushioned heel, a flexible sole, firm heel support, and arch supports that fit your feet. The toe box must provide room for the toes to work to prevent blisters. Several companies manufacture shoes designed for the sport of walking. Try one of these or one made for cross training or jogging but be sure it fits your foot. The shoe should never feel like it needs to be broken in. It should feel comfortable from day one.

Do you replace your worn-out shoes soon enough? A study at Tulane University found that all shoes, regardless of brand, price, or type of construction, lose most of their shock absorbency after 500 miles of use. This is a good reason for keeping records of your mileage. Take your old shoes with you when shopping for a new pair so that a knowledgeable salesperson can evaluate the wear pattern to help you choose a suitable shoe.

Technique and Safety Tips

Walking posture is erect but relaxed. To alleviate tension, the abdomen should be pulled in, the rib cage lifted, and the shoulders pulled down. This will help you keep relaxed and increase your endurance. Your arms should be bent at about a 90-degree angle, and your hands (loose fist) should swing slightly above your waist. Your arms counterbalance your leg motion. You may discover during your walk that your arms have dropped, resulting in a slower pace. Do you ever see joggers with their arms at their sides? Visualize that you are walking in a straight line. Hold your head up with the eyes focused ahead, watching the ground but not your feet. Your foot contact should be a heel roll to the ball of the foot and toes for pushing off. Resist the tendency to lean forward at the waist.

While you are walking, keep in mind these tips for a safe workout:

1. *Always carry some form of identification* (include pertinent medical information).
2. *Choose a safe time and place to exercise.* Take keys with you and lock the car and/or house.

Correct Walking Form

To check your form, have a friend watch you walk, or walk on a treadmill in front of a mirror. Here are the key points for good walking posture.

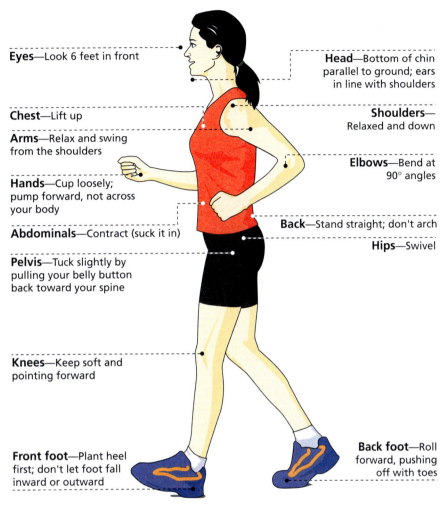

Eyes—Look 6 feet in front

Head—Bottom of chin parallel to ground; ears in line with shoulders

Chest—Lift up

Shoulders—Relaxed and down

Arms—Relax and swing from the shoulders

Elbows—Bend at 90° angles

Hands—Cup loosely; pump forward, not across your body

Abdominals—Contract (suck it in)

Back—Stand straight; don't arch

Hips—Swivel

Pelvis—Tuck slightly by pulling your belly button back toward your spine

Knees—Keep soft and pointing forward

Front foot—Plant heel first; don't let foot fall inward or outward

Back foot—Roll forward, pushing off with toes

Feet—Point toes forward, keeping feet parallel

3. *Plan your route carefully.* Use well-populated, well-lighted areas. Avoid areas that are dark and have dense shrubs and alleys.
4. *Know where you can get help along your route.*
5. *Use sidewalks or walk facing oncoming traffic, and walk in single file.*
6. *Obey traffic signals and signs.* Do not jaywalk.
7. *Keep alert at all times.* Give the right-of-way to cars. Don't assume the driver sees you.
8. *Wear bright, reflective clothing at dusk and at night.*
9. *Tell someone where you are going and when you think you will return.* Better yet, use the buddy system. It's more fun to walk with someone.
10. *Avoid dogs by selecting routes that are free of them.* The best advice is to ignore a barking dog and never walk between a barking dog and its human, especially if the human is a child.
11. *For the cleanest air, walk in the morning.* The air is more polluted at midday or later.
12. *Don't wear a headset;* you would be losing one of your most valuable sensory aids. If you wear a headset, keep volume low so that you can hear traffic or approaching strangers.
13. *Avoid peak traffic hours* unless you can use a jogging path or a sidewalk.

Tips for Increasing Walking Pace

What is your current walking pace? If you do not know, here is how you can measure your effort. Go to a quarter-mile track or measure 1 mile on a road with your car odometer. Time yourself walking for 1 mile. If it takes you 20 minutes, you are walking at 3 mph; if it takes you 15 minutes, you are walking a 4 mph pace; if it takes you about 13 minutes, you are walking at a 4.5 mph pace; if you do it in 12 minutes, you have reached a 5 mph pace. You can also calculate your speed by counting how many steps you take in one minute:

✔ 115 steps = 2.5–3.5 mph
✔ 125 steps = 3.0–4.0 mph
✔ 135 steps = 3.5–4.5 mph
✔ 150 steps = 5.0 mph

If you would like to increase your fitness walking pace try the suggestions in the Top 10 List "Techniques for Increasing Walking Pace."

Carrying hand weights and using walking poles, Powerbelts, and so on while fitness walking will increase the intensity of your workouts. Pumping your arms will accomplish the same effects. While the majority of healthy men and women can achieve a training heart rate with unaided walking, there are some people who may be too fit to achieve this threshold (e.g., young college students). Research shows that adding external weight to the body or involving the upper extremities during exercise can increase the intensity of walking.

For people who want to increase the overall intensity of their workout or make walking more of a total body workout, there are a variety of reasonably priced adjuncts to consider, such as weighted belts, gloves, vests, and walking poles (a.k.a. Nordic walking). They are safe and effective and can increase CRE and weight control benefits of a regular walking program. See Table 4-4.

When using the walking equipment described in Table 4-5, be aware that 50 to 70 percent of the increase in oxygen consumption and caloric expenditure comes from swinging the arms to a greater degree. In one study, for example, participants walked on a treadmill at 3.0 mph, and VO_{2max} was 15.9 ml/kg/min. Walking at the same speed while swinging the arms to chin height required 17.8 ml/kg/min. The addition of 2-pound weights further increased the oxygen cost to 18.9 ml/kg/min. Thus 63 percent of the increase above normal walking was attributed to the exaggerated arm swing. Swinging the arms may serve as a good intermediate step for increasing walking intensity without being encumbered with extra equipment.

How to Begin and Progress

Test your fitness using the 1-mile walk test described in Chapter 3. Then follow the appropriate level on the W.A.L.K.S. Program. After completing the "S" level, continue on the W.A.L.K.S. Maintenance Program for a lifetime of fitness.

Warm up for 5 to 10 minutes before starting the conditioning segment of your workout. The warm-up should be activity-specific, so for fitness walking begin gradually increasing the pace to that at your conditioning level.

TOP 10 LIST

Techniques for Increasing Walking Pace

1. *Pump your arms.* When your arms drag, the tendency is to slow down. Resist this. Keep your arms pumping and your legs will be forced to keep pace. Bend the arms to a full 90-degree angle; keep the shoulders low and relaxed (not raised).

2. *Heel walks.* Walk on your heels, with your toes off the ground. This stretches and strengthens your calves and especially your shins, training that puts power in your stride by helping you develop a stronger push-off and prevents the development of shin splints.

3. *Crossovers.* On a track, road, or sidewalk, practice walking along an imaginary straight line. Engage your hips by crossing your foot across the line with each step. This forces you to adopt the signature race-walking wiggle. Plus, extending your legs from your hips allows your pelvis to rotate forward so you can cover more ground with each step without overstriding.

4. *Use interval training.* Walk as fast as you can for 1 minute, then slow the pace for 4 minutes. Gradually increase the intervals by 1 minute every 2 weeks until you can do intense 4-minute intervals with only 1 minute at the slower pace.

5. *Simultaneously begin using the hard/easy system of training.* Go hard one day—either by taking a long walk or by doing intervals or hills—and easy the next. Practice at least 2 training days per week.

6. *Streamline your form.* Alter your strike to a straight-leg landing. When your heel touches the ground, the front leg should be straight. Your forefoot is flexed momentarily to land on the heel rather than the sole of the foot.

7. *Set "walk-to" targets.* Set a "walk-to" target a short distance in front of you (about 30 yards). Walk quickly to the target, reset the target, and walk fast to the new target. Keep resetting the walk-to targets throughout the route. Use mailboxes, driveways, road signs, and trees for targets. This technique helps keep you mentally involved in your fitness walking workout and helps you resist the tendency to stroll.

8. *Add bends and straightaways.* On a track, warm up for 10 minutes and then go your fastest on the straightaways, using the curves for slow recovery walks. Start with 6 to 8 laps, building to 15.

9. *Count steps.* Accelerate 100 steps five times in 30 minutes. This will teach your legs to move faster.

10. *Don't overdo it.* Limit speed workouts to twice a week so that sore muscles won't sideline you for the next day's walk.

TABLE 4-4	**Pros and Cons of Walking Equipment**	
Walking Equipment	**Pros**	**Cons**
Weighted Vests	• Form-fitting • Comfortable	• Minimal aerobic benefit • Expensive (compared with other equipment)
Wrist/Hand Weights	• Inexpensive • Easy to use • Moderate increase in intensity	• May elicit exaggerated blood pressure responses • No place to put the weight if you get tired • May increase incidence of overuse injuries
Walking Poles	• Excellent increases in intensity/caloric expenditure • Upper body muscular endurance increases • Puts less strees on knees	• May elicit a pressor response due to gripping poles • Not adjustable; different-height people need different poles • No place to put poles if you get tired
Powerbelts	• Excellent potential aerobic benefit • May increase muscular strength • Good for interval training • Resistance cords retract when not in use	• Higher levels may be too difficult to maintain • May elicit exaggerated blood pressure responses due to high degree of muscular effort

TABLE 4-5	**Heart Rate Increase, Oxygen Consumption, and Calorie Expenditures of Various Walking Equipment**		
Walking Equipment	**Heart Rate Increases (bpm)**	**Oxygen Consumption (ml/kg/min)**	**Calorie Expenditures (% of increase)**
Weighted Vests (5–10% of Body Wt)	3–7	1.3–2.5	3–10
Hand Weights/ Weighted Gloves (1–3 lb.)	6–13	1.5–4.0	5–15
Walking Poles	10–15	4.5–5.5	20–25
Powerbelts			
Base Unit	25–30	6.3–6.7	40–45
Powerpack 1	30–35	6.7–7.0	45–50
Powerpack 2	35–40	7.0–8.0	50–60
Powerpack 3	40–45	8.0–9.5	60–65

During the conditioning bout, always check your heart rate to be sure it stays within the target zone. Also use the RPE or talk test. Listen to your body and progress slowly for optimal results.

Cool down for 5 to 10 minutes after the conditioning bout. As in the warm-up, the cool-down should be activity-specific. Thus, reduce your pace, finishing with 5 to 10 minutes of slow walking.

For total fitness, stretch for flexibility. Improved flexibility is best achieved if it occurs at the end of the cool-down, when the muscles and joints are thoroughly warmed and pliable. Use flexibility exercises for your stretching routine.

Take each step on the chart and don't skip ahead. If the increase is too difficult, go back to the preceding level for a while. You should feel energized after your workout, not exhausted.

Variety

Adding variety to your walking workouts can keep you enthused about the activity for many years. Varying your walking routes gives you a change of scenery. Drive the car to a new area, park, and explore the surroundings during your workout. Mailing a letter, walking for an errand, taking window-shopping walks, and doing shopping

W.A.L.K.S. Program

Fitness Category	Starting Program
Low	W Level
Fair	A Level
Average	L Level
Good	K Level
Superior	S Level

W Level

Week	1–2	3–4	5–6	7–8	9–10	11–12	13–14
Warm-up (min.)	5–10	5–10	5–10	5–10	5–10	5–10	5–10
Conditioning bout (mileage)	1.00	1.25	1.50	1.75	2.00	2.25	2.50
Intensity % (target heart rate)	60–80	60–80	60–80	60–80	60–80	60–80	60–80
Cool-down (min.)	5–10	5–10	5–10	5–10	5–10	5–10	5–10
Frequency	3	3	3	3	4	4	4

A Level

Week	1–2	3–4	5–6	7–8	9–10	11–12	13–14
Warm-up (min.)	5–10	5–10	5–10	5–10	5–10	5–10	5–10
Conditioning bout (mileage)	2.00	2.25	2.50	2.75	3.00	3.25	3.50
Intensity % (target heart rate)	60–80	60–80	60–80	60–80	60–80	60–80	60–80
Cool-down (min.)	5–10	5–10	5–10	5–10	5–10	5–10	5–10
Frequency	3	3	3	4	4	4	4

L Level

Week	1–2	3–4	5–6	7–8	9–10	11–12	13–14
Warm-up (min.)	5–10	5–10	5–10	5–10	5–10	5–10	5–10
Conditioning bout (mileage)	3.00	3.25	3.50	3.70	3.75	4.00	
Intensity % (target heart rate)	60–80	60–80	60–80	60–80	60–80	60–80	60–80
Cool-down (min.)	5–10	5–10	5–10	5–10	5–10	5–10	5–10
Frequency	3	3	4	4	4	4	4

K Level

Week	1–2	3–4	5–6	7–8	9–10	11–12	13–14
Warm-up (min.)	5–10	5–10	5–10	5–10	5–10	5–10	5–10
Conditioning bout (mileage)	3.50	3.75	3.75	4.00	4.00	4.00	4.00
Intensity % (target heart rate)	60–80	60–80	60–80	60–80	60–80	60–80	60–80
Cool-down (min.)	5–10	5–10	5–10	5–10	5–10	5–10	5–10
Frequency	4	4	4	4	5	5	5

S Level

Week	1–2	3–4	5–6	7–8	9–10	11–12	13–14
Warm-up (min.)	5–10	5–10	5–10	5–10	5–10	5–10	5–10
Conditioning bout (mileage)	4.00	4.00	4.00	4.25	4.25	4.50	4.50
Intensity % (target heart rate)	60–80	60–80	60–80	60–80	60–80	60–80	60–80
Cool-down (min.)	5–10	5–10	5–10	5–10	5–10	5–10	5–10
Frequency	5	5	5	5	5	5	5

W.A.L.K.S. Maintenance Program (for a lifetime of fitness)

Warm-up:	5–10 min.
Conditioning bout:	3–5 miles per workout
Intensity %:	60–80
Cool-down:	5–10 min.
Frequency:	3–5 times per week
Weekly mileage:	9–25 miles

mall workouts can be fun. Walk with a friend, in a group, or by yourself for a change. Dogs make excellent walking companions. For a challenge, try an advanced exercise walking technique such as race walking, power walking, hill walking, or walking a fitness trail. Participate in a volksmarch, a competitive walking event, or join a Hashing Club (described in the "Jogging" section). Water walking (walking in waist-deep water) is popular in many areas; give it a try. Some people enjoy listening to music while exercising in a traffic-free area. Schedule walking meetings with coworkers. Train for a half-marathon (mini); see sample training program in the "Jogging" section. Try *Exercise Across the U.S.A.* (Lab Activity 4-6 on the book's website) for added incentives to keep walking. You won't become stale or bored with exercise if you vary your workouts.

Common Discomforts

As in running, most aches, pains, and injuries from walking occur from overuse. Listen to your body. Don't attempt to work through an injury. It will only aggravate the condition. The two most common walking complaints are shin splints and back-of-the-knee soreness. Refer to Chapter 8 for information about shin splints. Cut back on pace and distance until soreness subsides. Comfortable, well-fitting shoes will help prevent blisters. Consult a sports podiatrist if you suffer from foot problems such as calluses, bunions, heel spurs, ingrown toenails, high arches, flat feet, and an overly pronated foot. These conditions can be remedied but, if not corrected, may prevent you from fully enjoying your walking program.

INDOOR EXERCISE EQUIPMENT

(Including Stationary Bikes, Steppers, Treadmills, Ski Machines, Rowing Machines, and Elliptical Trainers)

Advantages/Disadvantages

When winter's plummeting temperatures, ice, snow, and chilly winds make outdoor exercise difficult, indoor exercise equipment may be for you. If it is too rainy, too hot, too dark, or unsafe to exercise outside, you can work out in the relative comfort and safety of a health club or your home. Indoor exercise equipment allows you to alternate indoor and outdoor workouts according to the weather, your schedule, and your mood.

Indoor workouts can be done on either your equipment at home or equipment in a health club. If you like working out with others, don't want to deal with equipment maintenance, and enjoy a variety of different types of exercise, a health club is a good place to start. At a club, you can try different types of equipment—bicycles, steppers, treadmills, skiers, rowers, and elliptical trainers—and see what you like best. If you can't seem to make time to get to the health club, with exercise equipment at home you don't have to go anywhere. You can exercise before or after work, be with your family, and read or watch TV at the same time. If you have children, you can keep an eye on them and won't have to hire a baby-sitter while you work out. The main advantage to working out at home is the convenience.

Disadvantages of home exercise equipment are that you have to decide what type of equipment and features you want, purchase it, make room for it in your house, perform your own maintenance, and find someone to repair it (or fix it yourself) if it breaks. You probably will be working out alone and may get bored with the same workout day after day. Also, if your enthusiasm wanes, the equipment may become a constant reminder of failed resolutions. However, working out in private is very appealing to many people. You know who used the equipment last, and for what you pay for a 1-year club membership, you can have your own equipment at home.

Advantages of working out at a health club include that you can switch from one type of equipment to another to avoid boredom or work different muscle groups; you can meet a lot of people; professionals are readily available to answer your questions; you don't have to buy, maintain, and repair the equipment; and you don't have to make space at home for it year-round.

Disadvantages of working out at a health club include that you will have to pay membership fees, schedule it in your day, have transportation, and at popular workout times possibly wait to get on some equipment.

What to Wear

You are working out inside, and so any comfortable workout gear will be fine; a T-shirt and shorts, supportive shoes, a water bottle, and a towel to wipe off sweat and you are ready to go.

Equipment

Equipment comes in two main types: aerobic and strength machines. Strength training information is covered in Chapter 6. This section will focus on aerobic equipment. Equipment ranges in price from a couple of hundred to several thousand dollars, depending on quality and options desired, but indoor exercise equipment need not be expensive. A jump rope, an exercise mat, elastic resistance bands, a step or a slide mat, and an aerobics video are low-budget. More costly exercise machines include steppers, cross-country ski simulators, climbers, treadmills, exercise bicycles, rowers, and elliptical trainers.

If you would like to work out at home and are not familiar with the variety of equipment available, join a health club for a 1- to 3-month trial period to try out and compare the different types. Then you will know what type of equipment you want to purchase and will be more familiar with the features available. Do not, however, expect a $200 home unit to function like a $2,000 health club model. Shop informed. Ask friends and family about equipment and features they like.

Be choosy. Avoid cheap equipment, which may be flimsy, noisy, unstable, or jerky and can make the whole workout experience so unpleasant that you'll soon use the machine as a coat rack. Shop for well-designed exercise equipment from a specialty retailer rather than from a TV infomercial or chain department store. The quality and durability will be worth the cost in terms of ease of use and maintenance. Think compact. Unless you have a lot of space, you probably will not want equipment that takes up a whole room. Steppers and exercise bicycles have the smallest "footprint" and are easily moved to the side when not being used. Think simple. Not much can go wrong with a jump rope, but plenty can go wrong with a flimsy treadmill. The more complicated a piece of equipment is to use and adjust, the more maintenance it needs. Many devices have timers, heart rate monitors, and ergometers that calculate your work output in calories.

Before you invest in home exercise equipment, try out several models and ask these questions:

1. How much will I use this? Do I enjoy this type of exercise?
2. Does the sales staff ask about my needs and fitness goals before helping me select equipment rather than automatically recommending the most expensive machine?

3. Does it have the features I want?
4. Is it easy to assemble?
5. If it breaks, how will I get it repaired? Can it be fixed locally?
6. What kind of warranty comes with it? What is the store's return policy?
7. Is it well-constructed of steel or alloy to last 10 or more years?
8. What kind of maintenance is needed, according to the manual?
9. Are the seats and grips comfortable, durable, and easily adjustable?
10. Does it work smoothly? How stable is it? Is it relatively quiet? Is it safe?
11. Where will I put it? How much space does it require?
12. Does the manual show how to use the equipment correctly and how to reach my target heart rate?
13. Do I need all the fancy gadgets, or will a more simple model do?
14. Can I get a workout with this machine that is intense enough for my current and future fitness levels?

Stationary Bikes

Advantages/Disadvantages

Most models work the lower body—primarily legs, hips, and buttocks—but some models have handlebars for exercising arms and shoulders. Some of the more expensive electronic models have programmed workouts such as interval training or hills to add variety. Upright models make efficient use of space, and you can read or watch TV as you exercise. They give you a good nonimpact workout that is easier on the joints than treadmills are. They are particularly good for overweight people who need to avoid extra stress on the back, knees, and ankles. Both upright and recumbent models are effective. Recumbent bikes, in which you sit back on a seat and pedal in front of the body, tend to be more expensive and need at least 6 to 7 feet of space but are easier on the back. Bicycle trainers, which put your regular bicycle on a stand with resistance to the rear wheel, require balance but are less expensive than stationary bicycles. Another model, popularized by Health Rider, does not involve pedaling; rather, you push on both pedals simultaneously as you pull on handlebars, exercising both upper and lower body muscles.

How to Select

A good machine is easy to adjust, moves smoothly, and feels stable. The seat should be comfortable and should adjust to your height. In many models, handlebars are also adjustable. The controls should be within easy reach, and the workload should adjust smoothly and easily. Look for a smooth, quiet ride; a sturdy frame; a wide, comfortable, adjustable seat; and an easy-to-read instrument panel. Cheaper models are made of flimsier metal; the resistance mechanism may be grabby, the seat less comfortable, and the whole device more "tippy."

Technique and Safety Tips

Proper seat height and pedaling cadence are the keys to avoiding knee problems. Seat height should be adjusted so that when you sit on the seat, your knee is almost fully extended on the downstroke. Also, keep the resistance moderate so that you maintain a cadence of about 60 to 100 rpm. Racers cycle at 80 to 100 rpm.

Steppers

Advantages/Disadvantages

Steppers primarily work the legs, hips, and buttocks and do not work the upper body. They take relatively little space and allow you to read or watch TV as you exercise. They may aggravate some knee problems. They tend to work the calves more than other types of equipment do.

How to Select

Steppers come with either dependent or independent pedals. With dependent pedals, as one goes down, the other goes up. The machine does some of the work for you because you are exercising one foot at a time. Independent pedal models, in which both feet have to be working at the same time, take a little more work to get the rhythm and coordination but give you a better workout. Hydraulic resistance mechanisms provide a fluid feel at an affordable price. High-end models have computerized interval resistance programs that can increase and decrease the workload through the exercise bout. Self-leveling pedals are a nice feature. Make sure pedals are big enough for you to balance on them comfortably. Some also come with poles for working the arms. Less expensive models are manually adjustable, so if you want to change resistance in the middle of a workout, you will have to get off and turn knobs or slide levers. They still give you a good workout, however, and so the lower price may be worth the minor inconvenience.

Technique and Safety Tips

Rest your hands lightly on the handlebars or railings for balance and take small steps at first. Stand tall and gradually begin to take deeper steps after you warm up. Do not lean on the railings or you will decrease the effectiveness of the workout.

Treadmills

Advantages/Disadvantages

Treadmills are popular and easy to use, giving you a good cardiovascular and lower body workout. They also tend to be used more than other types of equipment. However, they are noisy and more prone to breakdowns than other types of equipment. They also require a large space, about 6 by 4 feet, though you can purchase models that fold for storage. See Lab Activity 4-3 for sample workouts.

How to Select

✔ A motorized treadmill should have at least a 1.5-horsepower continuous-duty motor to be strong enough to maintain even speed. Two horsepower is even better.

✔ It should have a running belt that is at least 20 to 24 inches wide and a length of at least 48 inches.

✔ Look for a machine that will reach a top speed of at least 9 miles per hour. Even if you don't walk/run at this speed, higher speeds are useful for interval training.

✔ Ability to simulate at least a 10 percent incline is important for you to always be able to reach your target pulse.

✔ Look for a safety lock so a child cannot accidentally start the treadmill and an emergency shut-off button to cut power immediately.

✔ You need at least one handrail, preferably two for balance, and wide footrails. Also look for a wide two-ply rubber belt for durability on the running surface and some flexibility so that it gives a little with each stride.

Decide if you want a motorized or hand-crank incline and what other computerized features you desire, such as heart rate or calorie counting. Less expensive machines tend to have a shorter, narrower bed; lower horsepower; a faster starting speed; a lower top speed; a less durable one-ply belt; and fewer computerized features. They are also noisier, wear out faster, and may not keep the belt speed as consistent as the higher-end models do.

Nonmotorized treadmills are cheaper but move only with the pull of your feet on the belt, and they slow down if you do. They are better for walking than for running and may be harder on the joints than motorized treadmills, which move continuously at a preset speed.

Investigate the warranty Ask what's covered in the agreement, including parts and labor; who will service the treadmill; and length of coverage (average is 3 years).

Technique and Safety Tips

Start the machine at a slow pace. Straddle the belt, step with one foot a few times to get a feel for the speed, and then begin. Increase to normal speed as you warm up. Keep near the front of the belt at all times.

Ski Machines

Advantages/Disadvantages

Ski simulators can work both upper and lower body muscles and give you a smooth, nonimpact workout.

They do require a lot of space, up to 9 by 3 feet, but some models fold for storage when not in use. They are not suitable for people with balance problems that lead to dizziness or difficulty coordinating movements when standing. You can listen to music or watch TV, but you cannot read while you ski. Ski machines require practice to master the coordination but reward the effort with an excellent workout.

How to Select

Ski machines come in two basic types. One type, popularized by NordicTrack, has skilike rails onto which you place your feet. The rails glide back and forth on a track, and your hands alternately pull a cable. The other type has small platforms that slide back and forth on a track, and your hands usually pull on poles rather than cables. Cables are usually better than poles because they exercise your arms through a fuller range of motion, giving the muscles a better workout.

Like steppers, ski machines come in independent and dependent pedal models. Dependent pedal models are connected so that as one foot slides backward, the other automatically comes forward, producing a stiff-legged gait. Independent pedal models require more learning, but the gait is more natural. The muscles in both legs have to work with each stride, and you get a fuller workout. Look for skis that move smoothly, have a base long enough for your stride, and offer adjustable leg and arm resistance.

Technique and Safety Tips

Be forewarned that with a skier it may take several weeks to master the coordination, and they are not for anyone who has balance problems.

Rowing Machines

Advantages/Disadvantages

Rowers provide an excellent upper as well as lower body workout, toning the shoulders, back, arms, and legs. They do, however, require a lot of space, up to 8 feet by 3 feet. They can also be noisy, and you cannot read while working out.

How to Select

They come in piston and flywheel models. The piston models are cheaper and more compact, but flywheel models have smoother action. Some models give strokes per minute, total distance, time, and power output per stroke.

Technique and Safety Tips

Correct rowing technique takes practice to master and is important for avoiding back injury. Do not lean into the pull but keep upright throughout the range of motion.

Your legs, arms, and shoulders, not your back, should do much of the work, and your arms should move forward before you bend your knees. With a flywheel model, pull the bar into your abdomen, not your chin. The workout can be intense.

Elliptical Trainers

Advantages/Disadvantages

This machine simulates a combination of walking, running, and stair climbing in one motion. The workout is weight-bearing, but there is none of the jarring impact that occurs when you are exercising on pavement, a track, or a treadmill. The motion is even smoother than that of step machines. Physical therapists and athletic trainers love these machines because they allow athletes to continue their training regimen even while rehabilitating an overuse injury, such as Achilles tendinitis, runner's knee, shin splints, and even stress fractures. Elliptical trainers offer the same cardiorespiratory endurance and muscular benefits of running as well as providing refuge from Mother Nature's wrath and the dangers of traffic dodging.

Like all exercise machines, elliptical trainers have some drawbacks, though they are minimal. Because the muscles do not have to adjust for landing on the ground with each stride as they do with actual running, the overall muscle action (and thus, the overall workout), is not quite as intense on an elliptical trainer. The estimated

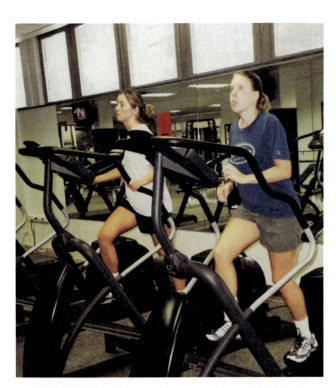

You will burn more calories if you let go of the handrails of treadmills and elliptical trainers and swing your arms.

overall workout benefit on an elliptical trainer is anywhere from 75 to 90 percent of that of a running workout. Ellipticals require minimal use of the arms and shoulders, and so they do not offer a total body workout. Elliptical trainers with armpole attachments reduce this drawback.

Ellipticals tend to be rather large machines, so they do not offer the mobility and storability offered by some other indoor exercise machines. Cost may be a drawback unless you can comfortably afford the $300 to $3,000 (health club model) price tag. Keep in mind that you get what you pay for.

How to Select

The elliptical trainer you select should have tension control that allows you to adjust and vary the resistance against the running ramps. The ramp elevation option on some machines is nice but not essential. You can get the same effect by running faster and/or adjusting the ramp resistance control to a higher tension setting. You may select a machine with arm poles similar to those on cross-country ski machines, thus allowing you to use them for an upper body workout. These are nice but not essential.

Experts recommend selecting a machine that has a read-out screen that shows information such as calories burned, time and distance run, and strides per minute.

A final piece of advice if you plan on buying an elliptical trainer: Try out a number of models before making a final decision.

Technique and Safety Tips

When you exercise on an elliptical trainer, you stand on two platforms, or ramps, "suspended" between wheel-gear and roller mechanisms. When you move your legs in a running motion, one ramp moves forward and slightly upward while the other ramp moves backward and slightly downward. You will leave your arms free (as in running) or hold on to the hand railing on the side of the machine.

Stand upright. Elliptical trainers can put pressure on the lower back if you lean forward or lean on the handrails while exercising. If you feel low back discomfort during or after the workout, check your posture. Feet that are too far apart can cause the hips to shift excessively, putting strain on the lumbar region. To stabilize, bring your feet closer together on the pedals.

How to Begin and Progress

Consult the owner's manual for guidelines specific to your exercise equipment regarding how to begin and progress. In general, treadmills and stationary bikes have the quickest learning curves, steppers run third, and ski machines and rowers require more balance and skill. However, for the time invested in the latter two, you can get a better upper body workout along with aerobic fitness, and so the time is well spent. Also, the rule of specificity applies, so if you are in great running shape but begin working out on a stepper or cycle, give yourself some time to build up to the same level of intensity and duration. If you are a beginner, start with 5 to 10 minutes, low intensity, 3 days the first week to get a feel for correct mechanics and how to use the equipment. Increase the workout by a couple of minutes each week. Pace your progress according to how you feel during and after the workout. If you feel tired and washed out, you are trying to progress too quickly and need to move back or maintain the same level until your endurance increases. If you feel good, you can continue to add a couple of minutes a week to each workout until you reach 20 to 30 minutes of continuous activity. To increase frequency, add an additional day each month until you are exercising up to 5 days a week at your target pulse. A suggested workout schedule follows:

Sample Beginning Program

Week	1–2	3–4	5–6	7–8	9–10	11–15
Warm-up (min.)	5–10	5–10	5–10	5–10	5–10	5–10
Conditioning bout (min.)	5–10	8–14	12–18	17–22	21–26	25–30
Intensity (target heart rate)	50–60	60–80	60–80	60–80	60–80	60–80
Cool-down (min.)	5–10	5–10	5–10	5–10	5–10	5–10
Frequency	3	3	3	3–4	3–4	3–5

IN-LINE SKATING

Advantages/Disadvantages

Modern skating has gone in-line. Instead of four wheels situated in box formation under the skate, the new skating gear has four urethane wheels positioned down the center of a supportive boot complete with brake pads. Skaters also need protective pads and a helmet to lower injury risk, which can be substantial.

Ice hockey players in Minnesota designed the first prototype for today's in-line skates. They enjoyed their dryland workouts so much that they began skating out of season for fun! The popularity of in-line skating exploded in the 1990s primarily because it is so easy to learn and convenient. People are no longer intimidated by the misconception that only the supercoordinated can skate on a single row of wheels.

In-line skating can be a competitive sport involving speed or fancy tricks, known as freestyle skating. Other sports, such as basketball and hockey, can be played on in-line skates, and skiers may cross train on in-line skates in the off-season. But the majority of in-line skaters do

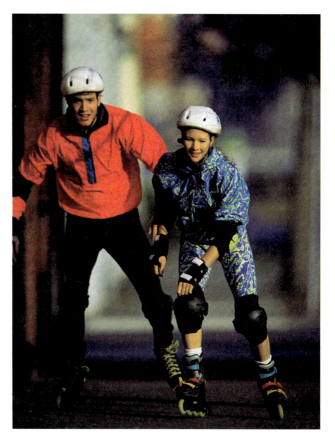

Wear protective gear every time you skate.

it primarily for fitness, recreational, social, or transportation purposes. Thirty-five percent of in-line skaters report using skates as a mode of transportation.

In-line skating has excellent potential for developing physical fitness, especially cardiorespiratory endurance and muscular endurance, plus it is invigoratingly fun. Vigorous and continuous striding can burn as many calories as jogging or cycling does. Skating is one of the best activities for improving balance and is ideal for cross training for any fitness activity. Serious skating increases muscular strength and endurance. It strengthens the musculature in the entire upper leg, including the hamstrings and quadriceps as well as the buttocks, hips, and lower back muscles. If you swing and pump the arms vigorously during skating, the biceps, triceps, and shoulder muscles can be strengthened and toned.

In-line skaters reap all the benefits of other forms of exercise: improved physical fitness; increased energy levels; lower blood pressure; weight control; relaxation; and a reduced risk of cancer, heart disease, and stroke. Physiological responses measured during in-line skating indicate that individuals with average fitness levels can achieve the appropriate exercise training effect on flat terrain, although the highly fit may need to skate uphill or skate fast to achieve the same benefit.

In-line skating does have a few drawbacks. This fun, aerobic, low-impact sport can be dangerous to skaters who don't wear helmets and protective pads or who do not learn safe starting and stopping techniques. If you have a fear of falling, suffer from osteoporosis, or have balance problems, in-line skating is not a good exercise choice. Another disadvantage with in-line skating is cost. In-line skates and the necessary safety gear can be expensive.

What to Wear

You can in-line skate in almost any kind of weather if you dress appropriately. Dress in layers when it's cool (removing outer garments as you warm up) and wear as little as decently possible when it's hot. You will be most comfortable skating in stretchy or loose-fitting clothes. The Lycra clothing worn by many runners is perfect. T-shirts are fine, and so are tights and bike shorts. Jeans are not usually comfortable and will bunch up under the knee pads or over the boot.

In-line skates are available in a spectrum of prices and styles. Before buying a pair, rent several types to see which one suits you. Talk to knowledgeable salespeople; tell them about your skating activity and the type of skating you are planning to do. The cost of a good pair of skates ranges from $100 to $400 or more. Add another $50 to $200 for the protective gear. To try on skates, bring a pair of absorbent socks that you plan to wear while skating. A sock that helps "wick" sweat away from the foot and aids in preventing blisters is a good choice. When you rent or buy your first pair of in-line skates, be sure to get a properly fitted helmet; knee and elbow pads; and wrist guards, specially designed gloves with extra padding at the palms. Treat protective gear like your seat belt; wear it every time you skate.

Necessary Gear

✔ *Skates:* Good in-line skates are not cheap. Expect to pay $100 to $400. The rule to follow is to buy the best possible skates you can afford. Originally, the skate boot was made from molded polyurethane, a lightweight but extremely sturdy material. But since 1994, the soft-boot in-line design skate boot has been the industry standard. The new boot fits like a hiking boot instead of a plastic ski boot. The fit should not be too tight or too loose. It should be flexible from the ankle up. It should allow some room for the toes (about one-fourth inch from the end of the longest toe to the end of the boot). In-line boots use laces, buckles, Velcro straps, or a combination of laces and buckles to tighten and secure the boot. The most effective and popular style is a boot that laces on the lower part and buckles on the ankle

for maximum support. Boots with vents to allow liberal air circulation are recommended. A foam liner, either built into the skate or an insert purchased separately, provides added comfort and helps prevent blisters. Look for liners with vents to aid breathability.

✔ *Helmet:* Select a helmet that provides a snug, comfortable fit. Look for approval by the two national helmet testing bodies, SNELL and ANSI.

✔ *Wrist guards:* This is a fingerless glove with a hard plastic splint running down the front. The plastic is curved slightly—not enough to hinder wrist and hand movement but enough to act as a shock absorber in the event of a fall.

✔ *Knee and elbow pads:* These are designed to prevent scrapes and bruises. Use only the style that has a hard plastic shield over the pad. Do not use cloth-covered pads from other sports, such as volleyball.

Technique and Safety Tips

Taking a few in-line skating lessons and studying an instructional video are the recommended methods for learning this sport. It is imperative to practice the following basic skills before you take to the street or trails: ready position, forward fall, forward stride and glide, basic turning, braking, and making emergency stops. Find a conveniently located paved area where you can go often to practice. It must be smooth and level with enough room to move about unobstructed. Empty parking lots and unused ball courts are ideal if they are free of pedestrians, debris, and bike traffic. Avoid hills until your skills are proficient. See Table 4-6 for some safety guidelines you need to follow.

TABLE 4-6	*Safety Guidelines for In-Line Skating*

1. Always wear full protective gear.
2. Achieve a basic skating level before taking to the road. Practice basic skills on a smooth, flat surface away from traffic.
3. Stay alert and courteous at all times.
4. Always skate under control.
5. Skate on the right side of paths, trails, and sidewalks.
6. Overtake pedestrians, cyclists, and other skaters on the left. Announce your intentions by saying, "Passing on your left."
7. Avoid water, oil, or debris on the trail and uneven, broken pavement.
8. Obey all traffic regulations.
9. Avoid areas with heavy automotive traffic.
10. Always yield to pedestrians.
11. Keep your gear in proper working order.

Skate Maintenance

In-line skates are relatively low-maintenance; that is one of the inviting aspects of the sport. You can put on your skates and get a good workout without much set-up or clean-up time. However, your skates will need occasional attention.

Tools   It's a good idea to put together a skate repair kit that can be carried in your skate bag. Be sure to choose components and tools that fit your particular model of skate. Your local skate shop can help you with the selection of components and tools.

Wheel Rotation or Replacement   The most common maintenance activity is rotation of the wheels. Wheels wear down while skating; therefore, to get maximum mileage, proper rotation is necessary. Rotation is changing the position of the wheels on the frame and turning the wheels over so the inside edges become the outside edges. To rotate your wheels, follow these directions:

Wheel in Position	Move to Position
1	3
2	4
3	1
4	2

Bearing Replacement   Bearings allow the wheels to spin smoothly and have the largest effect on the performance of the skate. Buy the best bearings you can afford. Each skate has two sets of bearings, one on each side of the wheel. ABEC bearings range from 1 to 7, with 1 creating the least amount of speed and 7 the greatest amount of speed. Fitness/recreation skaters usually use ABEC 3 bearings.

Brake Replacement   Brakes should be replaced when you have to lift your toe too high to be stable when stopping or when the bolt holding the brake in place begins to rub the ground. Loosen the bolt, remove the brake, and attach the new brake.

How to Begin and Progress

First, assess your fitness level by using the 1.5-mile timed run test described in Chapter 3. Remember that your current fitness level does not indicate your potential. Based on your fitness category, begin at the appropriate starting level. Progress through each level, one step at a time. Do not skip steps, and stay on each as long as necessary to adapt to that workload. Remember to monitor your pulse, and do not exceed your target heart rate range. Or, if you prefer, use the RPE to monitor your intensity level during the workout. Keep in mind the FITT prescription factors. Don't forget to warm up and cool down during each workout. To develop balanced fitness add 25 to 30 push-ups, 1 minute of abdominal curls, and 5 to 15 minutes of stretching per workout.

In-Line Skating Program	
Fitness Category	Starting Level
Low	1 or 2
Fair	3
Average	4
Good	5
Superior	6
Level	Skating
1	10–15 min.
2	10–20 min.
3	15–25 min.
4	20–40 min.
5	30–45 min.
6	45–75 min.

Variety

Adding variety to your skating workouts can keep you enthused about the sport for many years. Varying your skating routes gives you a change of scenery. Drive the car to a new area, park, and explore the area. Find new trails, paths, sidewalks, and parking lots on which to skate. Use your skates for transportation to and from school or work several days a week. Keep your skates in the trunk of the car and strap them on for a spontaneous workout when you see an opportunity (e.g., at lunchtime). Be sociable; skate with a friend or join a skating club. Pack a backpack with a water bottle and a snack for a longer than usual workout. Try speed skating, amateur racing, or freestyle or artistic skating, which is similar to ice figure skating. Extreme skating involves tricks, jumps, and ramps that might appeal to you. You won't become bored with exercise if you vary your workouts.

Common Discomforts

Each year more than 100,000 people are treated in hospital emergency rooms for in-line skating injuries. In-line skaters can reach speeds of 50 miles per hour or more, yet two-thirds do not wear protective clothing. Spontaneous loss of balance, falling due to debris or an irregularity on the skating surface, colliding with a fellow skater, and striking a stationary hazard, such as a tree, are the most common causes of falls by in-line skaters, studies show. Blisters, strains, sprains, and many other general complaints are addressed in Chapter 8.

Falling is the biggest concern when skating, and so you won't be surprised to learn that the number one injury site is the wrist. One-fourth of all skating injuries are injuries to the wrist, and over 40 percent of all these injuries result in fractures. "Skitching" can be deadly and should never be attempted. This is a popular activity in which a skater hooks on to a motor vehicle and attempts to hang on while coasting behind or beside the vehicle.

The U.S. Consumer Product Safety Commission (CPSC) and the International In-line Skating Association (IISA) recommend that a helmet, elbow and knee pads, and wrist guards with fingerless gloves be worn while skating to reduce the risk and severity of injuries, especially those involving the wrist.

JOGGING

Advantages/Disadvantages

Running is a simple way to develop cardiorespiratory endurance. You can do it alone, with a partner, or with a group. A good pair of running shoes is the only equipment you need. Finding a place to run is as simple as walking out your front door. Getting a full workout through running takes less time than do many other aerobic activities. It can be done in most types of weather, on vacation, or during a lunch break. As a weight-bearing exercise, jogging provides stress to the long bones, which aids in the maintenance of bone mineralization and decreases the risk of osteoporosis. Like other aerobic activities, jogging has positive benefits in terms of reducing obesity, stress, type 2 diabetes, and several heart disease risk factors.

Drawbacks to running include traffic, uneven pavement, and, occasionally, an aggressive dog. Trying to

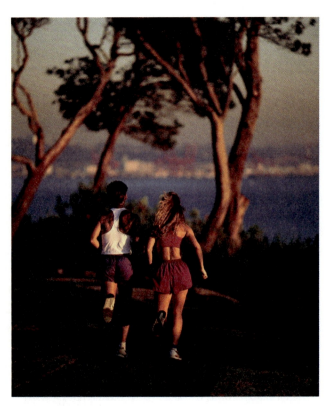

Vary your jogging workouts to avoid becoming bored and stale.

progress too quickly may cause impact problems such as shin splints and sore knees. Jogging is not for everyone. For individuals prone to musculoskeletal problems, low- or nonimpact activities such as bicycling and water exercise are less likely to precipitate injury. If you are overweight or out of shape, it may be best to start with a less intense activity, such as walking. Nonetheless, a carefully planned program of progressive activity enables many people to enjoy running as part of a fitness program.

What to Wear

You can run in almost any kind of weather if you dress appropriately. On hot days, wear as little as decently possible—shoes, socks, shirt, and shorts. For cooler weather, add layers: a long-sleeved T-shirt and tights or long pants. In cold weather, add a jacket or a turtleneck sweater and, to protect the ears and hands, a stocking cap and mittens. In wet weather, wear a cap with a brim to keep rain out of your eyes and rain-repellent clothing, if desired. Keep in mind that when you are running, you generate a great deal of body heat. When you are warmed up, it will feel about 20 degrees warmer than the actual temperature. A hot day would be 70 degrees or higher, a warm day 50 to 60 degrees, a cool day 30 to 40 degrees, and a cold day below freezing. High humidity on hot days and the wind-chill factor on cold days also should be considered (see Chapter 7).

A good pair of properly fitted running shoes is important in preventing injuries. When running, your foot strikes the ground with an impact of approximately three times your body weight. A well-made running shoe fitted by a trained salesperson can absorb shock and support the foot. A cheap pair of poor-quality shoes is no bargain if it leaves you with blisters or shin splints.

Technique and Safety Tips

Good running form is relaxed and mechanically efficient. Your energy goes into moving yourself forward and is not dissipated in extraneous movements. Maintain a relaxed, erect posture, head up, eyes looking ahead. Keep your shoulders relaxed and level, arms swinging freely from the shoulders, and hands unclenched, traveling between the hips and lower chest. Avoid hunching forward, your eyes watching your feet, your arms held stiffly or swinging across the midline of your body. Knees and feet should aim ahead, not to the center or side. Foot contact should be heel to ball or midfoot, not on the toes like a sprinter. Keep your stride length comfortable and effortless, with your foot landing under your center of gravity. Be careful not to overstride or bounce when you run. Stride length is a product of speed and leg strength. Unless you increase one of these elements, attempts to increase your stride length will waste energy. Breathe through your mouth and nose. It is hard to get enough air breathing through the nose alone.

While you are working on your running form, there are some safety guidelines you need to keep in mind:

1. *Before leaving home, let someone know your route and when you expect to return.* Carry identification.
2. *If you wear a headset, keep the volume low* enough so that you can hear approaching traffic.
3. *Keep alert.*
4. *If there is a sidewalk, jog on it.*
5. *If there is no sidewalk, run facing traffic on the extreme left edge or shoulder of the road.*
6. *Respect private property.* Do not run across lawns.
7. *Obey traffic signs and signals.* When crossing a street at the light, cross with the green light only.
8. *Maintain eye contact with motorists* whenever you cross in front of them.
9. *Give the right-of-way to cars.* Don't antagonize drivers even if they try your patience.
10. *If you run at night, wear light-colored clothing with reflective strips.*
11. *At night, do not run in unfamiliar areas.*
12. *Do not wear a vinyl sweat suit* while exercising, ever!

How to Begin and Progress

Begin at the level indicated by your cardiorespiratory fitness assessment (Chapter 3) and progress slowly. If you cannot complete a mile in 15 minutes, begin with walking briskly 15 to 30 minutes until your heart rate stays within the target range. When you can comfortably handle 2 miles in 30 minutes, you may begin the run/walk program. As in all activities, follow the FITT guidelines.

Run/Walk Program

Fitness Category	Starting Level
Low	1, 2, or 3
Fair	4
Average	5 or 6
Good	7 or 8
Superior	9 or 10

Level	Run	Walk	Repeats
1	–	15–20 min.	1
2	–	20–30 min.	1
3	30 sec.	30 sec.	8–12 plus 10- to 15-min. walk
4	1 min.	30 sec.	6–10 plus 10-min. walk
5	2 min.	30 sec.	4–10 plus 5- to 10-min. walk
6	4 min.	1 min.	4–6
7	6 min.	1 min.	4–5
8	8 min.	1–2 min.	3–4
9	12 min.	2 min.	2
10	20–30 min.	5 min.	1
11	up to 60 min.	–	1

Start at the level appropriate for your fitness category. Remember that your starting level does not indicate your potential. For each run/walk interval, begin with the lowest number of repeats indicated, and with each successive workout, add one repeat. When you can do the maximum number of intervals at one level, move to the next level. A 5-minute warm-up and 5-minute cool-down should accompany each workout. You may stay at one level as long as you need to or even move back a step if the beginning level is too difficult. If the workout has been appropriate, you should feel refreshed and relaxed, not exhausted, after exercise.

Variety

Much of the variety in running comes from running different routes and observing the changing scenery and seasons. If you run alone, you may wish to run occasionally with a partner or a group. Instead of taking a long run at a continuous pace, you might try *fartlek*, a Swedish term for *speed-play*. Fartlek mixes fast-paced runs, brief all-out sprints, and slow-paced recovery intervals. It is best done on uneven or hilly terrain such as a park or golf course. Interval training done once or no more than twice a week can add a change of pace. This alternates a fast-paced run over a predetermined distance with walking or a slow recovery jog. An example might be running 220 yards four to six times in 40 to 50 seconds with a 220-yard walk after each run. With interval training, you may vary the distance run, recovery interval, number of repetitions, and time or pace of the run. These workouts are usually done on the track but can be done on the road by running and then walking a set amount of time, running a certain number of telephone pole intervals, or selecting a long hill on your route and running up it several times. A fitness trail, or parcour, with exercise stations linked by a running trail, may be available at a local park or university, or you can make your own. To simulate a parcour on a regular running route, stop every 2 to 4 minutes to do a stretching or toning exercise (e.g., hamstring stretch, run 2 minutes, calf stretch, run 3 minutes, push-ups, run 3 minutes, abdominal curls, . . .).

Some activities are suitable for a small group. You can take a tennis or foam ball along to toss among some friends. You'll get quite a workout because this mixes sprinting and upper body exercise into the run. This is safer if your route has little traffic. Hashing is a popular club sport in the southern United States, Europe, and Russia. The idea is for a group to follow a marked course through an unfamiliar area. Elected group members meet at an earlier time to mark the route, usually with flour. Orienteering is popular in some areas. This is a cross-country type of activity in which participants navigate from point to point, using a map and compass, covering distances from 2 to 10 miles. Local fun-runs give you a chance to run with and meet other runners in a noncompetitive atmosphere. If you like competition, you can get information on road races from your local running club or athletic shoe store.

Common Discomforts

Most aches and pains in running do not occur suddenly. They are often from overuse—a long steady erosion that wears down the body. Many general complaints are addressed in Chapter 8. Specific to running, two additional discomforts, easily avoided, occasionally occur. If you run with shoes that are too short or don't fit well, in addition to developing blisters you could injure a toe. The toenail may turn black and possibly fall off. While painful, the condition is not permanent. The nail will grow back. If your thighs rub together when you run, you may suffer an abrasion. The solution is to apply petroleum jelly to the area and wear tights or shorts that cover your thighs.

WATER EXERCISE/AQUA AEROBICS

Advantages/Disadvantages

You don't have to know how to swim to get a vigorous workout in the water. You don't even have to get your head wet! As more people are discovering, exercising against water resistance in shallow water is a fine workout and great fun, especially with a group. Water exercise can be a social activity because you can carry on a conversation while working out. It is low-impact, and so joint problems are rare. The supportive effect of water buoyancy makes water exercise enjoyable and relaxing for individuals who have concerns about other forms of exercise. In chest-deep water, a person weighs only about a tenth of what he or she does on land. People who have arthritis or joint problems find that this buoyancy decreases stress to the joints, allowing a fuller range of motion than is possible on land. It is easy to individualize intensity levels so that you get a good workout, whatever your level of fitness.

Water has at least 12 times the resistance of air, and that number increases as movement speed increases. Thus, muscular conditioning improves, and in a time-efficient program as well. For example, biceps and triceps can be overloaded concentrically during the same exercise.

Hydrostatic (water) pressure pushes against the chest and body. This helps strengthen the breathing system and makes breathing on land easier. Hydrostatic pressure aids venous circulation and contributes to reduction in edema (swelling), which is especially helpful for expectant moms.

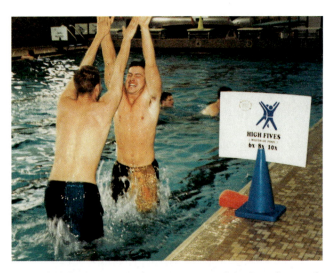

Nonswimming water workouts are one of the best forms of exercise because they build muscular strength and endurance as well as cardiorespiratory endurance. The faster you move, the harder your muscles work.

Water currents constantly challenge the trunk core muscles to maintain proper alignment when starting, stopping, and changing direction in the water. The abs have to work the entire time—a great plus.

Inclement weather is not a problem. Water exercise is cool even on the hottest summer days, and so heat stress is eliminated. It is also a comfortable indoor workout for rainy or cold winter days. If you are overweight and sensitive about exercising in public, the water covers you up so that you don't feel so self-conscious. Water exercise is also beneficial during pregnancy because of both decreased joint stress and decreased heat stress compared with other forms of exercise.

The drawbacks are few. You need access to a pool at a time when you can have a lane separate from lap swimmers. It is probably best to first join a class to learn the exercises and activities. Then you can work out on your own.

What to Wear

A comfortable swimsuit is all that is required. Some people also like to wear pool shoes to protect their feet when doing water running and walking workouts.

Technique and Safety Tips

Workouts may have a muscle toning emphasis or an aerobic emphasis or combine the two. In constructing workouts, maintain muscle balance by exercising all major muscle groups. Particularly emphasize stretching tight muscle groups (e.g., lower back, hamstrings, calves) and toning weak areas (e.g., abdominals, upper body). To overload, keep in mind that as in weight training, water adds resistance. The harder you push and pull, the more resistance you create and the more benefit you receive. In any activity, limit back hyperextension by keeping the abdominals firm while exercises are being performed. In the water, as on land, workouts must maintain a training heart rate for 20 to 30 minutes to produce aerobic benefit. Training heart rates for swimmers appear to be about 10 percent lower than those for land exercisers. This may also be true for other cardiorespiratory water exercise. To calculate an appropriate exercise intensity for water exercise, subtract 10 percent from your training pulse on land. Jogging in the water, aqua aerobics, and other vigorous activities can provide aerobic benefit if an adequate overload occurs. Several books that give examples of water exercises are available and are listed at the end of this chapter.

Whenever you exercise in the water, a few safety guidelines must be followed:

1. *Never work out in the water alone.* A lifeguard or workout partner, preferably one who can swim, should be present. Safety equipment, such as a life ring or a reaching pole, should also be available.
2. *Shower before entering the pool.*
3. *Do not go into the deep water unless you can swim.*
4. *Don't mix water and electricity.* If you like to exercise to music, keep electrical equipment away from the water and make sure that all electric outlets have ground-fault circuit interrupters that shut off the electricity if it contacts water. Better yet, use battery-powered equipment.
5. *Do not enter the pool if you have an open sore, infection, or rash.*
6. *Do all exercises through a full range of motion with slow, controlled movements.* Swinging or flinging movements can injure joints.
7. *Maintain good body alignment in walking and jogging.* Keep abdominals tight and hips tucked under and avoid excessive forward lean.

How to Begin and Progress

Water exercise workouts, like other aerobic programs, should incorporate a warm-up, conditioning period, and cool-down. The warm-up may be started on deck or in the water and may include a musculoskeletal (thermal) warm-up, stretching, and cardiorespiratory warm-up, transitioning smoothly into the conditioning bout. A thermal warm-up includes controlled movements using a gradually increasing range of motion and is designed to increase muscle temperature gradually. Prestretching exercises are designed to prepare muscles for activity and are generally held 5 to 10 seconds. A cardiorespiratory warm-up follows to transition the heart, lungs, and muscles gradually to an increased intensity level. Water exercise may involve many different activities—aerobic, muscle toning, and stretching. Recommendations on how to progress are given for the aerobic portion of the workout (e.g., water running) in terms of length of time at a training heart rate. Test your fitness by using the 500-yard water run test described in Chapter 3. Then follow the appropriate Water Exercise Program. Stay on each level as long as necessary; don't skip levels. Go back a level if the next feels too strenuous. Progress slowly, listen to your body, and follow the FITT factors. Monitor your THR or use the RPE.

Follow the conditioning bout with a 5- to 10-minute cool-down combining a period of gradually decreasing intensity exercise with stretching for flexibility.

Water Exercise Program

Fitness Category	Starting Level
Low	1
Fair	2
Average	3
Good	4
Superior	5 or 6

Level	Vigorous	Easy	Sets	Total Time
1	1 min.	30 secs.	8–12	10–18 mins.
2	2 mins.	30 secs.	6–8	15–20 mins.
3	4 mins.	30 secs.	4–6	18–27 mins.
4	6 mins.	30 secs.	3–4	19–26 mins.
5	8–10 mins.	1 min.	3	26–32 mins.
6	Continuous		1	30 mins. or more

Variety

Exercise with friends or with music. After mastering the exercises with only water resistance, you may wish to add kickboards, pull buoys, or other water exercise equipment to increase resistance. Vary the exercises and activities so that you don't do the same workout 2 days in a row. For example, an aerobic workout may involve, on different days, running or walking widths, aqua aerobics, step aerobics, water games, deep water running, treading and kicking drills, or circuit training. There are so many different things to do in the water that it is easy to add variety. Some examples of different types of workouts follow.

Muscular strength and endurance are built by performing repeats of exercises against resistance: side leg swings to tone inner thigh and outer hip, straight arm raises to tone deltoids, back leg swings to strengthen hamstrings and gluteus. A series of 8 to 12 exercises covering all major muscle groups can be performed for 1 minute each and repeated two to three times for a thorough muscular workout.

Water walking involves walking in waist- to chest-deep water fast enough to produce a target heart rate. Good body alignment during walking and jogging is important. Walk tall with abdominals pulled in and buttocks tucked in to avoid leaning forward. It is also essential, for muscle balance, to vary the walking movements. Variations include walking forward, backward, or

GUIDELINES FOR DEEP WATER JOGGING

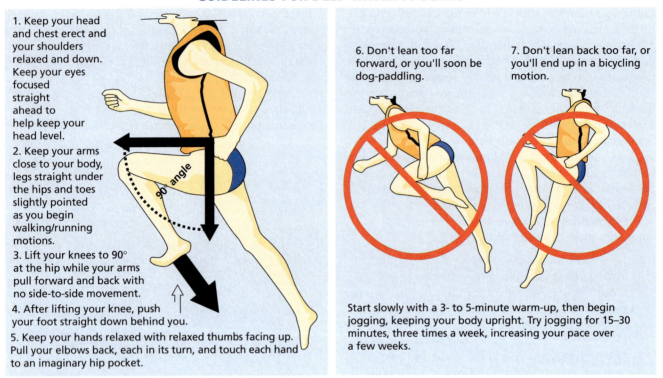

1. Keep your head and chest erect and your shoulders relaxed and down. Keep your eyes focused straight ahead to help keep your head level.

2. Keep your arms close to your body, legs straight under the hips and toes slightly pointed as you begin walking/running motions.

3. Lift your knees to 90° at the hip while your arms pull forward and back with no side-to-side movement.

4. After lifting your knee, push your foot straight down behind you.

5. Keep your hands relaxed with relaxed thumbs facing up. Pull your elbows back, each in its turn, and touch each hand to an imaginary hip pocket.

6. Don't lean too far forward, or you'll soon be dog-paddling.

7. Don't lean back too far, or you'll end up in a bicycling motion.

Start slowly with a 3- to 5-minute warm-up, then begin jogging, keeping your body upright. Try jogging for 15–30 minutes, three times a week, increasing your pace over a few weeks.

sideways and adding different arm variations, such as forward pulls, breaststroke, and backstroke.

Shallow water jogging is similar to water walking but is more intense, using a faster, bounding stride. A common error is running too much on the balls of the feet, which causes calf tightness. Try to press your heel to the pool bottom before pushing off on your toes.

Deep water jogging is a nonimpact workout. Exercisers may wear a flotation vest or belt and run, varying directions and arm movements. Deep water jogging without a flotation belt is strenuous. See the Guidelines for Deep Water Jogging above.

Interval training alternates high- and low-intensity workout segments. This can allow even the most athletic exerciser to get a vigorous workout. For example, you might alternate four laps of shallow water running with two laps of water walking.

Water aerobics, like land aerobics, puts exercise to music. Workouts may be choreographed or freestyle. Bench step workouts have also made the transition into the aquatic environment, with benefits similar to those in land workouts.

Plyometrics are vigorous jumping and bounding exercises that increase muscle strength and power. They are also aerobic. Examples include high jumps in place, bounding across the pool, and a series of high 2-foot hops. Because these are impact exercises, they can cause injury, are only for well-conditioned exercisers, and should be avoided if you have ankle, knee, or back problems. Water buoyancy lessens the risk of injury.

In circuit training, a series of exercises is performed for a certain number of repetitions or a given amount of time (e.g., 1 minute each of side leg circles, jumping jacks, push-ups, forward kicks). Exercises may be written on numbered cards placed around the pool edge, and as each exercise is completed, participants move quickly to the next exercise station. Exercises may stress one fitness component or several. A set of 8 to 12 exercises can be repeated, or time at each station can be increased to produce overload.

Flexibility exercises are often used as a part of a water exercise program. A static stretch is held 20 to 30 seconds or more for each major muscle group to increase range of motion. Occasionally, it is fun to try a water game for variety. Examples include shallow water polo, inner-tube water polo, water baseball, freeze tag, sharks and minnows, water basketball, and volleyball.

Common Discomforts

The most common discomforts water exercisers encounter are tight calves and blisters from running barefoot on the pool bottom. Blisters can be avoided by starting with only a few minutes of running in the pool and giving the feet time to toughen as you gradually progress in workouts. You could also wear pool shoes or clean sneakers during workouts. Calves tend to get tight because, due to buoyancy, most running and walking in the pool is done on the ball of the foot. Take care to stretch calves before and after the workout.

Frequently Asked Questions

Q. What is the Pilates Method of body conditioning?

A. The Pilates (pronounced puh-LAH-teez) Method was developed in the 1920s by physical trainer Joseph H. Pilates for rehabilitation for dancers. It is an exercise system that isolates and strengthens muscles without joint stress and without building bulk. It is a system of controlled exercises aimed at stretching and strengthening muscles of the back, buttocks, and abdomen for improved posture, better balance, relief of aches/pains, and increased flexibility. Pilates designed more than 500 specific exercises using five major pieces of unique apparatus. Instead of performing many repetitions of each exercise, more precise movements requiring proper control and form are used. All Pilates movements must generate from the "powerhouse" or the "core" (the abdomen, lower back, and buttocks). It can be tough on your back. Today's Pilates classes primarily use mat work, but classes featuring Pilates machines, which magnify resistance by using springs and pulleys, are also available.

   Conditioning sessions are done one to one with certified instructors or in closely supervised small groups. Instructors complete a rigorous certification program including extensive apprenticeship hours.

   It is not generally as meditative or focused on stress reduction as is yoga or Tai Chi. See General Resources for video information.

Q. Are yoga and Tai Chi really considered exercise?

A. Absolutely. In addition to enhancing balance, flexibility, and strength, these ancient disciplines can improve mood and provide some cardiovascular benefit. For example, an Australian study found that Tai Chi reduces heart rate, blood pressure, and stress hormones as effectively as brisk walking does. Yoga can decrease blood pressure; although traditional versions typically do not supply much aerobic benefit, newer "power yoga" classes incorporate standard yoga poses into a strenuous session that works both the heart and the lungs.

Q. How much benefit do I get from a sport like golf?

A. To get much benefit from golf, you will have to abandon the cart, since the major exercise is in the walking. In a Finnish study, middle-aged former golfers resumed their game, without carts, two to three times per week. After 5 months, they had increased their aerobic performance and endurance, raised their "good" HDL-cholesterol level, and lost an average of 3 pounds and nearly an inch from their waistlines.

Q. My hands swell when I'm fitness walking. Is this a problem? It feels funny and I don't like it.

A. Swelling in your hands is normal. When you swing your arms, the blood rushes down into your hands. It isn't harmful but it can be uncomfortable, especially if you wear rings. It's a good idea to take them off before you walk. To improve venous blood flow back to the heart and minimize swelling, keep your elbows bent at a 90-degree angle as you swing your arms. See "Correct Walking Form" in this chapter. You can also try squeezing your hands into fists from time to time as you walk. This helps push blood back from the fingers to the heart.

Q. During the winter and at other times when the weather is bad, I work out in the fitness gym. How can I avoid picking up a cold, flu, and other germs from the equipment?

A. These five simple tips can help you stay healthy at the gym all year long:
   • Keep your hands clean. After touching weights and machine hand rails, keep your hands away from your eyes, nose, ears, and mouth until you can wash them.
   • Take two towels, one for yourself and one to wipe down the machines and mats before you use them.
   • Cover up. The less skin-to-equipment contact you have, the better. Keep cuts clean and bandaged. Wear flip-flops in the shower.
   • Use your own mat in classes like yoga, etc.
   • Launder workout clothes after every workout.

Q. My fitness level has plateaued. What can I do to jump-start it?

A. To keep improving, change a variable in the FITT prescription every 4 to 6 weeks.
   • **F**requency: If you exercise three times a week and aren't seeing improvement, try adding another day.
   • **I**ntensity: Slowly increase your speed or incline when using cardio machines.
   • **T**ime: Add 10 percent to each workout, or add 5 minutes to each workout, or make one weekly workout twice as long.
   • **T**ype: Try a different cardio machine or take a class to add interest to your continuous, rhythmic exercise; add resistance training to your exercise program.

Q. What are the most common mistakes made by individuals who engage in aerobic exercise?

A. Here are the top 10 common mistakes made by individuals who engage in aerobic exercise:
   1. Rely upon "muscle burn" as an accurate indicator of exercise intensity. Your heart's response to the demands of exercise is not related to how much your muscles "burn" during physical activity. For a training effect to occur, individuals must exercise within their training heart rate zone. It is okay to use your perception of effort (i.e., rating of perceived exertion, or RPE).

2. Mistake neuromuscular difficulty as a meaningful barometer of training intensity. Even though individuals may find it relatively difficult to perform whatever combination of limb and trunk movements are involved in a particular activity (e.g., exercising on a cross-country skiing machine), it does not necessarily mean that they are achieving the desired training effect.

3. Work out at an inappropriate level of intensity. Getting the most out of your aerobic exercise efforts requires that you exercise within the appropriate training zone.

4. Engage in activities that place too much stress on the lower extremities. Some aerobic activities involve a greater degree of impact forces on the lower body of the exerciser than others do. Also, some individuals can withstand greater loads on their lower extremities than others. It is critical that you select your aerobic exercise modality wisely.

5. Worry more about the exercise clothes on their bodies than the footwear on their feet. The most important personal wear item of significant consequence while exercising is proper footwear.

6. Lean on the exercise machine while working out. Many individuals compromise the safety and quality of their aerobic workouts by excessively leaning on the handrails of whatever aerobic equipment they are using while exercising (e.g., treadmills, ellipticals, cross-trainers, or stair climbers).

7. Fail to warm up before exercising.

8. Fail to cool down after exercising.

9. Fail to get enough rest. Even though you may feel passionate about exercising, you need to give your body adequate rest from working out to provide it with the opportunity to recover from the physical demands you have placed upon it.

10. Rely upon aerobic exercise gimmicks marketed on television and the Internet. Geared to individuals who are wishfully looking for a quick, easy, and painless way to achieve the innumerable benefits of proper exercise, most of these items look too good to be true, and they are.

Q. My friends and I want to join a health club. What are some tips so we don't get ripped off?

A. Follow these seven tips on how to select a health club:

- Ask friends and family about local clubs, equipment, and advantages and disadvantages.
- Visit several clubs at times you would be going, such as after work, to see how crowded they are. Check out the bathrooms, locker room, pool, and weight room. All should be clean and well maintained. Equipment should be in good repair. Talk to the regulars to see how they judge it. See that it has the features and types of equipment you want to use.
- Professionals should be available to show you how to use the equipment correctly for the most effective workout and to avoid injury. Ask about instructor qualifications. Certification by a professional group demonstrates a commitment to quality instruction. Many national certifying organizations certify instructors in different activities. Some of these are the American College of Sports Medicine, YMCA, YWCA, International Dance-Exercise Association, Aerobics and Fitness Association of America, and National Strength and Conditioning Association.
- Look for a health club with at least 3 years of continuous operation. Call the local Better Business Bureau or your state or local consumer protection agency to check if any negative reports have been filed. Ask to see evidence of bonding from the club (this protects you if the club goes out of business).
- Membership fees are negotiable, so no matter what is printed on the brochure, negotiate!
- Start with a short-term membership. Only 10 percent of members are still working out after 3 months, so either pay on a monthly basis or sign up for a 3-month trial membership.
- Read the contract carefully before signing, making sure it covers everything you have discussed with the club employees. If you change your mind, most states have a 3-day cooling-off period during which you can void the contract and get a full refund.

Summary

Cardiorespiratory endurance is perhaps the most important component of health-related fitness. It is measured by VO_{2max}, your body's maximal ability to transport and utilize oxygen during exercise. VO_{2max} can be increased by training, and decreases with inactivity or aging. It is often measured in field tests such as the 1.5-mile run or 1-mile walk. Benefits of long-term cardiorespiratory fitness training include improvements in exercise capacity, exercise recovery, muscular fitness, weight management, cognitive function, and psychological well-being. Regular exercise also reduces risk of chronic diseases such as cardiovascular disease, high blood pressure, type 2 diabetes, and certain types of cancer. The FITT prescription factors for cardiorespiratory fitness can be applied to many different activities to produce high-level fitness. Intensity of exercise, measured by heart rate, is a key factor in developing cardiorespiratory endurance. The Karvonen equation can be used to determine an adequate target heart rate range to produce cardiorespiratory benefits in many fitness activities.

The exercise time requirements needed for health, weight management, and fitness are outlined in this chapter. How to use a pedometer to accumulate 10,000 steps is discussed.

The eight fitness activities in this chapter include aerobic dance, bicycling, fitness swimming, fitness walking, indoor exercise equipment, in-line skating, jogging, and water exercise/aqua aerobics. In each activity unit you found valuable information concerning taking part in the activity. Now you have the necessary tools to begin a program of aerobic activity—one you will enjoy and pursue for a lifetime. You will also have the satisfaction of knowing you are nurturing the most important habit you can adopt to safeguard your health. The ball is in your court. Select an activity and go to it. We wish you well.

General Resources

Collage Video Specialists, 5390 Main St. N.E., Dept. 1, Minneapolis, MN 55421, (800) 433-6769 (Pilates, yoga, Tai Chi)

Creative Instructors Aerobics Educational Videos, 2314 Naudain St., Philadelphia, PA 19146, (215) 790-9767 or (800) 435-0055

Dynamix Music Service, 733 W. 40th St., Suite 10, Baltimore, MD 21211, (800) 843-6499

IDEA Resource Library: Aqua Exercise, IDEA: The Association for Fitness Professionals, 6190 Cornerstone Court E., Suite 204, San Diego, CA 92121-3773

Muscle Mixes, P.O. Box 533967, Orlando, FL 32853, (800) 52-MIXES or (407) 872-7576

Optimal Health Clicker (888) 339-2067

Pedometers: Digi-Walker, www.digiwalker.com (888) 748-5377 Accusplit Eagle (800) 935-1996

Power Productions, P.O. Box 550, Gaithersburg, MD 20884-0550, (301) 926-0707 or (800) 777-BEAT (call for a free catalogue)

Powerbelts: Inergi Fitness, Norcross, GA (800) 797-2358

Resources for Walking Equipment: Wrist/hand/ankle weights: any large department and sporting equipment stores

Walking Poles: Exerstrider, Exerstrider Products Inc. Madison, WI (800) 554-0989

Weighted Vests: Smart Vest, Training Zone Concepts, Inc. Flint, MI (888) 797-8378

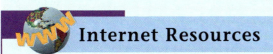

Internet Resources

Aerobics Fitness Association of America
www.afaa.com
Includes "Exercise Gets Personal," an interactive site where you can design a customized exercise program.

American College of Sports Medicine
www.acsm.org (800-846-5643)
Information on sports research, health and fitness, and aerobic exercise guidelines, along with a quarterly fitness newsletter. "Current Comments" gives information on a variety of exercise topics of recent interest.

American Council on Exercise
www.acefitness.org
Features 100 fitness fact sheets, free e-newsletters, and a variety of different fitness activities from bicycling to swimming.

American Heart Association
www.americanheart.org
Health tools include an exercise diary and a body mass calculator. Information includes exercise and fitness promotion for women, children, and seniors; information on how exercise affects heart health; exercise tips; and a health heart workout quiz.

American Volkssport Association
www.ava.org (800-830-9255)
Walking and hiking events sponsored by chapters throughout the United States.

Centers for Disease Control and Prevention
www.cdc.gov
Information on getting started in physical activity, exercise tips, links to other fitness resources, and health promotion for increasing physical activity in your school or community.

The Cooper Institute for Aerobics Research
www.cooperinst.org
Discover the latest fitness news, from aerobics to weight loss.

Digiwalker pedometers
www.digiwalker.com
Information on programs and how to purchase this pedometer.

Health Partners
www.healthpartners.com
Information on the 10,000 Steps movement.

International Dance-Exercise Association (IDEA)
http://www.ideafit.com
Information about certification and equipment.

Marathoning: Listings of marathons, training logs, charts, race results, and other helpful links.

Chicago Marathon Program (designed by Hal Higdon)
www.halhigdon.com/marathon

Galloway Program (designed by Jeff Galloway)
www.jeffgalloway.com

Marathon Guide
www.marathonguide.com

The National Strength and Conditioning Association
www.nsca-Lift.org (800-815-6826)
Information about new strength and conditioning research.

The President's Council on Physical Fitness and Sports
www.fitness.gov/challenge/challenge.html

Information on award programs such as Presidential Active Lifestyle Award (PALA). Site explains how to count steps using a pedometer.

Runner's World
www.runnersworld.com
Search for half-marathon/full-marathon schedules.

Shape Up America
www.shapeup.org
Provides information, programs, and tips on weight management.

Small Step
www.smallstep.gov
A U.S. Department of Health and Human Services website; helps people get started toward a more active and healthy lifestyle. Gives tips on eating healthier and getting more activity.

Bibliography

Armstrong, L., et. al. *ACSM's Guidelines for Exercise Testing and Prescription*, 7th ed., Mitchell H. Whaley, ed. Philadelphia: Lippincott Williams & Wilkings, 2006.

Barnes, D. E., et al. "A Longitudinal Study of Cardiorespiratory Fitness and Cognitive Function in Healthy Older Adults." *Journal of the American Geriatrics Society* 51 (April 2003): 459–465.

Bassett, D. L., Jr., P. L. Schneider, and G. E. Huntington. "Physical Activity in an Old Amish Community." *Medicine and Science in Sports and Exercise* 36, no. 1 (January 2004): 79–86.

Blair, S. N., et al. "Influences of Cardiorespiratory Fitness and Other Precursors on Cardiovascular Disease and All Cause Mortality in Men and Women." *JAMA* 276, no. 3 (July 17, 1996): 205–210.

Borg, G. "Psychophysical Bases of Physical Exertion." *Medicine and Science in Sports and Exercise* 14 (1982): 707.

"CDC Healthy Youth! Physical Activity." www.cdc.gov (August 17, 2005).

Cuddihy, T. F., R. P. Pangrazi, and L. M. Tomson. "Pedometers: Answers to FAQs from Teachers." *Journal of Physical Education, Recreation, and Dance* 76, no. 2 (February 2005): 36–40.

Franklin, B. A., and J. L. Roitman. "Cardiorespiratory Adaptations to Exercise." Roitman, Jeff, ed., *ACSM's Resource Manual for Guidelines for Exercise Testing and Prescription*, 4th ed. Philadelphia: Lippincott Williams & Wilkins, 2001.

Golding, L. A. "Convincing Adults to Exercise." *ACSM's Health & Fitness Journal* 8, no. 6 (November/December 2004): 7–11.

Hultquist, C. N., et al. "Comparison of Walking Recommendations in Previously Inactive Women." *Medicine and Science in Sports and Exercise* 37, no. 4 (April 2005): 676–683.

Karvonen, M., K. Kentala, and O. Mustala. "The Effects of Training on Heart Rate: A Longitudinal Study." *Annals of Medicine and Experimental Biology* 35 (1957): 307–315.

Klein, D. A., L. Burr, and W. J. Stone. "Making Physical Activity Stick: What Can We Learn from Regular Exercisers?" *ACSM's Health & Fitness Journal* 9, no. 4 (January/February).

Le Maurier, G. C. "Walk Which Way?" *ACSM's Health & Fitness Journal* 8, no. 1 (January/February 2004): 7–10.

Loupias, J., and L. Golding. "Deep Water Running: A Conditioning Alternative." *ACSM's Health & Fitness Journal* 8, no. 5 (September/October 2004): 5–8.

Melanson, E., J. R. Knoll, M. L. Bell, et al. "Commercially Available Pedometers: Considerations for Accurate Step Counting." *Preventive Medicine* 39 (2004): 361–368.

Miller, M. C. "Is Exercise a Good Treatment for Depression?" *Harvard Mental Health Letter* 19 (June 2003): 8.

Persinger, R., C. Foster, M. Gibson, et. al. "Consistency of the Talk Test for Exercise Prescription." *Medicine and Science in Sports and Exercise* 36, no. 9 (September 2004): 1632–1636.

"Prevalence of No Leisure-Time Physical Activity–35 States and the District of Columbia 1988–2002." www.jama.ama-assn.org 291, no. 14 (April 14, 2004): 1693–1694.

Rush, S. "Avoiding Exercise Related Fatigue." *ACSM's Health & Fitness Journal* 9, no. 2 (March/April 2005): 30–32.

Schneider, P. L., S. E. Crouter, and D. R. Bassett Jr. "Pedometer Measures of Free-Living Physical Activity: Comparison of 13 Models." *Medicine and Science in Sports and Exercise* 36, no. 2 (2004): 331–335.

Schneider, P. L., S. E. Crouter, O. Lukajic, and D. R. Bassett Jr. "Accuracy and Reliability of 10 Pedometers for Measuring Steps Over a 400-m. Walk." *Medicine and Science in Sports and Exercise* 35, no. 10 (2003): 1748–1779.

Sidman, M. S. "Count Your Steps to Health & Fitness." *ACSM's Health & Fitness Journal* 6, no. 2 (January/February 2002): 13–17.

Sinelnjkov, O., P. Hastie, A. Cole, and D. Schneulle. "Bicycle Safety Sport Education Style." *Journal of Physical Education, Recreation, and Dance* 76, no. 2 (February 2005): 24–29.

Thompson, D. L. "Improving VO2max." *ACSM's Health & Fitness Journal* 9, no. 5 (September/October 2005): 4.

Thompson, D. L. "VO2max: Links to Health and Performance." *ACSM's Health & Fitness Journal* 9, no. 4 (July/August 2005): 5.

Thompson, D. L. "VO2max: The Basics: Part I." *ACSM's Health & Fitness Journal* 9, no. 3 (May/June 2005): 5.

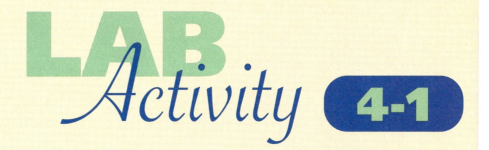

Name _____ **Class/Activity Section** _____ **Date** _____

Calculate Your Target Heart Rate (THR) Range

The target heart rate represents the intensity level at which you should exercise to produce cardiorespiratory benefits. This amount of exercise (overload) is enough to condition the heart, lungs, and muscles but is not overly strenuous. Monitoring intensity during a workout is done by measuring the heart rate. For fitness to occur, your heart rate must be raised to approximately 60 percent of the difference between the resting and maximal heart rates. An increase in heart rate equal to 80 percent of the difference between resting and maximal rates is a reasonable upper intensity level for most exercises. This is the target heart rate range (or training heart range). The Karvonen formula for calculating your target heart rate is as follows:

THR = (maximal HR* − resting HR**) × Intensity % + Resting HR

    *Maximal HR = 220 minus age

    **Resting HR = count your pulse at rest for 60 seconds

When estimating your target heart rate range, two factors are involved:

- Your age: _____ .
- Your resting heart rate (RHR): _____ .

Use these numbers in the formula that follows:

1. 220 − _____ = _____
         your age   (estimated maximal heart rate [MHR])

2. _____ − _____ = _____
     MHR (resting HR) HR reserve

3. _____ ×   0.60   + _____ = _____
    (HR reserve) (lower intensity) (resting HR) (lower target heart rate)

   _____ ×   0.80   + _____ = _____
    (HR reserve) (higher intensity) (resting HR) (higher target heart rate)

4. Target heart rate range is _____ to _____ beats per minute.

5. For a quick pulse check during exercise, my THR ÷ 10 is _____ to _____ beats.

Example: Jeff is 23 years old and has a resting heart rate of 72 beats per minute.

1. 220 − 23 = 197 MHR
2. 197 − 72 = 125 heart rate reserve
3. 125 × .60 = 75 + 72 = 147
   125 × .80 = 100 + 72 = 172
4. THR range is 147 to 172 beats per minute.
5. THR ÷ 10 is 15 to 17 beats.

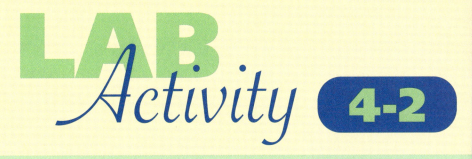

Using a Pedometer: "How Many Steps Do I Take?"

Wear your pedometer for one full "normal" or "typical" week. Put it on first thing in the morning and wear it until you go to bed at night. Before you go to bed, record your steps for that day. Read the section in this chapter about pedometer use and see Table 4-3, "Five Steps to Reach 10,000 Steps a Day." See the "One Mile Equivalent" section in Lab Activity 4-6 on the book's website for additional activities that can count toward your step goal.

1. Week 1: Steps I accumulated each day.

    Day/date _____   Steps = _____

    Day/date _____   Steps = _____

    Day/date _____   Steps = _____

    Day/date _____   Steps = _____

    Day/date _____   Steps = _____

    Day/date _____   Steps = _____

    Day/date _____   Steps = _____

    Total number of steps for Week One is _____

2. Divide by 7. This is your 7-day step average, also known as your **baseline activity level.**

What is your **7-day step average** or **baseline activity level?** _____

Any surprises?_____

_____

3. Weeks 2 and 3:

    • Calculate your **step count goal** using the 10% method. This is the number of steps you wish to add each day beyond your baseline activity level. Example: If your baseline activity level is 6,000 steps, an increase of 10% will be 600 steps (6,000 × .10 = 600). During Weeks 2–3 you would accumulate 6,600 steps per day. To progress, you would plan to add 600 steps every two weeks thereafter. (Example: Weeks 3–4 your goal would be to increase to 7,200 steps; Weeks 5–6 your goal would be to increase to 7,800 steps; Weeks 7–8 your goal would be to increase to 8,400 steps; and so on until you reach your ultimate goal of 10,000 steps or more.)

    What is your personal DAILY STEP COUNT GOAL for Week 2 and Week 3?

    _____ steps. (Your 7-DAY AVERAGE/BASELINE ACTIVITY × .10)

    OR

    • ALTERNATE METHOD: Calculate your personal 7-DAY AVERAGE or BASELINE ACTIVITY LEVEL using the 500-step method. Increase your 7-day average by 500 steps instead of using the 10% method. (Example: If your baseline is 6,000 steps, add 500 steps to set the goal for Weeks 2–3. This would be 6,000 + 500 = 6,500; Weeks 4–5 would be 7,000 steps; Weeks 6–7 would be 7,500; and so on until you reach your ultimate goal of 10,000 steps or more.)

LAB Activity ■ CHAPTER 4

What is your personal DAILY STEP COUNT GOAL FOR Week 2 and Week 3?

_____ steps. (Your 7-DAY AVERAGE/BASELINE + 500)

4. Calculate your personal activity goals using the 10% Method or the 500-Step Method for the next 12 weeks. Your instructor may prefer one method over the other. Use the attached pedometer log to record your daily activity.

   Weeks 2–3: _____ steps per day

   Weeks 4–5: _____ steps per day

   Weeks 6–7: _____ steps per day

   Weeks 8–9: _____ steps per day

   Weeks 10–11: _____ steps per day

   Weeks 12+ _____ steps per day

5. List specific strategies you plan to use in order to work toward your step goals.

PEDOMETER LOG

Name _____

Class/Activity Section _____

	Sunday	Monday	Tuesday	Wednesday	Thursday	Friday	Saturday	Weekly Average
Week of: ____ Goal: ____ Steps = ____ Miles = ____								
Week of: ____ Goal: ____ Steps = ____ Miles = ____								
Week of: ____ Goal: ____ Steps = ____ Miles = ____								
Week of: ____ Goal: ____ Steps = ____ Miles = ____								
Week of: ____ Goal: ____ Steps = ____ Miles = ____								

NOTE: Approximately 2,000 steps = 1 mile
List the specific strategies you use to work toward your step goals:
(make copies as needed)

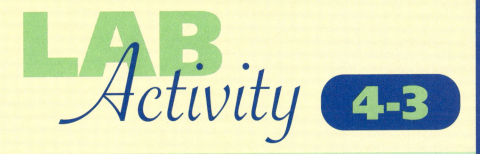

| Name _____ | Class/Activity Section _____ | Date _____ |

30-Minute Treadmill Workouts

Directions: These sample workouts are designed to expend more calories than will walking/jogging at a steady pace. Substitute any of the workouts into your normal exercise program one or two times per week. Note: Adjust your pace as needed.

1. Basic Intervals

Prolonged bursts of speed followed by shorter recovery periods.

Minutes	Speed	
	Jogging	Walk/Jog
0–5 (warm-up)	5.7 mph	3.3 mph
5–7	6.0	3.5
7–9	6.5	4.0
9–11	7.0	4.5
11–12	5.5	3.0
12–14	6.5	4.0
14–16	7.0	4.5
16–18	7.5	5.0
18–19	5.5	3.0
19–21	7.0	4.5
21–23	7.5	5.0
23–25	8.0	5.5
25–30 (cool-down)	5.7	3.3

2. Hills

Keep the same speed throughout the workout (a base pace is 6.0 mph for joggers and 3.5 mph for walkers) while gradually increasing the incline. Midway through the workout, gradually reduce the incline.

Minutes	Incline
0–5 (warm-up)	0.5
5–10	2
10–13	4
13–15	6
15–16	8
16–18	6
18–21	4
21–26	2
26–30 (cool-down)	0.5

3. Speed Ladder

Gradually increase speed until you are near maximum exertion. Note: This workout is intense. Take the pace down if needed.

| | Speed | |
Minutes	Jogging	Walk/Jog
0–5 (warm-up)	5.5 mph	3.4 mph
5–8	7.0	4.2
8–9	6.0	3.5
9–12	7.0	4.2
12–13	6.0	3.5
13–16	7.0	4.2
16–17	6.0	3.5
17–20	7.0	4.2
20–21	6.0	3.5
21–24	7.0	4.5
24–25	6.0	3.5
25–30 (cool-down)	5.7	3.4

4. Which of the three 30-minute workouts did you try? Did you try all three?

5. Which did you find most challenging, most enjoyable, easiest? Explain.

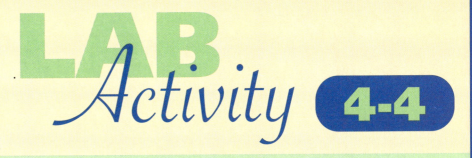

LAB Activity 4-4

Cardiorespiratory Exercise Log Sheet

(MAKE COPIES OF THIS FORM AS NEEDED)

	Week	Sun	Mon	Tues	Wed	Thurs	Fri	Sat	Total
1	Date:	_____	_____	_____	_____	_____	_____	_____	
	RHR:	_____	_____	_____	_____	_____	_____	_____	
	Distance/time/steps:	_____	_____	_____	_____	_____	_____	_____	_____
	Type of activity:	_____	_____	_____	_____	_____	_____	_____	
	EHR:	_____	_____	_____	_____	_____	_____	_____	
	Location:	_____	_____	_____	_____	_____	_____	_____	
2	Date:	_____	_____	_____	_____	_____	_____	_____	
	RHR:	_____	_____	_____	_____	_____	_____	_____	
	Distance/time/steps:	_____	_____	_____	_____	_____	_____	_____	_____
	Type of activity:	_____	_____	_____	_____	_____	_____	_____	
	EHR:	_____	_____	_____	_____	_____	_____	_____	
	Location:	_____	_____	_____	_____	_____	_____	_____	
3	Date:	_____	_____	_____	_____	_____	_____	_____	
	RHR:	_____	_____	_____	_____	_____	_____	_____	
	Distance/time/steps:	_____	_____	_____	_____	_____	_____	_____	_____
	Type of activity:	_____	_____	_____	_____	_____	_____	_____	
	EHR:	_____	_____	_____	_____	_____	_____	_____	
	Location:	_____	_____	_____	_____	_____	_____	_____	
4	Date:	_____	_____	_____	_____	_____	_____	_____	
	RHR:	_____	_____	_____	_____	_____	_____	_____	
	Distance/time/steps:	_____	_____	_____	_____	_____	_____	_____	_____
	Type of activity:	_____	_____	_____	_____	_____	_____	_____	
	EHR:	_____	_____	_____	_____	_____	_____	_____	
	Location:	_____	_____	_____	_____	_____	_____	_____	

Comments/goals:_____

_____

_____

Log Sheet

(MAKE COPIES OF THIS FORM AS NEEDED)

Name ______________________

Week __________ RHR __________ THR __________

Goals: ______________________

____

____

	Date	RHR	Distance/time/steps	HR (at end of workout)	Location	Comments
Sun						
Mon						
Tues						
Wed						
Thur						
Fri						
Sat						

Total __________

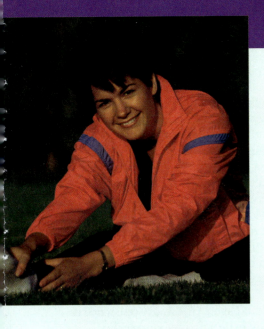

Chapter 5

Developing Flexibility

5

*Blessed are the flexible for they shall not
be bent out of shape.*
—Author unknown

Objectives

After reading this chapter, you will be able to:

1. Identify nine benefits of and five cautions for stretching.
2. Identify factors affecting flexibility.
3. Define two types of flexibility.
4. Identify four types of stretching.
5. Identify guidelines for flexibility development.
6. Define five principles of flexibility development.
7. Perform flexibility exercises for basic fitness.
8. Identify safe exercises from a list of safe and contraindicated exercises.
9. Give general guidelines for identifying exercises that increase risk of injury.
10. Explain how flexibility and muscular fitness contribute to wellness.

Terms

- active stretching
- collagen
- dynamic flexibility
- dynamic stretching
- elastic elongation
- elastin
- golgi tendon organ (GTO)
- inverse stretch reflex
- muscle spindle
- passive stretching
- plastic elongation
- proprioceptive neuromuscular facilitation (PNF)
- reciprocal innervation
- static stretching
- static flexibility
- stretch reflex

A Fit and Well Way of Life Online Learning Center www.mhhe.com/robbinsfitwell1e
Go to the Online Learning Center for chapter quizzes, outlines, flashcards, and additional lab activities.

*F*lexibility, the ability to move the joints through their full range of motion, is an important factor in achieving wellness throughout the life span. It enables us to reach, bend, twist, and perform movements without excessive tightness or stiffness. As children, we are naturally flexible, but as we age, flexibility tends to decrease. Disuse, injury, excessive body fat, and muscle imbalances are common factors associated with loss of range of motion. This chapter covers many aspects of flexibility—its benefits, types, cautions, principles, and guidelines. In addition, it highlights illustrated programs for developing this important component of fitness.

FLEXIBILITY

You can maintain youthful flexibility by incorporating stretching into your regular workouts. The flexibility exercises in this section are grouped as follows: a basic fitness flexibility program with exercises for joggers, walkers, aerobic dancers, cyclists, swimmers, and water exercisers and examples of PNF partner-assisted stretches. Contraindicated exercises, safer substitutes, and general rules for identifying common exercises that put back and joints at increased risk of injury are also discussed.

Benefits of Flexibility

Several benefits can be gained from flexibility development:

✔ *Decreased aches and pains.* Tight, inflexible muscles pull unevenly across joints, causing skeletal misalignment, poor posture, unnecessary fatigue, and muscle and joint pain. Stretching can alleviate these problems.

✔ *Enhanced ability to move freely and easily* and to perform activities such as bending down to tie your shoes, scratching your back, and turning to look back as you are driving.

✔ *Possible decreased risk of injury.* When tight muscles restrict the natural range of motion of a joint, the slightest unusual twist can cause a strain or pull, such as a strained hamstring. Inflexibility also is a precipitating factor in overuse injuries such as tendinitis, because inelastic muscles transfer excessive stress to even less pliable connective tissue.

Some research indicates that the importance of stretching in injury prevention may vary depending on the type of activity to follow. It may

be more important in activities involving vigorous jumping and bouncing (like soccer or basketball) in which the muscle-tendon unit undergoes high-intensity stretch-shortening cycles. It may be less important in activities with limited demands for stretch-shortening cycles (e.g., jogging, walking). While the effects of stretching in injury prevention are controversial and research has generally not shown that stretching before exercise decreases risk of injury, a long-term flexibility program designed to alleviate muscle tightness and imbalance can offer benefits. Excessively tight areas, identified by flexibility assessment, can be corrected and adequate flexibility restored for sports and daily activities. Many rehabilitation professionals would agree that injury resistance is best enhanced by including in your weekly workouts exercises designed to enhance both flexibility and strength as part of a balanced muscular fitness program.

✔ *Recovery from injury.* Athletic trainers and physical therapists commonly utilize stretching in injury rehabilitation programs. Research has shown that gentle stretching in a pain-free range of motion is important in shortening the rehabilitation period after injury. This enables a person to more quickly regain normal range of motion and return to activity.

✔ *Enhanced athletic performance.* In racquetball, golf, tennis, volleyball, and swimming, greater range of motion and ability to apply force through that range of motion can confer a winning edge.

✔ *Reversal of age-related flexibility declines.* We tend to lose flexibility as we age, partly due to age-related changes in connective tissue and muscle, partly due to decreasing levels of activity. A regular stretching program can improve flexibility at any age.

✔ *Improved posture, appearance.* We look and feel better when we carry ourselves tall with shoulders back, chest high, and back straight. Unfortunately, over time, we may tend to "sag into gravity" and develop a "hunched over" appearance with rounded shoulders, forward head, and sagging abdominals. Muscle tightness across the chest, hamstrings, and lower back coupled with weakness of opposing muscles can contribute to and perpetuate poor postural habits. Over time, poor posture tends to worsen and becomes harder to self-correct as muscle imbalances increase. Stretching to correct shortened muscles, along with strengthening the weak opposing muscles, can enhance posture and help a person "stand tall" naturally without continual conscious effort.

✔ *Decreased muscle soreness after exercise.* Research has shown that delayed-onset muscle soreness and stiffness that occur 1–2 days after exercise can be decreased by stretching the affected muscles.

✔ *It feels good.* Stretching reduces muscular tension, promoting relaxation.

Cautions

If carelessly done, stretching may cause injury. You must be careful not to overstretch, particularly when muscles are cold and tight. Stretching is not a competitive activity, so don't try to imitate the most flexible person in your class. Injured areas should be stretched with great care and not into pain, which risks reinjury. If you feel pain during stretching, particularly joint pain, stop!

While less flexible individuals may envy those who can do splits with ease, keep in mind that more flexibility is better only up to a point. There is concern that excessive flexibility, unless accompanied by muscular strength, may overstretch ligaments and tendons and increase joint laxity and susceptibility to injury. For this reason, it is wise to combine stretching with muscle strengthening for optimal fitness benefits.

Factors Affecting Flexibility

Several factors affect joint flexibility. These include joint structure, soft tissues (joint capsule, muscle, tendon), inactivity, muscle temperature, age, genetics, gender, obesity, injury, and neural factors.

Joint Structure

The range of motion of joints varies from one joint to another depending on joint structure, the joint capsule, and connective tissues of the muscle-tendon structures surrounding the joints. Some joints, like fingers or the elbow, are hinged for flexion and extension. Others, like the shoulder, a ball-and-socket joint, are more mobile and permit motion in several planes. The joint capsule is connective tissue that surrounds the joint and gives it stability while controlling mobility. If joint structure alone determined range of motion, stretching would not be effective as this is not amenable to change. However, stretching does affect the range of motion of soft tissues surrounding a joint.

Soft Tissues

Muscles and their fibrous sheaths of connective tissue, ligaments, tendons, and skin surrounding a joint also affect its range of motion. It is estimated that about 47 percent of a joint's total resistance to stretching is contributed by ligaments and the joint structure, about 41 percent from connective tissue, 10 percent from tendons, and 2 percent from skin. Muscle contains **elastin,** elastic fibers, and **collagen,** fibrous connective tissue. Like an elastic band, muscles temporarily lengthen when stretched, then return to their resting length. Most of the resistance to stretching that we feel comes from fibrous connective tissue within and covering muscles. Repeated stretching over time increases the ability of a muscle to be lengthened with less resistance.

Inactivity

Physically active individuals tend to be more flexible than sedentary individuals. Perhaps the most common cause of low flexibility is a sedentary lifestyle. With disuse, the body adapts to a limited range of motion. Muscles and connective tissue become less pliable, shorten and weaken, leaving a person more susceptible to injury.

Muscle Temperature

Stretching is easier and more comfortable if muscles have been warmed up first by large-muscle activity such as walking or light calisthenics. When muscles are cold, they are stiffer and more resistant to stretching. As muscle temperature increases, connective tissue becomes softer and resistance to stretching decreases by as much as 20 percent. Heat with stretching relaxes collagen fibers and allows increased elongation. Stretching alone does not warm up muscles. For this reason, increasing deep muscle temperature by adequate warm-up is probably more important in reducing risk of injury in the workout that follows than is stretching alone. Also, stretching during a cool-down may allow muscle collagen to restabilize toward its new increased length, making changes more permanent and longer lasting.

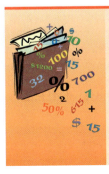

THE NUMBERS

25%	Amount of flexibility lost between the ages of 25 and 50.
70%	Number of adults who do not stretch for flexibility.
30%	Portion of adults who stretch 3 or more days per week.
2–3	Days per week of stretching recommended for good health.

Age

As we grow older, we tend to lose flexibility, related partly to decreasing levels of activity with age and partly to connective tissue changes due to aging. A regular program of stretching can counteract these flexibility declines. Research has shown that range of motion can be improved at any age, even in the 80s and 90s.

Genetics

Some people seem to be naturally more flexible than others, even "double-jointed" (they aren't, really). This may be due to inherited differences in joint structure and elasticity of connective tissue. While you may not be able to change your genetics, you can improve your flexibility within your genetically determined range of motion. People who have never been able to touch their toes may, for example, be able to get inches closer with practice but may never be able to wrap their palms around their feet without bending their knees.

Gender

Females tend to be more flexible than males throughout the life span. This may be due to gender-specific variations in joint structure.

Obesity

Excess body fat in and around joints and muscles can present a mechanical block to full range of motion. The excess tissue acts like a wedge, preventing full joint motion due to tissue approximation. Excessive muscle hypertrophy can likewise impede full joint range of motion.

Injury and Scar Tissue

Injury to muscles and joints results in decreased range of motion initially due to pain and guarding. Flexibility can be lost over time due to decreased use as the injury heals, causing muscles and connective tissue to tighten and weaken. Flexibility is also compromised by the formation of scar tissue, which is weaker and less elastic than the original tissues.

Neural Factors

When a muscle is stretched, **muscle spindles,** stretch receptors within the muscle cells, are stimulated. They sense the amount and speed of stretch, and if a muscle is overstretched or stretched too fast, they activate the stretch reflex to prevent injury. The **stretch reflex** causes the muscle to contract to prevent overstretching the joint.

The **golgi tendon organ (GTO),** another type of receptor located within the muscle tendon, detects the amount of tension in a muscle. When excessive tension is placed on the muscle, the GTO triggers the **inverse stretch reflex,** causing the muscle to relax to prevent injury. GTOs respond after the muscle spindles, and only if a stretch is sustained for 5 seconds or longer. The signal sent by the GTO overrides the signal by the muscle spindles, and causes the muscle to relax, underlining the effectiveness of sustained stretching. Muscle spindles and GTOs have opposite effects and both monitor and maintain the muscle-tendon unit in a safe range of motion.

Another neural factor affecting muscle is **reciprocal innervation.** Muscles work in pairs, and when one muscle contracts, through reciprocal innervation, its opposing muscle relaxes to permit movement. For example, during a biceps curl, the triceps relaxes to permit the biceps to shorten. This effect is incorporated into some stretching programs by consciously contracting a muscle to produce relaxation and increased range of motion in the opposing muscle group.

Types of Flexibility

There are two basic types of flexibility: static and dynamic. **Static flexibility** refers to the range of motion that can be achieved through a slow, controlled stretch. **Dynamic flexibility** is the range of motion achieved by quickly moving a limb to its limits.

Static stretching techniques are those in which you slowly stretch a muscle to the point of tension and hold, such as in holding a sitting hamstring stretch. The stretching force is provided by gravity or the force of one limb pulling on another. When a muscle is stretched and held at a constant length, after a period of time there is a gradual loss of tension and muscle lengthening. Static stretching is the most commonly used type of stretching. It does not activate the stretch reflex and is associated with limited muscle soreness. It does not increase muscle temperature, so some type of prior warm-up activity is recommended.

Dynamic stretching employs swinging or ballistic moves such as a high forward kick. Dynamic stretching is associated with increased muscle soreness and is not used much in personal fitness programs because of increased risk of injury. Dynamic exercises may be useful in preparation for athletic activities requiring such moves, but they carry increased risk that a muscle or joint could be overstretched, resulting in muscle or tendon tears and joint injury. Also, these exercises may initiate the stretch reflex, which may cause the stretched muscle to contract, limiting flexibility gains. While both types of stretching can increase flexibility, static stretching is preferred in health-related fitness programs because it is highly effective and carries little risk of muscle or joint strain.

Static and dynamic stretching may be performed actively or passively. With **active stretching,** you use your own muscle forces to stretch yourself. For example, you can stretch calves by sitting and pulling the toes back. With **passive stretching,** someone or something else assists with a stretch. The assist could be gravity, body weight, a strap, or leverage: for example, using gravity or a slant board to assist with a calf stretch. You relax the muscle you are trying to stretch and use the external assist to apply force. Both active and passive stretching improve flexibility, but passive stretching is more commonly used.

Guidelines for Flexibility Development

Flexibility exercises are part of a balanced fitness program. The goal is to develop and maintain an adequate range of joint motion for ease of movement in your daily activities. Flexibility gains are proportional to the overload applied: to the frequency, intensity, and time (duration) of stretching.

✔ *Frequency:* Stretch at least 2 to 3 days a week, daily if possible. Greater flexibility is produced by more frequent stretching.
✔ *Intensity:* Low-intensity stretching is best. Progress at your speed. Stretching is not competitive. Flexibility changes from day to day, and on some days you might not be able to stretch as far as you did the day before. Stretch slightly beyond the normal range of motion, to the point of tension, and hold. Do not force a stretch.
✔ *Time:* The ACSM recommends a 10- to 30-second stretch, though holding up to 60 seconds in a cool-down stretch can increase flexibility retention.
✔ *Repetitions:* At least four 10- to 30-second sustained stretches for each muscle group are recommended.

Depending on the number of stretches and length of repetitions, a flexibility session can last 10 to 30 minutes.

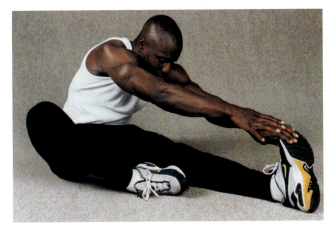

Flexibility gains are greatest during cool-down stretching.

TOP 10 LIST

Tips for Developing Flexibility

Everyone can benefit from flexibility. To maximize the results from the time invested, implement the following guidelines in your next stretching session:

1. *Warm up before stretching.* An increase in muscle temperature produced by fast walking, slow jogging, jumping jacks, or other large muscle exercises will make stretching safer and more productive. You are sufficiently warmed up when you begin to sweat.
2. *After warm-up, use stretching as preparation for activity.* While some feel that stretching during warm-up decreases the risk of injury in the activity that follows, there is no evidence that this is true. Warm-up stretching is different from a planned program of stretching for general flexibility. Warm-up stretching can be limited to what is essential, avoiding overstretching. Stretch the muscle groups used in the activity, hold at the point of tension for 10 seconds, and do not push for flexibility increases. Any gains will be minimal due to the tightening effect of the workout that follows.
3. *Stretch for flexibility during cool-down.* Muscles are warmest and most elastic at this point. Stretching is easier. More permanent changes in muscle lengthening occur with low-force, long-duration stretching if muscles are allowed to cool in a stretched position. Cooling muscles before releasing tension apparently causes muscle collagen (connective tissue), like stretched taffy, to stabilize toward its new stretched length.
4. *Stop at the point of tension, not pain.* Stretching to the point of pain, or until muscles quiver, can risk overstretching injury.
5. *Stretch slowly and evenly,* hold 10 to 30 seconds, and release slowly.
6. *Try to consciously relax* the target muscle as you stretch.
7. *Maintain a regular breathing pattern* as you stretch.
8. *Don't bounce.* A slow sustained stretch is more effective.
9. *Incorporate 8 to 12 stretches into your program.* Flexibility is specific to a joint, and so a well-planned program for general flexibility will contain one stretch for each major muscle group. Warm-up or cool-down stretching may contain fewer exercises because such stretching is activity-specific and has different goals. Pay particular attention to body areas that are least flexible and stretch them more often.
10. *Strive for muscle balance.* When stretching muscles on one side of a joint, stretch those on the other side as well; for example, if you stretch hamstrings, stretch quadriceps too.

Principles of Flexibility Development

Over time, a program of regular stretching can produce beneficial changes in muscle and joint range of motion. To develop an effective stretching program, several principles affecting flexibility development must be considered. These principles include progressive overload, specificity, reversibility, individual differences, and balance.

Progressive Overload

Improvement in joint range of motion can occur when sustained stretching produces elastic and plastic elongation. **Elastic elongation,** the temporary lengthening of soft tissue, occurs when muscle is stretched and returns to its resting length. Connective tissue within and surrounding muscle has both elastic and plastic properties. Longer or more intense stretching can produce **plastic elongation,** a semi-permanent lengthening of tissues. After a stretch is removed, elastic elongation reverses while plastic elongation remains. Plastic elongation is the goal of stretching programs. It is best obtained through static or slow, sustained stretching. The amount of plastic elongation is considered time-dependent and is proportional to the amount of force applied. If tissue is stretched to the point of tension but not pain (which may activate the stretch reflex) and held, the tissue will gradually relax, elongate, and less force will be required to maintain the new length. A prolonged stretch is needed to achieve plastic elongation.

Specificity

Flexibility is specific to a joint; that is, flexibility in one leg does not guarantee flexibility in the other leg, and flexibility in the shoulders does not ensure flexibility in the lower back. It is also specific to joint angles—a person who can do front splits may be less flexible in side splits.

Reversibility

Like any other fitness component, flexibility changes are reversible. If a person stops stretching, over time, range of motion will decrease back to levels sustained by daily activities. Gains from flexibility can be lost in as little as 3–4 weeks without stretching. On the other hand, flexibility can be maintained with stretching as few as 2–3 days per week.

Individual Differences

People vary in their ability to develop flexibility. Variations in proportions of collagen and elastin in muscle tissue, joint structure, length of muscles, and attachment points of tendons on bones may contribute to differences in joint range of motion as well as ability to increase that range. Within your genetic endowment, you do have potential for improvement. A regular stretching program can help you enhance and maintain your flexibility within your genetically determined range.

Balance

We often have muscles that are tighter on one side of the body (right-left or front-back). Pay attention to flexibility differences and work to improve them. Your hamstrings may be tighter on one side than the other. It is common for chest muscles to be tighter than the opposing upper back muscles, and lower back muscles are often tighter than abdominals. Spend more time stretching the tighter areas to alleviate the imbalance.

Flexibility Exercises for Basic Fitness

As part of a warm-up or cool-down, exercises A through F are important for runners, walkers, and aerobic dancers. Cyclists, swimmers, and water exercisers should add upper-body stretches G through I. If time is limited, save stretching for the cool-down. For basic fitness flexibility, perform the full program of exercises in Figure 5-1. Hold each one 10 to 30 seconds and repeat at least four times.

A. Hamstring stretch
   Sit and extend one leg in front, with the other bent and tucked as shown in diagram (a). Keeping shoulders erect, press abdomen forward. Hold. Repeat with other leg.
B. Lower back/hip flexor stretch
   Lie on your back with one leg straight and one bent. With hands behind thigh, press thigh toward chest. Keep extended leg straight. Repeat left.
C. Spinal twist (lower back and hip abductors)
   Sit with right leg extended, step left leg over right, and turn upper body toward left. Repeat on other side.

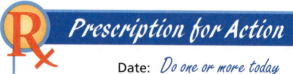

Prescription for Action

Date: *Do one or more today*

✔ While studying or reading the morning paper, sit on the floor and stretch hamstrings.
✔ While on the phone, do calf and quadriceps stretches.
✔ If you have a desk job, take a 5-minute stretch break every hour—do ankle circles, half head rolls, and shoulder stretches.
✔ After every hour of computer use, stretch wrists, back, and shoulders.
✔ While watching TV, stretch during commercials.

Prescribed by: *YOU*

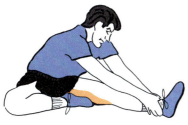

(a) Hamstring stretch

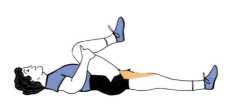

(b) Lower back/hip flexor stretch

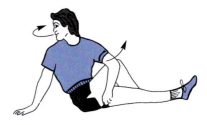

(c) Spinal twist

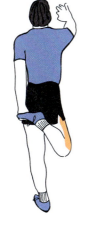

(d) Quadriceps stretch

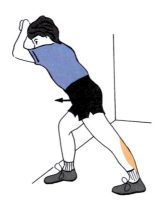

(e) Calf/Achilles stretch

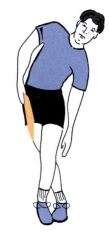

(f) Iliotibial band stretch

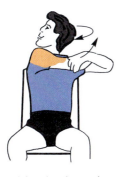

(g) Deltoid stretch

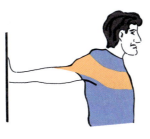

(h) Pectoral stretch

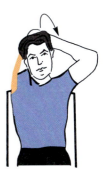

(i) Triceps stretch

FIGURE 5-1   Flexibility exercises.

D. Quadriceps stretch

    Stand with right leg bent at the knee. With left hand, pull right heel toward buttocks. Keep shoulders up, abdominals tight, and hips tucked under to prevent back hyperextension. Omit if you have knee problems.

E. Calf/Achilles stretch

    Standing in forward lunge position, toes pointing forward, press heel toward floor. Repeat with other leg. Bend back knee to stretch soleus.

F. Iliotibial band stretch

    Cross left foot over right, press hips to right. Repeat with other side.

G. Deltoid stretch

    Cross right arm in front of body and pull it in toward midline with left hand.

H. Pectoral stretch

    Place right hand on wall, with elbow extended but not locked. Twist shoulders left. Repeat with left arm.

I. Triceps stretch

    Pull left elbow behind head. Repeat right.

PNF Partner-Assisted Stretches

A type of static stretching called **proprioceptive neuromuscular facilitation (PNF),** a partner-assisted stretch often used by athletic trainers, is highly effective for increasing flexibility. It utilizes the nervous and muscular systems to facilitate stretching. It was developed by Herman Kabat, M.D., and two physical therapists in the 1940s for use on paralysis patients to improve flexibility and strength. PNF utilizes the inverse stretch reflex produced by golgi tendon organs to relax the target muscle and allow a greater stretch. It is thought that when the muscle is first stretched, then contracted, the GTO reflexes are stimulated, relaxing the muscle. To perform a PNF contract-relax stretch, you first perform a 10- to 30-second static stretch, then contract the muscle for 6 seconds to produce fatigue, and then relax while a partner stretches your limb for 10 to 30 seconds. The forced contraction fatigues the muscle and increases the muscle's ability to relax while being stretched.

Another type of PNF stretching called the *contract-relax-agonist contract* inserts a contraction of the opposing muscle group before the final stretch; e.g., in the hamstring stretch (a) below, after contracting hamstrings, the person would contract quadriceps, pulling the leg back as far as possible for about 10 seconds. If the quadriceps is contracted, through reciprocal innervation, the hamstring relaxes even more and can be passively stretched to a greater range of motion. Some research indicates that the contract-relax-agonist contract method is the most effective PNF technique.

Be sensitive to your partner's needs and flexibility levels. Be sure to communicate when more or less resistance or pressure is needed throughout each exercise. Work with the same partner throughout the series. Switching partners can lead to injury because of unfamiliarity with the flexibility limits of the person being stretched. Some examples of PNF stretches are illustrated in Figure 5-2.

A. Hamstring stretch
Lie on your back and lift one leg into the air. Partner supports ankle and knee in a static stretch. Next, keeping knee extended but not locked, push against your partner as he or she resists. Stretch and then relax as partner eases leg into a new stretch.

B. Inner thigh stretch
Sit with knees out and bottoms of feet together. Press down on knees in a static stretch. Next, partner kneels behind and resists on knees as you press them upward. Finally, relax as partner gently presses them toward the floor in a stretch.

C. Gluteal/lower back stretch
Sit cross-legged and stretch forward. Partner kneels behind you with hands on your upper back. Next, resist back against partner. Then stretch forward as partner assists.

D. Pectoral stretch
Sit cross-legged with fingers interlaced behind your head and back, supported by partner's thigh. Partner gently pulls your elbows back for 10 seconds and then resists as you attempt to pull them forward. Next, relax as partner gently stretches them back.

Other Programs for Enhancing Flexibility

Tai Chi and yoga are very old yet newly popular activities that can enhance flexibility and balance as well as reduce stress.

Tai Chi is an ancient Chinese exercise known for its slow, graceful movements. It originated as a self-defense activity but now is used to enhance standing balance, flexibility, lower-body strength, and neuromuscular control. It is a good exercise for people of all ages and can be enjoyed throughout the lifetime.

Yoga, which means to yoke or unite, is another ancient art with several branches, each with its own style. Hatha yoga is the most widely practiced in the United

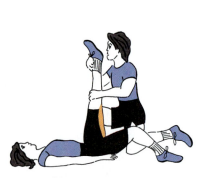
(a) Hamstring stretch

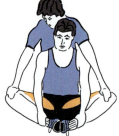
(b) Inner thigh stretch

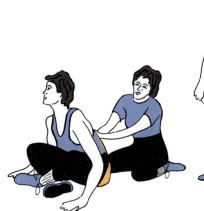
(c) Gluteal/lower back stretch

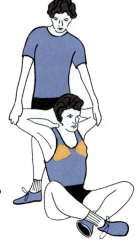
(d) Pectoral stretch

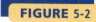 **FIGURE 5-2**   PNF partner-assisted stretches.

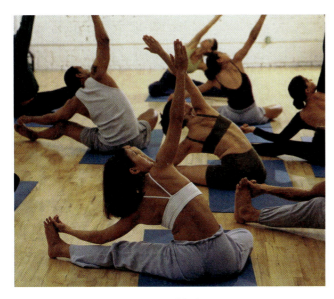

Yoga can improve flexibility and balance.

States. It involves using mental focus and coordinated breathing while assuming a series of physical postures. Some people do yoga to reduce stress, others to improve flexibility and balance. Different forms of yoga may be more vigorous or more relaxing, and so if one type doesn't appeal to you, there are others to investigate.

One way to get started in yoga or Tai Chi is to enroll in a class. Either can be learned at a beginning level in a few weeks of instruction, though mastery may take years. Instructional videotapes are available for home use and can be obtained at a video store. The yoga Sun Salutation, a series of yoga poses, is pictured and described in Lab Activity 5-2 for you to experience.

CONTRAINDICATED EXERCISES

A few stretching and toning exercises added to an aerobic program can promote balanced fitness by increasing flexibility in tight muscles and strengthening weak ones. However, not all conditioning exercises commonly done in classes or seen on videotapes are good for everyone. These potentially harmful exercises are labeled *contraindicated exercises* (Figure 5-3).

By studying people with aches and injuries, fitness experts have learned that some common stretching and toning exercises should be avoided. Others should be modified for safety and effectiveness. Be aware of which commonly done high-risk movements you should avoid and which high-benefit, low-risk exercises you should do instead. Here are some examples:

1. *Yoga plow:* Sometimes done as a back stretch, this exercise can injure discs, ligaments, and nerves in the neck and back. A better back stretch is a single- or double-knee tuck to the chest.

2. *Knee tuck to chest:* Hyperflexing the knee by pulling it to the body with the arms or hands placed on top of the tibia places undue stress on the knee joint. Note: The hand position should be *changed to hug the thigh rather than the shin.*

3. *Head roll:* Hyperextension can injure discs in the neck. Safer neck stretches include half-head rolls to the front, turning the head side to side so that the chin touches the right and left shoulders, and touching an ear to each shoulder.

4. *Hurdler stretch:* This stretch can cause groin pull, injure knee cartilage, and overstretch the medial collateral ligament—the one that helps stabilize the knee. It may also cause hip joint discomfort because the femur of the leg that is tucked behind is in a position of extreme rotation in the joint capsule. The alternative hurdler stretch safely stretches hamstrings.

5. *Full squat:* Excessive flexion or extension of the knee is dangerous. To strengthen the quadriceps, substitute half-knee bends for full squats, the duckwalk, deep lunges, and squat thrusts. Deep knee flexion exercises overstress knee ligaments and cartilage.

6. *Standing toe touch:* This exercise risks the straining of back ligaments. Limit forward flexion in a standing position. As your trunk dips below a 25- to 45-degree angle, the lower back muscles cease to work and the posterior ligaments joining bone to bone must support the load.

7. *Leg stretches at a ballet bar (or other high object):* These may be potentially harmful. When the extended leg is raised 90 degrees or more and the trunk is bent over the leg, it may lead to sciatica problems, especially when the exerciser has limited flexibility. Substitute the back and hamstring stretches suggested in 1, 4, and 6 in Figure 5-3.

8. *Leaning forward and twisting the trunk to the side:* These moves are particularly hazardous to the lower back, adding a shearing force to the stress on back ligaments. Avoid swinging hands and the trunk through the knees, windmill toe touches, waist circles, and elbow-knee lunges. There is no exercise you can do standing to tone your waist. The most effective exercise for reducing the waist is aerobic exercise and sensible nutrition. To tone oblique abdominals, the muscles that underlie the waist area, use twisting bent-knee abdominal curls. Lying on your back with heels close to your buttocks and crossing your arms across your chest (or with a hand touching each shoulder), curl the shoulders first toward the right knee and then toward the left knee.

9. *Double-leg lifts, straight-leg sit-ups, and low leg scissors:* These do little or nothing to tone the abdominals.

Don't	**Do**	**Explanation**

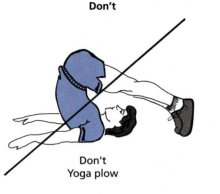

Don't
Yoga plow

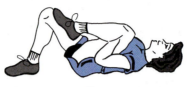

Do
Single-knee tuck to chest

1. *Yoga plow:* Sometimes done as a back stretch, this exercise can injure discs, ligaments, and nerves in the neck and back. A better back stretch is a single- or double-knee tuck to the chest.

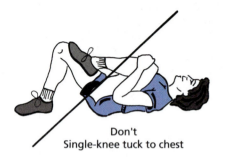

Don't
Single-knee tuck to chest

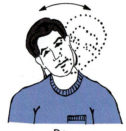

Do
Single-knee tuck to chest
Note: Hug the **thigh**, not the knee.

2. *Knee tuck to chest:* Hyperflexing the knee by pulling it to the body with the arms or hands placed on top of the tibia places undue stress on the knee joint. Note: The hand position should be *changed to hug the thigh rather than the shin.*

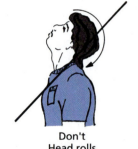

Don't
Head rolls

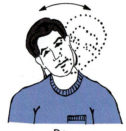

Do
Half-head rolls

3. *Head roll:* Hyperextension can injure discs in the neck. Safer neck stretches include half-head rolls to the front, turning the head side to side so that the chin touches the right and left shoulders, and touching an ear to each shoulder.

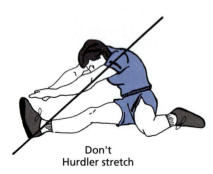

Don't
Hurdler stretch

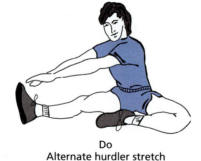

Do
Alternate hurdler stretch

4. *Hurdler stretch:* This stretch can cause groin pull, injure knee cartilage, and overstretch the medial collateral ligament—the one that helps stabilize the knee. It may also cause hip joint discomfort because the femur of the leg that is tucked behind is in a position of extreme rotation in the joint capsule. The alternative hurdler stretch safely stretches hamstrings.

 FIGURE 5-3   Contraindicated exercises.

They tighten hip flexors, which in most people are too tight already, causing lordosis (swayback). They may also cause lower back strain. The most effective exercise for toning abdominals is bent-knee abdominal curls in which the lower back stays on the ground while the shoulders curl forward about 3 inches. To avoid jerking on the head or neck, cross your arms across your chest or behind your head with a hand touching each shoulder.

Don't   **Do**   **Explanation**

Don't
Full squat

Do
Half-knee bend

5. *Full squat:* Excessive flexion or extension of the knee is dangerous. To strengthen the quadriceps, substitute half-knee bends for full squats, the duckwalk, deep lunges, and squat thrusts. Deep knee flexion exercises overstress knee ligaments and cartilage.

Don't
Standing toe touch

Do
Lying hamstring stretch

6. *Standing toe touch:* This exercise risks the straining of back ligaments. Limit forward flexion in a standing position. As your trunk dips below a 25- to 45-degree angle, the lower back muscles cease to work and the posterior ligaments joining bone to bone must support the load.

Don't
Ballet bar leg stretch

Do
Sitting hamstring stretch

7. *Leg stretches at a ballet bar (or other high object):* These may be potentially harmful. When the extended leg is raised 90 degrees or more and the trunk is bent over the leg, it may lead to sciatica problems, especially when the exerciser has limited flexibility.

FIGURE 5-3   Contraindicated exercises.   *(continued)*

10. *The swan arch, prone double-leg raises, and yoga cobra:* These produce excessive back hyperextension and possible back strain. In a prone position, raise your right arm and the opposite leg a few inches off the ground and then switch; this will strengthen the back safely.

11. *Donkey kicks or fire hydrants:* Done on hands and knees with the back hyperextended, these may

strain the lower back. To protect the back, hold your abdominals tight, round your back, and raise your leg no higher than 6 to 12 inches.

Your body is meant to move in many ways—to bend, twist, and stretch. Some people can do high-risk exercises for years with no ill effects. For others, after only a few repetitions, injury occurs. You may not know into which category you fit until it is too late. The problem is that

Don't	Do	Explanation

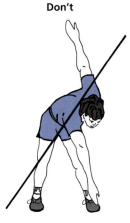

Don't
Windmill toe touches

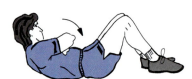

Do
Oblique abdominal curls

8. *Leaning forward and twisting the trunk to the side:* These moves are particularly hazardous to the lower back, adding a shearing force to the stress on back ligaments. Avoid swinging hands and the trunk through the knees, windmill toe touches, waist circles, and elbow-knee lunges. There is no exercise you can do standing to tone your waist. The most effective exercise for reducing the waist is aerobic exercise and sensible nutrition. To tone oblique abdominals, the muscles that underlie the waist area, use twisting bent-knee abdominal curls. Lying on your back with heels close to your buttocks and crossing your arms across your chest (or with a hand touching each shoulder), curl the shoulders first toward the right knee and then toward the left knee.

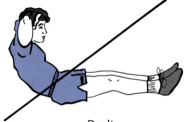

Don't
Straight-leg sit-ups

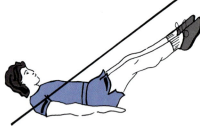

Don't
Double-leg lifts

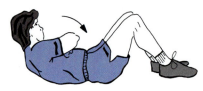

Do
Bent-knee abdominal curls

9. *Double-leg lifts, straight-leg sit-ups, and low leg scissors:* These do little or nothing to tone the abdominals. They tighten hip flexors, which in most people are too tight already, causing lordosis (swayback). They may also cause lower back strain. The most effective exercise for toning abdominals is bent-knee abdominal curls in which the lower back stays on the ground while the shoulders curl forward about 3 inches. To avoid jerking on the head or neck, cross your arms across your chest or behind your head with a hand touching each shoulder.

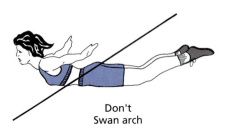

Don't
Swan arch

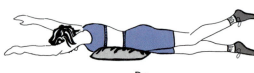

Do
Single arm/leg raises

10. *The swan arch, prone double-leg raises, and yoga cobra:* These produce excessive back hyperextension and possible back strain. In a prone position, raise your right arm and the opposite leg a few inches off the ground and then switch; this will strengthen the back safely.

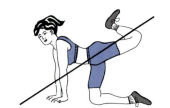

Don't
Donkey kicks

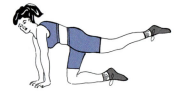

Do
Modified donkey kicks
(can be done with forearms on floor)

11. *Donkey kicks or fire hydrants:* Done on hands and knees with the back hyperextended, these may strain the lower back. To protect the back, hold your abdominals tight, round your back, and raise your leg no higher than 6 to 12 inches.

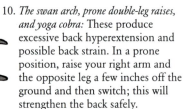

FIGURE 5-3   Contraindicated exercises.   *(continued)*

some movements increase risks to muscles, joints, and connective tissue. While you may need to do deep squats if you are a competitive weightlifter or a yoga plow if you are in a yoga class, these moves don't offer any special benefit for the fitness exerciser. Low-benefit, high-risk exercises should be minimized in programs designed to emphasize personal fitness. Follow these general rules when exercising:

1. Do not hyperflex the knee.
2. Do not hyperextend the knee, neck, or lower back.
3. Do not apply a twisting or lateral force to the knee.
4. Avoid holding your breath during exercise.
5. Avoid stretching long/weak muscles (e.g., abdominals) and avoid shortening already short/strong muscles (e.g., hip flexors). See common muscle imbalances in Table 8-2.
   a. Most people should avoid aggravating common postural faults: forward head, dorsal kyphosis (rounded upper back), medial rotations of the thigh, and pronation of the foot.
   b. Most people need to stretch the chest muscles, hip flexors, calves, hamstrings, lower back, and medial thigh rotators.
6. Avoid stretching any joint to the point of pain.
7. Be especially careful when using passive stretches with another person (unless the person is a physical therapist).
8. Avoid movements that place acute compressional forces on spinal discs, such as extending and rotating the spine simultaneously (e.g., trunk and neck circling and double-leg lifts).
9. Avoid movements that cause joint impingements or cartilage damage, such as arm circles in the palm-down position.
10. If the nature of your sport regularly requires the violation of good mechanics (baseball catcher assuming a deep squat position or gymnast performing double-leg lifts), make certain the muscles are as strong as possible to endure the stress.

Frequently Asked Questions

Q. Is it possible to become too flexible? Is that a problem?

A. It is possible for the muscles and connective tissue surrounding a joint to become too flexible. Joints are constructed to move within a certain range of motion. Excessive motion can damage tendons and ligaments and tear the joint capsule. Once a muscle has been stretched to its maximum length, further stretching will only loosen tendons and ligaments (which you do not want to stretch), which can cause joint instability and increase the risk of injury. There is a trade-off between flexibility and stability. The greater a joint's range of motion is, the less stable the joint is structurally and the more it must rely on the muscles supporting it to control the range of motion. For example, the shoulder has relatively high flexibility compared with the hip, which has greater structural stability. Shoulder dislocation is fairly common; hip dislocation is not. If the muscles and connective tissue become very extensible, there is a measure of safety as long as there is sufficient muscular strength to control the movement. For example, gymnasts are very flexible but also develop strength to control that range of motion. If you wish to develop greater than average flexibility for a sport or physical activity, it is important to strengthen the muscles that you stretch (and vice versa) for balanced fitness.

Q. What are the advantages and disadvantages of stretching with a partner?

A. On the plus side, stretching with a partner adds a social element that makes it more fun. It's a good way to get to know your classmates if you stretch with different people. You can relax while your partner stretches you, and so you may get a better stretch. On the minus side, you and your partner must communicate well to minimize the risk of overstretching and it takes longer than stretching alone. A good compromise is to do a few partner stretches along with individual stretches.

Q. If I am short on time, is it better to stretch before or after exercise?

A. When you stretch before exercise, the muscles tighten up again during the workout. After exercise, the muscles are warmer, more extensible, and stretching is easier. Also, if you stretch muscles during cool-down, the flexibility changes tend to be longer lasting (plastic elongation) than if you stretch before exercise.

Q. How important is stretching in my training program?

A. Research does not conclusively demonstrate that stretching prevents injury. However, we tend to lose flexibility and move more stiffly as we age, and regular stretching prevents this loss. Maintaining youthful flexibility can enhance your ability to perform daily activities, such as turning to look as you are backing up your car. It also enhances performance of athletic activities—making it easier to get a full stride as you run or a full reach in swimming. Being able to apply forces through a full range of motion gives more power to athletic skills.

Summary

Flexibility is an important asset in fitness and daily activities. It enhances the ability to move freely and easily, aids with posture and appearance, helps with recovery from injury, and can reverse joint stiffness and tightness that creeps up over time. Factors that affect flexibility include joint structure, soft tissues, inactivity, muscle temperature, age, genetics, gender, obesity or excessive muscle hypertrophy, injury and scar tissue, and neural factors. Flexibility gains are proportional to the overload applied, to the frequency, intensity, and time of stretching.

While static stretching is recommended for most fitness activities, dynamic stretches may be used for certain athletic activities, and both types may be done either passively or actively. Principles of flexibility development include progressive overload, specificity, reversibility, and balance. A series of stretches for basic fitness as well as PNF partner-assisted stretches were given. Some potentially harmful or contraindicated exercises that put joints at increased risk of injury, and guidelines for identifying them, were also discussed.

Internet Resources

American College of Sports Medicine
www.acsm.org
Information on sports research, health and fitness, aerobic exercise guidelines, and a quarterly fitness newsletter. "Current Comments" gives information on a variety of exercise topics of recent interest.

International Fitness Association
www.ifafitness.com
Provides information about physical fitness, strength training, types of stretching, and the physiology of stretching.

Bibliography

Alter, M. *Science of Flexibility,* 3rd ed. Champaign, IL: Human Kinetics, 2004.

Fredette, D. M. "Exercise Recommendations for Flexibility and Range of Motion." In J. L. Rothman, ed., *ACSM's Resource Manual,* 4th ed. Philadelphia: Lippincott Williams and Wilkins, 2001.

Humphries, B. E., L. Dugan, and T. L. A. Doyle. "Muscular Fitness." In L. Kaminsky, ed., *ACSM's Resource Manual for Guidelines for Exercise Testing and Prescription,* 5th ed. Philadelphia: Lippincott Williams and Wilkins, 2006.

Kurz, T. *Stretching Scientifically: A Guide to Flexibility Training,* 4th ed. Island Pond, VT: Stadion Publishing Co., 2003.

Lan C., J. S. Lai, and S. Y. Chen. "Tai Chi Chuan: An Ancient Wisdom on Exercise and Health Promotion." *Sports Medicine* 32 (April 2002): 217–24.

Mayo Clinic. "Flexibility: Stretching to Stay Limber." *Mayo Clinic Health Letter* 18 (February 2000): 4–5.

Wallace, J. "Principles of Musculoskeletal Exercise Programming." In L. Kaminsky, ed., *ACSM's Resource Manual for Guidelines for Exercise Testing and Prescription,* 5th ed. Philadelphia: Lippincott Williams and Wilkins, 2006.

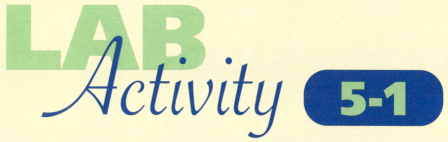

LAB Activity 5-1

Sample Flexibility Program

Equipment Needed:

Mat

Procedure

Read Chapter 5 and then complete these exercises as illustrated in Figure 5-1. Hold each stretch 10 to 30 seconds and repeat four times.

FLEXIBILITY EXERCISES

Exercise	Repetitions	Exercise	Repetitions	Exercise	Repetitions
A. Hamstring stretch	_____	D. Quadriceps stretch	_____	G. Deltoid stretch	_____
B. Lower back/hip flexor stretch	_____	E. Calf/Achilles stretch	_____	H. Pectoral stretch	_____
C. Spinal twist	_____	F. Iliotibial band stretch	_____	I. Triceps stretch	_____

Results

1. What are three things you learned about flexibility training by doing this program?

2. What did you learn about your flexibility levels in different body areas?

3. What did you like/dislike about this type of program?

A. Hamstring stretch

Sit and extend one leg in front, with the other bent and tucked as shown in diagram (a). Keeping shoulders erect, press abdomen forward. Hold. Repeat with other leg.

B. Lower back/hip flexor stretch

Lie on your back with one leg straight and one bent. With hands behind thigh, press thigh toward chest. Keep extended leg straight. Repeat left.

C. Spinal twist (lower back and hip abductors)

Sit with right leg extended, step left leg over right, and turn upper body toward left. Repeat on other side.

D. Quadriceps stretch

Stand with right leg bent at the knee. With left hand, pull right heel toward buttocks. Keep shoulders up, abdominals tight, and hips tucked under to prevent back hyperextension. Omit if you have knee problems.

E. Calf/Achilles stretch

Standing in forward lunge position, toes pointing forward, press heel toward floor. Repeat with other leg. Bend back knee to stretch soleus.

F. Iliotibial band stretch

Cross left foot over right, press hips to right. Repeat with other side.

G. Deltoid stretch

Cross right arm in front of body and pull it in toward midline with left hand.

H. Pectoral stretch

Place right hand on wall, with elbow extended but not locked. Twist shoulders left. Repeat with left arm.

I. Triceps stretch

Pull left elbow behind head. Repeat right.

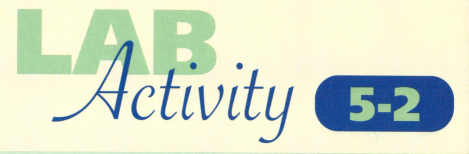

LAB *Activity* 5-2

Hatha Yoga Workout: Sun Salutation (or Salute to the Sun)

Introduction: The Sun Salutation, one of the most popular yoga routines, is a series of 12 postures (poses) performed in a single, graceful flow. Each movement is coordinated with the breath. Inhale as you extend or stretch, and exhale as you fold or contract. Complete the instructions below and answer the questions. The Sun Salutation is on the back of this page. This is a tear-out exercise that may be used anywhere.

1. Go through the Sun Salutation routine slowly several times. One complete routine consists of two sequences: one for the right side of the body, and one for the left. Concentrate on the proper order of the poses during this initial practice session.

2. Now practice the routine concentrating on inhaling and exhaling at the correct time.

3. Describe how the arms and shoulders feel after going through this yoga workout.

4. Were you able to step each leg up between the hands in one movement on the Lunge pose?

   Yes/No   Discuss:

5. Were you able to press the heels of the feet down to the floor on the Downward Dog pose?

   Yes/No   Discuss:

6. What is your evaluation of the Sun Salutation as a strength and flexibility exercise routine?

7. Is there any way to make this routine aerobic? If so, how?

8. How could this routine help with stress management?

Sun Salutation

1
Mountain

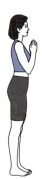

Stand with feet together, slightly pigeon-toed (big toes touching, heels apart), with your hands together, palm to palm, at heart level. Take several deep breaths. **Exhale.**

2
Slight Arch

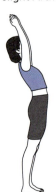

Inhale. Tighten buttocks, stretch arms upward, gently arching your back as far as feels comfortable and safe.

3
Standing
Forward Bend

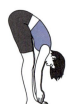

Exhale, while bending forward and downward, bringing your hands flat to the floor beside your feet, bending the knees if necessary. Touch head to knees, if possible.

4
Lunge

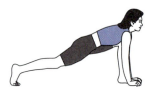

Inhale and step the right leg back in a wide backward lunge. Keep left foot between hands.

5
Plank

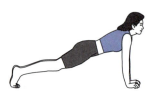

Exhale and step left leg back into plank. **Inhale.** Hold the position and breathe. Tighten abs.

6
Knees and Chest

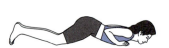

Hold your breath and lower the body in one unit, close to the floor. **Exhale** as you touch knees, chest, and chin to the floor. Lower hips, point feet and toes.

7
Cobra

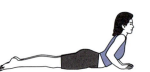

Inhale, lifting your chest toward the sky, with elbows slightly bent and pressed into your ribs. Straighten arms as much as feels comfortable.

8
Downward Dog

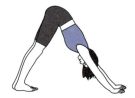

Exhale, tuck toes under lifting hips up and bringing the body into inverted V. Align head with arms. Press heels down.

9
Lunge

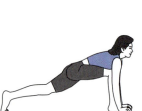

Inhale. Lift head and step the right foot up between hands.

10
Standing Forward
Bend

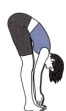

Exhale. Bring the left foot up and go into standing forward bend.

11
Slight Arch

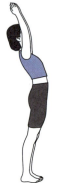

Inhale. Rise slowly. Tighten buttocks, lift arms overhead, and arch back.

12
Mountain

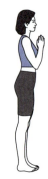

Exhale. Return to position number 1. Repeat the sequence, stepping with the left leg.

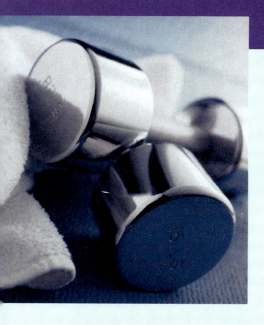

Chapter 6

Developing Muscular Fitness

Exercise is a gift you give yourself.
—Anonymous

Objectives

After reading this chapter, you will be able to:

1. Identify five benefits of and five cautions for resistance training.
2. Identify differences between training programs for strength and programs for muscular endurance.
3. Describe two basic types of muscular exercise and give an example of each.
4. Define three principles of resistance training.
5. Identify correct safety guidelines for weight training.
6. Describe four types of resistance training programs.
7. Explain how muscular fitness contributes to wellness.

Terms

- agonist
- antagonist
- atrophy
- concentric contraction
- constant resistance exercise
- dynamic (isotonic) exercise
- eccentric contraction
- fast-twitch muscle fiber
- hypertrophy
- isokinetic
- muscular power
- progressive overload
- repetition (rep)
- repetition maximum (RM)
- set
- slow-twitch muscle fiber
- static (isometric) exercise
- Valsalva maneuver
- variable resistance exercise

A Fit and Well Way of Life Online Learning Center www.mhhe.com/robbinsfitwell1e
Go to the Online Learning Center for chapter quizzes, outlines, flashcards, and additional lab activities.

At one time physical fitness programs consisted almost entirely of strength and flexibility exercises. Then, in the 1970s, aerobic activities rose to prominence. As a result, strength and flexibility exercises were swept into the role of supplemental activities and added to the main workout only if time permitted. As people flocked to gyms to do aerobics, they were exposed to weight training and began to value the benefits of muscular fitness. Today, as the emphasis on balanced fitness grows, muscular fitness is assuming new importance. It can enhance the ability to perform daily tasks and athletic performance. Muscular fitness makes it easier to perform routine activities such as carrying groceries upstairs, lifting a child, and moving the couch. It is perhaps the most important fitness component for older adults because muscular fitness is essential for carrying out activities of daily living that help maintain functional independence. Enhanced muscular fitness allows us to perform vigorous activities with less risk of straining muscles or connective tissue, and so it is important in the prevention and rehabilitation of injuries. This chapter covers muscular fitness benefits, cautions, principles, and guidelines along with illustrated programs for developing this important fitness component.

MUSCULAR FITNESS

Many people start muscular fitness programs to look better, feel better, shape and tone muscles, or increase lean muscle mass. At the same time, they increase muscular strength and endurance. In this section, we will examine benefits, muscle structure and function, general principles, safety, and specific exercise programs for muscular strength and endurance.

Resistance Training: Benefits and Cautions

An advantage of aerobic activities is their cardiorespiratory benefits. Resistance training can offer additional benefits whether your goal is health-related fitness or improved athletic performance.

Weight Control   The more muscle a person has, the higher his or her metabolism is and the more calories he or she burns, even at rest. This is one reason men can consume more calories without gaining weight than can women of equal size—the average male has roughly twice the muscle mass of the average female. Muscle is active, high-metabolic tissue, while fat is storage tissue. Resistance training increases muscle mass, which increases the rate at which you burn calories 24 hours a day, not just during the workout. This makes weight control easier. While women do not appear to gain as much muscle as men do from weight training, when differences in body size are taken into account, gains are comparable. Over a 4- to 6-month period, a man may gain 4 to 6 pounds of muscle, and a woman 2 to 3 pounds. Muscle is denser than fat and pound for pound takes up less space, and so as muscle is gained, if fat is lost, the result is a loss of unwanted inches. While aerobic exercise and a nutritious low-fat diet are the quickest ways to reduce body fat, weight training does offer advantages for long-term weight control.

Weight Gain   For those who wish to gain weight, increasing lean muscle mass, not fat, is a desirable goal, and there is no better way to do this than weight training. However, rate and quantity of muscle tissue gains vary from person to person because they are partially genetically determined. Those with a naturally tall, lean build tend to gain muscle more slowly than do those with a stockier build, and men gain faster than women do. A weight-gain program is outlined in the weight-training section for those who wish to increase lean weight.

Appearance   Developing a lean, well-toned body is the main reason many people exercise. If you feel that you need to lose weight but your body fat percentage is in the average range, reevaluate. Weight loss alone does not give a firm, well-toned appearance to flabby thighs or abdominals. Resistance training is the most effective way to shape and tone muscles, resulting in a trimmer appearance. Posture improves when agonist/antagonist muscles are in balance. Strengthening weak muscles and stretching tight, inflexible muscles help develop good body alignment so that you move more fluidly and feel and look better.

Time Economy   Instead of doing 50 leg lifts without weights, you can cut your workout time by adding resistance. Lift a weight heavy enough to produce fatigue in 8 to 12 repetitions and you will get more benefit in fewer lifts. For basic muscular fitness, a balanced resistance-training workout of 10 to 12 exercises takes approximately 30 minutes to complete. Despite what you may observe in the gym, more is not necessary. While body builders, competitive weightlifters, and other strength-event athletes work out much more than this, keep in mind that they have different goals. Health-related fitness levels can be developed and maintained in much less training time than is needed for competition.

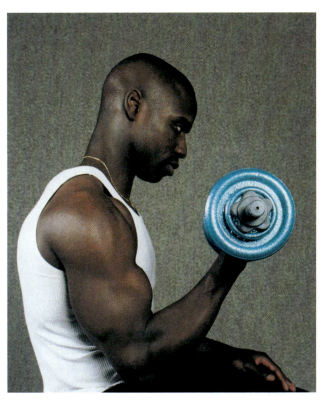

Resistance training is the most effective way to shape and tone muscles and is an important part of a balanced fitness program.

Energy   Performance and efficiency improve with resistance training—more work can be done with less effort as muscular strength and endurance increase.

Athletic Performance   Stronger muscles enable you to better control the forces of movement—self-generated and external—as well as your body position during activity. Improved muscular fitness contributes to skill-related components of balance, speed, power, coordination, and agility. All other things being equal, a strong person can run faster, jump higher, and throw a ball farther than can a weaker individual.

Injury Prevention   Aerobic exercises such as jogging and aerobic dance have the potential to cause injury through repetitive, forceful impact against unyielding surfaces. Strong, flexible muscles and connective tissue can better withstand the stress of many forceful landings during a workout. When ligaments, tendons, muscle, and bone are strengthened through muscular exercise, the risk of injury is decreased. Many aerobic activities tend to develop strength in only a few groups of muscles, leaving others weak. For example, jogging strengthens the quadriceps but leaves the hamstrings weak. Weak muscle groups are more susceptible to strains or pulls. A well-designed resistance-training program develops balanced, proportional strength in agonists (prime movers) and antagonists (opposing muscle groups). If injury does occur, it may be less severe and may heal more quickly if the muscle is well conditioned. A carefully designed program can also rehabilitate injuries to help you regain normal (or better) strength levels. For more detailed information on injury prevention, see Chapter 8.

Bone Strength   Resistance exercises decrease the risk of osteoporosis. This is important not only for the elderly but for young people as well. Osteoporosis may cause a fracture at age 60, but it starts much earlier—in the teens and 20s. You need good exercise and eating habits to build adequate bone density. The pull of muscles on bone in weight-bearing exercise stimulates development of increased bone density and bone quality and preserves existing bone. Research indicates that intensity of lifting is clearly related to bone mineralization. Lifting relatively heavy weights in a few repetitions may be more effective in increasing bone mass than is lifting a light weight many times.

Flexibility   Moving weights through a full range of motion, from full extension to full contraction, stretches and tones muscles. This is an important training technique to master to maintain flexibility. Muscles become short and tight if exercises are performed repeatedly through only a partial range of motion.

Balance   Strong, fatigue-resistant muscles mean better balance during static and dynamic activities not only in athletics but in functional activities for people of all ages. Studies have shown improvements in balance for

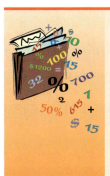

THE NUMBERS

80%	Adults who do not exercise for muscular strength or endurance.
30	Age at which the average person begins to lose muscle mass.
1–2%	Strength lost yearly after the age of 30.
20–30	Minutes of exercise needed to strengthen all major muscle groups.
2–3	Days per week of strength training recommended for good health.

elderly people participating in strength training. This may translate into improved gait stability, decreased risk of falls, and reduced frequency of hip fractures—even for people in their 80s.

Cardiovascular Health   Resistance training may enhance cardiovascular health by reducing several risk factors associated with cardiovascular disease. Studies have shown a decrease in resting diastolic blood pressure that is most significant in individuals with previously elevated blood pressure; decreases in exercise heart rate and exercise blood pressure; increased exercise tolerance; and modest improvements in blood lipid profile. Resistance training also has been shown to increase insulin sensitivity and decrease glucose intolerance in diabetic exercisers. Although little change in VO_{2max} occurs with traditional weight training, if a circuit weight-training program consisting of 10 exercises, 15 repetitions each, with a short (15 to 30 seconds) rest between is followed, modest improvements in VO_{2max} of 5 to 8 percent have been recorded.

Psychological Benefits   While many people begin an exercise program to improve appearance, many other less visible but equally important effects may result. Benefits in the emotional dimension of wellness from regular exercise include feeling better, decreased stress, decreased depression, and enhanced self-esteem and self-confidence.

Social Benefits   In addition to offering physical and psychological benefits, lifting with a partner or friend offers social benefits. There are many more opportunities for conversation and interaction when you work out with someone than when you watch a movie.

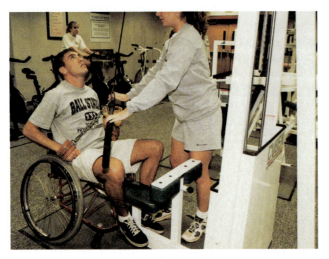

Resistance training benefits everyone. Greater muscular fitness improves performance of everyday activities and recreational and competitive sports.

℞ Prescription for Action

Date: *Do one or more today*

✔ While watching TV, use your exercise band during commercials.

✔ While sitting, do abdominal isometric contractions or press knees together hard for 6 seconds, 5–10 times, to tone inner thigh.

✔ Treat yourself with an exercise ball and video to add variety to your exercise program.

✔ Carry and load your own groceries; take the stairs instead of the elevator.

✔ If you usually use weight machines, make an appointment for instruction to enable you to try free weight exercises, and vice versa.

✔ Try a personal trainer for one session to check your lifting form and technique and get suggestions for improvement in your lifting program.

Prescribed by: *YOU*

Benefits at Any Age   Regardless of your age, you can benefit from resistance training. It is untrue that loss of strength is inevitable with age or that older people cannot gain strength. While the typical sedentary individual can lose up to 30 percent of his or her muscle mass between the ages of 20 and 70, this loss is more from atrophy due to disuse rather than from aging alone. Adequate levels of muscular strength are particularly important to older adults to maintain their functional independence and quality of life. Several studies including people in their 70s, 80s, and 90s participating in resistance training have shown that participants increased muscle mass, more than doubled their strength, and improved their functional mobility and ability to perform daily living activities.

Disadvantages and Cautions   Although resistance training has many benefits, it does have disadvantages. Resistance training is not a complete exercise program because it does not develop cardiorespiratory endurance. As in any physical activity, injury is possible if you are careless or ignore safety procedures. You may have trouble accessing equipment. Also, you can expect some mild muscle soreness during the first week of the program.

Individuals with cardiovascular problems or high blood pressure should seek medical guidance due to the tendency of blood pressure to increase during strength training. Those who have hernias, arthritis, or lower back problems should also seek medical clearance. Individuals with these health concerns may benefit from resistance training but should be aware that they may need special exercise modifications.

Avoid use of hand and ankle weights during jogging, high-impact aerobic dance workouts, and other activities involving running and jumping. Ankle weights may distort proper form, increase stress to legs and feet, and increase the risk of strains and sprains. While small increases in oxygen consumption and caloric expenditure result from using light weights, the same effect can be produced with less risk by exercising longer or harder.

When used with controlled form and rhythm in a muscle toning or walking program, however, light weights are beneficial for increasing heart rate and muscular fitness in the upper body. All in all, resistance training offers few drawbacks and many major advantages for the time invested.

Muscle Function

Muscles are made of individual muscle fibers bound together and sheathed in connective tissue. They end in a tendon that connects the muscle to a bone. An example is the Achilles tendon, which you can feel above your heel, connecting your calf to your foot. Muscle fibers can contract to shorten the muscle or relax and return to their resting length. They are also elastic. They can be stretched and will spring back to their resting length.

Muscle fibers are classified into types based on their endurance, speed of contraction, and ability to exert force. **Slow-twitch** (ST) **muscle fibers** have high aerobic capacity but low power and are recruited primarily for endurance-type activities such as jogging. **Fast-twitch** (FT) **muscle fibers** are able to contract more quickly and generate more force but fatigue relatively quickly. They are important for short-burst, powerful activities such as sprinting and jumping. ST fibers are recruited initially during muscular contraction, and FT fibers are recruited when weight training becomes more intense and requires greater speed or force. The ratio of ST to FT muscle fibers is genetically determined and varies from one person to another. Resistance training increases the size and strength of both fiber types as well as their ability to exert force.

Muscles cannot expand and push. Movement is produced as muscle contracts, shortens, and pulls on bones across a joint. As a muscle on one side of a bone contracts, muscles on the other side must relax to allow movement to occur. The contracting muscle that initiates movement is called the **agonist.** The opposing muscle is called the **antagonist.** In a biceps curl (Figure 6-1), the agonist is the biceps and the antagonist is the triceps. In a triceps extension, the roles reverse. What is the agonist in a hamstring curl? What is the antagonist?

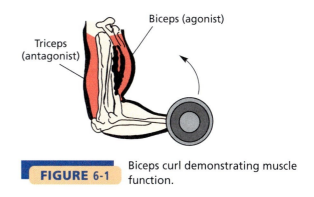

FIGURE 6-1   Biceps curl demonstrating muscle function.

Determinants of Muscular Fitness Gains

Gains in muscular fitness result from neurological and muscular adaptations. Dramatic strength gains early in a program are often due to a "learning effect"—that is, you learn how to lift weights more efficiently. Your body represses its self-protective reflexes and increases its ability to recruit muscle fibers fully when needed.

Your overall potential for the development of muscular fitness is determined by many factors, including the types, number, and size of muscle fibers you possess and how well your muscular system can recruit them during muscular effort. The more muscle fibers you have, the larger they are, and the better your system is at activating them during muscular effort, the greater your strength is. While the types and number of muscle fibers you possess are genetically determined, size and muscle fiber recruitment are a product of training.

Muscle Fiber Recruitment

When a muscle contracts, only the number of muscle fibers required for that momentary effort will shorten. Individual muscle fibers cannot contract partially. They are working as hard as possible or not at all. This is called the *all-or-nothing principle*. For example, when a biceps curl calls for a 50 percent effort, all fibers in the muscle do not contract at 50 percent effort; rather, a portion of the muscle's fibers contract fully while the remainder rest. After these first muscle fibers contract, fatigue slightly decreases their ability to apply force. On each subsequent contraction, more fibers must be recruited to continue to lift the same weight. After several muscle contractions, enough fibers are fatigued that the muscle temporarily can no longer generate the same effort in what is called *temporary muscular failure*. Muscle fibers increase strength only if they are stimulated by intensity of effort. If your goal is to develop maximal muscular strength, try to recruit, or activate, as many muscle fibers as possible by working a muscle to a state of temporary muscular failure. If you are working for health-related fitness levels, a less intense effort is adequate.

Muscle Atrophy and Hypertrophy

Muscles adapt to the load placed on them. When the load increases over time, muscular strength and endurance improve. When muscles are not used, they grow weaker, stiffen, and **atrophy,** or shrink in size. A dramatic example of muscle atrophy occurs when a person has an injured limb in a cast for several weeks. When the cast is removed, the muscles of the affected limb are noticeably smaller. Increasing amounts of exercise over time are necessary to rebuild muscle strength, size, and flexibility.

When muscles are stimulated by an increased workload, they grow stronger and muscle fibers experience **hypertrophy,** or increase in size. This increase occurs in both men and women and is proportional to muscle mass. The average man has about twice the muscle mass of the average woman, and so hypertrophy in men is more pronounced.

Gender Differences

Some women worry that they will develop big shoulders or massive, masculine musculature because of weight training. This myth is reinforced by televised images of women's body-building competitions. Be assured that shoulder width, like hip width, is influenced by genetics and that significant muscle gains require hours of strenuous weight lifting for many months. Dramatic muscle hypertrophy and masculinization also can occur with anabolic steroid abuse. Men have a greater potential for muscle hypertrophy than women do because men have higher levels of sex hormones such as androgen and testosterone, which promote muscle growth. Some of the strongest women athletes are gymnasts, who have very feminine physiques. Weight training is also popular with TV and movie stars who exercise to maintain a fit, toned appearance and help control weight. Be assured that massive muscles don't occur by accident or with a 20- to 30-minute muscle-toning workout twice a week.

Types of Resistance Training Programs

Two basic types of muscular exercise are static (isometric) and dynamic (isotonic). Different resistance programs have been developed for each type.

Static (Isometric) Exercise

Static (isometric) exercise is exercise in which the muscle contracts but does not change length and little or no movement occurs. If you pushed your palms together hard, your pectoral muscles would contract and try to shorten, but your arms would not move. An advantage of static exercise is that it requires little or no equipment and can be done almost anywhere—for instance, while sitting at a desk. However, these exercises are not widely

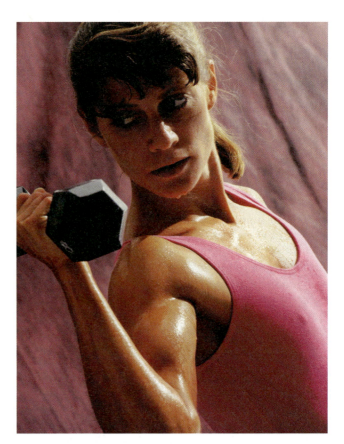

Weight training can help maintain a fit, toned appearance and control weight.

used because resistance is applied at only one point in your range of motion, and thus strength development is limited. Also, it is difficult to know how much force is being exerted, and so strength gains are not as easy to observe as they are when equipment is being used. However, static exercises can be useful in strengthening muscles after an injury, when dynamic movement would be painful or even increase injury.

Dynamic (Isotonic) Exercise

Dynamic (isotonic) exercise is exercise in which the muscle contracts and shortens and movement occurs. Most daily activities, such as pushing, pulling, and lifting, are dynamic. Dynamic exercise programs can be done with free weights, exercise machines, elastic resistance, or calisthenics such as crunches and push-ups. Dynamic exercise involves two types of muscle contractions: concentric and eccentric.

In a **concentric contraction,** a muscle shortens as it overcomes resistance. For example, a weight is lifted as the biceps contract during the lifting phase of a biceps curl. **Eccentric contraction** occurs when a muscle lengthens and contracts at the same time, gradually allowing a force to overcome muscular resistance; for example, the biceps contract eccentrically during the lowering phase of a biceps curl. Eccentric contraction is a beneficial component of strength development because it makes up half of the muscular effort. The same muscles are involved in eccentric and concentric contractions, and so lowering should be done in a smooth, controlled manner for maximal benefit and to prevent potential injury from dropping the weight.

Advantages of dynamic exercise are that it strengthens through a full range of motion, the load is measurable, and a variety of isotonic programs are available. Calisthenics, free weights, and machines such as Universal or Nautilus use dynamic exercise.

Two common types of dynamic exercises involve constant resistance or variable resistance. In **constant resistance exercise,** a constant resistance (weight) is used throughout the range of motion. However, the force needed to move the weight varies with leverage determined by the angle of the joint; that is, it increases or decreases as the load is moved through the range of motion. For example, with a biceps curl, it is easier to move the weight through the first and last thirds of the motion and harder through the middle third. The ability to lift a weight is limited by the amount of strength required to move it through this "sticking point."

In **variable resistance exercise,** the force needed to move the weight is changed to provide a maximum load throughout the range of motion. This requires special machines, such as Nautilus, that increase the resistance as the weight is moved through the ends of the range of motion where you are able to exert greater force.

Another type of dynamic exercise is **isokinetic,** in which the speed of movement is controlled. The advantage of isokinetic work is that the load applied mirrors the force exerted by the user while the speed remains constant. Isokinetic machinery often is used in rehabilitation and is not common in most fitness centers.

Both constant resistance exercise and variable resistance exercise are effective in developing muscular fitness. Different types of exercises and equipment have advantages and disadvantages, but the most important factor in fitness gains is a person's motivation and effort rather than the type of equipment used.

Principles of Resistance Training

Strength gains are proportional to the load applied and the frequency and intensity of effort. Basic principles of resistance training include progressive overload, specificity, and recovery.

Progressive Overload

Progressive overload is the most important principle of resistance training. To stimulate a muscle to increase strength or endurance, it must gradually be overloaded or forced to work at a higher than normal effort. Either the number of lifts (**repetitions**) performed or the amount of weight (load or resistance) must gradually be increased or recovery time between exercises must be decreased. Increasing the number of repetitions or decreasing rest increases muscular endurance. Increasing the weight lifted increases strength. General programs increase load and repetitions until a desired maintenance goal is reached.

You must exercise two to three times a week to improve muscular fitness. Significant strength gains require at least 8 consecutive weeks of training. To maintain strength, one intense workout is adequate for health fitness. Athletes will need to train at least twice a week to maintain fitness in the off-season.

Specificity

The speed of contraction, range of motion, amount and type of resistance, and number and type of exercise are a few of the variables that determine the results of strength training. If you desire a specific result, such as an increase in muscle mass, your program must be designed and executed to produce that result.

Recovery

Exercise stimulates a muscle to take in more protein and nutrients and undergo changes that increase its ability to contract forcefully. After a workout, you will be weaker, not stronger, due to fatigue. Improvement occurs during recovery, which gives the muscle fibers time to repair and grow. This requires more recovery time than for the cardiorespiratory system. Strength workouts are best done with 2 to 3 days of rest between sessions to allow recovery and improvement to occur. Lifting may be done more frequently, using a split routine with the upper body one day and the lower body the next.

Guidelines for Developing Muscular Fitness

In increasing muscular strength, endurance, or power, the key variables are resistance, repetitions, and speed. The purest example of strength is one maximal lift, and the closer a program comes to this, the greater the strength gains are. However, risk of injury is high when working at or near maximal levels. Athletes working to develop strength often exercise at 80 to 90 percent or higher effort a few (five to eight) times. Muscular endurance is enhanced by contracting repeatedly (e.g., one to two sets of 15 to 20 reps) with moderate (50 to 60 percent) effort.

There is some crossover effect between muscular strength and muscular endurance. Development of muscular strength also produces an increase in muscular endurance; for example, if you can lift a 100-pound weight 5 times, you can probably lift a 5-pound weight 20 times. However, muscular endurance does not enhance strength. If you can lift a 5-pound weight 20 times, you

TABLE 6-1	Guidelines for Resistance Training Programs			
	Muscular Endurance	**Health Fitness**	**Bodybuilding (Weight Gain)**	**Muscular Strength**
Frequency (workouts per week)	3–5	2–3	4–10	2–3
Resistance (% of 1 RM)	50–60%	70–75%	70–80%	80–90%
Repetitions	15–20	8–12	5–10	5–8
Sets	1–2	1–2	3–5	1–3
Rest between sets*	0.5–1 min.	1–2 min.	1–3 min.	2–4 min.

*Rest between sets may be decreased by alternating lifts using different body parts.

may not be able to lift a 100-pound weight even once. If you want to develop both muscular strength and endurance, a muscular strength program can provide double benefits.

Muscular power, a function of strength and speed, is the ability to apply force rapidly. Power is increased by performing a muscle contraction quickly, as in the plyometric exercises often used in athletics. While muscular power is not necessary for health-related physical fitness, it is an asset in many sports.

Guidelines for resistance training programs are summarized in Table 6-1. Optimal results can be obtained from any resistance training program, and risk of injury can be minimized if you follow the guidelines in Table 6-2.

Sequence

Ideally, first work large muscle groups and complex multiple joint exercises, ending with small muscle groups and isolated single joint exercises. It is difficult to exercise large muscle groups adequately if you have already fatigued the smaller supporting muscles. The suggested order of exercises is hips/legs, torso, arms, abdominals (see the sample weight-training program).

Form

✔ Never sacrifice form for weight. After progressive overload, correct exercise form is the most important (and most neglected) factor in

maximizing strength gains and minimizing the risk of injury. Improvement is more rapid if correct technique, not only quantity of weight, is emphasized.

✔ Always work through a complete range of motion for flexibility and maximum strength gains. Move from full extension without lockout to full flexion.

✔ Keep your back straight and abdominals tight to protect your lower back.

✔ When doing standing exercises, keep the knees slightly bent and the hips tucked under to support your back.

✔ Avoid "cheating," a breakdown in exercise form that occurs when extra muscles are used to complete the exercise, decreasing the load to the prime mover. Cheating occurs when the load is too heavy or you are fatigued. Remember: Quality of work is more important than the number of repetitions or amount of weight lifted.

Rest Between Sets

A **set** is a group of lifts followed by a rest period. For example, a person doing eight biceps curls has done one set of eight repetitions. A rest period between sets of an exercise should allow sufficient recovery so that good form can be maintained. This time will vary, depending on the intensity of lifting, with 1 to 2 minutes of rest recommended between sets of a health fitness program and 2 to 4 minutes between sets of a strength program. To make efficient use of time, you may alternate exercises on different body parts—for example, legs, then arms—so that one muscle group is recovering while you are working another.

Muscle Balance

Muscles work in pairs, and so it is important to strengthen muscles on both sides of a bone so that they pull evenly across joints and maintain body alignment. For example, if pectorals are stronger than upper back muscles, rounded shoulders result. When upper back muscles are strengthened, shoulders are naturally held erect. Tight lower back muscles opposed by weak, sag-

TABLE 6-2	Safety Guidelines for Resistance Training

1. Warm up before each workout and stretch afterward.
2. Use good technique—keep your abdominals tight, back straight, hips tucked under, knees relaxed.
3. Work each exercise through a full range of motion from full extension without lockout to full contraction.
4. Perform each exercise smoothly, with control. Do not swing the limbs or use momentum. Faster is not better.
5. Before you lift, inhale. Exhale on the exertion. Do not hold your breath.

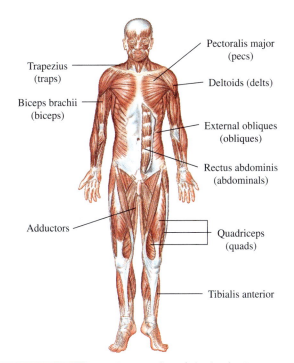

Trapezius (traps)

Biceps brachii (biceps)

Pectoralis major (pecs)

Deltoids (delts)

External obliques (obliques)

Rectus abdominis (abdominals)

Adductors

Quadriceps (quads)

Tibialis anterior

FIGURE 6-2A Major muscles of the body. Front. SOURCE: John W. Hole, Jr., *Human Anatomy and Physiology*, 4th ed. Copyright © 1987 Wm. C. Brown Publishers, Dubuque, Iowa. All Rights Reserved. Reprinted by permission.

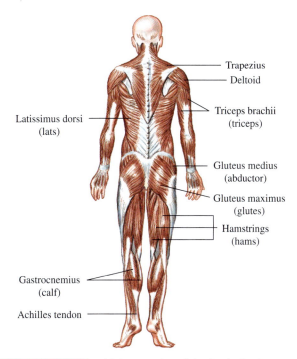

Latissimus dorsi (lats)

Gastrocnemius (calf)

Achilles tendon

Trapezius

Deltoid

Triceps brachii (triceps)

Gluteus medius (abductor)

Gluteus maximus (glutes)

Hamstrings (hams)

FIGURE 6-2B Major muscles of the body. Back. SOURCE: John W. Hole, Jr., *Human Anatomy and Physiology*, 4th ed. Copyright © 1987 Wm. C. Brown Publishers, Dubuque, Iowa. All Rights Reserved. Reprinted by permission.

ging abdominals pull the back into an exaggerated curve. This stresses lumbar vertebrae, increasing back fatigue and the risk of lower back pain. Well-toned abdominals support the back, improve appearance, and prevent back problems. Resistance programs must be planned to develop proportional strength in the following muscle pairs: biceps/triceps, pectorals/trapezius-rhomboids, abdominals/lower back, hamstrings/quadriceps, gastrocnemius/anterior tibialis, and deltoids/latissimus dorsi (Figures 6-2a and 6-2b).

Breathing

Exhale as you push or pull; inhale as you lower the weight. For example, on a biceps curl, exhale as you lift the weight and inhale as you lower it to the starting position. Holding your breath while you strain against a closed epiglottis is called the **Valsalva maneuver.** This can elevate blood pressure dangerously and cause dizziness or fainting.

Speed of Movement

Exercising in a smooth, controlled manner maximizes strength gains and reduces injuries. Take 2 seconds to lift (concentric or shortening contraction) and 2 to 4 seconds to lower (eccentric or lengthening contraction). Control the movement; do not fling, swing, or kick. Jerky movements will cause excessive wear and tear on your joints. Also, when you use momentum to perform an exercise, you apply force and develop strength only

through the first part of the movement. Lower a limb with the same control used to lift it. Do not drop weights with a crash. You are stronger lowering a weight than lifting it.

Resistance Training Programs

There are many types of resistance training programs. The type of program you select will depend on your goals and the type of equipment (if any) you plan to use. Four basic resistance training programs are shown in Table 6-3. Regardless of the type of program you select, you can keep track of your progress with the *Resistance Training Log* in Lab Activity 6-1 at the end of this chapter.

Weight Training

Weight training is a noncompetitive exercise program used to develop several health-related physical fitness components: muscular strength, muscular endurance, flexibility, and body composition. It differs significantly in its goals from the competitive sports of weight lifting and bodybuilding. Male, female, young, old, athlete, and fitness exerciser–all benefit from weight training. Beginners with low levels of muscular fitness benefit the most and will notice results more quickly than will experienced lifters. Weight training can build muscular fitness levels so that recreational, competitive, and daily activities are accomplished more easily, with less strain and fatigue.

TABLE 6-3   *Basic Resistance Training Programs*

	Machines	Free Weights	Elastic Band	No Weights
Legs	Leg press Leg extension Hamstring curl	Squats Lunges	Squats Leg extension Hamstring curl Side leg lift Inner thigh lift Three-way leg pointer	Wall sit Lunges Partner leg extension Partner hamstring curl Partner inner/outer thigh press
Ankles	Toe press	Calf raise	Toe press Toe lifts	Calf raise Partner foot flexion
Chest	Bench press	Bench press	Push-ups	Push-ups Dips Partner elbow press forward
Shoulders	Military press	Military press Shoulder shrugs	Deltoid raise	Partner overhead press
Back	Lat pull Rowing Back extension	Bent-over rowing Back extension	Lat pull Rowing	Partner lat pull Partner elbow press backward Core exercises
Abdominals	Abdominal curls	Abdominal curls	Abdominal curls	Core exercises
Arms	Triceps press Biceps curl	Triceps press Biceps curl	Triceps press Biceps curl	Push-ups Pull-ups Partner biceps curl

Equipment

For beginners, it really doesn't matter what type of equipment is used. A beginner will improve on almost any type of program as long as an adequate overload is provided. Two major types of equipment used in weight training are free weights and machines. Both have advantages and disadvantages:

✔ Free weights are far less expensive than machines, and so you can have your own set at home. Free weights cost about $100 on sale, double that if you add a padded bench and rack. Machines can cost upward of $500 to $5,000.

✔ You have more variety of exercises on free weights than on machines because you have the freedom to lift in so many different positions.

✔ Lifting with proper technique is crucial. A wrong move can cause injury with any lifting but particularly with free weights.

✔ To lift free weights safely, you must have a skilled spotting partner who can handle the weight in case you start to lose control.

✔ For muscular fitness development, free weights have an advantage over machines because they not only develop strength in the prime movers but also develop balance and coordination by strengthening other muscles required to balance and control the weight.

✔ Machines such as Nautilus and Universal are easy to use and safer than free weights because they guide your movements and control the weights. An advantage of Nautilus equipment is that it provides variable resistance, adjusting the load for strength variations throughout a lift.

✔ Because of the cost of machines, it is best to start your machine-workout program at a health club or gym.

✔ Proper lifting technique is easier to learn on machines, and you won't need a spotting partner.

✔ Loads can be changed quickly, and so the workout may take less time than with free weights.

For safety, convenience, and time, machines have the edge. Whether you use free weights or machines, always follow the safety guidelines in Table 6-4 to minimize risk of injury.

Weight Room Etiquette

Be aware of and follow common weight room etiquette guidelines while working out:

✔ Wipe sweat off benches after use.
✔ Rerack weights when you are done.
✔ Don't lie around on the equipment chatting between sets if people are waiting to use the machine. Let them work in between sets while you are resting.

TOP 10 LIST

Resistance Training Mistakes to Avoid

Resistance training is a great way to shape and tone muscles. If done wrong, however, it can elevate blood pressure and cause back strain, sore knees, or ankle sprain. Also, training mistakes slow your progress. Here are the most common errors to avoid:

1. *Holding your breath during lifting.* This can cause a dangerous increase in blood pressure. Exhale on exertion, inhale on release.
2. *Lifting too heavy a weight.* If you can't lift it with full range of motion with good form, lighten the load. Train, don't strain.
3. *Arching the back.* During the bench press or military press, this can strain back ligaments. Tighten abdominals and keep the back straight.
4. *Using momentum.* "Kicking" the weight up in the quadriceps extension or hamstring curl decreases the load through the full range of motion and slows progress. Bouncing or jerking a lift strains ligaments and indicates the weight is too heavy or you are getting too tired to lift smoothly.
5. *Doing reps too quickly.* Length of time a force is applied is a factor in muscle fitness. Lift for two to four counts and lower slowly for two to four counts for best results. Yes, it is harder than lifting fast. It takes fewer reps to get the same result compared to lifting fast.
6. *Not using full range of motion.* Strength is built only in the range of motion used. If you stop before the "sticking point," you are building muscle imbalances.
7. *Not wiping off sweat.* Sweat makes your grip slippery.
8. *Going too deep in squats or leg press.* This strains knee ligaments. Don't go below 90 degrees.
9. *Letting ankles roll out when legs are loaded.* This can cause ankle sprain. Keep ankles straight in squats or toe presses.
10. *Working only "problem" areas.* Or working the agonist but not its opposing antagonist. In other words, working biceps but not triceps or abdominals but not the back. This causes muscle imbalances, increasing risk of injury.

TABLE 6-4   *Safety Using Weights*

1. Never attempt to lift more than you know you can handle. Work out—don't show off.
2. Always make sure that the weight pins, bars, and collars are secure.
3. Don't lift weights alone. Always work with someone else.
4. Keep sweat wiped off your hands; it makes weights slippery.
5. When using free weights, work with a trained spotter.
6. Return all equipment to the proper place. Don't leave it lying around for someone to trip over.

If you exercised only problem areas, you would increase imbalances. Prime muscle movers, the muscle(s) mainly responsible for the joint movement, are listed and can be found in Figures 6-2a and 6-2b. The following exercises, listed in the order of large muscle groups and complex multiple joint exercises to isolated single joint exercises and small muscle groups, may be done on machines (Figure 6-3). Free weight exercises are also described and illustrated (Figure 6-4). If you plan to use machines, your first workouts should include learning how to adjust and efficiently use the equipment.

Weight Training Exercises

A. Leg press
Prime mover: quadriceps, hamstrings, and gluteus maximus
On leg press, sit on seat, adjust position to last slot or to a 90-degree knee angle.
Place feet squarely on pedals, press out smoothly (do not lock knees), and return to starting position.

B. Leg extension
Prime movers: quadriceps
Sit on bench with both feet under the rollers. Toe in slightly. Do not lie back.
Extend your legs, hold 1 second, and return to starting position.

C. Hamstring curl
Prime movers: hamstrings and gluteus maximus
Lie face down on the bench, hook both heels under the rollers. Position knees at the pivot point where the rollers attach to the bench. Pull up to 90 degrees, hold for 1 second, and return to starting position.

D. Toe press
Prime mover: gastrocnemius
On leg press station, place feet squarely on pedals, press out to full leg extension without knee lockout. Press with toes from flat-footed position to foot extension and return.

E. Bench press
Prime movers: pectorals and triceps
Lie on bench, head next to the machine. The grips should be lined up approximately with the

✔ Don't drop or bang the weights together. This can damage the equipment and increases the noise level unnecessarily.

Program for Health Fitness

A conditioning program should develop balanced strength. Many muscle strains occur because of weakness in the pulled muscle or its opposing muscle. A well-planned strength program prevents strength imbalances.

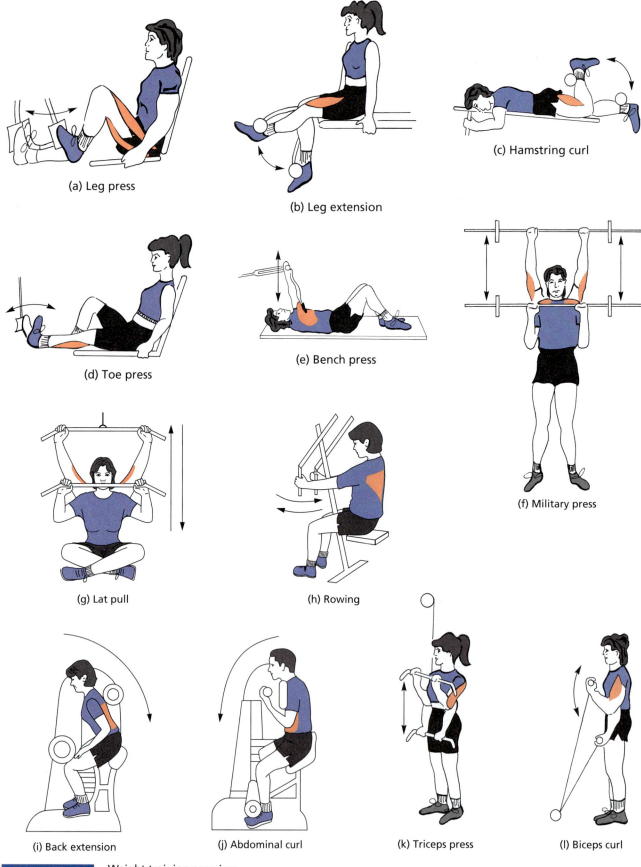

(a) Leg press

(b) Leg extension

(c) Hamstring curl

(d) Toe press

(e) Bench press

(f) Military press

(g) Lat pull

(h) Rowing

(i) Back extension

(j) Abdominal curl

(k) Triceps press

(l) Biceps curl

FIGURE 6-3   Weight training exercises.

shoulders. Place your feet flat on the bench with knees bent and back flat. Press to extension and return. If you tend to have shoulder problems, lower the bar to only 4 inches above your chest, then extend.

F. Military press
Prime movers: deltoids and triceps
Sit on the stool or stand with abdominals tight, back flat, and knees slightly bent. With shoulders close to handles, extend upward with arms until they are straight but not locked, then return.

G. Lat pull
Prime movers: latissimus dorsi
Grip bar directly above shoulders or at handles. Pull down until you are kneeling or sitting. From this position, pull down to chest and return.

H. Rowing
Prime movers: rhomboids, latissimus dorsi, and biceps
Sit on the machine with arms almost fully extended. Pull back as far as possible, drawing shoulder blades together. Return to starting position.

I. Back extension
Prime movers: erector spinae, gluteus maximus, and quadratus lumborum
Sit on the machine with back against upper back pad and feet under ankle rollers. Fasten hip belt if one is available, to keep hips from lifting or sliding out of position. Slowly extend trunk back fully and slowly return to starting position.

J. Abdominal curl
Prime movers: abdominals and hip flexors
Sit with pad on upper chest, knees flexed, and feet on footpad. Use seat belt if provided, to keep hips from lifting off seat. Flex trunk as far forward as possible. Return slowly to starting position.

K. Triceps press
Prime movers: triceps
Stand facing lat bar. With palms facing down, grasp the bar so that hands are shoulder width apart. Keep elbows at waist. Press down to extension and return.

L. Biceps curl
Prime movers: biceps
Stand facing the weights, hold bar with both hands, palms up. Flex arms until the bar meets shoulders. Return to starting position. Keep back straight, abdominals firm.

Free Weight Exercises These exercises (Figure 6-4) may be done with a set of barbells or hand weights. Practice each move without weights before attempting weighted sets. Free weights provide additional challenge over machines because balance and coordination are developed in addition to strength. Strict attention to lifting form is critical, because with free weights, a

moment's carelessness can cause an injury. Always work with an experienced spotter in case you have difficulty. When possible, use power/squat racks with adjustable supports for added safety. To protect the back, you need to keep abdominals firm, back straight. Breathe continuously; do not hold your breath.

A. Squat
Prime movers: gluteus maximus, quadriceps, and hamstrings
Start standing upright with the bar resting on your shoulders. Keep the head up, abdominals tight, back flat, feet a bit wider than your shoulders. With back straight, slowly lower hips until tops of thighs are parallel with the floor. Pause. Drive up with legs and hips to the starting position.

B. Lunge
Prime movers: gluteus maximus and quadriceps
Standing upright with the bar on the shoulders off the neck, abdominals tight, back flat, step forward (or backward) until the front thigh is parallel with the floor. The front knee should be over the ball of the foot. Keeping back straight, take a controlled step back to the starting position. Repeat with the opposite leg. This exercise requires considerable balance. You may wish to start first with dumbbells and progress slowly to use of a barbell.

C. Calf raise
Prime mover: gastrocnemius/soleus
Place bar on shoulders, position balls of feet on board and heels off board. Press up onto balls of feet, then lower with control. Knees straight tones gastrocnemius; knees bent tones soleus.

D. Bench press
Prime movers: pectorals and triceps
Lie with head and buttocks on bench, feet stabilized on ground for balance and safety. Grip about 4 inches wider than shoulders, palms under bar (pronated). Lower bar to chest. Focus eyes up to the sky; do not watch bar. Elbows should be directly under bar and forearms perpendicular to ground. Do not let bar slide to the neck. Press to extension, then return.

E. Military press
Prime movers: deltoids and triceps
Sit on bench or stand. With barbell on chest, press upward with arms until they are straight overhead but not locked, then return.

F. Shoulder shrug
Prime mover: trapezius
Holding barbell or two dumbbells, raise shoulders toward ears, pause, lower shoulders.

G. Bent-over rowing
Prime movers: rhomboids and latissimus dorsi
Stabilize one knee and hand on a bench; opposite hand holds the weight, and foot is flat on the floor. Pull elbow up and in toward the spine.

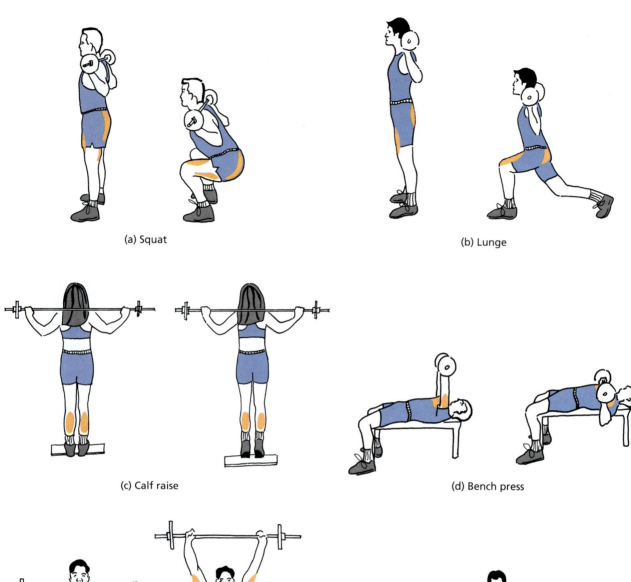

(a) Squat

(b) Lunge

(c) Calf raise

(d) Bench press

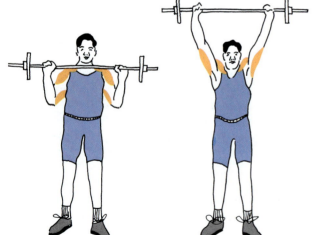

(e) Military press

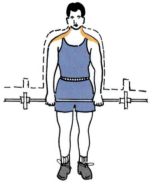

(f) Shoulder shrug

FIGURE 6-4   Free weight exercises.

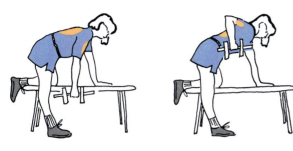

(g) Bent-over rowing

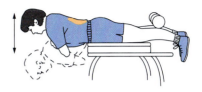

(h) Back extension

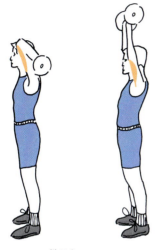

(i) Triceps press

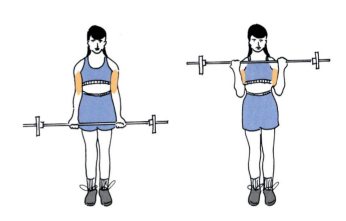

(j) Biceps curl

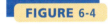 **FIGURE 6-4** Free weight exercises. *(continued)*

H. Back extension
   Prime movers: erector spinae, gluteus maximus, and quadratus lumborum
   Lie with your hips on the seat pad and ankles under the ankle rollers, arms crossed across chest. Slowly extend trunk to a horizontal position, hold 3 to 5 seconds, and slowly lower to starting position. After you can easily do 15–20 repetitions, you may increase resistance by holding light hand weights to your chest.

I. Triceps press
   Prime mover: triceps
   Standing with abdominals firm, feet apart for stability, grip the weight, palms up, and, keeping elbows near the ears, slowly lower bar behind the head. Pause, then press until elbows are fully extended.

J. Biceps curl
   Prime mover: biceps
   Grasp bar, palms up, holding bar about thigh level. Bend elbows, moving bar in an arc toward shoulders. Pause, then slowly return to starting position.

How to Begin and Progress

According to the ACSM, basic health fitness benefits can be obtained by lifting in a single set of 8 to 12 exercises. If time permits, you may choose to do multiple sets for optimal muscle fitness and muscle growth. A minimum of two to three intense workouts a week is recommended.

The first week, a beginner should lift for one set of 8 to 12 repetitions under the supervision of a trained professional. The first workouts should use light weights and concentrate on form, rhythm, and breathing. This will also minimize muscular soreness. The second week, an additional set can be added if desired, and the third week, a starting load can be established. Other weight training programs for goals of increasing muscular endurance, strength, or size are given in Table 6-1.

Establishing Your Workload

After several weeks of conditioning and working on lifting form, you may establish an appropriate workload. For each exercise find the maximum amount of weight you can lift once with good form (one **repetition maximum** or **1 RM**). In a general conditioning program, 75 percent of that weight will be your workload. In the workout, lift to fatigue at each station. If you can do fewer than 6 reps, the weight is too heavy. If you can do 12 or more reps at that load, the weight is too light. Increase or decrease the load in the next workout, if necessary. At the correct workload, the last 2 reps of each exercise should be difficult for you to do, and you should reach temporary muscular failure between 8 and 12 reps.

Increasing Your Workload

When you can do 12 reps, increase the amount of weight. If you can do at least 6 reps at the new weight, stay with that weight until you can do 12 reps. If, when you increase the weight, you cannot do at least 6 reps, drop back to your old weight and increase the number of reps each time until you can do 15. You should then be able to increase the weight and do at least 6 reps. In general:

- ✔ Increase only one variable at a time (reps, sets, resistance).
- ✔ Increase reps or sets first, then resistance.
- ✔ When increasing resistance, decrease reps.
- ✔ To increase muscular endurance, increase the number of reps or sets or decrease rest between sets.
- ✔ Increase the workload by no more than 5 to 10 percent each time.

Variety

You can incorporate variety into your workout by changing the workload, recovery period, number of sets, reps, rhythm, and number or order of lifts. Here are a few examples of different programs:

1. *Health fitness:* one to two sets of 8 to 12 reps at 70 to 75 percent 1 RM. Rest 1 to 2 minutes between sets.
2. *Muscular strength:* one to three sets of 5 to 8 reps at 80 to 90 percent 1 RM. Rest 2 to 4 minutes between sets.
3. *Muscular endurance:* one to three sets of 20 reps at 50 to 60 percent 1 RM. Rest 30 to 60 seconds between sets.
4. *Bone strength:* Two to three sets of 8 to 12 reps at 70 to 85 percent 1 RM. Rest 2 minutes between sets. Do two to three times per week.
5. *Eccentric emphasis (negatives):* Lift for two counts, lower for eight. Some experts say that lowering the weight is more important to strength development than is lifting it. This does tend to promote more muscle soreness. Strength increases occur with eccentric lifting alone, and because you can lower more weight than you can lift, you may need to increase resistance.
6. *Supersets:* Work opposite muscle groups immediately (triceps/biceps, hams/quads).
7. *Continuous set:* Lift to muscular exhaustion at your regular weight, lower one plate and lift to exhaustion, and continue to lower weight as you fatigue. This is a type of muscular endurance program. It is supposed to increase muscular definition. It can be done with machines but is difficult with free weights.
8. *Pyramid:* Lift 6 reps at 70 percent 1 RM, 4 reps at 80 percent 1 RM, 2 reps at 90 percent 1 RM, 1 rep at 100 percent 1 RM. This program emphasizes strength.
9. *Split routine:* Work upper body one day and lower body the next day or do pushers (e.g., quads, triceps) one day and pullers (e.g., hams, biceps) the next. You must work 4 to 6 days per week. This reduces total body fatigue but requires more time.
10. *Aerobic circuit:* A circuit is a group of exercises performed with little rest after each. Lighten weight to 40 to 60 percent of 1 RM. Lift quickly 30 seconds (15 to 20 lifts), then recover for 15 to 30 seconds, while switching to the next station and setting the weight. Alternate a leg station with an arm station as you proceed through the circuit. As the goal is aerobic conditioning, you may also include a jump rope, bench step, jumping jacks, or jogging in place station. Begin with one set of 10 to 12 exercises and work up to three sets, maintaining a target pulse. This is designed to strengthen the heart as well as develop muscular endurance. Be careful to maintain good form—it is easy to get sloppy and hurt yourself in this workout because the lifting rhythm is so quick.
11. *Muscle size (weight gain) program:* A bulk-up of three to five sets of 5, gradually increasing to 10 reps at 70 to 80 percent effort should be performed for several months to increase lean weight.
12. *Periodization:* Periodization involves changing training variables at regular time intervals while working for a specific event or fitness goal such as weight loss, increase in muscle mass, or muscular strength. The time period during which the training programs are cycled may be a year, a month, a week, or each workout. For example, a person may cycle workouts monthly: first month, muscular endurance; second, muscular strength; third, a split routine working on muscle size; and fourth, cross-training to recover from the other cycles. An advantage of periodization is that the variety of training helps develop balanced muscular fitness while preventing boredom, overtraining, and injury. Example: weeks 1–4: 2 sets of 15 to 20 reps; weeks 5–8: 3 sets of 5 to 8 reps; weeks 9–12: 5 sets of 5 to 10 reps; weeks 13–16: aerobic activities.

Common Discomforts and Training Errors

After lifting for a few weeks, you may notice a buildup of callus on your palms. If it bothers you, lifting gloves will offer some protection. If you experience nausea or light-headedness, stop and figure out the cause.

- ✔ Did you allow enough time since your last meal?
- ✔ Are you exhaling on the effort?
- ✔ Are you trying to progress too quickly?

If you experience pain, particularly joint pain, pay attention. It could be an early warning sign of injury. You may be lifting too heavy a weight or stressing your joints with poor form. Lifting too heavy a weight leads to poor form and increases the risk of injury. Jerking, straining, holding your breath, using momentum, bouncing, and arching the back are problems that need to be corrected. Have a professional check your form periodically to make sure you are not falling into bad habits.

Performance Aids

Many people take nutritional supplements or try other products that claim to increase strength, build muscle, or reduce fat. Unfortunately, most of these products do not live up to their advertised claims and are a waste of money, and some are even potentially dangerous.

Table 6-5 lists several performance aids used by weight trainers and their effects and side effects.

How to Shape and Tone Without Weights

There are many ways to develop muscular strength and endurance. While weight training is an excellent program, it is not always convenient. The programs described next can be done at home or while traveling. The abdominal and core strengthening, hip and thigh, and upper-body programs require no special equipment. Partner exercises add a social dimension to a workout. Elastic resistance produces results without bulky equipment, which makes it easy to exercise on a trip.

While weights add intensity to a workout, they are not always necessary when the goal is to shape and tone. Muscles develop firmness by working against a resistance, and that resistance can be your body weight. These programs emphasize muscular endurance rather than strength by increasing time in contraction or reps. Core trunk muscles in particular benefit from a muscular endurance routine because their function is one of endurance—sustained contraction. If you would like a total body program, combine this with the upper body routine that follows.

TABLE 6-5   *Performance Aids Promoted to Weight Trainers*

Substance	Advertised Claim	Effects/Side Effects
Amino acid and protein supplements	Muscle growth	May cause unbalanced protein metabolism, dehydration, gout, liver and kidney disease, calcium excretion
Anabolic steroids	Increased muscle mass, strength	Increased muscle mass, strength, aggression, testicular atrophy, acne, impotence, masculinizes women
Caffeine	Increased endurance	Increased endurance, nervousness, tremors
Chromium	Muscle growth	No effect on body composition or strength
Clenbuterol and beta 2 agonists	Increased muscle mass, cuts fat	Rapid heart rate, tremor, anxiety, headache, no proven effect on strength or endurance
Creatine monohydrate	Increased energy, muscle growth	Increased power in short-term high-intensity exercise, weight gain, muscle cramps, increased risk of heat stroke, decreased endurance
Ephedrine and other stimulants	Increased energy	Anxiety, tremor, cardiac arrhythmia. Increased risk of heat stroke due to cardiac and central nervous system effects
Growth hormone	Increased muscle size, strength	Slight increase in fat-free mass and water. No increase in strength or endurance. Acromegaly, diabetes, hypothyroidism
HNB (beta-hydroxy beta-methybutyrate)	Enhanced strength and body composition	No benefit for strength or body composition in trained individuals
Megadose vitamins	Increased energy, strength	No benefit. Excess water-soluble excreted. Excess fat-soluble can be toxic (see Chapter 10). Excess of one vitamin may decrease absorption of others

SOURCE: Randy Eichner, "Ergogenic Aids: What Athletes Are Using—and Why," *Physician and Sports Medicine* 25 (April 1997) 70; S. Powers and E. T. Hurley, *Exercise Physiology*, New York: McGraw-Hill, 2001.

Abdominal and Core Strengthening Exercises

Core trunk stabilizers include all the trunk muscles—the abdominals and the hip and back muscles—which support the body, hold us upright, absorb and transmit forces, and enable us to twist, turn, and bend. Trunk strength is important because it provides a base of stability and power from which the arms and legs work. Most functional movements originate in or rely on trunk stability for efficient performance. Weakness in the trunk musculature increases stress on joints, ligaments, and tendons; impedes performance; and increases the risk of injury. Strong core stabilizers make the body more efficient and decrease the risk of back pain or injury. They also improve posture, appearance, breathing, and athletic performance.

A set of strengthening exercises for abdominals (1–9), gluteus (10, 11), and back muscles (12, 13) is shown in Figure 6-5. The exercises should be performed at a

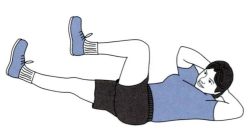

(1) Bicycle exercise

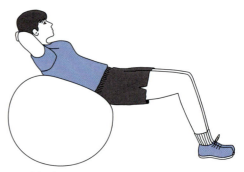

(2) Abdominal crunch on stability ball

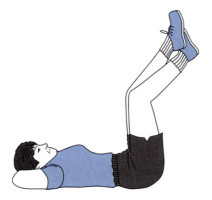

(3) Vertical leg crunch

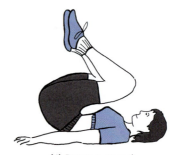

(4) Reverse crunch

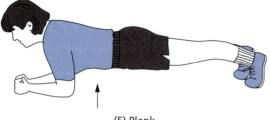

(5) Plank

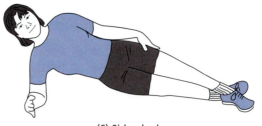

(6) Side plank

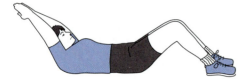

(7) Long arm crunch

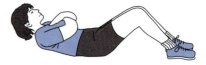

(8) Abdominal curl "crunch"

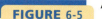

FIGURE 6-5 Abdominal and core strengthening exercises.

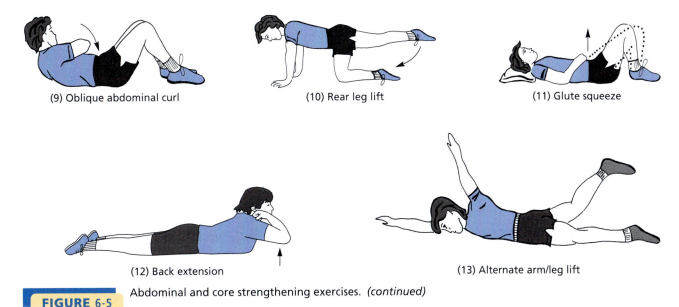

(9) Oblique abdominal curl   (10) Rear leg lift   (11) Glute squeeze

(12) Back extension   (13) Alternate arm/leg lift

FIGURE 6-5   Abdominal and core strengthening exercises. *(continued)*

slow, steady pace with equal effort in both directions. Lift two counts and lower two counts—don't just lift and fall out of the contraction. The abdominal exercises chosen include those listed as most effective in a study by Peter Francis at San Diego State University. Core muscles can be worked 3 to 5 days a week because they are endurance muscles designed for sustained contraction. You will want a mat or carpeted surface to work on.

1. Bicycle exercise
   Lie on your back with hands behind your head. Raise knees to a 45-degree angle and slowly do a bicycle pedaling motion as shown in Figure 6-5 (1). Touch right elbow to left knee and left elbow to right knee.
2. Abdominal crunch on stability ball
   Lie on stability ball with feet flat on floor, thighs and trunk parallel to floor. Cross arms behind shoulders or across chest; contract abdominals by raising trunk about 45 degrees. Spread feet apart for better balance. To work obliques more, bring feet closer together.
3. Vertical leg crunch
   Lie on your back with legs raised in the air, knees slightly bent and crossed at the ankles. Cross hands behind the shoulders to support the head. Keep chin lifted to prevent jerking the head. Lift the trunk and slowly lower.
4. Reverse crunch
   Lie on the back with ankles crossed, feet off the ground, and knees at about a 90-degree angle. Place arms on the floor beside your trunk. Press lower back to the ground, contract the abdominals, and rotate hips 1 to 2 inches. Your feet will lift slightly toward the ceiling with each contraction.

5. Plank
   Lie as in Figure 6-5 (5), face down, propped with elbows under chest, palms down. Lift up on toes and tighten back and abdominals, keeping body straight and head and spine neutral. Hold 10 to 60 seconds, rest, repeat. If a straight-back position is too difficult, begin with hips hiked up or hold the contraction a shorter amount of time. Do not let the hips sag.
6. Side plank
   Lie as in Figure 6-5 (6) on side with weight balanced between forearm, palm, and feet. Contract back and abdominals to hold body straight. Do not push hips out behind the body. Hold 10 to 30 seconds, rest, repeat on the other side. If a full-body position is too difficult, begin with the half-plank, balancing weight between knees and forearm. For an advanced version, try lifting the top foot in the air for 5 to 10 seconds.
7. Long arm crunch
   Lie on your back with knees bent and heels next to buttocks. Extend arms alongside your ears, chin raised, eyes focused on ceiling. Contract abdominals, keeping lower back to floor, lift shoulders as for a basic crunch, lower slowly.
8. Abdominal curl "crunch"
   Lie on your back with knees bent, heels next to buttocks. Place hands across chest or behind shoulders. Keep eyes focused on ceiling, chin up and about a fist's distance from your chest. Contract your abdominals; do not jerk your head forward as you curl. Keeping lower back on the ground, curl shoulders up 3 inches and slowly lower.

9. Oblique abdominal curl
   Lie on the back as for the basic crunch but add a twist, bringing right elbow toward left knee, then left elbow toward right knee. Elbow does not have to touch knee.

10. Rear leg lift (gluteus)
    On hands and knees, hollow abdomen and round back to protect it. Extend right leg to the rear. Tense gluteus. Raise and lower leg slowly six to eight counts. Repeat left.

11. Glute squeeze
    Lying on back with knees bent, squeeze gluteus hard, raising hips no more than 3 inches from floor. Do not arch back. Hold for a count of five, relax, repeat.

12. Back extension
    Lie on your stomach with feet on the floor, head neutral, hands touching shoulders. Slowly lift head, shoulders, and chest. Hold 5 to 10 seconds, then slowly lower. Variation: Squeeze shoulder blades in toward spine while holding trunk lift.

13. Alternate arm/leg lift
    Lie on your stomach with arms extended in front. Raise right arm while lifting left leg. Hold 5 to 10 seconds. Repeat on other side. Keep head neutral.

Hip and Thigh Exercises

These exercises (Figure 6-6) will not burn calories as aerobic work will, and so if you want to remove inches, diet and aerobic exercise are still important. Also, fat will not burn off only in the area exercised. While you can't spot reduce fat, say, in the thighs by doing leg lifts, you can spot tone flabby muscles. Be patient and you may begin to see a difference in 8 to 12 weeks. You do not need to count repetitions. Select one exercise for each body area and perform it for 1 minute. Start with one set and build up to two sets, 3 days a week. Variations are given to add variety to your program. If you wish to add intensity without purchasing weights, a sand-filled sock can be tied on as an ankle weight. You will want a mat or carpeted surface to work on.

A. Outer hip (hip abductors)
   1. Lying side leg lift
      Lying on one side, head resting on arm and lower leg bent for balance, slowly raise and lower top leg.
      Variations: This can be done standing. Keep foot level and leg lifting directly to side, not toward front.
   2. Kneeling side leg lift
      Take a hands and knees position with one leg extended to side.
      Tighten abdominals and round back to protect it. You may also support weight on one forearm if desired. Tense hip and raise and lower leg slowly no higher than 6 inches.
      Variations: Circle leg forward, then reverse.

B. Inner thigh (thigh adductors)
   1. Inner thigh lift
      Lying on left side, raise and lower left leg, keeping foot turned to side (not upward). Repeat right. To increase resistance, press gently

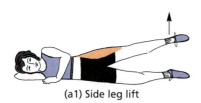

(a1) Side leg lift

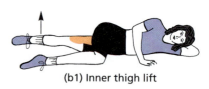

(b1) Inner thigh lift

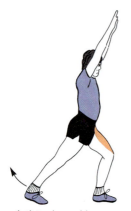

(c1) Backward lunge

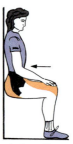

(c2) Wall sit

FIGURE 6-6   Hip and thigh exercises.

on left calf with right foot as you raise and lower leg or add an ankle weight.

2. Plié
   Standing with feet 3 feet apart and knees bent, place hands lightly on inner thighs. Press thighs against hands, pulling in hard for a count of five. Repeat.

C. Quadriceps, hamstrings

1. Backward lunge (quadriceps and hamstrings)
   Keeping shoulders erect and weight centered over right foot, step back and touch lightly with left foot and then return to starting position. Repeat. Switch legs after 1 minute of reps.

2. Wall sit (quads)
   Hold a sitting position with back against a wall for balance. Keep hips above knee level.

Upper Body Exercises

Upper body exercises can improve appearance by straightening rounded shoulders, firming upper arm muscles, and toning pectorals that underlie and support the breasts. You do not need to count repetitions. Select one exercise for each body area and repeat for 1 minute. If you wish to increase resistance, bricks, books, or cans of food can serve as hand weights. Upper body exercises are illustrated in Figure 6-7.

A. Push-up (pectorals/triceps)
   These may be done standing, with hands against a wall and feet placed about 3 feet away from the wall (easiest), on the floor with knees bent (medium), or with weight supported on hands and feet (hardest). Keep abdominals firm and hips slightly flexed to support back. Lower to right angles of arms and then press back to arm extension.
   Variations: Keeping hands close emphasizes triceps. Keeping hands wide increases pectoral strengthening.

B. Dip (pectorals/triceps)
   Dips are an alternative way to tone the same muscle groups that push-ups tone. They may be done on a dip bar or using chairs. With weight

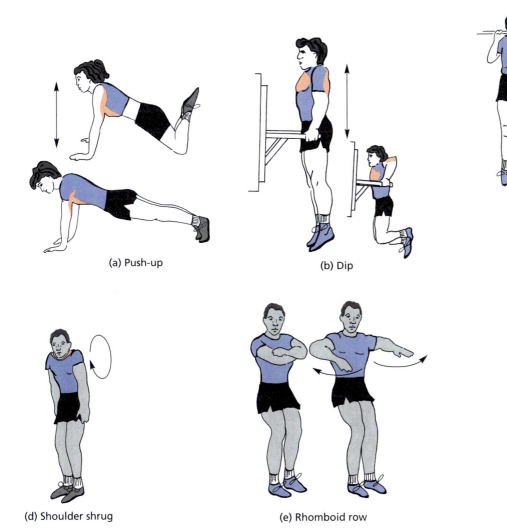

(a) Push-up   (b) Dip   (c) Negative pull-up

(d) Shoulder shrug   (e) Rhomboid row

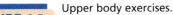

FIGURE 6-7   Upper body exercises.

evenly distributed between bars or two sturdy chairs, place a hand on each. Bend knees or extend legs so that weight is on arms, not feet. Bend arms to right angles and return to extension.

C. Negative pull-up (latissimus dorsi/biceps)

Negative pull-ups offer the same benefits as full pull-ups for upper back and arms. Stand on a chair if necessary to grasp a pull-up bar with arms flexed. SLOWLY lower yourself to a count of five. As you gain strength over several weeks, try to start with a few full pull-ups and finish with negatives.

D. Shoulder shrug (trapezius)

Shoulder shrugs can tighten upper back muscles to reduce rounded shoulders. Combine this with pectoral stretches for best results. Rotate shoulders in full circles—up-back-down—working to pull shoulder blades together.

Variations: Add resistance by holding a weight in each hand.

E. Rhomboid row (rhomboids)

Rhomboids are muscles that pull the shoulder blades back, down, and together. These also need to be strengthened to reduce rounded shoulders. With arms slightly below shoulder level, elbows bent, pull elbows fully back, squeezing shoulder blades together, and hold for a count of five. Rest two counts. Repeat.

Stability Balls

The stability ball is a large inflatable rubber ball also known as a Swiss ball, fitness ball, or balance ball. It has long been used in physical therapy because it introduces an element of instability to which the body naturally responds by contracting core trunk muscles to keep the spine in neutral alignment and stay balanced over the ball. It can be used in a fitness class or at home for a variety of exercises to increase muscular fitness, core strength, posture, and balance, because you must maintain a stable trunk throughout each exercise. To start, you can use it for abdominal crunches, obliques, and back extensions. You can also sit on the ball and exercise with hand weights to build core strength and balance. Many stores offer introductory videos or DVDs along with the equipment so that you can learn to use it in an effective manner.

Stability Ball Exercise Guidelines

✔ To choose a ball size—when you sit on the ball, your knees should be at a 90-degree angle and your thighs parallel to the floor.

✔ The ball should be inflated so that it is firm but can still contour to your body. Do not inflate it until it is "hard."

✔ It is important to maintain good posture while working out. Keep your abdominals tight to protect your lower back. Avoid back and neck hyperextension.

✔ Do each exercise slowly.

✔ If you have never used a ball, start with sitting on the ball and rocking the hips, then try the easiest skills like back extension or bridging. Place the ball against a wall or keep your hands and/or feet on the floor for stability.

✔ Attempt more difficult skills only after mastering the easier exercises.

✔ Strength exercises should be done for 8–12 repetitions.

Stability Ball Exercises   Here are 10 exercises that you can do with a stability ball. They are illustrated in Figure 6-8.

1. Push-up (pectorals, triceps)

Kneel facing the ball. Roll forward to lie on top of the ball. Reach forward, placing your hands on the floor. Walk your hands out until the ball is under your thighs. Tighten your abdominals, keeping your body straight. Bend your elbows, then lower your upper body toward the floor. Your body should be straight from shoulders to ankles. Push back to the starting position. To increase difficulty, roll the ball back so only your shins or feet are resting on it.

2. Knee tuck press (deltoids, triceps)

Kneel on the stability ball and place hands on the floor. Bend your elbows, then lower your upper body toward the floor. Push up from this position.

3. Shoulder roll-out from knees (back extensors, rectus abdominis)

Kneeling on the floor, place hands on the stability ball. Roll it forward and back, keeping back straight and abdominals tight.

4. Back wall squat (quadriceps, gluteus maximus, hamstrings)

Stand and press the ball against a wall with your back. Position feet shoulder width apart and forward as if you are going to sit in a chair. Bend your knees, rolling the ball down until your knees are at a 90-degree angle and your thighs are parallel to the floor. Keeping your back pressed against the ball, hold for five counts. Straighten your knees and return to the starting position.

5. Ball transfer (rectus abdominis)

Lie on your back with hands resting on the floor and grip ball between your ankles. Curl the pelvis to lift the ball off the floor into the air, reach up, and transfer it to your hands, then back to your ankles.

6. Prone knee tuck (rectus abdominis)

Place shins on the stability ball and hands on the floor. Roll the ball back away from your hands, keeping shoulders aligned with hands,

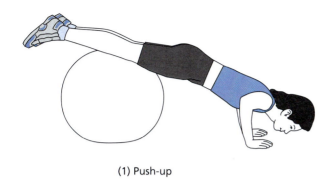

(1) Push-up

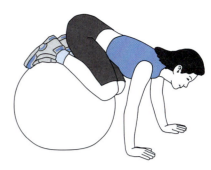

(2) Knee tuck press

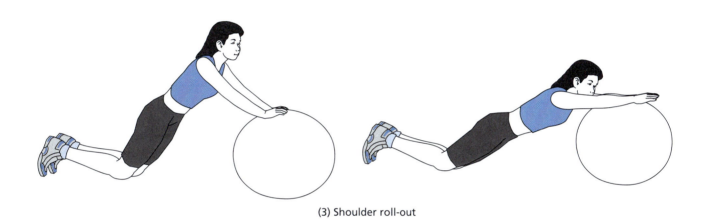

(3) Shoulder roll-out

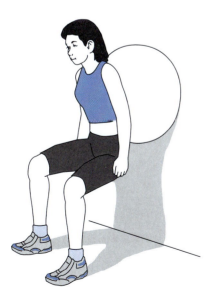

(4) Back wall squat

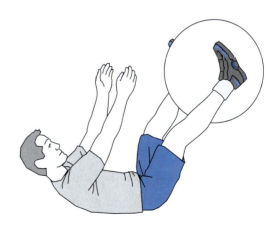

(5) Ball transfer

FIGURE 6-8   Stability ball exercises.

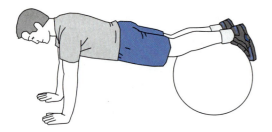

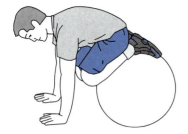

(6) Prone knee tuck

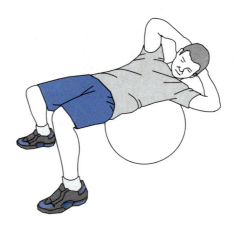

(7) Oblique curl

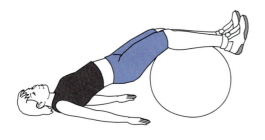

(8) Bridge

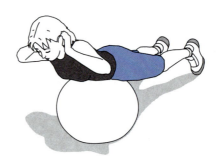

(9) Back extension

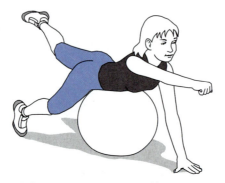

(10) Prone opposite arm and leg raise

FIGURE 6-8   Stability ball exercises. *(continued)*

abdominals tight, body straight. Extend legs, then bend knees in toward your chest and roll the ball forward until your knees are at your chest. To increase difficulty, try from a bent elbow position on the floor.

7. Oblique curl (rectus abdominis, external and internal oblique abdominals)

   Lie with the top of the ball beneath the center of your back, feet spread wide on the floor for stability. Rotate hips to one side and slowly curl the right side of the upper body toward the left leg. Return to starting position; repeat alternating sides.

8. Bridge (back extensors, gluteus maximus, hamstrings)

   Lie on your back with legs on the ball, hands resting beside you on the floor. Slowly lift hips until your back is straight and weight is on your upper back. Pause, then return slowly to the starting position. Avoid pressing the neck into the floor or arching the back. To make it easier, place ball under knees. To make it harder, place under heels.

9. Back extension (back extensors)

   Lie prone with hips on the ball, feet on the floor and trunk slightly flexed. Arms may be at your sides or behind shoulders. Tighten your upper back, slowly raising shoulders until the spine is straight or slightly extended. Keep head neutral to avoid neck hyperextension. Hold, then relax slowly to starting position. Repeat.

10. Prone opposite arm/leg raise (back extensors, gluteus maximus, hamstrings, deltoids)

    Lying prone on the ball, extend right leg behind you, foot touching floor. Keep head neutral. Reach in front with the left arm, raising it close to your ear. Lift the arm and leg slowly at the same time, pause as you reach extension, then lower slowly. Repeat alternating sides.

Pilates

Pilates is a program that originally was used by dancers to improve core muscle strength, balance, muscle control, and flexibility. It now is being offered in fitness centers and is enjoyed by many exercisers for its health benefits. Development of strength and control in abdominal and back muscles is important for preventing back pain. Pilates emphasizes proper breathing, correct spinal and pelvic alignment, and concentration on smooth, flowing movement. It incorporates a series of group mat exercises and Pilates exercise equipment that uses springs to create resistance. If you are interested in trying Pilates, many fitness centers offer introductory sessions and many fitness retailers have videos or DVDs available for home use.

Elastic Resistance

Elastic resistance exercise was developed in the 1950s. It was originally used by physical therapists who gave patients surgical rubber tubing to add resistance to rehabilitative exercise programs. Elastic bands and tubing are lightweight, portable, and readily available at fitness centers and medical supply companies. They are inexpensive but do not last forever and need to be replaced as they wear out. Safety tips are listed in the Top 10 "Tips for Elastic Resistance Exercise." They come in different strengths, based on the thickness of the elastic. Thin bands are best for beginners and for upper body work. Thicker bands are useful for lower body work. Two thin bands can be used in place of one thick band. The principles of form, rhythm, and breathing apply here as for any strength training program. Elastic resistance exercises are illustrated in Figure 6-9.

Elastic Resistance Exercises

A. Squat (gluteus maximus, quadriceps, hamstrings, biceps)

   Step on the band with feet about shoulder width apart and hold ends of the band low enough to feel moderate tension. Slowly squat until hips are just above knees, bending elbows to maintain tension in the band. Return to standing.

B. Leg extension (quadriceps)

   Tie band around ankles. Lie back, knees bent and feet on floor. Keeping knees and thighs together, straighten knee, lifting the foot as high as possible. Release slowly and repeat. Change legs.

C. Hamstring curl (hamstrings, gluteus maximus)

   Place the band around ankles. Lie face down with arms under the chin or hands under hips. Bending knee, slowly lift one foot. Release slowly, maintaining some tension in the band. Repeat. Change legs.

D. Side leg lift (hip abductors)

   Place the band around both legs—around ankles is hardest, around knees easiest. Lying on right side, torso supported by arms, slightly bend lower leg for support. Keep hips facing forward and lift upper leg. Lower, keeping tension on the band, and repeat. Change sides.

E. Inner thigh lift (thigh adductors)

   Place band around left arch and right ankle. Lie on right side with trunk supported by arms. Lift bottom leg slowly, hold briefly, lower slowly, repeat. Switch sides.

F. Three-way leg pointer (gluteus maximus, gluteus medius, quadriceps).

   Place band around ankles. Place hand on wall for support. Keeping abdominals firm and back straight, pull foot back, return, to the side, return, and forward, return. Repeat with other leg.

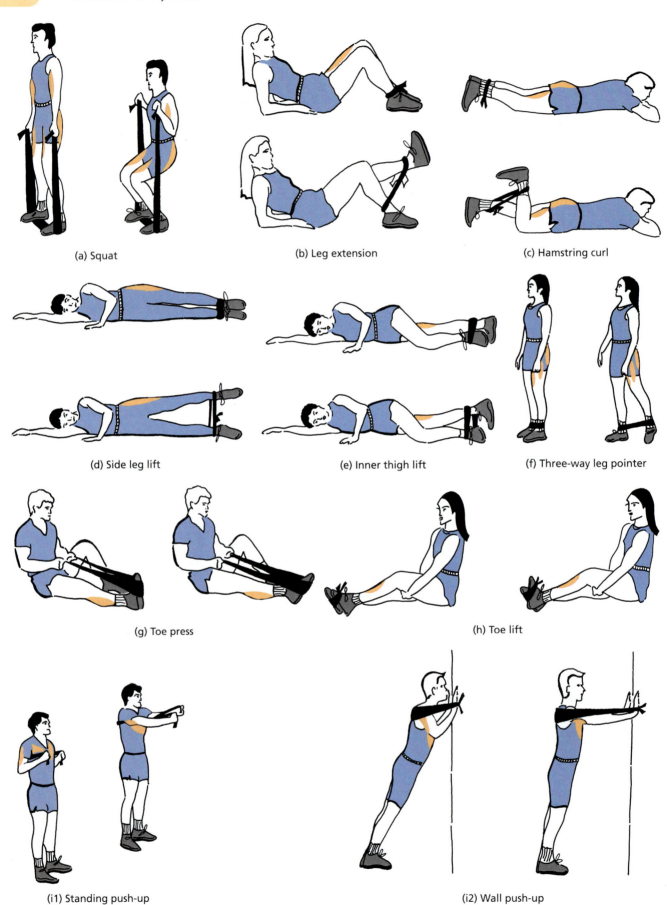

(a) Squat

(b) Leg extension

(c) Hamstring curl

(d) Side leg lift

(e) Inner thigh lift

(f) Three-way leg pointer

(g) Toe press

(h) Toe lift

(i1) Standing push-up

(i2) Wall push-up

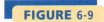

FIGURE 6-9   Elastic resistance exercises.

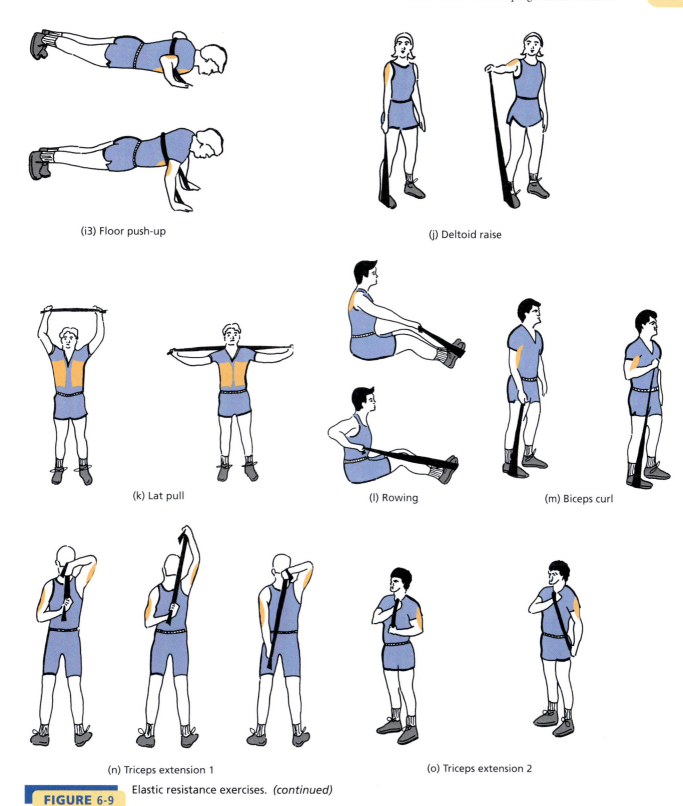

(i3) Floor push-up

(j) Deltoid raise

(k) Lat pull

(l) Rowing

(m) Biceps curl

(n) Triceps extension 1

(o) Triceps extension 2

FIGURE 6-9   Elastic resistance exercises. *(continued)*

TOP **10** LIST

Tips for Elastic Resistance Exercise

Exercising with elastic bands has its risks as well as its benefits. To maximize your results and minimize the risk of getting snapped by an elastic band, follow these tips:

1. *Check the band for tears before every workout.* Do not use it if it shows cracks or tears because it may break.
2. *Point the band away from your face.* Never point it toward another person.
3. *Keep a towel handy to wipe off sweat.* Sweat makes the band slippery.
4. *Leave slight tension on the band between reps.* This maximizes muscle toning. Do not let the band go slack.
5. *Wear socks.* This prevents the band from biting into the ankles in leg exercises.
6. *Men may want to wear exercise pants.* This will prevent the band from ripping out leg hair.
7. *Keep the wrist in line with the forearm.* Wrist hyperextension, a common mistake in lat pulls and bicep curls, stresses the carpal joints of the wrist.
8. *Stretch the band slowly and release slowly.* Use a controlled rhythm—pull 2 seconds, hold briefly, release 2 seconds. Begin with 30 seconds of repetitions and work up to 1 minute for each exercise. One to two sets is a good goal.
9. *Progress to a stronger band.* Or add a second band to progress when the workout gets too easy (eventually it will).
10. *Powder the band lightly with cornstarch after use to keep it in good condition.*

G. Toe press (gastrocnemius, soleus)

Holding ends of band, place around ball of foot. With knee straight, slowly press through ball of foot from extension to flexion and back (gastrocnemius). To emphasize soleus, repeat with knee slightly bent.

H. Toe lift (tibialis anterior)

Tie band around arches. Place heels about 6 inches apart forward to back. Keeping one foot pointed, pull toes of the other foot back toward your face. Relax. Repeat on both feet.

I. Push-up (pectorals, biceps)

Three styles of push-ups are described here from easiest to most challenging. Use the style appropriate for your current strength level.

1. Standing push-up: Wrap the band around your back and under your arms. Bend elbows and grasp ends of band. Extend arms forward, then return slowly.

2. Wall push-up: Tie ends of the band together and wrap around your shoulders and under palms, with hands about shoulder width apart. Place feet about 3 feet from the wall. Extend arms, then return.
3. Floor push-up: Trap ends of the band under hands. Keep abdominals tight and back straight to protect it as you bend and extend arms.

J. Deltoid raise (deltoid, triceps)

Place one end of band under foot and hold the other end by your hip. Standing with good posture, lift arm to shoulder level, lower slowly.

K. Lat pull (latissimus dorsi)

Hold band overhead, elbows extended but not locked. Pull arms apart to shoulder level. Be careful not to get hair caught in band.

L. Rowing (rhomboids)

With band around arches and knees extended, grasp band about mid-shin. Pull elbows back and try to bring shoulder blades together. Release slowly.

M. Biceps curl (biceps)

Place one end of band under foot, grasp other end low, and, keeping elbow at your side, curl right arm to shoulder. Slowly release.

N. Triceps extension 1 (triceps)

Standing with good posture, grasp both ends of band behind your back. Extend upper arm toward ceiling, pause, then slowly release, pressing lower hand toward hip.

O. Triceps extension 2 (triceps)

Standing with good posture, grasp ends of band. Press lower hand toward hip, pause, then slowly release. Do both arms.

Partner Resistance Exercises

Exercising with a partner can be both challenging and enjoyable. Partner communication and sensitivity to your levels of strength and fatigue are important. The partner must vary resistance for different muscle groups and increase resistance during the eccentric part of each contraction. While many of these exercises can be done without equipment, to add variety, you may wish to try them using a towel to pull on (biceps curls) or a broomstick (overhead press). This is a balanced program of four lower body and five upper body exercises. You may either count reps or perform each exercise for a minute and work up to two or three sets (Figure 6-10).

A. Leg extension (quadriceps)

Sit on a bench or chair. Move one leg from flexion to full extension and back as partner resists by pressing on front of lower leg.

B. Hamstring curl (hamstrings, gluteus)

Lie face down while partner straddles your back and places a hand on each ankle. Bend knees and curl calves toward buttocks as your partner resists.

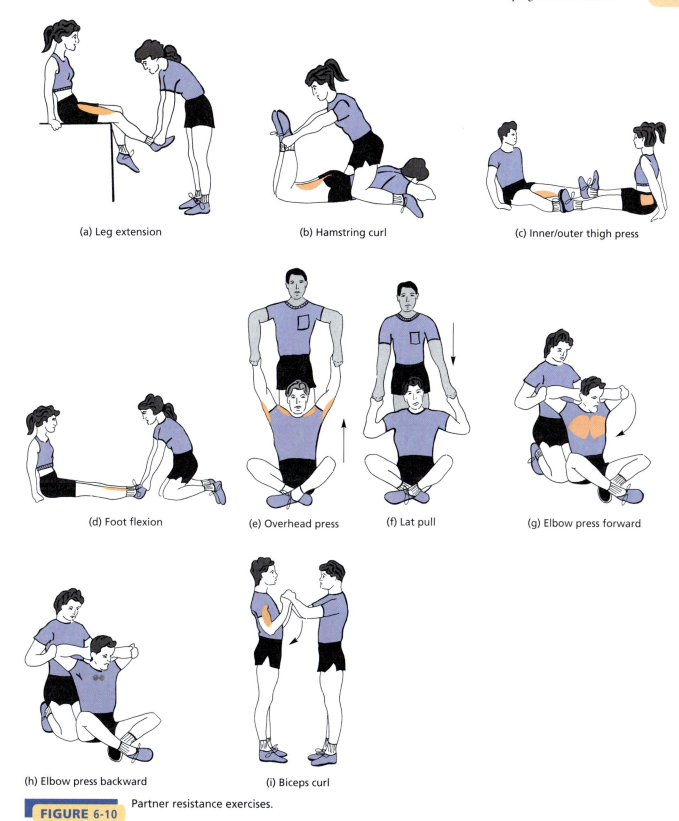

(a) Leg extension

(b) Hamstring curl

(c) Inner/outer thigh press

(d) Foot flexion

(e) Overhead press

(f) Lat pull

(g) Elbow press forward

(h) Elbow press backward

(i) Biceps curl

FIGURE 6-10   Partner resistance exercises.

Continue the resistance as you return to the starting position.

C. Inner/outer thigh press (thigh adductors and abductors)

Sit, facing each other, legs forward, hands behind hips for balance. One partner places both feet inside the other's feet and presses outward as the other partner resists by pressing inward. Switch positions after six to eight reps.

D. Foot flexion (anterior tibialis)

Sit with legs extended. Partner kneels and presses down on top of both feet as you flex them and then return to extension.

E. Overhead press (deltoids, triceps)

Sit with hands at shoulder level, palms up. As partner resists, press up toward ceiling and then return to starting position.

F. Lat pull (latissimus dorsi)

Sit and reach high overhead to grasp partner's hands. As partner resists, pull down to shoulder level and slowly return to starting position.

G. Elbow press forward (pectorals)

Sit with elbows out and hands touching shoulders. As partner resists at the elbows, pull them in toward your midline and return to starting position.

H. Elbow press backward (rhomboids)

Sit with elbows out or with arms crossed. Partner sits behind, pressing on your elbows as you press back, pulling shoulder blades together. As partner continues resistance, return to starting position.

I. Biceps curl (biceps)

Stand, palms facing upward. Partner resists on your palms as you curl arm from extension to flexion and back. This may also be done holding a towel in one hand in front of body. Partner sits or kneels facing you, resisting on other end of towel as you curl your arm.

Frequently Asked Questions

Q. Should I eat more protein to build muscle if I weight train?

A. Research has shown that the primary fuel for muscle is carbohydrate, in the form of glycogen. The American Dietetics Association (ADA) does not support the belief that the protein needs of a weight lifter are greater than average. The body is unable to store extra protein, and excess protein is converted to fat, not used to build muscle. The average American already consumes 1½ to 2 times the RDA of protein. Excess protein can also promote dehydration and loss of calcium, which can increase risk of osteoporosis. The ADA states that a balanced diet will supply all the protein a weight trainer needs. Exercise scientists and dieticians agree that if you want to build muscle, you should concentrate on a well-balanced diet combined with resistance training.

Q. How good is the abdominal equipment shown in TV infomercials?

A. There is no piece of equipment that tones abdominals better than the abdominal exercises in Figure 6-7. Before you rush out to buy the newest advertised piece of abdominal gear, ask yourself if you will use it regularly. Be skeptical of any equipment that promises effortless results, spot reduction, burning more calories, or greater weight loss than other methods. While you can spot tone, you can't wear the fat off just one body area. Loss of abdominal fat requires regular exercise that works the whole body as well as cutting back on calories. Before you decide, go to a gym or fitness center and try out various types of equipment to see what you like and what meets your needs.

Q. How can I tone my lower abdominal muscles?

A. Based on electromyographic studies of people doing various types of abdominal and core exercises, people cannot selectively recruit upper versus lower abdominal muscles. The rectus abdominis acts as a sheet and contracts as a whole. During certain exercises, like leg lifts, a person may feel greater fatigue in the lower abdominal region because the iliopsoas "hip flexor" is being worked, and it originates below the lower abdominal region. A person can selectively train transverse abdominals, which connect hip-to-hip, by contracting the abdominals, trying to pull the navel toward the spine, holding for 5 seconds, and repeating four to five times.

Q. What do I do if I hit a plateau in weight training?

A. While initial progress may be rapid, after about 6 months of strength training, a plateau is common. If you have been doing the same program for months, it is time to vary the routine. You may benefit from changing the sequence of exercises so that muscles are fatigued in a different order. You can replace some of the exercises with one that strengthens the same muscle group (e.g., fly instead of chest press or squats instead of leg press). If you have been lifting more than 12 repetitions of a weight, increasing the intensity and dropping the number of repetitions will make the muscles work harder. Also, make sure that you are giving your muscles sufficient recovery time, at least 48 hours between workouts.

Q. Why should I add resistance exercises to my exercise program?

A. Strength training is an important part of a balanced fitness program. Stronger muscles help prevent injury, improve your ability to participate in sports, and prevent loss of muscle fibers that begins around age 25.

Q. Does strength training decrease risk for osteoporosis?

A. Bones are living tissue, constantly remodeling to the stresses placed on them. Without weight-bearing exercise, bones demineralize. They require the regular stimulus of weight-bearing exercise to take up bone mineral. Walking and jogging using the resistance of body weight are excellent leg and hip-bone strengtheners. Weight training at an intensity of 70 to 85 percent of 1 RM, two to three sets of 8 to 12 repetitions, 2 to 3 days per week has been shown to produce a gradual increase in bone density, which decreases risk of osteoporosis. Like muscle, the rule is "use it or lose it."

Q. Which is better, free weights or machines?

A. It depends on your goals. A beginner will improve with overload from either system. Machines are safer and you don't need a spotter, but they are expensive to buy or you need access to a gym. With free weights, you need a spotter for safety, but they are inexpensive, and so you can have a set at home. Free weights allow a greater variety of exercises than do machines and develop balance, timing, and muscular fitness, and so many athletes prefer them. If you have access to both, start with machines, and as you gain strength, gradually work in a few free weight exercises to see which you like better.

Q. I just started a weight-training program. How long until I see results?

A. Rate of improvement varies with individuals—some gain quickly, others more slowly. If you are lifting 2

to 3 days a week using a general program of one to two sets of 8 to 12 reps at 75 percent of 1 RM, you may begin increasing reps or load within 3 to 4 weeks. The most rapid gains are seen in the first 6 months, but people can continue to improve for years. Other factors affecting rate of improvement include good nutrition, adequate recovery between workouts, and sufficient sleep.

Q. Should I take creatine to help build muscle mass? Is it safe?

A. Creatine supplements appear to enhance performance in repeated bursts of maximal activities such as weight lifting. Research is ongoing to see if it really increases muscle mass or weight due to water retention. Potential adverse effects include muscle cramps, diarrhea and gastrointestinal pain, and dehydration and kidney dysfunction. Long-term effects on other sites, including the brain, heart, liver, and reproductive organs, are not known. Creatine is considered a dietary supplement and not a drug, and so a manufacturer's claims of performance and safety do not have to be substantiated by the U.S. Food and Drug Administration.

Q. I have been doing 100 abdominal crunches a day for 6 weeks, and still my abdominals aren't flat. Why? They feel really strong and tight.

A. A layer of fat often overlays the abdominals, giving them a rounded appearance. Crunches will strengthen the abdominals, making them feel firm. If you are overweight, diet will help reduce the fat layer to get the results you seek. If you are of normal weight, check your posture—habitually standing with an overarched lower back will make the abdominals protrude even if they are firm.

Q. When I stop exercising, will my muscles turn into fat?

A. No. Muscle and fat (adipose tissue) are made up of different types of cells. Lack of exercise allows muscles to atrophy and turn flabby. Without exercise, a person burns fewer calories and may add pounds of fat. Muscle tissue can no more be turned into fat tissue than a cat can be turned into a dog!

Summary

Muscular strength and muscular endurance exercises are a vital supplement to a regular program of aerobic exercise. They can enhance appearance by improving the shape, firmness, and tone of muscles. Enhanced posture, decreased risk of lower back pain, greater ease of movement, improved athletic performance, and more energy are benefits. While injury is possible in any exercise program if safety guidelines are ignored, sensible strengthening programs decrease the risk of injury for those who participate in health-related fitness programs or athletics.

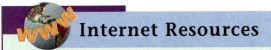

Internet Resources

American College of Sports Medicine
www.acsm.org/sportsmed
Provides information on sports research and health and fitness, aerobic exercise guidelines, and a quarterly fitness newsletter. "Current Comments" gives information on a variety of exercise topics of recent interest.

American Council on Exercise
www.acefitness.org
Has fitfacts information sheets on over 100 different health and fitness topics, health and fitness tips, fitness questions and answers, healthy recipes, and a free monthly e-newsletter on health and fitness topics.

ExRx.net
www.exrx.net
Exercise information including weight training, fitness testing, bodybuilding, anabolic steroids, and weight management.

National Strength and Conditioning Association
www.nsca-lift.org
Provides research-based information on strength training and conditioning for improving fitness and athletic performance.

Bibliography

Adams, K. J. "Strength, Power and the Baby Boomer." *Current Comment from the American College of Sports Medicine* (January 2002) www.acsm.org

Ahmed, C., et al. "Relations of Strength Training to Body Image among a Sample of Female University Students." *Journal of Strength and Conditioning Research* 16 (December 2002): 645–648.

American College of Sports Medicine. *ACSM's Guidelines for Exercise Testing and Prescription,* 5th ed. Philadelphia: Lippincott Williams & Wilkins, 2006.

American College of Sports Medicine. "Selecting and Effectively Using Free Weights" (2003). www.acsm.org

Anders, M. "New Study Puts the Crunch on Ineffective Ab Exercises." *ACE Fitness Matters* (May/June 2001): 9–11.

Baldi, J. C., and N. Snowling. "Resistance Training Improves Glycaemic Control in Obese Type 2 Diabetic Men." *International Journal of Sports Medicine* 24 (August 2003): 419–423.

Banz, W. J., et al. "Effects of Resistance versus Aerobic Training on Coronary Artery Disease Risk Factors." *Experimental Biology and Medicine* 228 (April 2003): 434–440.

Cole, A. J. "Lumbar Stabilization Exercises" (June 6, 2001). www.spine-health.com

Conley, M. S., and R. Rozenel. "Health Aspects of Resistance Exercise and Training." *Strength and Conditioning Journal* 23 (December 2001): 9–23.

Consumer Reports. "A Safer, Livelier Way to Strengthen Your Body's Core Muscles." *Consumer Reports on Health* (April 2005): 8–10.

Cussler, E. C., et al. "Weight Lifted in Strength Training Predicts Bone Change in Postmenopausal Women." *Medicine & Science in Sports & Exercise* 35 (January 2003): 10–17.

Deschenes, M. R., and W. J. Kraemer. "Performance and Physiologic Adaptations to Resistance Training." *American Journal of Physical Medicine and Rehabilitation* 81 (November 2002): S3–16.

Evetovich, T., and K. Eversole. "Adaptations to Resistance Training." In L. Kaminsky, ed., *ACSM's Resource Manual for Guidelines for Exercise Testing and Prescription,* 5th ed. Philadelphia: Lippincott Williams and Wilkins, 2006.

Field Notes. "Neurosurgeons Link Supplements to Heatstroke Deaths." *The Physician and Sports Medicine* 30 (September 2002): 32.

Fleck, S. J., and W. J. Kraemer. *Designing Resistance Training Programs,* 3rd ed. Champaign, IL: Human Kinetics, 2003.

Follin, S. L., and L. B. Hansen. "Current Approaches to the Prevention and Treatment of Osteoporosis." *American Journal of Health-System Pharmacy* 60 (May 2003): 883–901.

French, L., et al. "Prevention and Treatment of Osteoporosis in Postmenopausal Women." *The Journal of Family Practice* 51 (October 2002): 875–882.

Gotshalk, L. A., et al. "Cardiovascular Responses to a High-Volume Continuous Circuit Resistance Training Protocol." *Journal of Strength and Conditioning Research* 18 (November 2004): 760–764.

Haff, G. G., et al. "Carbohydrate Supplementation and Resistance Training." *Journal of Strength and Conditioning Research* 17 (January 2003): 187–196.

Hakkinen, A. "Effectiveness and Safety of Strength Training in Rheumatoid Arthritis." *Current Opinion in Rheumatology* 16 (March 2004): 132–137

Hoffman, J. "Resistance Training and Injury Prevention." *ACSM Current Comment* (May 2002). www.acsm.org

Hubal, M., et al. "Variability in Muscle Size and Strength Gain after Unilateral Resistance Training." *Medicine & Science in Sports & Exercise* 37 (June 2005): 964–972.

Humphries, B. "Strength Training for Bone, Muscle and Hormones." *Current Comment from the American College of Sports Medicine* (July 2001). www.acsm.org

Izquierdo, M. "Once Weekly Combined Resistance and Cardiovascular Training in Healthy Older Men." *Medicine & Science in Sports & Exercise* 36 (March 2004): 435–443.

Kell, R. T., et al. "Musculoskeletal Fitness, Health Outcomes and Quality of Life." *Sports Medicine* 31 (December 2001): 863–873.

Kemmler, W., et al. "Exercise Effects on Fitness and Bone Mineral Density in Early Postmenopausal Women: 1-Year EFOPS Results." *Medicine & Science in Sports & Exercise* 34 (December 2002): 2115–2123.

Kraemer, W. J., and N. A. Ratamess. "Fundamentals of Resistance Training: Progression and Exercise Prescription." *Medicine & Science in Sports & Exercise* 36 (April 2004): 674–688.

Kraemer, W. J., J. S. Volek, and S. J. Fleck. "Chronic Musculoskeletal Adaptations to Resistance Training." In J. L. Rothman, ed., A*CSM's Resource Manual,* 4th ed. Philadelphia: Lippincott Williams & Wilkins, 2001.

Kraemer, W. J., et al. "Changes in Muscle Hypertrophy in Women with Periodized Resistance Training." *Medicine & Science in Sports & Exercise* 36 (April 2004): 697–708.

Kraemer, W. J., et al. "Effects of Concurrent Resistance and Aerobic Training on Load-Bearing Performance and the Army Physical Fitness Test." *Military Medicine* 169 (December 2004): 994–999.

Leetun, D. T., et al. "Core Stability Measures as Risk Factors for Lower Extremity Injury in Athletes." *Medicine & Science in Sports & Exercise* 36 (June 2004): 926–934.

Mayo Clinic. "Sarcopenia." *Mayo Clinic Health Letter* 20 (February 2002): 7.

Mayo, M. J., et al. "Exercise-Induced Weight Loss Preferentially Reduces Abdominal Fat." *Medicine & Science in Sports & Exercise* 35 (February 2003): 207–213.

Mendes, R. R., et al. "Effects of Creatine Supplementation on the Performance and Body Composition of Competitive Swimmers." *Journal of Nutrition Biochemistry* 15 (August 2004): 473–478.

O'Connor, D. M., and M. J. Crowe. "Effects of b-Hydroxy-b-Methylbutyrate and Creatine Monohydrate Supplementation on the Aerobic and Anaerobic Capacity of Highly Trained Athletes." *Journal of Sports Medicine and Physical Fitness* 43 (March 2003): 64–68.

Radim, J., et al. "Associations of Muscle Strength and Aerobic Fitness with Metabolic Syndrome in Men." *Medicine & Science in Sports & Exercise* 36 (August 2004): 1031–1037.

Rosario, E. J., et al. "Comparison of Strength-Training Adaptations in Early and Older Postmenopausal Women." *Journal of Aging and Physical Activity* 11 (November 2003): 143–155.

Shoepe, T., et al. "Functional Adaptability of Muscle Fibers to Long-Term Resistance Exercise." *Medicine & Science in Sports & Exercise* 35 (June 2003): 944–951.

Vincent, K. R., et al. "Strength Training and Hemodynamic Responses to Exercise." *American Journal of Geriatric Cardiology* 12 (February 2003): 97–106.

Visser, M., et al. "Muscle Mass, Muscle Strength, and Muscle Fat Infiltration as Predictors of Incident Mobility Limitations in Well-functioning Older Persons." *Journals of Gerontology A: Biological Sciences and Medical Sciences* 60 (March 2005): 324–333.

Wallace, J. "Principles of Musculoskeletal Exercise Programming." In L. Kaminsky, ed., *ACSM's Resource Manual for Guidelines for Exercise Testing and Prescription,* 5th ed. Philadelphia: Lippincott Williams and Wilkins, 2006.

Wescott, W. *Building Strength and Stamina,* 2nd ed. Champaign, IL: Human Kinetics, 2003.

Yoshimura, N. "Exercise and Physical Activities for the Prevention of Osteoporotic Fractures: A Review of the Evidence." *Nippon Eiseigaku Zasshi* 58 (September 2003): 328–337.

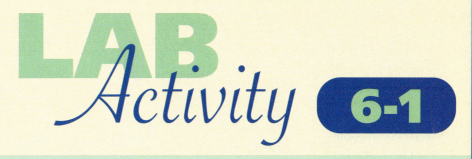

Resistance Training Log

Exercise	Seat/Pad	Date																	
		Reps/Sets																		
		Reps/Sets																		
		Reps/Sets																		
		Reps/Sets																		
		Reps/Sets																		
		Reps/Sets																		
		Reps/Sets																		
		Reps/Sets																		
		Reps/Sets																		
		Reps/Sets																		
		Reps/Sets																		
		Reps/Sets																		
		Reps/Sets																		
		Reps/Sets																		
		Reps/Sets																		
		Reps/Sets																		
		Reps/Sets																		

LAB Activity ■ CHAPTER 6

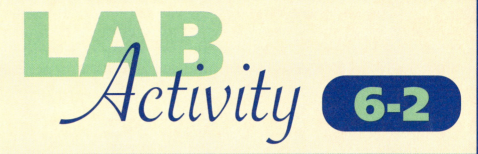

Weight Training Experience

Equipment Needed:

Weight training machines or free weights

Purpose

To experience a weight training program

Procedure

Read the "Weight Training" section and then select one of the weight training programs listed and perform the exercises using a weight that you can lift 8 to 12 repetitions for one to two sets. As this is an introductory session, use light weights and concentrate on correct form, rhythm, and breathing. If you want to perform and compare the two types of programs, rest 1 day between workouts for best results. If assigned by your instructor, track your weight training program on the Resistance Training Log.

WEIGHT TRAINING EXERCISES

(Choose one program)

Machines	Weight	Repetitions	Free Weight	Weight	Repetitions
A. Leg press	_____	_____	A. Squat	_____	_____
B. Leg extension	_____	_____	B. Lunge	_____	_____
C. Hamstring curl	_____	_____	C. Calf raise	_____	_____
D. Toe press	_____	_____	D. Bench press	_____	_____
E. Bench press	_____	_____	E. Military press	_____	_____
F. Military press	_____	_____	F. Shoulder shrug	_____	_____
G. Lat pull	_____	_____	G. Bent-over rowing	_____	_____
H. Rowing	_____	_____	H. Back extension	_____	_____
I. Back extension	_____	_____	I. Triceps press	_____	_____
J. Abdominal curl	_____	_____	J. Biceps curl	_____	_____
K. Triceps press	_____	_____			
L. Biceps curl	_____	_____			

Results

1. What are three things you learned about weight training by doing this program?

2. If you tried both types of weight training, how did they compare? Which did you prefer and why?

3. What did you learn about your strength levels in different muscle groups?

Weight Training Exercises

A. Leg press
    Prime movers: quadriceps, hamstrings, and gluteus maximus
    On leg press, sit on seat, adjust position to last slot or to a 90-degree knee angle.
    Place feet squarely on pedals, press out smoothly (do not lock knees), and return to starting position.

B. Leg extension
    Prime mover: quadriceps
    Sit on bench with both feet under the rollers. Toe in slightly. Do not lie back.
    Extend your legs, hold 1 second, and return to starting position.

C. Hamstring curl
    Prime movers: hamstrings and gluteus maximus
    Lie face down on the bench and hook both heels under the rollers. Position knees at the pivot point where the rollers attach to the bench. Pull up to 90 degrees, hold for 1 second, and return to starting position.

D. Toe press
    Prime mover: gastrocnemius
    On leg press station, place feet squarely on pedals and press out to full leg extension without knee lockout. Press with toes from flat-footed position to foot extension and return.

E. Bench press
    Prime movers: pectorals and triceps
    Lie on bench, head next to the machine. The grips should be lined up approximately with the shoulders. Place your feet flat on the bench with knees bent and back flat. Press to extension and return. If you tend to have shoulder problems, lower the bar to only 4 inches above your chest, then extend.

F. Military press
    Prime movers: deltoids and triceps
    Sit on the stool or stand with abdominals tight, back flat, and knees slightly bent. With shoulders close to handles, extend upward with arms until they are straight but not locked and return.

G. Lat pull
    Prime mover: latissimus dorsi
    Grip bar directly above shoulders or at handles. Pull down until you are kneeling or sitting. From this position, pull down to chest and return.

H. Rowing
    Prime movers: rhomboids, latissimus dorsi, and biceps
    Sit on the machine with arms almost fully extended. Pull back as far as possible, drawing shoulder blades together. Return to starting position.

I. Back extension
    Prime movers: erector spinae, gluteus maximus, and quadratus lumborum
    Sit on the machine with back against upper back pad and feet under ankle rollers. Fasten hip belt if one is available, to keep hips from lifting or sliding out of position. Slowly extend trunk back fully and slowly return to starting position.

J. Abdominal curls
    Prime movers: abdominals and hip flexors
    Sit with pad on upper chest, knees flexed, and feet on footpad. Use seat belt if provided, to keep hips from lifting off seat. Flex trunk as far forward as possible. Return slowly to starting position.

K. Triceps press
Prime mover: triceps
Stand facing lat bar. With palms facing down, grasp the bar so that hands are shoulder width apart. Keep elbows at waist. Press down to extension and return.

L. Biceps curl
Prime mover: biceps
Stand facing the weights, hold bar with both hands, palms up. Flex arms until the bar meets shoulders. Return to starting position. Keep back straight, abdominals firm.

Free Weight Exercises

A. Squat
Prime movers: gluteus maximus, quadriceps, and hamstrings
Start standing upright with the bar resting on your shoulders. Keep the head up, abdominals tight, back flat, feet a bit wider than your shoulders. With back straight, slowly lower hips until tops of thighs are parallel with the floor. Pause. Drive up with legs and hips to the starting position.

B. Lunge
Prime movers: gluteus maximus and quadriceps
Standing upright with the bar on the shoulders off the neck, abdominals tight, back flat, step forward (or backward) until the front thigh is parallel with the floor. The front knee should be over the ball of the foot. Keeping back straight, take a controlled step back to the starting position. Repeat with the opposite leg. This exercise requires considerable balance. You may wish to start first with dumbbells and progress slowly to use of a barbell.

C. Calf raise
Prime mover: gastrocnemius/soleus
Place bar on shoulders, position balls of feet on board and heels off board. Press up onto balls of feet, then lower with control. Knees straight tones gastrocnemius; knees bent tones soleus.

D. Bench press
Prime movers: pectorals and triceps
Lie with head and buttocks on bench, feet stabilized on ground for balance and safety. Grip about 4 inches wider than shoulders, palms under bar (pronated). Lower bar to chest. Focus eyes up to the sky; do not watch bar. Elbows should be directly under bar and forearms perpendicular to ground. Do not let bar slide to the neck. Press to extension, then return.

E. Military press
Prime movers: deltoids and triceps
Sit on bench or stand. With barbell on chest, press upward with arms until they are straight overhead but not locked, then return.

F. Shoulder shrug
Prime mover: trapezius
Holding barbell or two dumbbells, raise shoulders toward ears, pause, lower shoulders.

G. Bent-over rowing
Prime movers: rhomboids and latissimus dorsi
Stabilize one knee and hand on a bench; opposite hand holds the weight, and foot is flat on the floor. Pull elbow up and in toward the spine.

H. Back extension
Prime movers: erector spinae, gluteus maximus, and quadratus lumborum
Lie with your hips on the seat pad and ankles under the ankle rollers, arms crossed across chest. Slowly extend trunk to a horizontal position, hold 3 to 5 seconds, and slowly lower to starting position. After you can easily do 15–20 repititions, you may increase resistance by holding light hand weights to your chest.

I. Triceps press
Prime mover: triceps
Standing with abdominals firm, feet apart for stability, grip the weight, palms up, and, keeping elbows near the ears, slowly lower bar behind the head. Pause, then press until elbows are fully extended.

J. Biceps curl
Prime mover: biceps
Grasp bar, palms up, holding bar about thigh level. Bend elbows, moving bar in an arc toward shoulders. Pause, then slowly return to starting position.

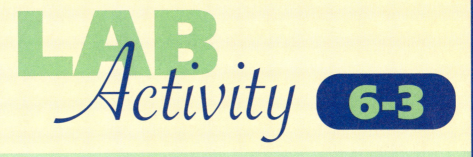

LAB Activity 6-3

Abdominal and Core Strengthening Workout

Equipment Needed:

Floor mat or carpeted surface
Stability ball

Procedure

These exercises are presented in Chapter 6, Figure 6-5. You can add or delete exercises depending on your goals. They should be performed at a slow, steady pace with equal effort in both directions.

ABDOMINAL AND CORE STRENGTHENING EXERCISES

Exercise	*Repetitions*
1. Bicycle exercise	_____
2. Abdominal crunch on stability ball	_____
3. Vertical leg crunch	_____
4. Reverse crunch	_____
5. Plank	_____
6. Side plank	_____
7. Long arm crunch	_____
8. Abdominal curl "crunch"	_____
9. Oblique abdominal curl	
10. Rear leg lift	_____
11. Glute squeeze	_____
12. Back extension	_____
13. Alternate arm/leg lift	_____

Results

1. What are three things you learned about abdominal and core strengthening by doing this program?

2. What did you learn about your muscular endurance levels in different muscle groups?

ABDOMINAL AND CORE STRENGTHENING EXERCISES

Exercise Instructions

1. Bicycle exercise

    Lie on your back with hands behind your head. Raise knees to a 45-degree angle and slowly do a bicycle pedal motion as in the figure. Touch right elbow to left knee, left elbow to right knee.

2. Abdominal crunch on stability ball

    Lie on stability ball with feet flat on floor, thighs and trunk parallel to floor. Cross arms behind shoulders or across chest; contract abdominals by raising trunk about 45 degrees. Spread feet apart for better balance. To work obliques more, bring feet closer together.

3. Vertical leg crunch

    Lie on your back with legs raised in the air, knees slightly bent and crossed at the ankles. Cross hands behind the shoulders to support the head. Keep chin lifted to prevent jerking the head. Lift the trunk and slowly lower.

4. Reverse crunch

    Lie on the back with ankles crossed, feet off the ground, and knees at about a 90-degree angle. Place arms on the floor beside your trunk. Press lower back to the ground, contract the abdominals, and rotate hips 1 to 2 inches. Your feet will lift slightly toward the ceiling each contraction.

5. Plank

    Lie face down, propped with elbows under chest, palms down. Lift up on toes, tighten back and abdominals, keeping body straight, head and spine neutral. Hold 10–60 seconds, rest, repeat. If a straight-back position is too difficult, begin with hips hiked up, or hold the contraction a shorter amount of time. Do not let the hips sag.

6. Side plank

    Lie on side with weight balanced between forearm, flat palm, and feet. Contract back and abdominals to hold body straight. Do not push hips out behind the body. Hold 10–30 seconds, rest, repeat on the other side. If a full-body position is too difficult, begin with the half-plank, balancing weight between knees and forearm. For an advanced version, try lifting the top foot in the air for 5–10 seconds.

7. Long arm crunch

    Lie on your back with knees bent, heels next to buttocks. Extend arms alongside your ears, chin raised, eyes focused on ceiling. Contract abdominals, keeping lower back to floor, lift shoulders as for a basic crunch, lower slowly.

8. Abdominal curl "crunch"

    Lie on your back with knees bent, heels next to buttocks. Place hands across chest or behind shoulders. Keep eyes focused on ceiling, chin up and about a fist's distance from your chest. Contract your abdominals; do not jerk your head forward as you curl. Keeping lower back on the ground, curl shoulders up 3 inches and slowly lower.

9. Oblique abdominal curls

    Lie on the back as for the basic crunch, but add a twist, bringing right elbow toward left knee, then left elbow toward right knee. Elbow does not have to touch knee.

10. Rear leg lift

    On hands and knees, hollow abdomen and round back to protect it. Extend right leg to the rear. Tense gluteus. Raise and lower leg slowly, six to eight counts. Repeat left.

11. Glute squeeze

    Lying on back with knees bent, squeeze gluteus hard, raising hips no more than 3 inches from floor. Do not arch back. Hold for a count of five, relax, repeat. This may also be done with legs extended, feet on stability ball, back on floor.

12. Back extension

    Lie on your stomach with feet on the floor, head neutral, hands touching shoulders. Slowly lift head, shoulders, and chest. Hold 5–10 seconds, then slowly lower. Variation: Squeeze shoulder blades in toward spine while holding trunk lift.

13. Alternate arm/leg lift

    Lie on your stomach with arms extended in front. Raise right arm while lifting left leg. Hold 5–10 seconds. Repeat on other side. Keep head neutral.

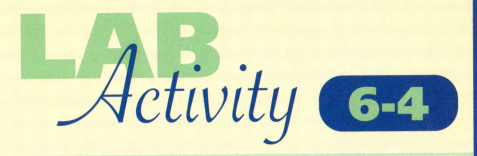

LAB Activity 6-4

Stability Ball Workout

Equipment Needed:

Stability ball

Procedure

Read the stability ball section in Chapter 6 and review Figure 6-8. Do these exercises slowly for best results.

STABILITY BALL EXERCISES

Exercise	*Repetitions*
1. Push-up	_____
2. Knee tuck press	_____
3. Shoulder roll-out	_____
4. Back wall squat	_____
5. Ball transfer	_____
6. Prone knee tuck	_____
7. Oblique curl	_____
8. Bridge	_____
9. Back extension	_____
10. Prone opposite arm and leg raise	_____

Results

1. What are three things you learned about abdominal and core strengthening by doing this program?

2. What did you learn about your muscular endurance levels in different muscle groups?

STABILITY BALL EXERCISES

Here are 10 exercises that you can do with a stability ball. They are illustrated in Figure 6-8.

1. Push-up (pectorals, triceps)

    Kneel facing the ball. Roll forward to lie on top of the ball. Reach forward, placing your hands on the floor. Walk your hands out until the ball is under your thighs. Tighten your abdominals, keeping your body straight. Bend your elbows, then lower your upper body toward the floor. Your body should be straight from shoulders to ankles. Push back to the starting position. To increase difficulty, roll the ball back so only your shins or feet are resting on it.

2. Knee tuck press (deltoids, triceps)

    Kneel on the stability ball and place hands on the floor. Bend your elbows, then lower your upper body toward the floor. Push up from this position.

3. Shoulder roll-out (back extensors, rectus abdominis)

    Kneeling on the floor, place hands on the stability ball. Roll it forward and back, keeping back straight and abdominals tight.

4. Back wall squat (quadriceps, gluteus maximus, hamstrings)

    Stand and press the ball against a wall with your back. Position feet shoulder width apart and forward as if you are going to sit in a chair. Bend your knees, rolling the ball down until your knees are at a 90-degree angle and your thighs are parallel to the floor. Keeping your back pressed against the ball, hold for 5 counts. Straighten your knees and return to the starting position.

5. Ball transfer (rectus abdominis)

    Lie on your back with hands resting on the floor and grip ball between your ankles. Curl the pelvis to lift the ball off the floor into the air, reach up, and transfer it to your hands, then back to ankles. Return to starting position.

6. Prone knee tuck (rectus abdominis)

    Place shins on the stability ball and hands on the floor. Roll the ball back away from your hands, keeping shoulders aligned with hands, abdominals tight, body straight. Extend legs, then bend knees in toward your chest and roll the ball forward until your knees are at your chest. To increase difficulty, try from a bent elbow position on the floor.

7. Oblique curl (rectus abdominis, external and internal oblique abdominals)

    Lie with the top of the ball beneath the center of your back, feet spread wide on the floor for stability. Rotate hips to one side and slowly curl the right side of the upper body toward the left leg. Return to starting position; repeat alternating sides.

8. Bridge (back extensors, gluteus maximus, hamstrings)

    Lie on your back with legs on the ball, hands resting beside you on the floor. Slowly lift hips until your back is straight and weight is on your upper back. Pause, then return slowly to the starting position. Avoid pressing the neck into the floor or arching the back. To make it easier, place ball under knees. To make it harder, place under heels.

9. Back extension (back extensors)

    Lie prone with hips on the ball, feet on the floor and trunk slightly flexed. Arms may be at your sides or behind shoulders. Tighten your upper back, slowly raising shoulders until the spine is straight or slightly extended. Keep head neutral to avoid neck hyperextension. Hold, then relax slowly to starting position. Repeat.

10. Prone opposite arm and leg raise (back extensors, gluteus maximus, hamstrings, deltoids)

    Lying prone on the ball, extend right leg behind you, foot touching floor. Keep head neutral. Reach in front with the left arm, raising it close to your ear. Lift the arm and leg slowly at the same time, pause as you reach extension, then lower slowly. Repeat alternating sides.

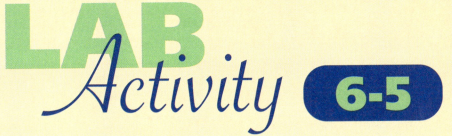

Name _____   **Class/Activity Section** _____   **Date** _____

Elastic Band Workout

Equipment Needed:

Elastic bands

Purpose

To experience a strength-training workout with elastic bands

Procedure

Read the "Elastic Resistance" section and then perform the exercises for 8 to 12 repetitions for one to two sets. As this is an introductory session, concentrate on correct form, rhythm, and breathing. See the handy pullout illustrating these exercises at the back of this text. If assigned by your instructor, track your program on the Resistance Training Log.

ELASTIC BAND EXERCISES

Exercise	*Repetitions*	*Exercise*	*Repetitions*
A. Squat	_____	G. Deltoid raise	_____
B. Leg extension	_____	H. Lat pull	_____
C. Hamstring curl	_____	I. Rowing	_____
D. Side leg lift	_____	J. Biceps curl	_____
E. Inner thigh lift	_____	K. Triceps extension	_____
F. Push-up	_____		

Results

1. What are three things you learned about resistance training with elastic bands by doing this program?

2. What did you learn about your strength levels in different muscle groups?

Elastic Resistance Exercises

A. Squat (gluteus maximus, quadriceps, hamstrings, biceps)

   Step on the band with feet about shoulder width apart and hold ends of the band low enough to feel moderate tension. Slowly squat until hips are just above knees, bending elbows to maintain tension in the band. Return to standing.

B. Leg extension (quadriceps)

   Tie band around ankles. Lie back, knees bent and feet on floor. Keeping knees and thighs together, straighten knee, lifting the foot as high as possible. Release slowly and repeat. Change legs.

C. Hamstring curl (hamstrings, gluteus maximus)

   Place the band around ankles. Lie face down with arms under the chin or hands under hips. Bending knee, slowly lift one foot. Release slowly, maintaining some tension in the band. Repeat. Change legs.

D. Side leg lift (hip abductors)

   Place the band around both legs—around ankles is hardest, around knees easiest. Lying on right side, torso supported by arms, slightly bend lower leg for support. Keep hips facing forward, lift upper leg. Lower, keeping tension on the band, and repeat. Change sides.

E. Inner thigh lift (thigh adductors)

   Place band around left arch and right ankle. Lie on right side with trunk supported by arms. Lift bottom leg slowly, hold briefly, lower slowly, repeat. Switch sides.

F. Push-up (pectorals, biceps):

   Wrap the band around your back and under your arms. Bend elbows and grasp ends of band. Extend arms forward, then return slowly.

G. Deltoid raise (deltoid, triceps)

   Place one end of band under foot and hold the other end by your hip. Standing with good posture, lift arm to shoulder level, then lower slowly.

H. Lat pull (latissimus dorsi)

   Hold band overhead, elbows extended but not locked. Pull arms apart to shoulder level. Be careful not to get hair caught in band.

I. Rowing (rhomboids)

   With band around arches and knees extended, grasp band about mid-shin. Pull elbows back and try to bring shoulder blades together. Release slowly.

J. Biceps curl (biceps)

   Place one end of band under foot, grasp other end low, and, keeping elbow at your side, curl right arm to shoulder. Slowly release.

K. Triceps extension (triceps)

   Standing with good posture, grasp both ends of band behind your back. Extend upper arm toward ceiling, pause, then slowly release, pressing lower hand toward hip.

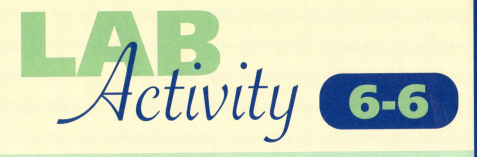

Partner Resistance Workout

Equipment Needed:

Floor mat or carpeted surface
Partner
Towel or broomstick

Procedure

These exercises are presented in Chapter 6, Figure 6-10. You can add or delete exercises depending on your goals. They should be performed at a slow, steady pace with equal effort in both directions. Perform 6–8 repetitions or about 1 minute of each exercise.

PARTNER RESISTANCE EXERCISES

Exercise	*Repetitions or time*
A. Leg extension	_____
B. Hamstring curl	_____
C. Inner/outer thigh press	_____
D. Foot flexion	_____
E. Overhead press	_____
F. Lat pull	_____
G. Elbow press forward	_____
H. Elbow press backward	_____
I. Biceps curl	_____

Results

1. What are three things you learned about abdominal and core strengthening by doing this program?

2. What did you learn about your muscular fitness levels in different muscle groups?

A. Leg extension (quadriceps)

Sit on a bench or chair. Move one leg from flexion to full extension and back as partner resists by pressing on front of lower leg.

B. Hamstring curl (hamstrings, gluteus)

Lie face down while partner straddles your back and places a hand on each ankle. Bend knees and curl calves toward buttocks as your partner resists. Continue the resistance as you return to the starting position.

C. Inner/outer thigh press (thigh adductors and abductors)

Sit, facing each other, legs forward, hands behind hips for balance. One partner places both feet inside the other's feet and presses outward as the other partner resists by pressing inward. Switch positions after six to eight reps.

D. Foot flexion (anterior tibialis)

Sit with legs extended. Partner kneels and presses down on top of both feet as you flex them and then return to extension.

E. Overhead press (deltoids, triceps)

Sit with hands at shoulder level, palms up. As partner resists, press up toward ceiling and then return to starting position.

F. Lat pull (latissimus dorsi)

Sit and reach high overhead to grasp partner's hands. As partner resists, pull down to shoulder level and slowly return to starting position.

G. Elbow press forward (pectorals)

Sit with elbows out and hands touching shoulders. As partner resists at the elbows, pull them in toward your midline and return to starting position.

H. Elbow press backward (rhomboids)

Sit with elbows out or with arms crossed. Partner sits behind, pressing on your elbows as you press back, pulling shoulder blades together. As partner continues resistance, return to starting position.

I. Biceps curl (biceps)

Stand, palms facing upward. Partner resists on your palms as you curl arm from extension to flexion and back. This may also be done holding a towel in one hand in front of body. Partner sits or kneels facing you, resisting on other end of towel as you curl your arm.

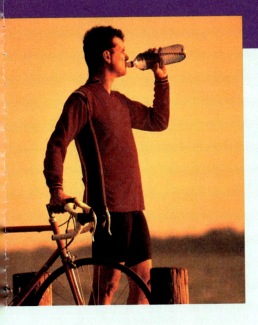

Chapter 7

Exploring Special Exercise Considerations

*Obstacles are those frightful things you see when
you take your eye off the goal.*
—Hannah More, English author

Objectives

After reading this chapter, you will be able to:

1. Identify the physiological bases for differences in men's and women's exercise performance levels.
2. List the similarities in men's and women's responses to exercise.
3. Identify correct recommendations for exercise during pregnancy.
4. Describe exercise addiction.
5. Describe how exercise affects disease resistance.
6. Identify recommendations for safe exercise in hot and cold weather.
7. Identify the best replacement fluids to prevent dehydration during exercise in hot weather.
8. Identify the effects of a regular program of exercise on the aging process.
9. Identify correct recommendations for exercise for individuals with chronic health conditions such as arthritis, asthma, diabetes, hypertension, and osteoporosis.

Terms

- amenorrhea
- dysmenorrhea
- endorphins
- electrolytes
- estrogen
- exercise addiction
- female athlete triad
- hemoglobin
- hyperthermia
- hyponatremia
- hypothermia
- Kegel exercises
- menarche
- oligomenorrhea
- sarcopenia
- stress incontinence

A Fit and Well Way of Life Online Learning Center www.mhhe.com/robbinsfitwell1e
Go to the Online Learning Center for chapter quizzes, outlines, flashcards, and additional lab activities.

This chapter brings together several concerns related to exercise participation. Eight major areas are addressed: similarities and differences in men's and women's exercise performance, females and exercise, males and exercise, exercise addiction, exercise and disease resistance, environmental considerations, aging and physical activity, and exercise and chronic health conditions. With increased knowledge of these special exercise considerations you will have a greater understanding of how to participate in and enjoy physical exercise throughout your life span. Be motivated to do so by these words—"Don't wait for your ship to come in. Row out to meet it."

SIMILARITIES AND DIFFERENCES IN MEN'S AND WOMEN'S EXERCISE PERFORMANCE

While performance levels may differ, men and women respond to exercise in a similar manner. Although women have approximately 20 percent lower maximal oxygen uptake than men (due to smaller heart size), with exercise they show similar rates of improvement. Performance levels differ for several reasons.

- ✔ *Strength:* Due to hormonal changes during puberty, a woman adds fat because of estrogen, while a man's muscle mass doubles because of testosterone. In fact, women have half as much or more muscle to move their weight and more inactive fat weight to carry. In addition, men's greater muscle mass gives them 30 to 40 percent greater strength. See "The Numbers" later in this chapter.
- ✔ *Performance and endurance:* Physically the male heart and lungs are larger than those of the female. The larger male heart and lungs produce higher stroke volumes and vital capacities than those of females do. Men also have more **hemoglobin** (the oxygen-carrying component in red blood cells) in their arterial blood than do women. Both the larger heart size and more oxygen in the blood result in greater cardiac output and greater maximal oxygen uptake. These factors give males advantages in terms of performance and endurance.
- ✔ *Heat tolerance:* Women have a higher body temperature at rest than men, fewer sweat glands, lower sweat production, and a propensity to start sweating at higher temperatures than do men. A woman's greater amount of adipose tissue (fat) serves as insulation and inhibits heat dissipation. The implication of these differences is that women have less tolerance to heat than men. As a result, women are more subject to heat stress than men and have to work relatively harder than men to achieve similar workloads under higher levels of heat conditions.

Even though women are at a disadvantage in terms of physical performance, they benefit equally from aerobic exercise in terms of fitness improvement. Training effect benefits such as loss of fat from deposit areas, increased bone density, and decreased exercise heart rates are similar for men and women. When differences in body size are taken into account, fitness gains for men and women are *essentially* the same.

Some women fear that exercise will make them develop large or bulky muscles or a masculine appearance. This is not likely unless a woman is using anabolic steroids and spending many hours doing extremely strenuous weight training. A person's potential for muscular development is genetically determined by levels of the sex hormone testosterone, and women have only one-tenth as much of this hormone as men. While women, like men, vary in their potential for muscular size development, what most women want from exercise is exactly what they will gain: decreased fat; increased lean body tissue; and firmer, toned muscles.

FEMALES AND EXERCISE

Once the sight of a female training on the road or competing in a race was sufficiently unusual that people would stop and stare. As late as 1965 women were threatened with banishment from international competition if they ran races longer than 1.5 miles, and it was 1984 before the first women's Olympic marathon took place. As the interest in fitness as a lifestyle has grown, so has the number of women participants in aerobic activities and athletics. Now that large numbers of females have adopted a physically active lifestyle, research has provided us with new information about topics of special interest to women.

Menstruation

Is it safe to exercise during menstruation? Yes. Menstruation is only one small part of the ongoing female reproductive cycle. In the past women sometimes used this as an excuse to avoid exercise, but now women are encouraged to follow a normal routine during all parts of the reproductive cycle. Research indicates that physical activity has little or no effect on the average woman's menstrual cycle. Accordingly, no restriction should be placed on the physical activity level of the average

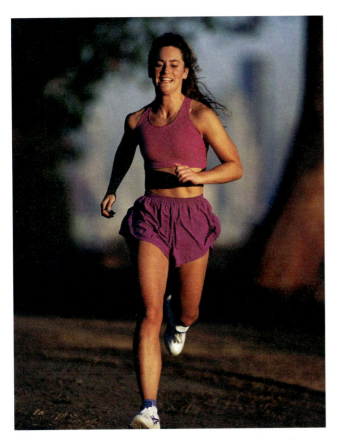

More women are discovering the joys of physical activity.

℞ *Prescription for Action*

Date: *Do one or more today*

✔ Make a list of reasons why you didn't exercise outside last winter and ways you can counter this during the cold months this year.
✔ Get up during TV commercial breaks and do 30 seconds (about the length of one commercial) of each of the following exercises:
  • jumping jacks (or jog in place)
  • push-ups
  • abdominal curls or planks
  • squats
✔ Show your grandparents or another older person how to use an exercise band.
✔ Weigh yourself before and after your workout today and see how much water you lost.
✔ Write down three reasons why you will want to exercise across your life span.
✔ Keep a log of how much water you drink today.
✔ Keep a log of how much calcium you get today.

Prescribed by _____*YOU*_____

woman at any phase of her cycle. The way women experience menstruation varies greatly. Most feel no different than usual; some may experience abdominal and leg cramps, backache, or mood swings, particularly during the first 2 days of the menstrual flow.

Dysmenorrhea, or painful menstruation, is probably neither caused nor cured by exercise. However, there is some evidence that enhanced fitness leads to a reduction in menstrual complaints, although this is still being researched. Some studies indicate that exercise decreases mood swings and relieves depression, anxiety, and irritability. Excess body water lost through perspiration can reduce weight gain due to water retention, relieving premenstrual bloating and edema. While no specific exercises cure severe cramps, participation in a program of regular exercise has been shown to decrease the frequency of minor menstrual cramps. This is perhaps due to increased abdominal tone, increased circulation to the uterus, or increased levels of pain-relieving **endorphins.**

Menstruation should be treated as a normal physiological function, not an illness. As long as she is comfortable, a woman should continue her regular exercise program. For women who want to look and feel their best, exercise is beneficial at any time of the month.

Studies indicate that young girls who exercise vigorously may experience a delay in **menarche,** the start of the menstrual cycle, decreasing their risk of cancer later in life. While the average American girl experiences

menarche between 11 and 12 years of age, those who train vigorously experience the first menstrual cycle at an average age of 15½, the same as the average age for menarche 100 years ago. This delay may be natural and even desirable, because it reduces the body's lifetime exposure to **estrogen**, a female sex hormone. The more menstrual cycles a woman has over her lifetime, the longer her exposure to estrogen and the greater her risk of cancer of the breast and reproductive organs. In addition, women who exercise tend to be leaner, thus producing less potent estrogen. In one study, women who had been athletic in high school and college had half the incidence of breast and reproductive cancer in later life compared with sedentary women. In fact, a sedentary lifestyle is considered a primary risk factor for cancer.

Menstrual abnormalities such as **oligomenorrhea** (infrequent or irregular menses) and **amenorrhea** (absent menses) occur in about 2 to 5 percent of the general population of women and in up to 28 percent of women athletes. In athletes, the prevalence appears high in sports that require greater intensity, frequency, and duration of training (e.g., distance running and swimming) or sports that emphasize low body weight or involve competition by weight class (e.g., dance, gymnastics, boxing, wrestling). Numerous factors, physiological and

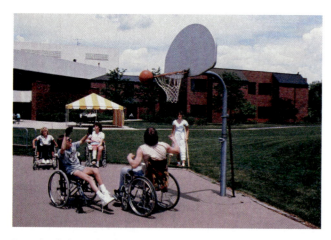

Everybody benefits from physical activity.

psychological, including change in diet or inadequate diet and physical and emotional stress, may affect menstruation abnormally (for example, stressors such as heavy athletic training and competition acting synergistically with other stressors in life). In athletes, the vast majority of cases of amenorrhea stem from an imbalance between activity level and nutritional intake. For example, a female student who menstruates during her off-season may lose her periods once preseason training begins because of increases in her activity level without corresponding increases in her nutritional intake. Her body can't sustain all its functions without adequate calories and nutrition, and reproduction mechanisms are the first to shut down.

Exercise-induced oligomenorrhea and amenorrhea are rare in women doing moderate amounts of exercise as part of a fitness program. They are more common among those whose menstrual cycles started late, past age 15, or who had a history of irregularity before starting exercise programs. Although no specific body fat percentage has been associated with the development of exercise-induced amenorrhea, the evidence suggests that decreased fat levels may lead to decreased production of one form of estrogen. Thus, as fat percentages decrease, estrogen levels decline, and the evidence of amenorrhea increases. Some scientists have suggested that the critical body fat level may be as low as 13 percent or that there may be no such critical level. If such a critical fat percentage does exist, it probably varies widely from individual to individual.

The focus of research is on how all the factors mentioned here may affect the hypothalamus, thereby influencing the production of important regulatory hormones relative to menstruation and metabolism, including estrogen, epinephrine, and corticoids. Whatever the cause, exercise-induced amenorrhea is considered reversible. Normal menstrual cycles resume with as minor a change in lifestyle as a 10 percent decrease in exercise, improved nutrition, or a weight gain of 4 to 5 pounds.

Also, exercise-induced amenorrhea does not seem to affect long-term fertility. While a woman with amenorrhea does not experience a regular menstrual cycle, it is still possible for her to ovulate and become pregnant. She should not rely on this for birth control and should continue her regular birth control method if pregnancy is not desired. Any active woman should be aware of her normal menstrual cycle and should discuss any irregularities with her physician to rule out conditions such as thyroid disorders, ovarian cysts, brain tumors, and pregnancy.

Female Athlete Triad

Some female athletes and other physically active women who are underweight and nonmenstruating are being diagnosed as victims of the **female athlete triad**. This is a life-threatening syndrome marked by three disorders:

✔ Disordered eating habits (inadequate food, energy intake insufficient to meet metabolic demands)
✔ Amenorrhea (for more than three months)
✔ Osteoporosis

Sports can be a win-win activity for young women. Research shows that exercise builds strong bones, helps control weight, and improves mood. It also reduces the risk of developing serious illnesses such as heart disease and breast cancer. But it also comes with risks such as female athlete triad.

Societal pressure on females to have an unrealistically low body weight fuels this condition. Fitness professionals who work with physically active females

TOP 10 LIST

Who's at Risk for Osteoporosis?

Although no one is immune to osteoporosis, the following factors increase one's risk:

1. Female
2. Postmenopausal
3. Amenorrheic
4. Small-boned
5. Eating a diet low in calcium
6. Alcohol, tobacco and caffeine use
7. Eating a diet high in protein
8. A sedentary lifestyle and/or getting only low-impact exercise
9. Medications (including prednisone)
10. A family history of osteoporosis

Note: Some vegetarian diets also increase the risk.

should learn ways to prevent, recognize, treat, and reduce its risks.

The problem has caught the attention of the International Olympic Committee Medical Commission, which recently developed a consensus statement on the dangers and possible treatments, and the National Collegiate Athletic Association, which published a coach's handbook on the topic.

The female athlete triad is not limited to college or elite athletes. It occurs in high school and middle school girls as well as other women who are physically active. Any woman, even if she is in her 40s, who has disordered eating and becomes amenorrheic will lose bone. A woman who has been amenorrheic for several years can have the bones of a 70- or 80-year-old woman.

Bone loss also can occur in men who have eating disorders. Those at risk are athletes in sports in which body weight is important, such as running, wrestling, and ski jumping. There is no triad for men at this time.

The problem begins when women do not consume enough calories for their activity levels; their energy deficits may disrupt their menstrual cycles. Estrogen, which is critical for preserving bone, drops to the level of post-menopausal women. At the same time, inadequate nutrition leads to other hormonal changes that inhibit the ability to build bone. With restrictive dieting, women often limit calcium-rich dairy products and other important nutrients for bone health. Such behaviors are especially harmful during the teen years up until about age 21 because women at those ages are still building bone.

No one knows how long women can go without menstruating before they experience bone loss, but going three months without a period is considered extremely dangerous. The weakened skeletons of athletes (or other physically active woman) can lead to fractures, especially in the legs, hips, and pelvis.

Amenorrhea often can be reversed with an increase in calories or a decrease in physical activity. Bone density does increase with a resumption of normal estrogen levels, but it does not appear to recover fully. Active young women who have not been menstruating regularly should have a bone-mineral density test, discuss low-dose estrogen replacement therapy with a physician, and consume a calcium intake of 1,500 mg/day (about 5 cups of milk). See the Top Ten list "Who's at Risk for Osteoporosis?"

Pregnancy

Is exercise advisable during pregnancy? How much? What are the benefits? Are there limitations or cautions to keep in mind? Are some exercises better than others?

Pregnancy is a natural and normal physiological function, not an illness. A pregnant woman is not fragile. Although she should always discuss her exercise plan with her physician, evidence keeps rolling in that exercise is more than just okay for a pregnant woman—it is good for both her and her baby. General advice for a healthy woman having an uncomplicated pregnancy is to continue her regular exercise program, being careful not to get overtired. If she has not been exercising before pregnancy, this is not a time to begin a crash program. A 20- to 30-minute walk, 3 to 4 days per week, is a program a doctor might approve. Throughout pregnancy, to keep the effort aerobic, a woman should use the "talk test." She should be able to carry on a conversation while exercising without getting out of breath. In early pregnancy, if exercising seems to require more effort, decrease the intensity and duration. Pregnant women should be counseled not to undertake excessive physical activity in a hot climate to which they are not acclimated. A gradual weight gain, which is natural and desirable, is likely to increase stress to joints, ligaments, and muscles. Also, muscles and connective tissues become more lax as they gradually undergo hormonal changes. Increases in the pregnancy hormone relaxin help facilitate the baby's birth but make the pregnant woman more susceptible to strains and sprains. Therefore, during late pregnancy and the early postdelivery period, vigorous increases in flexibility should not be pursued.

In the fifth to sixth month of pregnancy, due to increasing weight and joint flexibility, impact activities may become uncomfortable. At this time, many women switch to low- or no-impact exercises such as walking, swimming, and stationary cycling. While some women continue their normal exercise program to the day of delivery with no ill effects, don't feel guilty if you feel a need to cut back. Toward the end of pregnancy, if you fatigue easily and exercise seems to require more effort, it is natural to decrease the activity level. After the first trimester it is not advised to do exercises that require lying on your back. This position can block the blood supply to the uterus (by compressing the aorta and/or the vena cava), resulting in depression of the fetal heart rate. Throughout pregnancy, a woman needs to listen to her body and adjust her exercise level to maintain comfort.

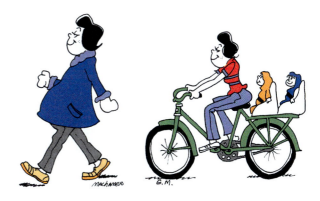

Exercise during and after pregnancy has many advantages.

TABLE 7-1   ACOG Guidelines for Exercise During Pregnancy and Postpartum

1. Regular exercise (at least three times per week) is preferable to intermittent activity. Competitive activities should be discouraged.
2. Vigorous exercise should not be performed in hot, humid weather or when you have a fever.
3. Ballistic movements (jerky, bouncy motions) should be avoided. Exercise should be done on a wooden floor or a tightly carpeted surface to reduce shock and provide a sure footing.
4. Deep flexion or extension of joints should be avoided because of connective tissue laxity. Activities that require jumping, jarring motions, or rapid changes in direction should be avoided because of joint instability.
5. Vigorous exercise should be preceded by a 5-minute period of muscle warm-up. This can be accomplished by slow walking or stationary cycling with low resistance.
6. Vigorous exercise should be followed by a period of gradually declining activity that includes gentle stationary stretching. Because connective tissue laxity increases the risk of joint injury, stretches should not be taken to the point of maximum resistance.
7. Heart rate should be measured at times of peak activity. Target heart rates and limits established in consultation with a physician should not be exceeded. Use the "talk test" to gauge exercise intensity. Slow down if you cannot comfortably maintain a conversation during exercise.
8. Care should be taken to rise gradually from the floor to avoid a sudden drop in blood pressure. Some form of activity involving the legs should be continued for a brief period.
9. No exercise should be performed while lying on the back after the first trimester. This slows blood flow back to the heart and decreases its output. Also, avoid *motionless standing,* which may also decrease heart output.
10. Exercises that employ the Valsalva maneuver should be avoided.
11. Caloric intake should be adequate to meet not only the extra energy needs of pregnancy but also those of the exercise performed.
12. Maternal core temperature should not exceed 38°C (101°F).
13. Liquids should be taken liberally before and after exercise to prevent dehydration. If necessary, activity should be interrupted to replenish fluids.
14. Women who have led sedentary lifestyles should begin with physical activity of low intensity and advance activity levels gradually.
15. Activity should be stopped and the physician consulted if any unusual symptoms appear. (See Table 7-2.)

Specific pregnancy exercise guidelines from the American College of Obstetricians and Gynecologists are listed in Table 7-1. Also review Table 7-2.

There are many reasons exercise is important during pregnancy. The physiological changes of pregnancy place a great demand on the body. Labor and delivery are perhaps the most physically demanding events a woman will experience. Exercise can maintain optimal fitness, enabling a woman to control weight gain, improve muscle tone, improve posture, decrease backache, and decrease constipation. Exercise can also aid in increasing energy, increasing psychological well-being, managing stress, enhancing sleep at night, and regaining a prepregnancy figure.

While fitness is no guarantee of a quick labor or easy delivery, endurance and increased capacity to deal with the physical stress of childbirth are assets that come from fitness. A fit mother can enjoy a quicker recovery from childbirth and can regain her normal fitness and activity levels in less time than can the unfit.

Stress Incontinence

Stress incontinence, an involuntary leakage of urine when you laugh, cough, sneeze, or exercise, is a common problem, particularly in women over 30 who have given birth. During pregnancy and birth, these muscles become weakened and stretched. One solution is to wear a sanitary pad, but a better approach is to strengthen the perineal muscles that control this function. The pelvic floor is a hammocklike muscle layer attached at the front and back of the pelvis. It supports the

TABLE 7-2   Reasons to Discontinue Exercise and Seek Medical Advice During Pregnancy

1. Any signs of bloody discharge from the vagina
2. Any "gush" of fluid from the vagina
3. Sudden swelling of the ankles, hands, or face
4. Persistent, severe headaches and/or visual disturbance; unexplained spell of faintness or dizziness
5. Swelling, pain, and redness in the calf of one leg (phlebitis)
6. Elevation of pulse rate or blood pressure that persists after exercise
7. Excessive fatigue, palpitations, chest pain
8. Persistent contractions (more than six to eight per hour) that may suggest onset of premature labor
9. Unexplained abdominal pain
10. Insufficient weight gain during the last two trimesters

pelvic organs, including the bladder, uterus, and rectum. Kegel exercises, named after the Los Angeles physician who developed them, strengthen the pelvic floor muscles and may prevent or cure stress incontinence. As a side benefit, many women report increased pleasure during intercourse.

Kegel Exercise

Kegel exercises are done by contracting the perineal muscles, which surround the bladder neck and vagina. To learn the exercise, when urinating stop and start the

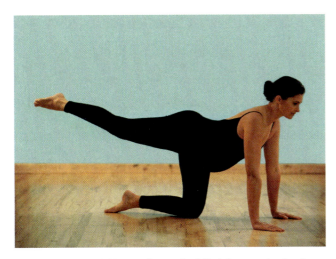

No exercise should be performed while lying on the back after the first trimester.

flow. Hold the contraction for 3 to 4 seconds during the stop phase. The muscle action you take to do this when urinating is the action you must take when doing Kegel exercises. You can do these exercises anytime—contract hard and then release. Do 10 in a row, and work up to five sets of 10 daily. These exercises should be done before, during, and after pregnancy.

Postpartum: Getting Back into Shape

Giving birth and coping with the demands of a new baby are both joyful and stressful for a new mother. The main problem in resuming exercise is not fatigue or shortness of breath, which might be expected, but finding someone to watch the baby while the mother takes a well-deserved break. Postpartum recovery times vary greatly. If the delivery has been normal, walking is encouraged in the hospital the day after delivery. This can be continued when the woman returns home. Rest, good nutrition, and a progressive walking program will make recovery faster than will complete inactivity or resuming prepregnancy activity levels too soon. You should not rush into impact activities such as jogging or pursue flexibility increases until you have given loosened joints (due to the hormone relaxin) a chance to recover—6 to 16 weeks. Abdominal curls are important for toning overstretched abdominal muscles and preventing back problems. Also, do Kegel exercises to strengthen pelvic floor muscles.

A nursing mother needs to avoid fatigue and dehydration, which may reduce milk production. Drink fluids liberally, and nap when the baby does to ensure adequate rest. Wear a good supportive bra, with pads to control leaks, and nurse before exercise for greater comfort. There is no conflict between nursing a baby and doing moderate exercise. Both help a mother regain her prepregnancy figure.

Breast Support

Does bouncing cause breasts to sag? Some believe that breast movement stretches the skin and ligaments that support the breasts. There is no evidence to support this claim; the main culprits are genetics and pregnancy. Still, a good bra makes exercise more comfortable by reducing breast movement during activity. The best designs flatten breasts to redistribute their mass across the chest wall. This results in less mass for gravity to affect. Racerback and crossback straps prevent slippage off the shoulder. Certain designs are more suited to small-breasted women, while others are more comfortable for large-breasted exercisers. A woman should try different styles to decide what is best for her. A good exercise bra should (1) limit breast movement, (2) have wide straps that do not slip off the shoulders, (3) have a wide band at the bottom to prevent the bra from riding up, (4) have no rough seams or uncovered fasteners to prevent chafing, and (5) be made of nonabrasive materials and be seamless or at least have seams that do not cross the nipple area.

MALES AND EXERCISE

Participation in sports and physical activities no longer ends with graduation from high school or college. Large numbers of men are continuing or beginning lifetime exercise programs.

Exercise appears to lower the hormonal levels of males as it does that of females. In one study, testosterone levels of men who ran 40 miles a week averaged 30 percent less than the levels of nonexercisers. The runners' levels were still in a normal range, and the effect was reversible. Sperm count and libido were not affected. While it may lower hormonal levels, overtraining is not associated with decreased fertility in male athletes unless it is accompanied by anorexic behavior and a high-stress lifestyle.

A more common male fertility problem results from constantly wearing tight undershorts. For the testicles to maintain normal sperm production, they must be a few degrees cooler than normal body temperature. Their position outside and slightly away from the body accomplishes this. When the testicles are overheated by consistently being held close to the body, sperm production temporarily decreases. A switch to boxer shorts solves the problem.

Male bicyclists have additional concerns. Males who ride for extended periods (i.e., 2 to 3 hours or more) have an increased risk of reduced perineal (crotch) area circulation. It is caused by compression of the bike saddle. This can lead to pain, numbness, and, in severe cases, male impotence. Females are not exempt from this problem. Reduced perineal circulation in females may result in sexual and urinary tract dysfunction. Male bicyclists traveling over rough terrain may also experience pain and injury to the testicles. The following tips will help avoid these problems:

✔ Level the seat or point the nose downward to reduce pressure on the perineum.
✔ Lower the seat so that the legs support more weight. (Knees should bend slightly at the bottom of the pedal stroke.)
✔ Avoid handlebar extensions because they place more body weight on the nose of the seat.
✔ Stand up and pedal every 10 minutes to encourage blood flow in the perineum.
✔ Rise out of the seat when going over bumps.
✔ Avoid crush injuries involving the top tube by riding a bike of proper size. The top tube of a mountain bike should be 3 to 4 inches below the crotch when one is standing over it; for road bikes, clearance should be 1 to 2 inches.
✔ Consider replacing a narrow racing-style saddle with a wider seat or a seat designed to reduce compression on the perineum. Special seats are available for males.
✔ Switch to a recumbent bike.

EXERCISE ADDICTION

Exercising is unconditionally great for the body, the soul, and the mind, right? Almost, but not quite. Even the most benign or beneficial elements can cause harm when taken to an extreme. Although exercise is highly recommended for health and vigor, it is not protected from this universal truth. When a commitment to exercise crosses the line to dependency and compulsion, it can create physical, social, and psychological havoc for those involved.

A "positive addiction" can be a healthy adaptation to the barriers to exercise in life because commitments to work, family, and other healthy pursuits must compete with time to work out. Sometimes the line between commitment and compulsion is crossed. There can be a negative side to exercise that gradually, insidiously takes over from the positive.

Exercise addiction is not just another term for overtraining syndrome. Healthy athletes training for peak performance and competition can experience overtraining symptoms, the short-term result of too little rest and recovery. **Exercise addiction,** in contrast, is a chronic loss of perspective of the role of exercise in a full life. A healthy athlete and an exercise addict may share similar levels of training volume. The difference is in the attitude and the consequences. An addicted individual isn't able to see value in unrelated activities and pursues the activity even when it is against his or her best interest.

The exercise addict has lost balance, allowing exercise to become overvalued compared to elements widely recognized as giving meaning to a full life (e.g., school, work, friends, family, community involvement). When emotional connections are passed up in favor of additional hours of training; when injury, illness, and fatigue don't stop a workout; when all free time is consumed by training–*exercise addiction* is the diagnosis. Withdrawal symptoms such as anxiety, irritability, and depression, which appear when circumstances prevent exercise, are the warning signs of addiction.

To the addict, there is no exception to the rule "the more the better." Anything that interferes with the quest for more exercise is resented.

The paradox inherent in exercise addiction is the blurred boundary between what is healthy, admirable, and desirable and behavior that is over the edge and dependent. The addict answers poor performance with more exercise and less rest. A healthy athlete looks at the big picture and adjusts training programs, allowing for rest and recovery among the training variables.

Remember that working out should always have an element of play. If exercising loses all aspects of fun, something has gone wrong. The most competitive athletes still love their sport. They love it because it gives pleasure, not because it has become a compulsive need. Take the self-assessment in Table 7-3 to see if you are losing your perspective on exercise.

TABLE 7-3	Are You Addicted to Exercise?

Directions: Rate yourself as honestly as you can on the following checklist.

Yes	No	
____	____	1. I have missed important social obligations and family events in order to exercise.
____	____	2. I have given up other interests, including time with friends, to make more time to exercise.
____	____	3. Missing a workout makes me irritable and depressed.
____	____	4. I feel content only when I am exercising or within the hour after exercising.
____	____	5. I like exercise better than sex, good food, or a movie–there's almost nothing I'd rather do.
____	____	6. I work out even if I'm sick, injured, or exhausted. I feel better when I get moving.
____	____	7. In addition to my regular exercise schedule, I exercise more if I find extra time.
____	____	8. Family and friends have told me I'm too involved in exercise.
____	____	9. I have a history (or family history) of anxiety or depression.

Scoring: If you checked yes on three or more of the statements, you may be losing your perspective on exercise.

EXERCISE AND DISEASE RESISTANCE

During exercise, 75 to 85 percent of the energy produced is released in the form of heat, producing an increase in body temperature. Much of this heat is dissipated at the skin, but body temperature still is elevated during exercise. This regular increase in body temperature, it is speculated, is inhospitable to some viruses and might decrease the incidence of viral infections in exercisers. Moderate exercise also has been found to boost the immune system. However, overtraining leading to exhaustion might weaken the system and increase susceptibility to colds and minor infections. Studies on the relationship between the immune system and physical exercise have produced contradictory results. Nonexercisers who start a new program of intense exercise, exceeding their individual exercise limits, or who exercise sporadically may experience weakened immunity for a brief period. Highly trained athletes may weaken their immune systems with acute, exhaustive exercise. Of course, psychological and emotional stress may play important roles here, too—whether it be the anxiety felt by the new, out-of-shape exerciser or by the athlete competing for a championship. Few people exercise so strenuously that they need to worry about any possible adverse effects on immunity. The problem for most Americans is too little exercise rather than too much. For anyone in doubt, a consistent and regular program of moderate exercise is a key component of overall health and well-being, including the immune system. However, the optimal level of exercise for each individual's immune system is unknown.

Should you exercise when you have a cold or feel ill? Many professionals recommend that you decrease the intensity and frequency of workouts or take some days off when you have a cold or feel one coming on. Illness affects lung and heart function as well as skeletal muscles. As a result, performance may be reduced. Some people find that exercising when they have a mild cold makes them feel better. Illnesses vary in severity and people react differently to them, so listen to your body. If you only have a minor head cold and otherwise feel fine, it is probably acceptable to work out. Avoid exercise to the point of exhaustion. Avoid exercise if you have the flu, have a fever, feel achy, feel extremely tired, are heavily congested, or have swollen glands. Exercise does not cure illness. The old adage that "you can sweat out a cold" with exercise is untrue. When you recover from illness, do not start exercising at the same level as before. Give yourself a few days to build back to normal levels.

ENVIRONMENTAL CONSIDERATIONS

Exercising in the Cold

Your friends think you're crazy for sharing a narrow roadway with cars that spray you with slush as you exercise on a chilly winter day. Walking, running, and cycling are more complicated in the winter. Still, there is something liberating about a good workout on an icy winter day. Cold weather workouts can be invigorating, comfortable, and safe if you follow these tips:

1. *Layer clothing*: Dress in several thin layers so that you can remove or add a layer as needed. Wool and polypropylene clothing wick moisture away from the skin to keep you dry. The outer layer of clothing should be breathable and windproof.

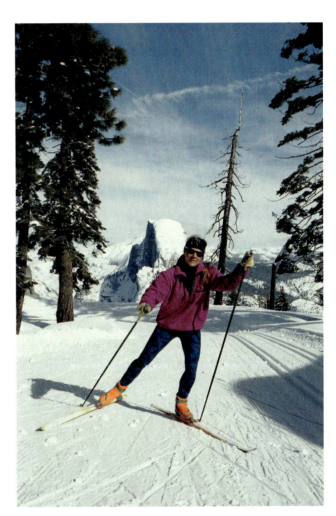

There is no possibility that you will freeze your lungs or throat. The air is warmed as it passes through your mouth and throat. Wear a mask or scarf over your nose and mouth if the cold air bothers you.

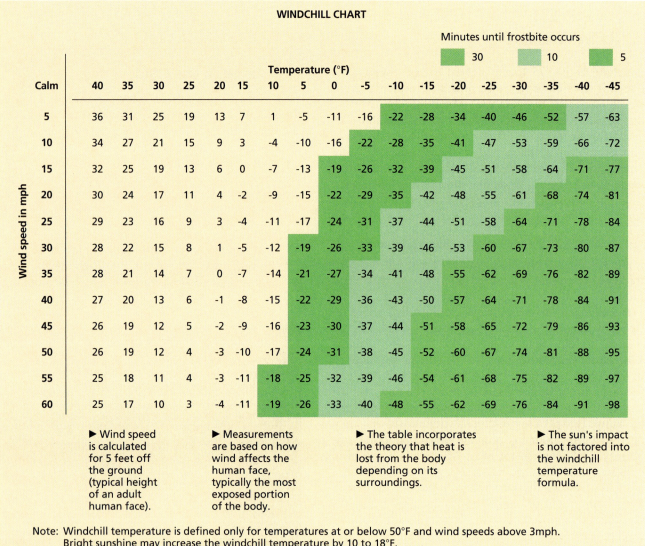

WINDCHILL CHART

Minutes until frostbite occurs

| | 30 | 10 | 5 |

Temperature (°F)

Calm	40	35	30	25	20	15	10	5	0	-5	-10	-15	-20	-25	-30	-35	-40	-45
5	36	31	25	19	13	7	1	-5	-11	-16	-22	-28	-34	-40	-46	-52	-57	-63
10	34	27	21	15	9	3	-4	-10	-16	-22	-28	-35	-41	-47	-53	-59	-66	-72
15	32	25	19	13	6	0	-7	-13	-19	-26	-32	-39	-45	-51	-58	-64	-71	-77
20	30	24	17	11	4	-2	-9	-15	-22	-29	-35	-42	-48	-55	-61	-68	-74	-81
25	29	23	16	9	3	-4	-11	-17	-24	-31	-37	-44	-51	-58	-64	-71	-78	-84
30	28	22	15	8	1	-5	-12	-19	-26	-33	-39	-46	-53	-60	-67	-73	-80	-87
35	28	21	14	7	0	-7	-14	-21	-27	-34	-41	-48	-55	-62	-69	-76	-82	-89
40	27	20	13	6	-1	-8	-15	-22	-29	-36	-43	-50	-57	-64	-71	-78	-84	-91
45	26	19	12	5	-2	-9	-16	-23	-30	-37	-44	-51	-58	-65	-72	-79	-86	-93
50	26	19	12	4	-3	-10	-17	-24	-31	-38	-45	-52	-60	-67	-74	-81	-88	-95
55	25	18	11	4	-3	-11	-18	-25	-32	-39	-46	-54	-61	-68	-75	-82	-89	-97
60	25	17	10	3	-4	-11	-19	-26	-33	-40	-48	-55	-62	-69	-76	-84	-91	-98

Wind speed in mph

▶ Wind speed is calculated for 5 feet off the ground (typical height of an adult human face).

▶ Measurements are based on how wind affects the human face, typically the most exposed portion of the body.

▶ The table incorporates the theory that heat is lost from the body depending on its surroundings.

▶ The sun's impact is not factored into the windchill temperature formula.

Note: Windchill temperature is defined only for temperatures at or below 50°F and wind speeds above 3mph. Bright sunshine may increase the windchill temperature by 10 to 18°F.

FIGURE 7-1   Windchill chart. Source: National Weather Service.

2. *Avoid overheating*: Don't overdress or you'll overheat. You should feel a little cool until you warm up. Do take the windchill factor into account when preparing for a workout (Figure 7-1).

3. *Avoid overexposure*: There is a possibility of frostbite if you don't dress properly. Frostbite can occur on outer body areas such as the fingers and toes when your skin temperature drops below 32°F. Frostbite can easily be avoided by covering exposed areas and by getting inside and warming up if any body parts feel numb or tingly. **Hypothermia** is a life-threatening condition in which body temperature drops to a dangerously low level. Medical attention should be sought immediately.

4. *Protect exposed parts*: Fingers and toes receive the smallest blood supply and experience winter's chill fastest. Mittens are more effective than gloves, which allow cold air to circulate around the fingers. On extremely cold days it may be advisable to wear two pairs of socks or a thermal insole if the feet get too cold. Exposed ears or face can become windburned or chapped. To avoid discomfort, wear a hat and spread a thin layer of petroleum jelly on exposed skin areas.

5. *Work with the wind*: Plan out-and-back workouts, heading into the wind on the way out so that you can return with the wind to your back. Not only will you appreciate the push when you're tired, you'll be less likely to be chilled by your sweat during the return.

6. *Exercise with caution:* Winter weather changes the safety rules for outdoor exercise: Fewer daylight hours, icy roads, and snowy nights lower visibility

TABLE 7-4	*Heat Illnesses*	
Condition	**Symptoms**	**Immediate Care**
Heat cramps	Painful muscle spasms (calf is common) Sweaty skin Normal body temperature	Isolate cramps: Direct pressure to cramp and release, stretch muscle slowly and gently, gentle massage, ice
Heat exhaustion	Profuse sweating Cold, clammy skin Flu-like symptoms Dizziness Weak, rapid pulse Shallow breathing Headache Normal or slightly above normal temperature	Move individual out of sun to a well-ventilated area Place in shock position (feet elevated 12–18°) Gentle massage of extremities Give cool water to drink Remove extra clothing and cool the skin with water or a fan Reassure May apply wet towels Refer to physician or call EMS
Heat stroke (this is an extreme medical condition)	No perspiration Dry skin Very hot Temperature as high as 106°F Skin color bright red or flushed (African American–ashen) Rapid strong pulse Unresponsiveness (may be confused, stagger, or be agitated)	Transport to hospital quickly (call EMS) Remove as much clothing as possible without exposing the individual Cool quickly, starting at the head and continue down the body (use any means possible–fan, hose down, pack in ice) Wrap in cold, wet sheets for transport Treat for shock (place in a semireclining position)

for drivers. Exercise at midday as often as possible. Avoid high-volume traffic areas, wear bright clothing, and be prepared for potential hazards by remaining alert. Wear waffled or ridged shoe soles to provide extra traction on icy roads.

7. *Stay motivated*: Winter exercising demands greater personal motivation than exercising at any other time of the year. Winter holidays, less daylight, and poor weather can disrupt a routine. To maintain enthusiasm, set realistic wintertime goals to work toward. Don't worry about your pace. Between the slick footing and the heavy clothing, it's prudent to run relaxed. Just go fast enough to stay warm.

8. *Be safe*: Tell someone your route and when you expect to be back. Better yet, go with a friend.

Don't hesitate to mix your usual exercise with other activities–cross-country skiing or sledding in snow country, aerobics, stair climbing, indoor cycling, or water exercise if you crave a break from the cold. Your heart will benefit as long as you stay in your training zone, and the cross-training will work new muscle groups.

Exercising in the Heat

Given a couple of weeks and plenty of water, the human body can adapt well to exercise in the heat. Hot weather workouts make the body work harder than it does in cool weather. The heart must pump enough blood not only to fuel working muscles but also to carry heat to the skin to be dissipated, reducing work capacity. Drinking plenty of cold fluids is critical to maintain sweating, your body's air-conditioning system. The body can acclimatize to heat but not to dehydration. Overexertion in hot weather, particularly when coupled with dehydration, can lead to heat cramps; heat exhaustion; heatstroke; or **hyperthermia**, a life-threatening condition in which the body's temperature rises to a dangerous level. Particularly susceptible are people who are over 40, are out of shape, are overweight, have heart disease, or have previously experienced heat injury. See Table 7-4 for symptoms and care of heat illnesses.

When performing endurance exercise, men and women have similar responses in terms of adaptability to hot weather. Both genders are equally susceptible to heat stress, and both respond by acclimatization. To exercise safely when the weather is hot and humid, follow the Top 10 "Guidelines for Hot Weather Exercise" and postpone the workout when the Heat Safety Index is in the danger zone or above (Figure 7-2).

Heavy Sweating During Exercise

One of the hazards of exercising in hot, humid weather is dehydration caused by excessive loss of body water in the form of sweat. Overheating while exercising indoors at any time of the year can be as dangerous as outdoor exercise due to low levels of air movement. Sweat cannot evaporate effectively, and this may result

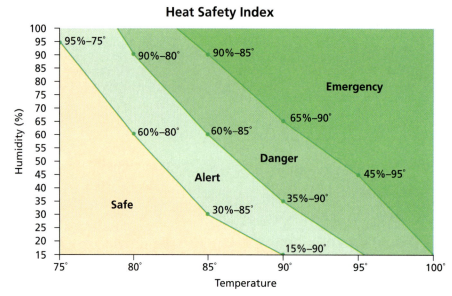

FIGURE 7-2 Heat safety index. Source: Ball State University Weather Station, Department of Geography.

in a heat illness. Dehydration disturbs cellular fluid and electrolyte balance, thus interfering with muscular contraction. Water losses of as little as 2 to 3 percent of body weight have been shown to impair exercise performance, reduce the amount of time a person can exercise, reduce cardiac stroke volume (volume of blood pumped out with each heartbeat), and reduce cardiac output (the amount of blood pumped by the heart over time). Water loss can also interfere with the body's ability to regulate internal temperature, resulting in overheating, which can be deadly.

Sweat is primarily water, but a number of major **electrolytes** (essential minerals in the form of salts) and other nutrients may be found in varying amounts. Sodium, chloride, and potassium are the predominant electrolytes found in sweat. They help maintain normal body fluid volume and are involved in nerve impulse transmission and muscle contraction (this includes the heart muscle).

Electrolyte Replacement

Is profuse sweating likely to create an electrolyte deficiency? No. That is not likely to occur even during prolonged exercise, such as marathon running. This is not to say that electrolyte replacement is not important and that electrolyte deficiency is impossible. After prolonged exercise with heavy sweating, the body's stores of electrolytes are diminished and could eventually become deficient. However, with a normal diet, it is difficult to create an electrolyte deficiency.

Salt tablets are not recommended to replace lost sodium and chloride because these electrolytes are abundant in a normal diet. Tablets may be prescribed for

TOP 10 LIST

Guidelines for Hot Weather Exercise

1. Respect the heat. Hot, humid, sunny weather can be deadly.
2. Monitor weather conditions before exercising and adjust your workout accordingly. Postpone exercise when heat safety index is in the danger zone or above.
3. Drink plenty of fluids to avoid dehydration (see Figure 7-3).
4. Weigh yourself before and after a workout. A sudden loss of weight may signal dehydration.
5. Wear loose-fitting clothing that allows air to circulate and expose as much skin to the air as possible to promote sweat evaporation.
6. Wear light colors because they reflect rather than absorb sunlight.
7. When acclimating to warmer weather in the spring, decrease exercise intensity and duration. Allow 2 weeks to acclimate to normal exercise levels.
8. Check with your doctor about the effects of any medications you take because some can reduce heat tolerance.
9. Do not wear vinyl or rubber sweat suits to lose body weight. They can lead to dehydration and death.
10. Stop exercising at the first sign of heat illness. See Table 7-4.

those who cannot replace them through normal dietary means. Keep in mind that diets high in sodium have been associated with high blood pressure. Citrus fruits, fruit juices, and bananas are foods recommended for electrolyte replacement.

Fluid Replacement: Water or Sports Drinks?

Rehydration (replacing body fluid volume) is critical to safe, effective exercise involving heavy sweating indoors or outside. For years we were told that water is the best drink to replace fluids, because that is mainly what you lose when you sweat during a hard workout. But science is dynamic, and conventional wisdom sometimes becomes history in the light of new discoveries. Water is still considered one of the most effective ways to rehydrate and works fine for the fitness exerciser and those exercising for less than 1 hour. Also, water is convenient and free. New information, concerning exercise of *1 hour or more*, now gives the slight edge in fluid replacement to electrolyte-containing beverages such as the popular sports drinks. This is the case because fluids containing electrolytes are more readily retained in the body's tissues. Why? Because plain water tends to increase urination slightly so that fewer fluids remain in the body's tissues. Also, when fluids taste good (as sports drinks do), they are more readily consumed. Thus the intake is increased. Due to these new findings, many commercial beverages have been produced to help in the process of rehydrating the body. These drinks are commonly known as carbohydrate-electrolyte replacement solutions (CES) or sports drinks. Other than water, the major ingredients in these solutions are carbohydrates in the form of glucose and/or sucrose and some of the major electrolytes. The glucose/sucrose content varies with the different brands, ranging from 1 percent to over 10 percent. Studies have shown that sports drinks containing carbohydrates boost endurance and energy as well as help delay fatigue during exercise. Select a sports drink carefully. Drinks with high carbohydrate concentrations are slow to empty from the stomach, interfering with rehydration, and can cause bloating and nausea. Avoid sports drinks containing carbohydrate concentrations higher than 8 percent (4 to 8 percent works best). Experiment during training to find out if you can handle one of these drinks. You should drink early and frequently during your workouts. Don't do anything new for competitive events. If you are a competitive athlete or marathoner or if you are exercising for several hours at a time in hot humid weather, the fluid of choice for most effective rehydration or prevention of dehydration is a sports drink (not to exceed 8 percent carbohydrate concentration). Water is the next best fluid, followed by fruit juices diluted with 50 percent water. All three are preferable to caffeinated sodas. Caffeine promotes urination, and the carbonation gives you a feeling of being fuller than you are. This information, which gives sports drinks a slight edge in terms of rehydration, does not mean that drinking water is not a good way to replace lost fluids.

Whatever you drink, drink it cold. Cold drinks are better than warm ones because they help cool down the core temperature of the body and empty from the stomach faster. Athletes/exercisers drink substantially more when fluids are cold. See the Fluid Pyramid in Figure 7-3 for fluid replacement guidelines.

Water: Are Americans Dehydrated?

Probably not. New research has reexamined the old question of how much water we should consume daily. Until recently it was believed that most Americans were dehydrated and in danger of all kinds of health problems because of that. Is there anyone on the planet who has not heard of the longtime standard health rule "drink at least eight 8-ounce glasses of water every day"? That's 64 ounces! Where did that advice originate? Is this the recommendation today?

The "eight 8-ounce glasses rule" originated from a 1945 Food and Nutrition Board report recommending 1 milliliter of water for every calorie consumed, averaging eight cups for a 2,000-calorie diet. The medical community at the time bought into that report, and the notion that the body needs at least eight 8-ounce glasses of water a day became a firmly established rule.

Later research found no evidence to support the notion that it is mandatory to consume eight 8-ounce

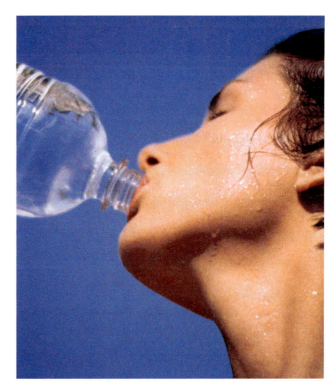

A regular intake of low-fat dairy products, lean meats and fish, along with fresh fruits and vegetables can also supply water needed by the body.

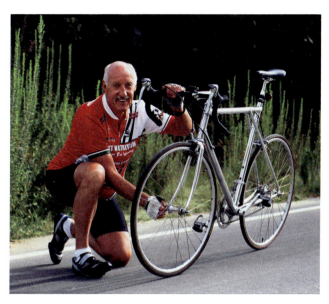

Studies show that people who exercise are less likely to suffer from dementia and Alzheimer's disease. Additional blood flow to the brain may help flush away the plaque.

- ✔ Diabetes
- ✔ Osteoporosis
- ✔ Depression and anxiety
- ✔ Falls and broken bones
- ✔ Some kinds of cancer
- ✔ Alzheimer's disease

We now feel that these health problems are more related to physical inactivity. The body adapts to whatever load is placed on it, and the ability to do work is reduced if the load lessens. Attitudes are changing. Older adults, encouraged by their doctors and by research revealing the benefits of exercise, are biking, swimming, jogging, lifting weights, and walking in ever-increasing numbers. We know that older adults (even up to age 100) are remarkably responsive to exercise, reaping health benefits. As the health-conscious baby-boom generation matures, its members are likely to redefine the concept of aging.

Aging and Performance

Some say, "Growing old isn't so bad if you consider the alternative." James Dean's "Live fast, die young, and leave a good-looking corpse" does have its proponents, but they are quickly weeded out of the genetic pool. At birth, we each have an 80-plus-year warranty, but the maintenance is up to us. Just like any machine, the human body grows less efficient as it ages. The decline in aerobic fitness among the sedentary is about 1 percent every year after age 25. Decreases in strength, flexibility, and endurance and increased body fat proportion with age are often accepted as a natural part of the aging process. These changes may be common, but they are not inevitable. The most significant factor contributing to declines in physiological capacity at any age is *lack of regular exercise*. The "use it or lose it" rule applies. As much as 50 percent of the functional decline seen in aging is related to disuse and can be prevented with regular aerobic exercise. Unused muscles atrophy, lose elasticity, and grow weak. Ligaments and tendons shorten and tighten, decreasing range of motion and causing aches and pains as they pull across joints. As muscle tissue atrophies, basal metabolism drops, resulting in an increase in body fat even when a person is not eating enough to maintain adequate nutritional levels.

Other adverse changes that occur with aging can also be favorably affected by exercise. For example, exercise can enhance insulin sensitivity, reduce blood pressure, and improve psychological well-being.

Osteoporosis has become a national health priority—one in two women and one in four men over the age of 50 will have an osteoporotic fracture in their lifetime. (See "The Numbers.") As the population ages, osteoporosis here and around the world will result in an

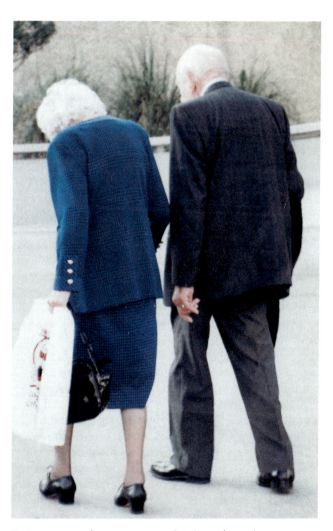

Postmenopausal women can maintain and may increase their bone density by regularly doing weight-bearing and resistance exercise.

THE NUMBERS

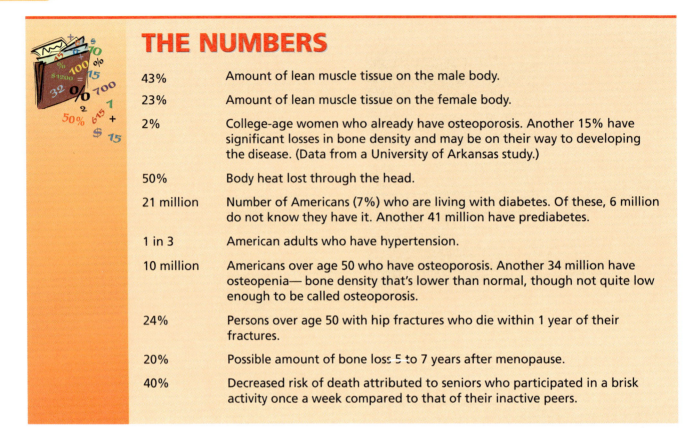

43%	Amount of lean muscle tissue on the male body.
23%	Amount of lean muscle tissue on the female body.
2%	College-age women who already have osteoporosis. Another 15% have significant losses in bone density and may be on their way to developing the disease. (Data from a University of Arkansas study.)
50%	Body heat lost through the head.
21 million	Number of Americans (7%) who are living with diabetes. Of these, 6 million do not know they have it. Another 41 million have prediabetes.
1 in 3	American adults who have hypertension.
10 million	Americans over age 50 who have osteoporosis. Another 34 million have osteopenia— bone density that's lower than normal, though not quite low enough to be called osteoporosis.
24%	Persons over age 50 with hip fractures who die within 1 year of their fractures.
20%	Possible amount of bone loss 5 to 7 years after menopause.
40%	Decreased risk of death attributed to seniors who participated in a brisk activity once a week compared to that of their inactive peers.

epidemic of life-diminishing, life-threatening fractures. To develop optimal bone strength and mass and ward off osteoporosis, women need adequate amounts of calcium in the diet, estrogen in the bloodstream, and weight-bearing exercise in their lifestyle. Exercise acts synergistically with estrogen to develop bone strength. Inactivity accelerates bone mineral loss and increases the risk of osteoporosis. Bone mass usually peaks between the ages of 25 and 30 and then gradually declines. The decline is hastened by menopause. While exercise alone cannot prevent osteoporosis, it may help premenopausal women build their bone densities so that they enter menopause ahead of the game. Ideally, women and men should exercise early in life to build bone and later in life to keep it strong. Weight-bearing exercise and strength training that stresses the bone help increase bone content, which is better increased by a combination of the two than by strength training alone. Once osteoporosis has developed, women and men should still be encouraged to exercise except while a fracture is healing. Men also are affected by osteoporosis, but at later ages than women. Studies show that men and women 60 and older who train with weights, exercise bands, and resistance machines several times a week can quickly double their total body strength. See the exercise band photo. This helps fight osteoporosis by keeping skeletons sturdy. Also, such strength gains have major implications for maintaining independence in

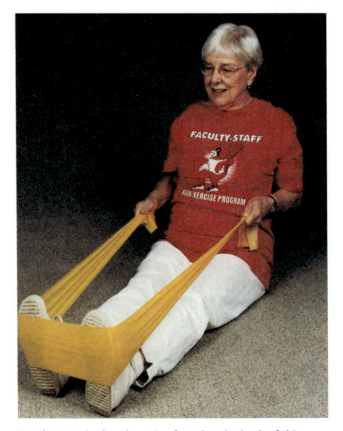

Use the exercise band routine found at the back of this book. Proper strength training offers numerous benefits to people of all ages and fitness levels.

later years. Muscle weakness can advance to the stage where an elderly individual cannot do common activities of daily living. Household tasks such as getting out of a chair, sweeping the floor, and taking out the trash may become impossible. Reduced functional ability may then increase the chance of nursing home placement. Lifelong exercise may also help protect the elderly against falls and the devastating effects of hip fractures. It's never too late to start exercising. Starting late in life is far preferable to not starting at all.

While aging is unavoidable, declines in functional capacity with age are not inevitable. How you age is largely up to you. Cardiologist George Sheehan has said that growing older isn't so bad; it is inactive people who give aging a bad name.

As one physician observed, "So many things we think are linked to aging . . . actually have to do with lifestyle. Exercise produces a 40-year age offset. A fit person of 70 is the equal of an unfit person of 30 in regard to bones, muscles, heart, brain, sex, and everything else. I see an immense energy in old people who continue [exercise]." Exercise intensity appears to be the key to getting the greatest benefit. A group of master athletes (ages 40 to 75) studied over an 18-year period showed no significant decline in aerobic capacity if they maintained training intensity. *For most elderly fitness exercisers, however, an exercise intensity of 50 to 70 percent maximal heart rate reserve is considered adequate.*

The effect of true nonpreventable aging involves a gradual loss of the speed and vigor with which we do activities, but it should not prevent us from doing them. As one older runner observed, "I can do everything I used to. It just takes longer to do it and longer to recover."

Exercise is adult play. At what point was our childhood eagerness to get out and romp replaced by hours of sitting in front of the TV watching others play? Whether aging is an extension of a full and active life or a gradual wasting away is determined by how you choose to live your life.

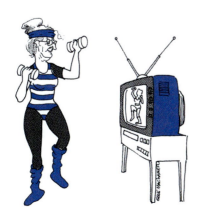

Exercise slows the aging process.

TOP 10 LIST

List of Benefits of Exercise for Older Adults

1. Helps maintain the ability to live independently and reduces the risk of falling and fracturing bones.
2. Increases energy and helps the individual perform daily routines with greater ease.
3. Helps control joint swelling and pain associated with arthritis.
4. Helps maintain healthy bones, muscles, and joints.
5. Enhances cardiorespiratory function and improves peripheral circulation; decreases the risk of arteriosclerosis and other circulatory problems.
6. Reduces constipation.
7. Reduces symptoms of anxiety and depression and fosters improvements in mood and feelings of well-being.
8. Helps people with chronic, disabling conditions improve stamina and muscle strength.
9. Reduces the risk of dying from coronary heart disease and of developing high blood pressure, colon cancer, and diabetes.
10. Improves a person's posture, decreases backache, enhances appearance, and helps control weight.

Does Exercise Increase Life Span?

While the length of your life may have a strong genetic component, study after study has shown that exercise helps lower the risk of major chronic diseases and premature death. Research conducted at the Cooper Institute for Aerobics Research in Dallas found that exercise of *moderate* intensity improved the overall *quality* of life (e.g., enhanced the ability to perform daily tasks, helped with weight control, enhanced psychological well-being) and perhaps increased the *quantity* of life by postponing a heart attack or stroke. A second study, part of the famous ongoing research on male Harvard alumni, reported that exercise of moderate intensity improved the quality of life but that it took exercise at a *vigorous* intensity level to add years to one's life. The Harvard men who had expended at least 1,500 calories a week in vigorous physical activity had a 25 percent lower death rate than did sedentary men. Vigorous activity was defined as fast walking, jogging, playing singles tennis, swimming, and performing heavy, sustained household chores. Studies such as these illustrate that any exercise has health benefits, but more exercise, enough to give your heart and lungs a real workout, is better. While a healthful lifestyle is no guarantee of a longer life, it does stack the odds in your favor.

Are you ever "too old" to begin exercise? No! While the overall impact you can make on the quality of your life is greater if you start exercising young and continue throughout life, there is no age at which the benefits of exercise stop. The older you are, the more you need exercise. Instead of searching for the "fountain of youth," Ponce de Leon would have been better off to dock his ship and remain on land—to start a walking program. The Top 10 List "Benefits of Exercise for Older Adults" identifies the benefits of exercise for older adults.

EXERCISE AND CHRONIC HEALTH CONDITIONS

The general FITT principles of exercise prescription apply to individuals with and without chronic disease. Also, it is essential to include flexibility and strength training exercises in all well-designed exercise programs. However, certain conditions may require differences or modifications in exercise programming in order to maximize effectiveness, avoid complications, and increase enjoyment of the activity. Each of the following conditions is highlighted with a brief overview and special exercise considerations to ensure safety and enjoyment: arthritis, asthma, diabetes, hypertension, and osteoporosis. If you have any of these conditions, it is important to check with your physician before participating in an exercise program. Have your doctor fill out the Exercise Clearance Form in Chapter 3.

Arthritis

Arthritis and rheumatoid disease cause muscle weakness, fatigue, pain and stiffness, and swelling in joints and other supporting structures of the body such as muscles, tendons, ligaments, and bones. The two most common forms are osteoarthritis and rheumatoid arthritis. Fourteen percent of Americans have arthritis and rheumatoid disease. Osteoarthritis is a degenerative joint disease that typically affects the knees, hips, feet, spine, and hands. Rheumatoid arthritis is a chronic, systemic inflammatory disease that affects the synovial membranes of joints. The complications of arthritis may lead to a less active lifestyle.

Scientists stress that physical activity of the type and amount recommended for health has not been shown to cause or worsen arthritis. While rest is important during flare-ups, lack of physical activity is associated with increased muscle weakness, joint stiffness, reduced range of motion, and fatigue.

The goals of an exercise program for people with arthritis are to preserve or restore range of motion and flexibility around affected joints; increase muscle strength and endurance; and increase cardiorespiratory endurance conditioning to improve mood and decrease health risks associated with a sedentary lifestyle.

Recommendations/modifications for exercise for those with arthritis include:

✔ Begin slowly and progress gradually.
✔ Avoid rapid or repetitive movements of affected joints.
✔ Perform flexibility exercise one to two times daily, using pain-free range of motion exercises. These can be done on land or in water such as a pool, hot tub, or warm bath. Physicians should provide specific stretches to be done instead of saying, "just stretch." Yoga and Tai Chi are good activities for increasing flexibility.
✔ Perform cardiorespiratory endurance exercise initially in short bouts (i.e., 10 minutes each time). Work up to 30 minutes. Performing three 10-minute sessions per day is also acceptable. Aquatic, walking, and cycling activities are advised.
✔ Perform resistance training two to three times per week. Do not exercise with pain.
✔ Include functional lifestyle activities (e.g., climbing stairs, standing up from a sitting position, buttoning clothes) daily.
✔ Avoid exercise during flare-ups.
✔ Stop exercise if you have continuing joint pain that lasts more than an hour after exercise, unusual fatigue, increased weakness, decreased range of motion, or increased joint swelling.
✔ Morning exercise may not be advised for those with significant morning stiffness.

Asthma

Years ago, it was thought that strenuous physical activity was dangerous if you had asthma, but now we know better. Exercise is not only safe if done properly; it is an integral part of treatment. Studies have shown that physically fit people have fewer attacks, need less medication, and lose less time from work or school. Seventeen million Americans are living with asthma.

Activities that involve short, intermittent periods of exertion such as volleyball, baseball, half-court basketball, and tennis are generally well-tolerated by individuals with asthma. Activities that involve continuous exertion such as jogging, field hockey, and cycling as well as cold weather sports (e.g., cross-country skiing, ice skating, jogging in winter) may be less well-tolerated. However, with proper precaution, most people with asthma are able to fully participate in these activities. Swimming is well-tolerated because of the warm, moist air environment. Other beneficial activities include both indoor and outdoor cycling, aerobics, walking, or running on a treadmill.

To make sure asthma doesn't interfere with your ability to exercise, keep it under control. If your doctor has prescribed medications for daily use, use them faithfully. Take necessary steps to control allergies. Visit the doctor on a regular schedule for instructions about monitoring your condition at home and be sure to report any problems promptly.

People with well-controlled asthma can exercise following the FITT prescription for exercise outlined in Chapter 4. For balanced fitness, strength training and flexibility components should also be included. Follow the guidelines described in Chapter 5 and Chapter 6. However, if your asthma is exercise-induced, pay special attention to avoiding environmental "triggers" such as cold, dry, dusty air and/or inhaled pollutants and chemicals. Even if your asthma is well-controlled, you may develop coughing, shortness of breath, chest pain, or nausea if you exercise without taking precautions. Do not exercise during an acute asthma attack; wait until the symptoms have subsided. For safe exercise participation follow these guidelines:

✔ Exercise regularly. Acute attacks are more likely if you exercise only occasionally.

✔ Warm up and cool down thoroughly.

✔ Avoid exercising in cold, dry air. In the winter, work out indoors, or if you are active outside, cover your mouth and nose with a scarf or breathing mask to warm the air you breathe.

✔ Don't exercise on days when your symptoms are bothersome, such as when you are wheezing or coughing.

✔ Avoid areas where air pollution is high (e.g., near highways or during high-traffic times of the day). On days when pollution is worse than normal or the pollen count is particularly high, exercise indoors or not at all.

✔ If your doctor recommends it, use medications as prescribed before exercising.

✔ If you develop symptoms during exercise, don't try to push your way through them. Stop what you are doing and follow the directions on your inhaler. If this doesn't bring relief within 15 to 20 minutes, seek medical help.

Diabetes Mellitus

Diabetes mellitus (both type 1 and type 2) is a chronic disease characterized by the body's inability to produce insulin or use the hormone properly. See Chapter 9 for expanded information about diabetes, especially Table 9-5. The treatment goal for diabetes is blood glucose control, which includes exercise, diet, and medications.

TOP 10 LIST

Exercising with Diabetes

1. Get proper medical advice before starting an exercise program.

2. Monitor blood glucose levels before, during, and after exercise, especially in the early stages of exercise training. Check twice prior to exercise, 30 minutes before and immediately before; and every 20 to 30 minutes during prolonged exercise. **If your blood glucose level is 300 mg/dl or higher, do not exercise**.

3. Don't exercise when you are sick. Exercising when you are sick can make your blood glucose levels fluctuate dramatically, and it may take longer to get well.

4. Keep fluid levels well up before, during, and after exercise, especially during hot weather. Dehydration can affect blood glucose levels and heart function.

5. Be aware of signs of hypoglycemia (low blood glucose) even several hours after exercise. Have a carbohydrate-based snack or drink handy.

6. Exercise 1 to 2 hours after a meal.

7. Avoid injecting insulin in a muscle that is about to be used for exercise.

8. Wear correct footwear. Peripheral vascular disease is relatively common in diabetics, and this often affects the feet.

9. Exercise at the same time each day. Exercising at a similar time, intensity, and duration each day helps you get to know your own blood glucose response to exercise training.

10. In case of emergency, wear an identification bracelet or shoe tag while exercising.

If you have diabetes, one of the best things you can do for yourself is to stay active. Before beginning an exercise program, diabetic individuals should undergo an extensive medical evaluation, particularly for the cardiovascular, nervous, renal (kidney), and visual systems because they are at high risk for diabetic complications.

Exercise increases vulnerability to two major diabetes-related problems: hypoglycemia (a rapid drop in blood glucose level) and foot sores (caused by peripheral vascular disease). Hypoglycemia is initially characterized by sweating, hunger, dizziness, anxiety, a rapid heart rate, and tremor. Without proper attention, the sufferer may lose consciousness and go into shock. Foot sores that are not properly treated can rapidly worsen, sometimes within a matter of hours, and lead to infection. Severe cases may require amputation. Individuals with advanced diabetic neuropathy should choose low-impact activities like swimming, rowing, water exercise, and cycling rather than high-impact ones like jogging. Everyone with diabetes should inspect the feet for signs of irritation before and after exercise. Activities like scuba diving and rock climbing can be dangerous if there is any possibility of hypoglycemia.

Diabetics with retinopathy and nephropathy should avoid activities that sharply raise blood pressure. To strength train, use light weights and multiple repetitions and avoid lifting high weights for low repetitions. Avoid exercise that causes jerky motions (e.g., bouncing on a trampoline); increases eye pressure (e.g., scuba diving or mountain climbing); or places your eyes below the level of your heart (e.g., toe touching).

With proper training, most diabetics can exercise as much as they wish. Follow the FITT prescription for cardiorespiratory endurance fitness and include flexibility and strength-training components for balanced fitness. See the Top 10 List "Exercising with Diabetes."

Hypertension

Hypertension (or high blood pressure) is defined as a blood pressure (BP) equal to or exceeding a systolic BP of 140 mm Hg and/or a diastolic BP of 90 mm Hg. Hypertension is one of the most prevalent forms of cardiovascular disease. It is the major contributor to strokes, heart attacks, congestive heart failure, peripheral vascular disease, and kidney failure. The risk of many of these diseases increases at levels of blood pressure well below the diagnostic threshold of 140/90 mm Hg. Therefore, lowering blood pressure may benefit individuals with any elevation above optimal levels. See Chapter 9 for important blood pressure information.

The American College of Sports Medicine advises that exercise should be the cornerstone of therapy for the prevention, treatment, and control of high blood pressure. Most aerobic, resistance, and flexibility types of exercise are recommended, but the primary form of exercise should be the aerobic type. The FITT prescription for cardiorespiratory endurance exercise should be adhered to but with the following adaptations:

✔ The preferred intensity of the aerobic exercise should be at the moderate-intensity level (below 70 percent HRR) because it appears to reduce BP as much as, if not more than, exercise at higher intensities. Walking, cycling, and swimming are good choices. The intensity level of running may be too intense.

✔ The preferred frequency of the aerobic exercise is 7 days per week because BP is lowered for several hours after a single bout of exercise. Lowering BP just a few days per week with aerobic exercise is not sufficient.

Additional special exercise guidelines for those with high blood pressure include:

✔ Do not exercise if resting systolic BP is greater than 200 mm Hg or diastolic BP is greater than 110 mm Hg.
✔ Vigorous activities done with high force, such as sprinting, rowing, or heavy lifting or straining, are not advised for hypertensive individuals.
✔ Downhill skiing may exaggerate an elevated BP response from the cold and elevation.
✔ Be aware of heat. Some BP medications impair the ability to regulate body temperature or can cause dehydration.
✔ Cool down. Extend the cool-down period because some BP medications may cause BP levels to drop after abruptly stopping exercise.
✔ Weight loss, even a few pounds, helps to lower BP.

Resistance training should not be the only or main mode of exercise for individuals with hypertension, but it should be combined with an aerobic exercise program. Use lower resistance (i.e., 30 to 60 percent of maximal effort) with higher repetitions (i.e., 12 to 15 repetitions). Follow these guidelines when performing resistance exercise:

✔ Avoid isometric types of exercise.
✔ Do not hold your muscle at the point of full muscle contraction.
✔ Avoid "holding" your breath while exercising, especially during resistance types of exercise.

Osteoporosis

Osteoporosis literally means "porous bone." It is a skeletal disease characterized by low bone mass, increased bone fragility, and increased risk for bone fracture. Osteoporotic fractures commonly occur in the hip, spine, and wrist but can occur at other sites. Osteoporosis is a silent disease in that a fracture is frequently the first indication of bone loss. Osteoporosis has a debilitating effect on independence and quality of life, especially for older adults. Risk factors for osteoporosis are family history, female gender, estrogen deficiency, low weight, dietary factors, prolonged use of corticosteriods, and physical inactivity. Bone mass attained early in life is perhaps the most important determinant of lifelong skeletal health. Young women who suffer from female athlete triad are at risk of bone loss and osteoporosis. Exercise can positively affect peak bone mass in children and adolescents, maintain or even modestly increase bone mass in adulthood, and assist in minimizing age-related bone loss in older adults. See the Aging and Physical Activity section in this chapter.

How does exercise help prevent osteoporosis? If bones are not used, they weaken. Studies on astronauts and injured athletes have shown that even well-conditioned

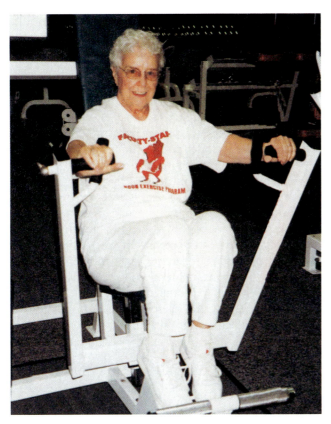

You don't stop playing because you grow old. You grow old because you stop playing. Strength training becomes increasingly important with age. Older adults need lighter weights with more repetitions and more time between sessions to recover.

individuals suffer from a reduction in bone mass and density during prolonged periods of inactivity. The detrimental results of little or no activity may be heightened as we get older. When force or stress is applied to a bone, the bone bends. This sets up a cascade of events that stimulates cells to strengthen the bone. The bone can adapt to stress or the lack of it by forming or losing mass. For the bone to become bigger and more dense, the stress must be above and beyond normal levels. The bone will continue to grow and adapt until it is restructured to handle the new imposed stress.

Each bone in the body must be stressed to grow strong. If the leg bones are stressed by running and jumping, the arm bones will not benefit unless they too are stressed with specific exercises (e.g., weight lifting). Thus a good exercise program to prevent and treat osteoporosis involves all of the major muscle and bone groups in the entire body.

Young bone is more responsive to exercise stress than old bone is. Given that approximately 60 percent of the final skeleton is built during adolescence, vigorous physical exercise during childhood and adolescence is more important than at any other time in life.

If you already have osteoporosis or low bone density consult your doctor before starting an exercise program. Depending on the status of your condition, your doctor may or may not recommend certain exercises and will inform you of precautions that are necessary when you exercise or perform regular activities. Avoid exercise when a fracture is healing. Use extreme caution when performing exercise that involves the following movements, as they may be dangerous:

- ✔ *Forward bending.* Avoid activities and exercise that involve bending forward excessively at the waist because they increase the risk of compression fractures of the vertebra.
- ✔ *Heavy lifting.* Avoid heavy lifting, especially when bending forward at the waist. This may include lifting loads of laundry, bags of groceries, or exercise weights.
- ✔ *Twisting.* Twisting movement can place unusual force on your spine. Golfing and bowling are two common sports that involve twisting and may be harmful. Check with your doctor about whether you can safely participate in these sports.
- ✔ *High-impact activities.* Activities that involve higher-impact movements, sudden stops and starts, and abrupt weight shifts put too much stress on your spine and can lead to falls and knee injuries. Such activities include sprinting, soccer, racket sports, volleyball, and basketball.

Sometimes you cannot avoid certain movements such as bending forward or reaching overhead. But you can use caution and practice good posture and body mechanics to decrease risk of injury.

If you don't have osteoporosis and are otherwise healthy, exercising to prevent osteoporosis is generally safe. Once osteoporosis has developed, exercise is still encouraged except while a fracture is healing. The following types of exercises are recommended for osteoporosis prevention:

1. *Weight-bearing and impact exercise.* Weight-bearing exercise means your bones and muscles are working against gravity as you exercise. These involve activities you do on your feet with your bones supporting your weight. Examples include brisk walking, jogging, skipping, jumping rope, stair-climbing or step-type exercises, racket sports, aerobic dance, dancing, hiking, and team sports. *Swimming and bicycling are not weight-bearing* because your body is supported by the water or the bike rather than your legs. Recent research reveals that for many, walking may not adequately stress the bones to improve their strength. Activities with more impact and higher intensity may be necessary. This would not be the case for frail elderly though. For osteoporosis prevention,

weight-bearing/high-impact activities are best and weight-bearing/low-impact activities are good but less so. This latter category includes low-impact aerobics and most cardiovascular machines (stair climbers, rowers, elliptical trainers, treadmill walking). Yoga and Pilates are non-impact and are activities that are least beneficial for osteoporosis prevention.

2. *Strength training*. Strength training uses resistance, such as free weights, weight machines, resistance bands, and water activities to strengthen muscles. Strength training activities for the legs, abdomen, and back should be emphasized to improve lower-body strength and posture to help prevent falls and broken bones. Because of the increase in gravitational force on bone in a weight-bearing position, strength training exercises performed on the feet are considered to be more effective at stimulating bone than machine-based exercises performed in a seated position. In the on-the-feet weight-bearing position, there is an increased load at the hip and greater demand for postural control and balance, which in turn optimizes bone health. Also recommended are push-ups and exercises performed on the feet (with or without hand weights) such as the forward, backward, and sideways lunge; squat; chair raise; heel and toe raise; stepping; and jumping.

3. *Back-strengthening*. Back-strengthening exercises should be included in exercise programs for the treatment and prevention of osteoporosis. Strengthening the muscles of the back may help improve the health of people with osteoporosis and low bone mass by improving posture and decreasing risk of compression fractures caused by the stooped posture commonly seen in people with the disease. Exercises that gently arch the back, the opposite direction of a stooped posture, can strengthen back muscle while minimizing back stress. See the Exercises for the Lower Back pullout at the back of the book.

Frequently Asked Questions

Q. Can I work out when I have a cold or upper respiratory infection?

A. It depends. Studies suggest that *moderate* exercise training (at 70 percent HRR) during an upper respiratory infection (URI) does not appear to extend the length or increase the severity of the illness. However, exercising during a URI should be considered carefully. Use the following guidelines to decide if it is okay for you to exercise during a cold or URI.

- If you are not experiencing extreme tiredness, malaise, fever, or swollen lymph glands, you may safely exercise at an intensity level lower than that of your regular workouts.
- Also, perform a "neck check." Assess cold symptoms and classify them as either above or below the neck. If symptoms are "above the neck" (i.e., runny nose, sneezing, or scratchy throat), you may exercise at a lower intensity. Exercise is not advised when you have "below the neck" symptoms (i.e., fever, aching muscles, productive cough, vomiting, or diarrhea).
- If you begin feeling better during the workout, increase the intensity of the workout accordingly.

Q. True or false? All alcoholic beverages are dehydrating.

A. False. Although nonalcoholic beverages are recommended for rehydration, especially when you are exercising or working in hot weather, beer, many mixed drinks, and wine are fairly diluted, and so they add to the total fluid intake. Concentrated alcoholic beverages such as vodka and brandy, if drunk undiluted, are very dehydrating.

Q. True or false? "Oxygenated" water, which is infused with 5 to 10 times as much oxygen as regular water, will help your muscles and improve your performance. So will vitamin-enriched water.

A. False and false. Studies have shown that oxygenated water does not improve aerobic performance or increase oxygen levels in the blood. The only way to get oxygen into the blood and muscles is through the lungs. Vitamin-enriched waters and those containing herbs also will not improve performance or benefit your health in any way. However, sports drinks containing low levels of sugar and sodium can help conserve carbohydrate stores and delay fatigue during a prolonged workout.

Q. Does exercise affect the cognitive ability of older adults?

A. Yes. Older adults who stay fit may be better equipped to deal with situations that require quick or multitask thinking. Research reveals that active seniors have increased executive control function (ECF). ECF is a type of complex thinking needed to handle a sudden unexpected change (such as a car darting into your lane) and in multitasking situations (such as talking on the telephone and checking e-mail simultaneously). Fit seniors have sharper thinking, a reduced risk of cognitive decline, and improved motor preparation. So do fit *young* people.

Q. What is **sarcopenia**?

A. Pronounced sark-ko-PEEN-ya, this is a word you are likely to hear more often. It means not only loss of muscle and strength but also decreased quality of muscle tissue. Most people lose 20 to 40 percent of their muscle tissue as they get older. Strength training can restore muscle mass and strength or at least slow this loss.

Q. Is it ever too late to start strength training?

A. No. In several recent studies, even elderly nursing home residents saw marked improvement after undertaking an 8-week program that significantly improved their balance, strength, and walking speed. It also helped lower cholesterol.

Summary

Exercise is meant to be enjoyed throughout life. Regardless of gender or age, the body improves with use and degenerates with disuse. People don't wear out; they rust out. For the greatest benefit from an exercise program, it is helpful to be aware of special concerns, such as how to exercise safely in hot and cold weather and how to avoid high-risk exercises. You have learned in this chapter that women respond to exercise the way men do but perhaps a little slower and to a lesser extent, and, with a physician's approval, pregnant women can safely exercise. This means training principles are approximately the same, regardless of gender. You have also learned that water is a fine rehydrater after exercise but that sports drinks are recommended for rehydration after prolonged exercise (60 to 90 minutes) and profuse sweating. Sports drinks contain electrolytes, which enhance fluid retention, contain carbohydrates, delay the onset of fatigue, and boost energy, and they taste good, which increases the likelihood that we will drink more when working out. You now understand that moderate exercise intensity strengthens the immune system and that unfortunately for some, exercise can become addictive. As you adjust to a physically active lifestyle, you will find that the benefits far outweigh the effort involved. Exercise will become a habit, and you will begin to look forward to your workout as an important part of your day.

Let the words of Don Ardell inspire you to maximize your potential to be the best you can be: "Excellence ain't easy. If it were, everyone would be doing it and it would be ordinary. Know that, in lots of ways, the deck is stacked against anyone who wants to excel. Do it anyway."

 ## Internet Resources

AARP Webplace
www.aarp.org
Lists healthy aging resources.

Administration of Aging
www.aoa.dhhs.gov
Department of Health and Human Services site that contains links on aging-related topics.

Alzheimer's Association
www.alz.org
Learn about what you can do to maintain a healthy brain.

American Diabetes Association
www.diabetes.org
Has an exercise section with FAQs. Also has information about cycling and walking events.

Arthritis Foundation
www.arthritis.org
Has information on health and exercise tips concerning arthritis. Also provides tips about living with arthritis and the latest research.

Cooper Institute for Aerobics Research
www.cooperinst.org
Provides information about exercise research.

Health A to Z
www.healthatoz.com
Includes health and medical search engines.

Healthfinder
www.healthfinder.gov
Consolidates official government health resources and offers links to over 500 health sites.

Mayo Clinic/Mayo Health Oasis
www.mayoclinic.com or www.mayohealth.org
A complete health and wellness library. Search by major subject area.

Medline Plus
www.medlineplus.gov
Provides healthy aging information.

National High Blood Pressure Education Program
www.nh/bi.nih.gov
Learn how to lower high blood pressure.

National Institute on Aging
www.nih.gov/nia
Provides information on healthy aging and aging concerns.

National Osteoporosis Foundation
www.nof.org
Gives information and exercises.

National Osteoporosis Society
www.nos.org.uk
Provides information and exercises and will answer questions.

National Women's Health Information Center
www.4women.gov
Contains women's health information.

Shape Up America
www.shapeup.org
Run by former surgeon general C. Everett Koop. Dedicated to educating and empowering consumers to improve their health.

Bibliography

Armstrong, L., et al. *ACSM's Guidelines for Exercise Testing and Prescription,* 7th ed. Mitchell H. Whaley, ed. Philadelphia: Lippincott Williams & Wilkins, 2000.

Brandon, J. L., L. W. Boyette, A. Lloyd, et al. "Resistive Training and Long-Term Function in Older Adults." *Journal of Aging and Physical Activity* 12, no. 1 (January 2004): 10–28.

Colcombe, S. J., A. F. Dramer, K. I. Erickson, et al. "Cardiovascular Fitness, Cortical Plasticity, and Aging." *Proceedings of the National Academy of Sciences* 101, no. 9 (March 2, 2004): 3316–3321.

Dembo, L. K. McCormick. "Exercise Prescription to Prevent Osteoporosis." *ACSM's Health and Fitness Journal* 4, no. 1 (January/February 2000): 32–38.

Dipietro, L. J. Dziura. "Exercise: A Prescription to Delay the Effects of Aging." *The Physician and Sports Medicine Journal* 28 (October 2000): 77–78.

Gulati, M., H. R. Black, and L. J. Shaw. "The Prognostic Value of a Nomagram for Exercise Capacity in Women." *The New England Journal of Medicine* 353, no. 5 (August 4, 2005): 468–475.

Jones, J. C., and R. Debra. "International Guidelines for Training Physical Activity Instructors of Older Adults: An Update." *Journal of Aging & Physical Activity* 12, no. 4 (October 2004): 463–479.

Kalapotharakos, V., M. Michalopoulou, et al. "The Effects of High- and Moderate-Resistive Training on Muscle Function in the Elderly." *Journal of Aging & Physical Activity* 12, no. 2 (April 2004): 131–143.

Kamijo, Y., K. Lee, and G. Mack. "Active Cutaneous Vasodilation in Resting Humans during Mild Heat Stress." *Journal of Applied Physiology* 98 (January 2005): 829–837.

Lee, I., M. C. Hsieh, and R. S. Paffenbarger. "Exercise Intensity and Longevity in Men: The Harvard Alumni Health Study." *Journal of American Medical Association* 273, no. 15 (April 19, 1995): 1179–1184.

Leibman, B. "Breaking Up. Strong Bones Need More Than Calcium." *Nutrition Action, Center for Science in the Public Interest* 32, no. 3 (April 2005): 1–8.

Loland, N. "Exercise, Health, and Aging." *Journal of Aging & Physical Activity* 12, no. 2 (April 2004): 170–184.

Manore, M. A. "Feeding the Active Female: Part II." *ACSM's Health & Fitness Journal* 9, no. 5 (September/October 2005): 26–28.

Slawta, J. N., and R. Ross. "Exercise for Osteoporosis Prevention." *ACSM's Health & Fitness Journal* 8, no. 6 (November/December 2004): 12–19.

U. C. Berkeley Wellness Letter. "Bone Density." June 2003.

Wilson, S. "An Ignored Epidemic." *Athletic Management* 15, no. 3 (April/May 2003): 47–58.

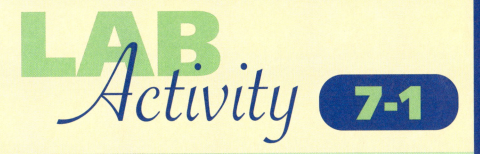

Exploring Special Exercise Considerations Challenge

1. Your sister's gynecologist just told her she is pregnant. Knowing you are taking a college fitness/wellness course, she asks you for advice concerning the fitness walking program she began 2 months ago to help her get back into shape and lose a few pounds. Give her three or four tips.

2. At dinner, two of your friends were debating whether to use a popular sports drink to replace the sweat they expected to lose in the July 4 12-mile run, which they estimated would take *more* than 1 hour to complete. The July 4 festivities are tomorrow, with the race beginning at noon in Old Town and ending at the top of Heartbreak Hill. What advice would you give them?

3. Your grandparents (age 65) were advised by their neighbor to stop that "foolish" exercising, slow down, and start acting their age. They ask you your opinion about this advice. What can you tell them about the benefits of staying physically active?

4. In Speech 101, your topic for the final exam speech is "The Difference Between Men's and Women's Exercise Performance Levels: Are They More Alike Than Different?" List three similarities and differences you want to highlight in your speech.

5. Take the "Are You Addicted to Exercise?" self-assessment in this chapter. How many "yes" statements did you check? _____ Discuss your assessment score. Have a friend you think may be becoming addicted to exercise also take the self-assessment in this chapter. How can you help a friend who may be becoming addicted to exercise?

6. Many of my friends are afraid to exercise outside during cold weather because they might freeze their lungs. How do you respond to that?

7. Your grandmother has been diagnosed with osteoporosis, and your grandfather has been taking medication for hypertension for several years. They want to begin an exercise program. List three or more dos and don'ts for each condition for them to follow.

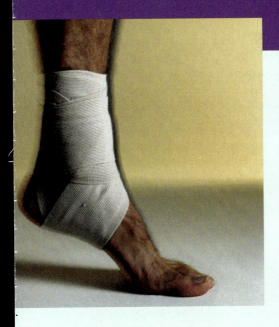

Preventing Common Injuries and Caring for the Lower Back

An ounce of prevention is worth a pound of cure.
—Anonymous

Objectives

After reading this chapter, you will be able to:
1. Identify four main reasons injuries occur.
2. Give three tips for avoiding an overuse injury.
3. Explain how muscle weakness and inflexibility contribute to injuries.
4. Identify four common muscle imbalances.
5. List and explain the general recommended treatment for common injuries (P.R.I.C.E.).
6. Describe the basic causes and treatment of ankle sprain, blisters, bursitis, chafing, heel spur syndrome, iliotibial band syndrome, muscle cramp, muscle soreness, muscle strain, patellofemoral syndrome, plantar fasciitis, shin splints, side stitch, stress fracture, and tendinitis.
7. Identify the symptoms of injury that indicate the need for medical attention.
8. Explain two vital components of rehabilitation needed to resume activity safely without injury.
9. Identify the two most important keys to preventing lower back pain.
10. Describe exercises recommended to reduce the risk of lower back pain.

Terms

- blisters
- bursitis
- cramp
- heel spur
- iliotibial band
- intervertebral disc
- ischemia
- ligament
- orthotics
- overpronation
- overuse
- patellofemoral syndrome
- plantar fasciitis
- P.R.I.C.E.
- pronation
- shin splint
- side stitch
- sprain
- strain
- stress fracture
- tendinitis
- tendons
- underpronation

A Fit and Well Way of Life Online Learning Center www.mhhe.com/robbinsfitwell1e
Go to the Online Learning Center for chapter quizzes, outlines, flashcards, and additional lab activities.

*Y*ou walk into your first jogging class, eager to improve your fitness. You have not exercised regularly, and you hope this class will help you get in shape. Your instructor begins with a warm-up and an easy jog around campus. After your run, you feel great and invigorated. The next morning, you wake up and your whole body aches. You don't remember having been run over by a truck. "What should I do now? Withdraw from class? Stay in bed? Buy stock in Ben-Gay? When will I be able to move again?"

Participation in fitness activities offers many benefits. These benefits far exceed the risk of injury. When you exercise, you intentionally use certain muscles to increase their strength and endurance. As your body adapts to these efforts, you may experience minor aches and soreness. Physical activity also carries some risk of overuse or injury. Fortunately, many of these discomforts are minor, and you will be able to continue or quickly resume your workouts. Everybody is built differently and varies in physical potential, so "listen to your body" to improve your personal fitness level safely—and avoid the pain of injury. This chapter discusses how to prevent injuries, how to recognize their signs and symptoms, and what treatments are recommended. It also examines how to maintain a healthy back, because chronic back pain is a common problem. Finally, factors that affect the musculature of the spine and ways to avoid lower back injury are covered.

INJURY PREVENTION

Prevention is the key to reducing the frequency of injuries. Ninety percent of injuries include slow wear and tear, strains, sprains, and inflammations. Understanding the causes of injuries allows you to stop minor problems before they turn you into the "walking wounded." Prevention is far more conducive to wellness than is any patch and repair job. There are four main reasons injuries occur:

1. *Overuse:* doing too much too soon or too often, causing a breakdown at the weakest point—ankle, Achilles tendon, shin, knee, or back.
2. *Footwear:* wearing improper or worn-out shoes.
3. *Weakness and inflexibility:* muscles so weak or tight that the slightest unusual twist strains them.

4. *Mechanical problems:* the result of biomechanical/anatomical problems (the way the foot hits the ground, body build, etc.) or using poor form while exercising.

An individually adjusted workload, well-made and well-kept shoes, supplemental toning and stretching exercises, and mechanical improvements will prevent the majority of injuries.

Overuse

To improve or maintain fitness, you must overload, or push beyond normal demands. Progressive overload following the guidelines in Chapter 3 is necessary and good to a point, but you must be able to recover between workouts. The goal is to exercise so that you improve but not so much that you cause **overuse**, excessive overload leading to injury or illness (Figure 8-1). Overuse problems commonly occur at the beginning of a new exercise program and account for the majority of injuries. It is estimated that 25 to 50 percent of athletes visiting sports medicine clinics have sustained overuse injuries. The first 2 months of a new program are the most critical. The body and muscles must be given time to adapt to the new demands gradually.

Set realistic goals early in a fitness program. Your instructor will help you determine an appropriate entry-level conditioning program and progression. Gradually increase your exercise intensity and duration to attain your personal goals. For example, if you have never participated in aerobics, your first goal may be to perform 10 minutes of continuous aerobic exercise even though other members of the class may work out 25 or 30 minutes. Try not to compete or compare yourself with friends who may be able to exercise for a longer duration or at higher intensity. You will be able to catch up in time, but if you attempt to keep up with them before your body is ready, you risk an overuse problem.

A good rule of thumb when building your program is to increase the duration of the workout no more than 10 percent weekly. A beginner should not jump from a 20-minute workout up to 40 minutes. Also, do not increase both intensity and duration during the same week. This principle holds true in aerobics, lap swimming, water exercise, bicycling, fitness walking, and jogging. Studies show an increasing injury rate with increasing weekly jogging distance beyond 20 miles per week. Many fitness buffs and athletes have a feeling of invulnerability. They think their bodies can adapt to increased exercise workloads without any problem. Realize that more is not always better. By allowing your body to adjust gradually to new exercise demands, you will greatly reduce the risk of suffering an overuse injury. See Table 8-1 for symptoms of overtraining, overuse, and chronic fatigue.

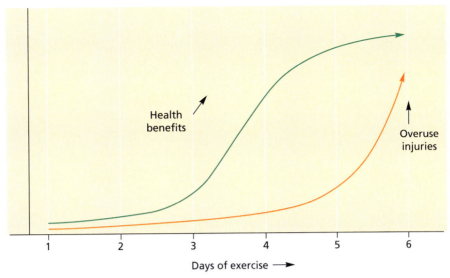

Health
benefits

Overuse
injuries

Days of exercise →

FIGURE 8-1 Overload is good up to a point. Overuse may cause injury. Health benefits accrue rapidly with 3 to 5 days per week of exercise. The risk of injuries increases with more than 5 days per week of exercise.

THE NUMBERS

17,000,000	Average annual number of Americans who sustain an exercise-related injury.
500	Miles of use in which your shoes will maintain their ability to absorb shock.
85%	Americans affected by low back pain at some time in their lives.
82%	Injuries that occur in the lower extremities.
78%	Injuries that are attributable to overuse.
10%	Maximum amount of time to safely increase exercise weekly.

Consider alternating an impact activity with a low-impact or nonimpact activity. This alternation gives the muscles a period of rest and recovery and switches the demands to a new muscle group. It is repetitive stress on the body that causes problems. Some people enjoy alternating activities because it adds variety and develops total body fitness better than any single activity can. It also gives specific muscles and joints a chance to rest and recover. For example, water exercise or bicycling is a good supplement to an impact exercise such as jogging.

It is crucial that you listen to your body during and after exercise. After a great workout, if you feel a little soreness, it should gradually decrease over the next hour. However, if you develop excessive soreness or pain, cut back in the next workout, try a different activity, or take a day off. The importance of rest is often overlooked. When you are fatigued, you are most susceptible to injury.

If you are getting the right amount of exercise, you should look good, feel good, and be alert and productive. Too much exercise, like too little, can be unhealthy.

After a workout, you should get enough rest to be fully recovered by the next workout. Rest is probably the most neglected aspect of fitness. Fitness does not occur during exercise alone but results from the proper combination of training and recovery. Exercise provides the overload that stimulates that improvement. During the rest period between workouts, the body adapts to the demands made on it. When the recovery is adequate, you will begin the next workout feeling strong and energetic. If you feel tired and washed out, rest will do you more good than exercise will. Pay attention to your water intake. Dehydration can be a major contributor to fatigue. Drink plenty of water daily—especially if you exercise in a hot climate. Also keep in mind that exercise isn't the only source of overstress. Chronic fatigue can result in part from other aspects of daily life, such as poor nutrition; emotional tension; job, social, or family problems; and lack of sleep.

There is a difference between the pain of injury and the pain of hard effort. The concepts of "no pain, no

TABLE 8-1	*Symptoms of Overtraining, Overuse, and Chronic Fatigue*

SIGNS IN YOUR TRAINING

- Persistent soreness and stiffness in joints, tendons, or muscles
- Labored breathing during a workout of normal intensity
- Performance decline or cutting sessions short
- Recovery taking longer
- Persistent lethargy, fatigue, and unusual lack of interest in exercise

SIGNS IN YOUR LIFE

- Increased tension, anger, irritability
- No interest in activities you usually do
- Poor concentration (general clumsiness, tripping, poor auto driving)
- Not sleeping well

SIGNS IN YOUR HEALTH

- Increased infections and colds
- Increases of six to eight beats per minute in morning resting pulse
- Swelling or aching lymph glands in neck, underarm, or groin area
- Skin eruptions in nonadolescents
- Constipation or diarrhea
- Loss of appetite
- Chronic thirst
- Cuts and scars taking a long time to heal
- Inexplicable weight changes, either up or down
- Anemia or amenorrhea (in women)

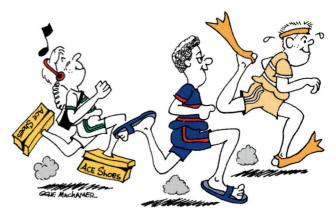

GENE MACHAMER

Improper footwear increases risk of injury.

gain" and "going for the burn" are useful in athletics but inappropriate for fitness exercisers whose goal is health, not athletic performance. Pain is the body's natural way of informing you that something is wrong. Pain may be localized or generalized. However, pain is a subjective response, and each individual tolerates it differently. Do not try to exercise through pain or injury. Previous injury is a strong risk factor for future injuries. Allow time for healing and correct mechanical problems before resuming activity.

Footwear

While many injuries are due to overuse, that is only part of the problem. Wearing improper or worn-out shoes places added stress on your hips, knees, ankles, and feet—the sites of up to 90 percent of sports injuries. The feet are the most abused and neglected part of the body. Good footwear can prevent many injuries and is the best investment you can make in an exercise program. Each time your foot hits the ground when you are jogging, the force of impact is three to five times your body weight. Your feet, ankles, shins, knees, hips, and lower back must absorb a tremendous amount of stress. If the stress is too

great, breakdown occurs at the weakest link in the chain. A well-fitted pair of shoes is the first line of defense against impact injuries.

Shoes should provide good shock absorption, support, and stability yet maintain a reasonable degree of flexibility. Your foot will naturally roll inward from outer heel contact to big toe pushoff when you jog; therefore, the heel counter (the rigid plastic insert in the shoe's heel) must be firm to prevent excessive heel movement. The bottom of the shoe must have good traction to prevent slipping. Shoes are manufactured to be used for a certain number of miles, and they can lose their cushioning ability even if the uppers still look good. Each step compresses the sole, causing it to flatten and gradually lose shock absorbability. Exercise shoes typically lose about one-third of their ability to absorb shock after 400 to 500 miles of use. The upper part of the shoe stretches and weakens, decreasing lateral support. This happens so gradually that you may not notice it until you try on a new pair of shoes. With less cushioning and support, there is a greater chance of injury. If you wear the shoes 5 to 10 hours a week during exercise (walking, jogging, aerobics, etc.), you should probably replace them every 6 months to retain adequate cushioning. Runners would be well advised to keep a log of their mileage as a reminder of when to buy new shoes.

Weakness and Inflexibility

Sit down with your feet extended in front. Slowly reach toward your toes. Can you touch them without bending your knees? Many exercisers who neglect flexibility exercises cannot pass this test for minimal flexibility. Their legs are too tight, and this increases susceptibility to muscle and tendon injuries. Aerobic activities are great for the cardiorespiratory system, but they alone do not develop balanced fitness. They tend to shorten and tighten muscles that are used repetitively, leaving opposing, relatively unused muscles weak. This can lead to muscle imbalance. If some muscles are too tight, joint

TABLE 8-2 Common Muscle Imbalances

The rule of thumb in avoiding injuries is to *stretch* the muscles that are tight and *strengthen* the opposing muscles that are weak.

Tight	Weak
Gastrocnemius (calf)	Tibialis anterior (shin)
Quadriceps (front of thigh)	Hamstrings (back of thigh)
Erector spinae (lower back)	Abdominals (stomach)
Pectorals (chest)	Rhomboids (upper back)

movement is restricted. Table 8-2 lists some common muscle imbalances. The solution to this problem is to stretch the tight muscles and strengthen the weak ones. A balance of strength and flexibility is important in injury prevention.

Incorporate a basic stretching routine into each workout, preferably during the cool-down. (See Chapter 5 for recommended flexibility exercises.) Stretch gently, placing only slight tension on the muscles. Hard stretching or bouncy movements may activate the stretch reflex. This causes the muscle to contract involuntarily and shorten—exactly the opposite of what you're trying to do—to protect itself from injury. Concentrate on event-specific exercises. For example, if you are a swimmer, you will want to spend additional time stretching the shoulders and arms. If jogging or aerobics is your activity, concentrate on stretching the hamstrings, quadriceps, lower back, and calf. Abdominal curls are an important supplement to any fitness workout. Strong abdominals and a flexible lower back are critical in preventing lower back problems.

Mechanics

Structural weaknesses, mainly affecting the legs, knees, ankles, and feet, are often revealed when a beginner starts a new exercise program or when overuse occurs. Biomechanical difficulties often arise in the feet. The foot is a marvelous structure of 26 bones, with almost double that number of ligaments and muscles. It strikes the ground about 80 to 90 times a minute during exercise. When a weak foot pounds the ground several thousand times a day, the potential for injury is great. Slight **pronation** of the foot is natural—that is, your foot will roll inward slightly after the outer edge of the heel strikes the ground. All bodies are not created equal, and so different foot types, gait styles, and body mechanics vary in susceptibility to injury. For example, knock knees or flat feet may cause **overpronation**—too much inward roll when the foot should be pushing off (Figure 8-2). This twists the foot, shin, and knee and can cause tendinitis, plantar fasciitis, or knee strain. Observing the wear pattern on your shoes can help you select a shoe designed for your specific mechanics. Set your shoes on a flat surface. If they tilt inward and if there is excessive shoe wear on the inside of the forefoot, your feet may overpronate. If, in contrast, the outside of the shoe is overstretched and tilts outward and there is excessive wear on the outside of the shoe, your feet may pronate too little. **Underpronation** is insufficient inward roll of the foot upon contact. People with high arches and tight Achilles tendons tend to underpronate. When the foot hits the ground, it does not roll inward enough to absorb the shock of impact, increasing the risk of shin splints, stress fractures, iliotibial band syndrome, tendinitis, and plantar fasciitis. Underpronation causes excessive wear on the outside of the shoe sole.

Moderate pronation problems can be corrected through wise shoe selection. Most exercise shoes are designed to limit overpronation, not eliminate all inward rotation. A person who overpronates needs motion-control shoes with a straight or semicurved last and features that limit pronation. The best shoe for an underpronator has a curved last to allow normal pronation. Employees in many sports shoe stores are trained to help you select a proper shoe. If discomfort persists, you may want to consult a physician or podiatrist who will check your foot mechanics. He or she may prescribe **orthotics**,

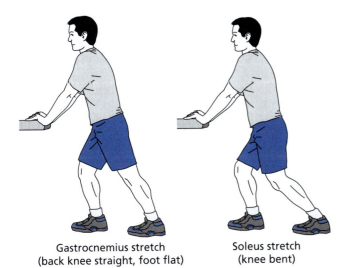

Gastrocnemius stretch
(back knee straight, foot flat)

Soleus stretch
(knee bent)

Good calf flexibility reduces the risk of Achilles tendinitis, plantar fasciitis, and shin splints.

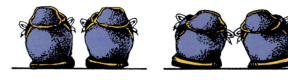

Underpronation

Overpronation

FIGURE 8-2 Underpronation and overpronation.

TOP **10** LIST

Tips for Preventing Injuries

1. *Warm up.* Walking, slow jogging, or gentle calisthenics the first 5 to 10 minutes of your workout will transition your muscles, heart, and metabolism into a higher gear. You're ready when you feel warmer and begin to break a sweat.

2. *Progress slowly.* Overuse—doing too much, too hard, too soon—is the leading cause of injury. Increase your workload by no more than 10 percent per week. Alternate hard with easy workout days and get sufficient rest between workouts.

3. *Work out regularly.* Sporadic exercise invites injury. Your muscles need several weeks to adjust to the stresses of exercise. Exercising every other day is safer and more effective than weekend workout binges that leave you stiff and sore.

4. *Cool down.* Walk around or continue your exercise at a lower pace for a few minutes to give your heart and respiratory rates a chance to transition back toward resting. You will feel better than you will if you stop suddenly and will avoid a potentially serious drop in blood pressure or even fainting from blood pooling in the extremities.

5. *Stretch for flexibility.* This is most effective during the cool-down, when muscles are warm and pliant, stretching is easier, and the effects on flexibility are longer-lasting (see Chapter 5).

6. *Try cross training.* Combining aerobic, strength, and flexibility exercises in your weekly program develops balanced fitness and avoids the one-dimensional stresses of doing only one type of workout. In other words, running is a fine aerobic activity, but it tightens hamstrings and calves and doesn't do much for the abdominals or upper body. Alternate high- and low-impact activities. Adding stretching daily and strengthening twice a week keeps the muscles in better shape, can reduce injury risk, and can improve the running.

7. *Drink water before, during, and after exercise.* Loss of water through sweat keeps you cool but can be dehydrating if fluids aren't replaced. Drinking enough water to match fluid lost through sweat is especially important in hot weather, when risk of heat illness is increased. Drinking a couple of cups of water 1 to 2 hours before exercise, and 8 oz. or more every 20 to 30 minutes during exercise will help. Also, weigh yourself before and after exercise. Any weight loss is due to loss of fluid (1/2 pound = 8 oz. of water) that needs to be restored. See Chapter 7 for additional information on fluid replacement for active people.

8. *Modify workouts in extreme heat or cold.* In hot spells, shift to early or late workouts, and try noon during cold weather. Pay attention to how you feel and ease back on workout intensity and duration until you acclimatize or until the weather improves.

9. *Pay attention to pain.* Pain is a signal that something is wrong. Trying to work through an injury will prolong or worsen it. If something begins to hurt or if you're not recovering from one workout to the next, cut back, switch activities, or take a couple of days off to give yourself a chance to mend. Resume activity at a lower intensity and progress gradually.

10. *Wear good, well-fitted shoes.* They are your first line of defense against impact injuries. Choose those appropriate for the activity and replace them every 400 to 500 miles or before the soles become compressed.

---

shoe inserts molded to your foot, to correct abnormalities. They allow the foot to operate mechanically efficiently. They are highly effective for alleviating excessive foot under- or overpronation.

Regardless of your body type, pay attention to form when participating in any aerobic activity. Participants in aerobic dance, water exercise, bicycling, and step aerobics and even those using stair-climbing and cross-country skiing machines need to understand the proper mechanics of each activity. In this way, many injuries and discomforts can be avoided. You will find technique and safety tips for a variety of aerobic activities in Chapter 4. You may also want to refer to the contraindicated exercises listed in Chapter 5.

The body is a marvelous mechanism. Considering its complexity, it is a wonder it doesn't break down more often. Exercise is vital to maintain wellness. Illness and injury are less common in those who maintain peak performance through regular exercise than it is in those who exercise sporadically. Even when injuries do occur, few are debilitating. Many simply cause some inconvenience. For a summary, see the Top 10 List "Tips for Preventing Injuries." If we can't prevent all injuries, it is important to be able to recognize the signs and symptoms of the most common ones. This gives you an opportunity to take corrective action in the early stages and limit downtime.

P.R.I.C.E.

Acute injuries to muscles, joints, and tendons are often accompanied by swelling. Swelling causes pain and decreased range of motion. Rapid recovery requires keeping the swelling to a minimum. The aim of treatment is to assist the healing process. The recommended treat-

TABLE 8-3	*Recommended Treatment for Common Injuries*

P	=	Protect from further injury
R	=	Rest to allow healing and avoid tissue irritation
I	=	Ice to reduce pain and swelling
C	=	Compress with a wrap to control swelling
E	=	Elevate to reduce swelling

ment for many injuries, whether mild or severe, is protect, rest, ice, compress, and elevate, or **P.R.I.C.E.** (see Table 8-3).

P = Protect

The classic advice of old-time coaches was to "run it off." On the contrary, it is important to protect the injured area from further tissue damage. Don't let the problem get worse. Look for the cause of the injury and remedy the situation. A medical professional might recommend that a more severely injured limb be protected with crutches, a splint, or a sling. The aim is to minimize irritation, tissue bleeding, inflammation, and pain and provide optimal healing conditions.

R = Rest

The injured area should be rested for 24 to 72 hours or more, depending on the severity of the injury. A few days of rest from the activity in which the problem occurred might be sufficient to protect irritated tissue from reinjury while healing from a minor strain. Switching to a different activity, such as swimming, cycling, or deep water running, can rest a sore area and maintain your conditioning. A minor complaint can become a major

problem if you keep aggravating the situation. Healing progresses more rapidly when stress to the area is reduced. Frequently, people will start back into their usual activity before they are ready and reinjure themselves. Wait until most of the pain and swelling have subsided and you have regained 80 percent of your normal range of motion compared with the uninjured side. If you are unable to exercise for a week, when you return to your usual workout routine, reduce your duration, frequency, and/or intensity by at least 25 percent. Do not resume your normal workout level until you are free of pain during and after exercise.

I = Ice

Apply ice to the injured part immediately. A convenient way to apply ice is to put ice cubes or crushed ice in a plastic freezer bag and place it on the injured area. A pound bag of frozen peas or corn also works well. You may apply the ice directly to the skin without risking freezing the skin. The ice may make the injured part ache for the first 5 to 10 minutes. Keep it on! When the area feels numb, discontinue the ice. This will give immediate pain relief and reduce inflammation and tissue damage.

How long will you need to leave the ice on? It varies with the amount of fat and muscle in the area being treated. Apply ice for about 10 minutes to areas with little fat and muscle, like fingers and toes. Apply the ice for 15 to 30 minutes to larger areas like an ankle or knee. Areas with a lot of fat and muscle, like a thigh, may need to be treated for up to 30–45 minutes for greatest effectiveness. Allow the area to rewarm for 45 minutes to an hour before icing again. What about frozen gel packs?

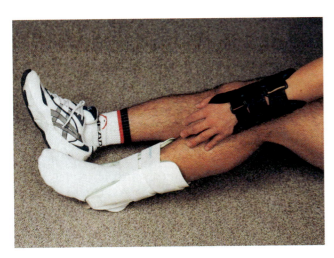

For a serious injury, a medical professional may recommend a splint to protect and rest the area while healing.

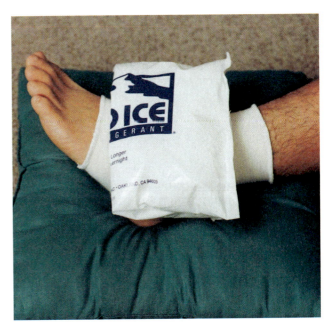

P.R.I.C.E. To transmit cold effectively, wet the elastic wrap before applying ice to the injury.

Gel packs should be left on for only about 10 minutes because they are much colder than ice packs and have potential to cause tissue damage (frostbite). Ice is preferred because it melts as it cools, and it is not likely to cause tissue damage. Ice the injured area every 3 to 4 hours for 48 to 72 hours or longer if pain and swelling persist. Ice should not be used by anyone who has diabetes, sensitivity to cold, or a medical condition with reduced blood flow to the arms or legs. These individuals need to seek medical advice for care of minor injuries.

If you feel mild discomfort when exercising and suspect an overuse injury such as tendinitis, you should apply ice to the tender areas right after you work out and reapply it several times a day for the next 48 hours or longer if pain lingers. Remember: You can never go wrong with ice. Sports medicine physician Francis G. O'Connor states, "Ice is indicated as long as inflammation persists—from the onset of the injury, through rehabilitation, and into sports return."

C = Compress

When not icing the injury, wrap the part with an elastic wrap to prevent fluid buildup in the injured area. Wrap it snugly but not tightly enough to interfere with circulation. If the part starts throbbing, the wrap may be on too tight. Remove the wrap and reapply it more loosely. Do not sleep with the wrap on.

E = Elevate

Raise the injured area above the level of the heart whenever possible. This will reduce the swelling by combating the effect of gravity pulling blood and fluids down to the injured area. Most people with an injured ankle or knee will place it on a pillow for elevation when going to sleep. However, you may move during the night and lose the elevation. Instead, place three or four books under the mattress to raise it approximately 6 to 8 inches.

HEAT AND PAIN RELIEVERS

Many people mistakenly apply heat to an acute injury. Heat applied too early stimulates blood flow and increases swelling and inflammation. Stick with ice for at least the first 48 to 72 hours or more after an injury, and only then, *after swelling has completely subsided*, should heat be applied. At that point heat may speed healing, relax muscles, and reduce stiffness. Either dry heat (heating pad or lamp) or moist heat (a hot bath, whirlpool, hot-water bottle, damp heat pack) will do. Apply the heat for 10 to 20 minutes, two or three times a day. You can also use it for 5 to 10 minutes before exercising to reduce stiffness.

Over-the-counter liniments and balms are popular methods for producing a warm feeling in muscles. The effect of these products is only superficial—the active ingredients stimulate sensory nerve endings in the skin to produce a sensation of heat. This has no healing effect and may mask the pain.

Aspirin or ibuprofen (such as Motrin or Advil) can reduce the pain and inflammation of minor sprains, strains, and tendinitis. Acetaminophen (such as Tylenol) is less helpful because it has no anti-inflammatory effect. Do not use anti-inflammatories to mask pain so that you can continue to work out—this will worsen an injury. Do not use the maximum recommended dose of these pain relievers more than 2 or 3 consecutive days because they increase risk of stomach bleeding. Consult your doctor before using any drugs.

COMMON INJURIES

In pursuit of wellness, you may occasionally push yourself beyond the current capabilities of your structure. Finding and keeping your peak is a challenge and part of a process of learning about your body's unique strengths and weaknesses. While some acute injuries are obvious, others can creep up slowly and gradually worsen. If, in your zeal to experience peak performance, you develop an athletic ailment, it will usually be minor and you will be able to resume activity within a few days. Here we will discuss the potential causes of, symptoms of, and treatments for the most common injuries listed alphabetically. Table 8-4 gives a summary of these common injuries, their symptoms, and their treatments.

Ankle Sprain

A **sprain** is a partial or complete tear of a **ligament**, the fibrous connective tissue that binds bones together to form a joint. A sprain is most often a result of a sudden force, typically a twisting motion that surrounding muscles are not strong enough to control. Both ankles and knees are vulnerable to sprains. An ankle sprain will produce swelling and tenderness on the outside of the ankle. The amount of swelling depends on the severity of the injury. In severe cases, discoloration or bruising will develop. Range of motion in the ankle may be decreased by swelling and pain. P.R.I.C.E. for the first 72 hours is the best treatment for sprains. It is extremely important to control the amount of swelling in the joint in order to return to activity quickly. Strong, flexible muscles help protect against sprains. For example, to prevent ankle sprain, strengthen ankles with flexion, inversion, and eversion exercises. High-top shoes or a commercial ankle wrap will not reduce the risk of reinjury and can provide a false sense of confidence. When you start back into activity, progress gradually. A sprained ankle can take 1 to 2 months to heal.

TABLE 8-4   *Common Injuries, Symptoms, and Treatments*

Injury	Symptoms	Treatment
Ankle sprain	Pain, swelling, tenderness on the side of the ankle	P.R.I.C.E., anti-inflammatories Move in pain-free range, strengthen when pain and swelling subside
Blisters	Small fluid-filled skin swelling at a site of friction	Remove source of irritation, protect area, do not pop unless painful, use antiseptic and bandage, leave skin in place
Bursitis	Pain, swelling, loss of movement near a joint	Rest area, ice, anti-inflammatories
Chafing	Skin irritation from friction	Remove source of irritation Protect with petroleum jelly, clothing, or bandage
Heel spur	Pain underneath heel	Rest, anti-inflammatories, heel pad in shoe, calf stretch
Iliotibial band syndrome	Snapping, pain on side of hip or knee	Rest from causative activity, ice, iliotibial band stretch
Muscle cramp	Muscle spasm, tightness, and pain	Gently stretch and massage muscle Drink fluids, rest or decrease intensity of activity, increase dietary calcium and potassium
Muscle soreness	Muscle aching with movement 1 to 4 days after increased exercise	Hot shower to area, gentle stretching, heat, anti-inflammatories help somewhat
Muscle strain	Tightness, sharp pain, swelling Weakness, loss of use Usually began during activity	Rest from activity that caused strain, ice, stretch and strengthen after pain decreases
Patellofemoral syndrome	Knee pain, stiffness walking up and down stairs or after sitting	Ice, strengthen quadriceps
Plantar fasciitis	Heel or arch pain Usually worse in morning	Ice, stretch arch, heel lift, arch support, stretch calf
Shin splints	Pain in lower third of front of lower leg	Rest from activity that caused injury, ice, stretch calves, strengthen anterior tibialis
Side stitch	Pain in side during activity	Stop activity, stretch side, press on sore area
Stress fracture	Pinpoint pain, swelling along bone	See physician Discontinue causative activity until healed
Tendinitis	Swelling, tightness, pain with movement near a joint where muscle attaches to bone	Rest from causative activity, ice, gentle stretching when pain abates

Blisters

Blisters are a common problem, especially for beginning exercisers. They are an accumulation of fluid under the skin due to excess friction. They are usually a problem only if they become infected or cause you to limp. The most common areas for blisters are the bottom of the foot, the sides of the big and little toes, and the back of the heel. Blisters can be prevented by eliminating the friction that causes them. Wear 100 percent acrylic (Orlon) socks. Acrylic is best at dissipating moisture and preventing blisters from forming. Cotton socks produce twice as many blisters, and even worse is a cotton-acrylic blend. One trick for preventing a blister is to apply a piece of duct tape over an irritated area *before* a blister forms. Never wear new shoes for a workout without first breaking them in by walking around in them at home for a few days. Should a blister be opened? Some say no; let the fluid reabsorb into the system because an open blister invites infection. Others say to pop the blister if it is painful and causes you to limp. The best treatment is to apply a donut pad and lubricant to the blister to reduce friction and pressure. To prevent blisters, some runners wear their socks inside out to avoid the abrasion of the rough interior seam. It may also help to wear two socks on the affected foot—a thin nylon sock inside an acrylic sock. If the blister is lanced, do not remove loose skin, and keep the area clean to prevent infection. Consult your physician if you think it may be infected.

Bursitis

Bursitis is inflammation of a bursa, a fluid-filled sac that lies between tissues and allows tendons, ligaments, muscles, and skin to glide smoothly over one another during activity. There are over 150 bursae, but the most commonly affected lie in the knee, elbow, shoulder, and hip. When a bursa becomes irritated because of overuse or training, it begins producing extra fluid and the sac swells, often within 24 hours, causing pain in the affected area. The recommended treatment is to protect the area, rest from activity, ice, compress with an elastic bandage to reduce swelling, and take anti-inflammatory medication. Do not wrap the knee tightly, however, as this could lead to blood clots by compressing the large vein behind the joint.

Chafing

When skin rubs against skin or against clothing, it becomes irritated and can crack and bleed. The most common problem areas are between the thighs, under the armpits, and on the nipples (runner's nipples). While chafing can happen to anyone, its frequency increases with greater body fat percentage. Treat chafing by applying petroleum jelly to the affected area. To prevent chafing, select clothing of smooth, nonabrasive material with few or well-covered seams. Synthetics are best. Avoid cotton because it stays wet, causing friction.

Avoid clothing that is tight or that bunches under the arms or between the legs. Wearing tights or knee-length exercise shorts can protect chafed thighs. Nipple chafing can be decreased by going shirtless in warm weather or by applying petroleum jelly and adhesive bandages to the nipples. Women should select a good exercise bra that has flat or covered seams.

Heel Spur

A **heel spur** is a bony growth on the underside of the calcaneus (heel bone) at the insertion of the plantar fascia. The pull of fascia on the heel can remodel the bone into a spur pointing toward the toes. Heel spurs are common and are not necessarily the sign of a problem. They do not always cause pain unless there is significant fat pad atrophy or unless they are caused by chronic irritation of the plantar fascia at its insertion. The heel pain of plantar fasciitis is sometimes associated with a heel spur. Treatment involves rest; anti-inflammatory medications; and insertion of a heel pad in the shoe to protect the heel, alleviate inflammation, and distribute impact during activity.

Iliotibial Band Syndrome

Tightness, burning, snapping, and pain on the side of the knee or hip may be related to inflammation of the **iliotibial band**, a long tendon that begins in the buttocks, runs down the side of the thigh, and attaches to the side of the lower leg just below the knee. Common in runners, an overtight iliotibial band may become inflamed from the friction of rubbing against the outer knee or hip bone as the knee repetitively flexes and extends. This is primarily an overuse injury and can be treated with decreasing or changing activity, ice, anti-inflammatories, and stretching the iliotibial band, hamstrings, and quadriceps (see stretches in Figure 5-1).

Muscle Cramp

A **cramp** is a sharp, involuntary muscle contraction. It may occur during exercise or at rest. The calf is the most common area for a muscle cramp to occur, but cramps may occur anywhere in the body. Muscle cramps may be caused by fatigue, which causes the nervous system to overstimulate muscles. Cramps may also be related to a strength imbalance, an electrolyte imbalance, or dehydration. Occasionally, low levels of circulating calcium or potassium in the blood can contribute to cramps. Cramps can be treated with fluid intake and with gradual stretching of the muscle. A calf cramp may be treated by extending the foot to a 90-degree angle. Occasionally, gentle massage may help.

Muscle cramps may be prevented by taking precautions when exercising in the heat. Wear light, loose clothing; drink water freely; gradually acclimatize yourself to the heat; and exercise during the cooler hours of the day. Improve fitness gradually and get plenty of potassium and calcium in your diet. Extra salt is not needed. A regular program of stretching may also help prevent muscle cramps.

Muscle Soreness

Muscle soreness is discomfort or tenderness after an increase in workout level. It may be fairly mild and usually is just a reminder that you had a good workout. For example, a person who has not recently lifted weights will develop muscle soreness following the first workout. There is no real pain but rather a mild achiness with movement of the major muscle groups used in the activity. After several sessions of the same activity, soreness will diminish or disappear. Duration of activity and eccentric (lengthening) contractions are highly correlated with muscle soreness. For example, running downhill repeatedly will produce more quadricep soreness than will an equal amount of flat or uphill running. Muscle soreness is thought to be caused by microscopic tears or spasms of the connective tissue. There is no long-term damage from this. Muscle soreness may develop immediately or over a 24- to 36-hour period following unaccustomed exercise and will usually disappear within 2 to 4 days. Other than following a sensible progression in

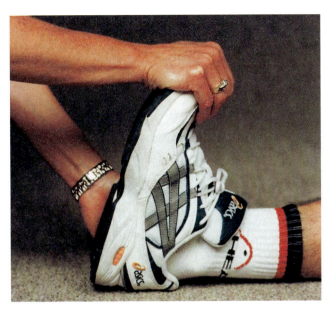

A calf cramp may be relieved by extending the foot and stretching the calf.

activities and intensity, there is no real prevention for muscle soreness. This is a normal response to an increase in exertion and part of an adaptation process that causes muscles to recover and build, leading to greater strength and endurance. There is little that can be done for mild muscle soreness. While stretching is beneficial for flexibility, it has little effect on reducing soreness. If there is sharp pain rather than soreness during activity, the problem may be a muscle strain.

Muscle Strain

A muscle **strain** is a tear of muscle fibers or a tendon and is sometimes referred to as a *pull*. Symptoms include sharp pain, weakness with possible loss of function, spasm or extreme tightness, and tenderness to the touch. There are many different causes, but it most often results from a violent contraction of the muscle. A strain may be caused by fatigue, overexertion, muscle imbalance or weakness, or electrolyte or water imbalance.

A strain may range from mild (more painful than just soreness) to a complete rupture of the muscle. The muscles most likely to be affected are the hamstrings, gastrocnemius, Achilles tendon, erector spinae, groin, and the rotator cuff muscles of the shoulder. Rest, ice, and anti-inflammatories are used to treat muscle strain. Reduce or eliminate activity until the injury starts to heal. The severity of the injury and which muscle is injured will affect the recovery time. The hamstrings usually take the longest to heal and rehabilitate. If the strain is severe, it will heal with a significant amount of scar tissue. Scar tissue is not elastic like muscle, and so stretching and strengthening exercises are important to return to normal function. To prevent strains, complete a full

warm-up before working out, take care not to overdo it, and work toward balancing strength and flexibility in opposing muscles.

Patellofemoral Syndrome

Pain around and under the kneecap, along with knee stiffness, is characteristic of **patellofemoral syndrome**. Symptoms include a dull pain when walking up and down stairs or after sitting with the knees bent for a period of time ("theater sign"), and occasionally mild swelling or a feeling that the knee is "giving way." Patellofemoral syndrome is associated with overuse, worn-out shoes, always running in the same direction on the track, excessive downhill running, and rapid ballistic movements such as those done in aerobics. One common cause is structural. Wide hips tend to make the quadriceps pull the kneecap out against the femur, producing inflammation. Loose kneecaps or a quadriceps muscle not strong enough to keep the patella in its groove also may lead to patellofemoral syndrome. The knee will not get better if you continue your activity during the injury.

Rest, ice, and anti-inflammatories are the conventional treatments for this injury. If the knee swells significantly, see a physician. Swelling may indicate a major problem that will take much longer to heal.

To prevent recurrence, the knee must be rehabilitated. Low-impact activities are recommended to strengthen muscles, for example, swimming and bicycling. To stabilize the knee and assist in correcting the tracking mechanism of the patella, strengthen the quadriceps. Stretching should increase hamstring and iliotibial band flexibility. In severe cases, surgery may be indicated.

Plantar Fasciitis

Plantar fasciitis causes heel or arch pain. It is most painful when a person takes the first few steps in the morning, but in severe cases, pain may continue throughout the day. It results from inflammation of the plantar fascia, a long thick band of connective tissue on the underside of the foot that attaches the base of the calcaneus to the base of the toes. Inflammation may result from excessive impact, worn shoes, or poor foot mechanics. Anatomical problems frequently cause plantar fasciitis— tight Achilles tendon, high arches, flat feet, or excessive pronation. Also, with age and repeated weight-bearing stress, the fat pad under the heel becomes flattened and less shock-absorbent. Rest, anti-inflammatories, calf stretching, ice, and arch supports or heel cups are the recommended treatments. Rolling a can of chilled soda or a frozen plastic bottle of water back and forth under the arch is a good way to apply cold to the area. Orthotics are often recommended to reduce symptoms in persistent/recurrent cases of plantar fasciitis.

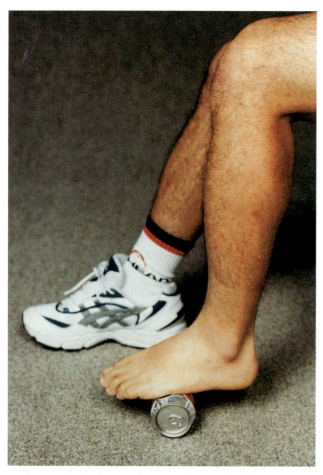

To treat plantar fasciitis, roll a cold can of soda under your arch to ice and stretch the fascia.

Shin Splint

A **shin splint** refers to pain in the front of the lower leg (shin). Early signs are acute burning pain or irritation in the lower third of the anterior tibialis. This may progress to slight swelling, redness, warmth, and inflammation. A variety of factors contributes to shin splints. They often come early in an exercise program and are particularly common in those who are out of shape, overweight, wide-hipped, knock-kneed, or duck-footed. Working out on very hard or very soft surfaces can bring on shin splints even if a person is well conditioned. Switching from a hard to a soft surface or vice versa, excessive mileage, improper footwear, poor foot mechanics, running on a road slope, and running in the same direction all the time on an indoor track may cause them. Women, particularly those who wear high heels, are affected nearly three times more often than are men.

Shin splints may be a sign of a long arch problem in the foot. As the long arch begins to sag, it stretches lower leg muscles and causes pain. Another cause is a muscle imbalance between the strong calf muscle and the weak anterior tibialis, which may lead to inflammation of the membrane between the tibia and the fibula. This imbalance can be corrected with toe pulls to strengthen the anterior tibialis and by stretching the calf (see the photos in this chapter). These should be done each workout. If mechanical problems are not corrected, shin splints tend to recur.

To treat shin splints, switch to a low- or nonimpact activity and rub ice on the affected area for 15 to 20 minutes three to four times a day. Aspirin therapy may be in-

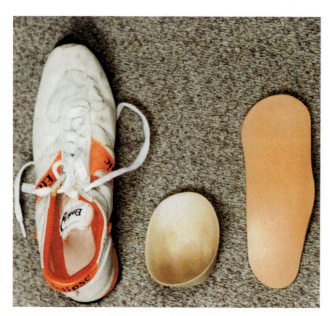

Orthotics or heel cups may reduce symptoms in persistent cases of plantar fasciitis.

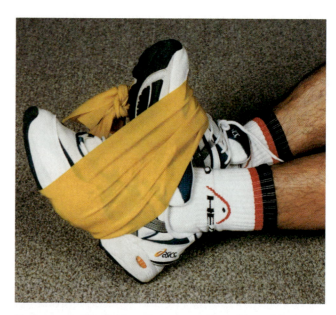

To decrease risk of shin splints, strengthen shins with a set of 15 to 20 toe pulls twice a week using an elastic band.

dicated for a few days to reduce inflammation. If the pain is persistent, consult a physician to rule out a stress fracture.

Side Stitch

A **side stitch** is a sharp pain just under the ribs, typically on the right side. It may result from participating in vigorous activity before the body has had a sufficient warm-up. It may be related to a lack of conditioning, weak abdominals, shallow breathing, consuming a meal too near the time of exercise, dehydration, excessive exercise intensity, or **ischemia** (inadequate oxygen) to the diaphragm. Side stitches tend to occur in unfit or new exercisers. Better conditioning brings more efficient blood flow and oxygen delivery to the respiratory muscles. To prevent side stitches, warm up well, increase exercise intensity gradually, and avoid eating 1 to 2 hours before a vigorous workout. Side stitches can be treated by stopping activity and stretching, massaging, or pressing on the painful area. After cessation of the activity for a few minutes, the pain and spasm should subside. Taking a deep breath may also break the spasm. Once the pain has dissipated, activity may resume.

Stress Fracture

A **stress fracture** is a microscopic break in a bone caused by overuse. While it can occur anywhere in the lower legs and feet, it is most common at the end of the tibia near the ankle and in the metatarsals of the feet. Unlike a broken bone, which occurs with a distinct traumatic event, a stress fracture is the result of cumulative overload that occurs over many days or weeks. Overtraining and overly rapid increases in training are the major causes. Bone is living tissue that adjusts to the exercise force demands placed on it. As force is applied, bone will remodel itself to handle the force better. If too much force is applied, the bone may fracture before it can successfully remodel. Running excessive mileage, overdoing impact aerobics, wearing worn-out shoes, exercising on hard surfaces such as asphalt or concrete, and having poor foot mechanics may cause a stress fracture. Because they have smaller, lighter bones, women are more susceptible to stress fractures than are men. Especially when combined with hard training, an inadequate intake of calcium and vitamin D can predispose one to the onset—and recurrence—of stress fractures.

A stress fracture may be confused with a case of severe shin splints, but stress fractures are more likely to cause pinpoint pain on the sore bone. Stress fractures are difficult to detect clinically. Frequently, they will not show up on an X ray until 3 to 4 weeks after the onset of symptoms. A bone scan can detect a stress fracture much earlier in the injury because it reveals the active bone for-

mation that occurs while the fracture is healing. The pain of a stress fracture will not go away with conventional treatments (ice, ultrasound) or medication. Only rest will decrease the pain.

The best treatment for a stress fracture is rest from the activity that caused it. This does not mean elimination of exercise altogether. Nonimpact activities such as riding a bicycle and swimming are good alternatives during the healing phase. Depending on the severity of the stress fracture, activity may be resumed within 2 to 6 weeks of diagnosis. "Running through the injury" is not recommended. This may lead to a nonunion fracture of the bone and a 6- to 8-week recovery period in a cast.

Tendinitis

Anytime you see "-itis," think inflammation. **Tendinitis** is the inflammation of a tendon from repetitive stress. Common signs of inflammation include pain, redness, heat, and swelling. **Tendons** are the fibrous cords that connect muscles to bones. They are vulnerable to inflammation because the force of muscle contractions is transmitted through them. The most commonly affected in runners, walkers, and aerobic dancers is the Achilles tendon, which connects two calf muscles, the gastrocnemius and soleus, to the back of the heel bone. Other areas commonly affected are the knee, shoulder, and elbow ("tennis elbow"). When a tendon is inflamed, normal daily activities, such as opening a door and walking up the stairs, can be painful. Tendinitis is often brought on by muscle tightness or increasing the workload too quickly. Achilles tendon problems are often due to tight calf muscles. When the foot flexes to push

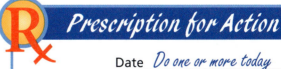

Prescription for Action

Date *Do one or more today*

✔ Check the inner side of the midsole of your shoes for wrinkles, which indicate they have been compressed by daily impact and need to be replaced.
✔ While waiting in line, clasp hands behind your back and pull elbows back to strengthen postural muscles.
✔ While watching TV, do 20 to 30 abdominal crunches or 5 to 10 back extensions.
✔ Put on your favorite music and do the back exercise program in this chapter.

Prescribed by: _____*YOU*_____

off, the powerful Achilles tendon pulls the heel up. If the calf is too tight, it yanks the heel up prematurely, stressing the Achilles tendon. Rest from the activity that caused the injury and stretching the calves to alleviate tightness are recommended. Over-the-counter anti-inflammatory medications (ibuprofen, aspirin) may also help. It may take 2 to 3 weeks to heal and rehabilitate completely. Continuing activity will only delay healing. Meanwhile, you may include alternative activities to maintain fitness. A regular program incorporating stretching and strengthening can help prevent tendinitis.

WHEN TO SEEK MEDICAL HELP

Not all injuries can be self-treated. If symptoms are severe or if self-treatment is not working, you need professional medical treatment. You should seek medical assistance for an injury if you experience any of the following symptoms:

1. The injury is extremely painful or the pain has not decreased in intensity within a day or two. You are unable to bear complete weight on that part or are unable to walk more than three or four steps without significant pain.
2. There is joint pain lasting more than 2 days or significant tenderness when you press on a specific spot in a joint, muscle, or bone, such as a bony part of the foot.

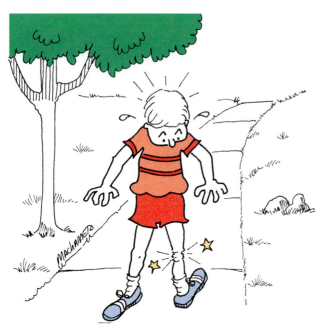

When in doubt, see a physician.

3. There is a loss of strength or range of motion (compared with the uninjured side) and loss of the ability to do normal tasks.
4. The limb gives way when you try to use it.
5. You heard a distinct "pop" or "snap" when the injury occurred.
6. The injured area, compared with the uninjured side, looks misshapen or has unusual lumps (other than swelling).
7. There is numbness or tingling in the injured area, which may indicate nerve compression.

Once injured, whom should you see? Your family doctor will be able to treat common sprains and strains. However, there are other sports injury specialists who can help. Table 8-5 describes some of these specialists.

Communicating with a doctor is an important step in assuming an active role in your health care. Be sure to tell the physician everything that happened leading up to the injury: what you felt, signs and symptoms, and any additional information to aid in diagnosing the injury. Do not feel rushed or intimidated by confusing terminology and tests. You are the consumer and are paying for the doctor's time and services. Do not rely on

TABLE 8-5	*Injury Specialists*

Physical therapists: These therapists are licensed by the state to administer rehabilitative techniques—from massage to strength and flexibility exercises. Many states require a doctor's referral before visiting a registered physical therapist.

Athletic trainers: Many colleges, universities, and sports medicine clinics have athletic trainers who have extensive knowledge of and experience in dealing with injuries. They are highly trained and must pass rigorous written and practical examinations to become certified.

Sports medicine clinics: Because sports medicine is a rapidly growing field, many communities and medical centers have specialized sports medicine clinics. Many clinics have "walk-in" hours and are likely to include some of the specialists already mentioned as part of their staffs.

Orthopedists: These M.D.s with specialized surgical training treat injuries to any part of the musculoskeletal system. Many specialize in athletic injuries.

Podiatrists: These D.P.M.s (doctors of podiatric medicine) treat foot-related problems common to fitness-related injuries. Though not M.D.s, they receive special training and are state-licensed. They can prescribe medications, design orthotics, and perform some surgeries.

Chiropractors: These D.C.s (doctors of chiropractic), believing that the alignment of the spine and proper nerve function are essential to body functioning, use manual manipulation and other physical therapy techniques to relieve pain and structural disorders.

the nurse, the receptionist, or a friend to explain your injury and treatment. Make sure you completely understand everything you must do to speed your recovery.

GETTING BACK INTO ACTION

There are three steps to getting back into action after an injury. First, move the injured part as early as possible, within a pain-free range, to regain flexibility. This motion will increase circulation and reduce stiffness and swelling. As you are able, work all the motions of a joint. For example, in an ankle injury, move the ankle up and down, in and out, 10 to 20 times, three to four times a day. Gradually increase the range of motion. If after moving the part you feel pain, it should subside within 1 hour. Apply ice and reduce the amount of repetitions in the next session. You may be doing too much too soon.

Second, after obtaining at least 80 percent pain-free range of motion, begin to build strength. Gradually increase the strength of a part to equal that of the uninjured side. You can use partner resistance, free weights, rubber tubing, or weight machines. If possible, work under the supervision of a qualified physical therapist or another rehabilitation professional, especially in the early stages of rehabilitation, because this is when you are most susceptible to reinjury.

Third, gradually work your way back to your former activity level. Do not expect to start where you stopped. Frequently, exercisers will try to begin working out at their previous level after merely reducing swelling and pain. Healing may not yet be complete. The result is often reinjury because the weakened area is unable to withstand the stress. Overload should be gradual, with the realization that *more* is not always *better*. If in doubt, start at the lowest level for your activity in Chapter 4 and increase that time by no more than 10 percent per week.

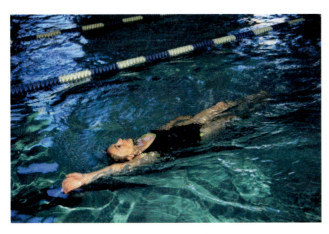

While recovering from an injury, switching to a nonimpact activity such as swimming can maintain your aerobic fitness.

While recovering from an injury, participating in a nonimpact activity such as deep water running, swimming, or stationary cycling can maintain endurance.

CARE OF THE LOWER BACK

Without question, back pain is one of the most common conditions affecting Americans—second only to the common cold as a reason for seeing a physician. Eighty percent of Americans will experience back pain sometime in their lives. Back pain affects a largely youthful population, with the first back pain episodes afflicting people in their 20s and 30s. One of the main contributors to this epidemic of poor back health is our sedentary lifestyle (and spending hours hunched over a computer or working at a desk). Fortunately, most back pain is preventable with exercise, good posture, and good lifting mechanics.

Ways to Avoid Lower Back Pain

Why does back pain occur? How can risk of back injury be reduced? We often take a healthy back for granted until something goes wrong. Back problems are rarely caused by a single, isolated factor. The 32-year-old computer programmer who hurts his back while pulling the lawn mower chain prefers to blame the lawn mower. His condition may actually be a result of several years of abuse and neglect. The pull on the lawn mower chain merely "triggered" the condition. During high school and college years, our bodies are relatively flexible. As we age, muscles begin to shorten and tighten, decreasing flexibility, especially in the back. Combine this with possible weight gain and declining overall fitness and it becomes evident why back pain afflicts millions. With few exceptions, back problems can be prevented with improved fitness, living and work habits, and posture.

The most important key to preventing lower back pain is maintaining strong abdominal muscles and back flexibility. Studies show that people who are physically fit have almost 10 times less back pain. Many of those who suffer back pain are overweight and have weak, sagging abdominals and short, tight back muscles. This puts the back into an overarched position, placing additional stress on the spinal column. Maintaining normal weight and keeping abdominal muscles strong and tight reduce strain on the spine. Strong abdominals keep the pelvis and spinal column stabilized in a normal position. At the same time, it is important to keep the opposing back muscles and hamstrings flexible. People with chronic back problems need to stretch and strengthen regularly, using the exercises in Figure 8-3. Exercise, not rest, is recommended for most people with back problems.

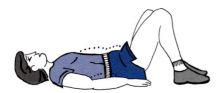

1. Pelvic tilt. Lie on back, knees bent. Press small of back firmly down to floor by tightening the abdominal muscles. Hold for a count of five.

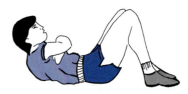

2. Abdominal curl. Do a pelvic tilt and, while holding this position, curl head and shoulders up until shoulder blades have been lifted from the floor. Hold briefly. Lower slowly.

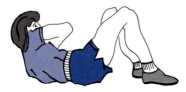

3. Oblique abdominal curl. Do a pelvic tilt and, while holding this position, curl head and shoulders up, twisting right shoulder toward left knee. Hold briefly. Lower slowly. Repeat on other side.

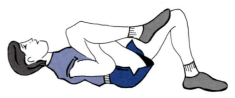

4. Low back stretch. (a) Lie on back. Pull one knee toward chest. Hold for a count of five. Repeat with other leg. (b) Double knee pull. Pull both knees to chest; hold for a count of five.

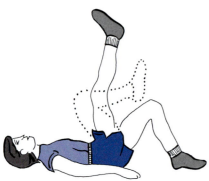

5. Lying hamstring stretch. Lie on back. Bring knee toward chest and extend leg toward ceiling. Flex foot. (You may grasp the back of your thigh with your hands.) Hold 20 seconds. Repeat with other leg.

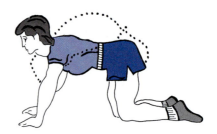

6. Cat stretch. Start on all fours. Round the back upward like a cat. Tighten abdominals. Hold for 5 seconds. Relax and return to starting position. Do not let back sag.

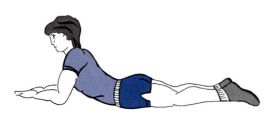

7. Upper back lift. Lie on your stomach with forearms flat on the ground. Tighten abdominals. Lift upper body by using back muscles. Do not press with arms. Hold for a count of five.

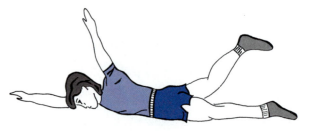

8. Alternate arm/leg lift. Lie on your stomach with arms extended in front. Raise one arm overhead toward ceiling while simultaneously lifting the opposite leg. Hold for a count of five. Repeat with the other arm and leg.

FIGURE 8-3   Exercises for the lower back.

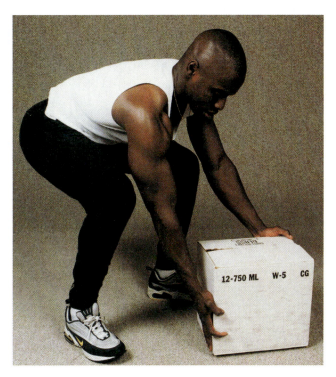

Correct lifting technique.

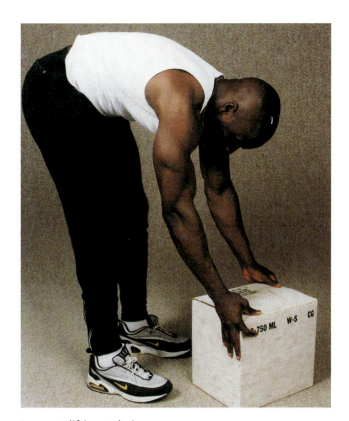

Incorrect lifting technique.

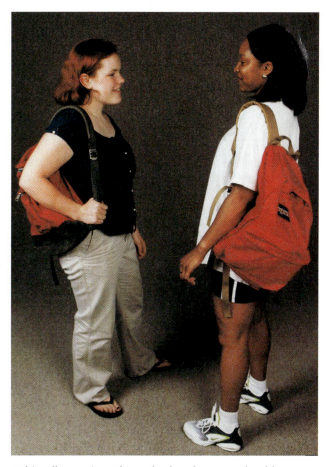

Habitually carrying a heavy backpack on one shoulder may cause back pain.

Sleeping position plays a role in back health. The one-third of your life you spend sleeping should help, not harm, your back. This makes it important to select a firm but not extremely hard mattress. Sleeping on a mattress that is too hard will leave the back unsupported. Sleeping on a sagging mattress places the back in an unbalanced position. Water beds, properly adjusted, may provide satisfactory back support as an alternative to a traditional mattress.

The fetal position is the best sleeping position for maintaining a healthy back. Lie on your side, pull your knees up to your chest, and put a pillow between your knees. This will round the lower back and alleviate back stress. If you must sleep on your back, place a pillow or similar object under your knees to relax the lower back. Sleeping on your stomach increases the arch of the back, shortening the back muscles. Placing a small pillow, or even your arm, under your pelvic bone (abdomen) may help reduce strain on your back.

To decrease back stress when getting out of bed, roll to one side and sit up sideways, using your arms to help.

This will eliminate using all your back and abdominal muscles to get out of bed. This tip is especially helpful if you currently have a back problem.

Good lifting mechanics can reduce the risk of lower back injury. When lifting a heavy weight, bend your knees as if sitting down; keep your head up and looking straight ahead. Your trunk should be held as erect as possible to maintain a neutral spine, and you should use the large muscles of the buttocks and legs to lift. It is also important not to let the knees pass the toes as you squat in order to avoid excessive knee stress. Combining lifting with a twisting force is one of the most common causes of back injury. Instead, lift the object and pivot with your feet rather than your waist.

Keep your body close to the object. Standing far away from the object will place undue stress on the lower back. Lift with your back straight rather than bent at the waist. When carrying heavy objects such as books, backpacks, and groceries, try to distribute the load equally and close to the body. Do not carry a backpack on one shoulder, as this puts uneven stress on back muscles and is a common cause of back pain. Finally, obtain help when lifting heavy objects. See the Top 10 List "Ways to Improve Back Health."

Back Tips for Sitting, Standing, and Driving

Many Americans spend the majority of their time behind desks or in cars. Sedentary jobs and lifestyle make us vulnerable to back pain. How can you maintain a healthy back if you spend a lot of time sitting at a desk? Sit close to your work and keep your hips and knees at a 90-degree angle. Your head should be positioned in line with your shoulder, and your chin should be parallel to

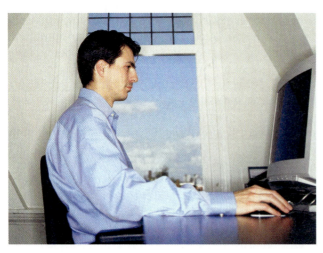

If you spend a lot of time behind a desk, sitting with good alignment can reduce the risk of back, neck, and shoulder pain.

TOP 10 LIST

Ways to Improve Back Health

1. *Stretch and strengthen.* Weak, tight muscles invite injury. Strengthen the abdominals with abdominal curls and do back stretching/strengthening exercises to maintain a strong, flexible spine (see Figure 8-3).

2. *Use good sitting posture.* Sitting for hours hunched in front of a computer screen can overstress back muscles. Sit erect, knees level with hips, feet flat on the floor. Add a towel roll behind your back to maintain the natural spinal curve.

3. *Use good standing posture.* To decrease back stress, stand with one foot elevated a few inches on a box to relax the back.

4. *Change positions frequently.* When sitting, take frequent breaks—1 to 2 minutes every 30 to 60 minutes. Stand up, stretch, move around. When standing, vary your body position and shift weight frequently.

5. *Use good sleeping posture.* Sleep on your side with knees bent and a pillow between your knees to relax your back. If you prefer sleeping on your back, put a pillow under your knees to reduce back stress. Avoid sleeping on your stomach.

6. *Use good lifting techniques.* Stand close to the object and bend your knees as if sitting down, keeping the back straight and head up. Tighten your abdominals and lift with your legs, keeping the object close to your body. Avoid bending from the waist and twisting as you lift.

7. *Don't overdo it.* Know your limits. Weekend bouts of yard work, such as 2 to 3 hours of gardening and raking the lawn on Saturday and playing 2 hours of basketball when you've been sitting behind a desk all week overstress the back. Spread out the work and play in shorter bouts over a few days to give your muscles a chance to adjust.

8. *Keep active.* Maintaining a base of fitness throughout the week enables you to go canoeing, play ball, or do that yard work on the weekend with less risk of a stiff, sore back compared with being a couch potato.

9. *Manage your weight.* Carrying extra pounds in front increases the load your back must support. Losing weight decreases back stress 24 hours a day.

10. *Distribute the load.* Habitually carrying a heavy bag, books, or backpack on one side creates uneven spinal stresses. Evenly distribute the load or switch sides to even out the stresses.

the floor. This will straighten the lower back and prevent slouching. When you sit in a chair, place both feet on the floor. If the chair is too low, it will increase your back curvature excessively. Use a chair that supports your back in its normal slightly arched position, or you can place a small pillow or towel against your lower back. Remove this low-back support for a few minutes every half hour to allow your back to change position.

Maintain good posture while driving, especially when driving long distances. Sitting for extended periods in an automobile is a common cause of back pain. To maintain normal spinal curvature, place a small pillow between your lower back and the seat. Sit close enough to reach the accelerator and steering wheel without slumping.

If your job requires long periods of standing, you can minimize stress on the back by putting one foot on a low stool. Frequently shift your weight from one leg to the other. Some occupations put unusual physical stress on the back. Dentists, nurses, and musicians may sit, lift, or move in twisted, awkward positions.

Wearing high-heeled shoes is unhealthy for the lower back. This shortens the Achilles tendon and hamstrings, throws the back into an overarched position, and overstretches the abdominals. Wear low-heeled shoes to maintain back health.

A common cause of pain farther up the spine is holding the phone between your ear and shoulder, which is usually done to free the hands. When your neck is scrunched to one side frequently throughout the day, it can cause headaches and neck and upper back or shoulder pain. If you use the phone a lot, to prevent neck and shoulder problems, try this:

✔ Buy an inexpensive phone rest that holds the receiver on your shoulder so that you don't have to twist your neck.
✔ Use a clipboard to secure your papers so that your hands are free.
✔ Try a speaker phone or headset.
✔ Hold the phone in the hand opposite the one you usually write with and make a conscious effort to avoid twisting your neck.

If you must sit, stand, or work in one position for an extended time, get up, stretch, and walk for several minutes. You will feel better, and your back will benefit from the change.

Not to be overlooked is the effect of emotional stress on back health. Stress produces tension, which increases sensitivity to pain, which creates more stress. The stress → tension → pain cycle can exacerbate the symptoms of any injury. Stress reduction and relaxation techniques can play an important role in the treatment of low back problems and other injuries.

Lower Back Injuries

The lower back is made up of many tiny ligaments that hold the vertebrae together from the skull to the tailbone. A sudden twisting force can injure these ligaments. There are also several groups of muscles, called the *erector spinae muscle group*, that parallel the spinal column. These muscles may be injured by lifting a heavy weight, excessively bending and twisting, or sleeping on a sagging mattress.

If your back aches, press the sore area with your fingers. If this does not cause pain, the injury is probably deeper. For sore, achy back muscles, lie on a bag of crushed ice or a cold pack for 20 minutes, or alternate 20 minutes of ice with 20 minutes of heat. If you have back pain, what symptoms indicate that you should see a physician? If the pain is severe, doesn't decrease with a few days of home treatment, radiates from the back into the buttocks or legs, or is accompanied by numbness or tingling, it may indicate an **intervertebral disc** injury. The intervertebral disc is a cushion that separates the bony vertebrae. Discs are filled with fluid and are flexible through early adulthood but thin and lose their resiliency as we age. A ruptured intervertebral disc may compress nerves, causing pain down the buttocks and legs. Consult a physician who specializes in back pain for these injuries.

Core Exercises for Lower Back Health

Research has shown that 80 percent of patients with back discomfort who visit physicians have no underlying organic disease. Most of these patients are deficient in strength and flexibility of core postural muscles of the trunk. There are several exercises you can do to maintain a healthy back. We recommend the exercise routine in Figure 8-3. These exercises focus on core strengthening for the abdominals *and* stretching and strengthening the back. Practice this series daily to get the best results. The exercises can easily be included as part of your exercise warm-up or cool-down routine. These exercises should not cause any pain, numbness, or tingling in the back and legs. If they do, discontinue them and consult your specialist.

Other exercise programs that can develop muscular fitness in core stabilizers include Pilates and stability ball exercises. Yoga and Tai Chi may also reduce back pain by increasing flexibility and reducing stress. For information on these exercise programs and additional core stability exercises, see Chapters 5 and 6.

Frequently Asked Questions

Q. I was told that I shouldn't pedal backward on an indoor cycling machine. Why not?

A. Pedaling backward can increase risk of knee injuries. When you pedal, the greatest pressure is exerted in the middle of the downstroke. Pedaling forward, this occurs in front of your body with your foot in the 3 o'clock position, a mechanically stable and safe position for the knee. Pedaling backward, the greatest force occurs in the 9 o'clock position, where the knee is less mechanically stable, putting you at increased risk of injury.

Q. A friend of mine who often had leg pain while running was diagnosed with chronic compartment syndrome. I never heard of that before. What is it?

A. Compartment syndrome causes a cramping pain, tightness, and swelling during exercise when pressure within the muscles builds to excessive levels. It is most common in the lower leg but can occur in the forearms and hands. Muscle groups are covered by a tough membrane called fascia which does not easily expand. Within these fascial compartments are nerves and blood vessels. Exercise increases muscle volume due to increased blood volume, and in some individuals this causes an increase in compartmental pressure. This increased pressure impairs capillary blood flow, decreasing oxygen to the tissues, and can damage blood vessels, muscles, and nerve cells.

Compartment syndrome can be acute or chronic. Acute compartment syndrome, often caused by a traumatic injury, is a medical emergency and can cause permanent injury unless promptly treated. Chronic compartment syndrome is not a medical emergency. It often occurs in one leg and can cause numbness or difficulty in moving the foot. While symptoms usually resolve within minutes to hours after stopping activity, they can linger and worsen over time in those who ignore the symptoms and continue the activity. This is usually treated surgically, with several small incisions in the muscle fascia to allow tissue expansion.

Q. Every time I start a running program, I get shin splints. What can I do to keep this from happening next time?

A. First, check your shoes. Are they less than 6 months (500 miles) old, and are they good running shoes? Well-cushioned shoes designed for the stresses of running are your first line of defense against impact injuries. If your shoes are okay, the problem may be overuse—doing too much too soon. Many beginners, in their zeal to get in shape, try to run a mile in the first workout and increase from there. Start with several weeks of walking. Once you can walk 2 to 3 miles without discomfort, alternate jogging and walking. Review the progression in Chapter 4 and do not try to progress faster. Try the shin-strengthening exercise in Chapter 6 and stretch the calves. Consider alternating days of running with cycling or another nonimpact activity and do not try to run through the shin splints. If your shins start to ache, switch to a nonimpact activity until they heal. When you start back after a layoff, decrease your workout by 25 to 50 percent, do more walking, and build back slowly.

Q. Which is better for an injury—heat or ice?

A. Ice is the treatment of choice for any acute injury. It decreases pain, limits swelling, and penetrates deep tissues better than heat does. Heat applied too early can increase swelling. Once swelling has subsided, heat can be relaxing and can decrease stiffness.

Q. I've been working out for 4 months and am not doing anything different. Why are my knees starting to bother me?

A. Are you wearing the same shoes you started with? If so, it is time to replace them as the soles compress over time, leaving you with less cushioning. Check your workout—are you running on hard surfaces, constantly going the same direction on a track or crowned roads, or repeatedly stepping up on curbs with the same leg? Finally, outside of workouts, have you added any new activity such as weekend yard work or carrying unaccustomed loads? Switch to a nonimpact activity for a few days to give your knees a chance to recover, then modify your workouts to reduce excessive impact or repetitive stresses on your knees.

Q. My joints pop and crack a lot when I move. Is there something wrong with them?

A. Joints can be noisy for a lot of reasons, mostly benign. If there is pain or swelling along with the popping, see your physician. If your joints feel fine, a little noise is common and harmless.

Q. I've read that wearing magnets can relieve back pain. Do they work?

A. Every year a new fad comes along, promising results that don't pan out. The body has natural healing ability, so if you buy a product and get relief, it is easy to attribute it to that product when you would have gotten better without it. A randomized, double-blind crossover study of chronic back pain patients found no difference in pain relief between those using real and sham magnets. Don't waste your money.

Q. Does exercise cause arthritis?

A. No. Exercise increases joint lubrication, helps joint range of motion, and strengthens muscles that support joints. Gentle range-of-motion and low-impact aerobic exercises are recommended as a way to decrease the stiffness and pain of arthritis, either rheumatoid or osteoarthritis. Osteoarthritis from joint wear and tear is common in those over 40, may have a hereditary component, and can be brought on by joint injury, jogging, or doing other high-impact activities that stress aging joints. So if arthritis runs in your family or if you have had joint injuries, it is even more important to keep your joints strong and flexible with regular exercise such as walking, swimming, and stretching.

Summary

Much soreness and injury can be prevented. Stretching, strengthening, proper warm-up, sensible progressions, and avoiding overuse are the keys. It is better to block injuries at the source than to pay doctors' fees to treat breakdowns. The pursuit of excellence involves learning to balance your strengths and weaknesses and cooperating with your body instead of assaulting it.

You can prevent lower back problems with proper care and treatment. Maintain leg and back flexibility, strengthen abdominals, use correct lifting mechanics, and reduce sources of lower back stress. This is all within your control.

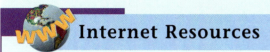

Internet Resources

About.com Sports Medicine
  http://sportsmedicine.about.com
Includes articles about sports, sports medicine, injury prevention, diagnosis, and treatment.

American Academy of Family Physicians
  www.familydoctor.org
Check out the patient site with information on all types of conditions, including common sports injuries and their diagnosis, treatment, and prevention.

American Academy of Orthopaedic Surgeons
  www.aaos.org
Contains information about orthopedic conditions, including sports injuries and their diagnosis, treatment, and prevention.

American College of Sports Medicine
  www.acsm.org/sportsmed
Has information on sports research and health and fitness, aerobic exercise guidelines, and a quarterly fitness newsletter.

"Current Comments" gives information on a variety of exercise topics of recent interest.

Medline Plus: Sports Injuries
  www.nlm.nih.gov/medlineplus/sportsinjuries.html
Covers sports injuries, screening, prevention, frequently asked questions, and treatment options.

The Physician and Sports Medicine
  www.physsportsmed.com
Contains articles on exercise, nutrition, injury prevention, personal fitness, and rehabilitation.

Virtual Sports Injury Clinic
  www.sportsinjuryclinic.net
Includes self-help advice and a virtual diagnosis for common sports injuries. Also covers rehabilitation, stretching, and strengthening for injury prevention.

Bibliography

Adams, W. B. "Treatment Options in Overuse Injuries of the Knee: Patellofemoral Syndrome, Iliotibial Band Syndrome, and Degenerative Meniscal Tears." *Current Sports Medicine Reports* 3 (October 2004): 256–260.

American Family Physician. "Running: Avoiding Running Injuries" (January 2003). www.aafp.org

Anandacoomarasamy, A., and L. Barnsley. "Long Term Outcomes of Inversion Ankle Injuries." *British Journal of Sports Medicine* 39 (March 2005): e14.

Cohen, R. S., and T. A. Balcom. "Current Treatment Options for Ankle Injuries: Lateral Ankle Sprain, Achilles Tendinitis, and Achilles Rupture." *Current Sports Medicine Reports* 2 (October 2003): 251–254.

Connolly, D., et al. "Treatment and Prevention of Delayed Onset Muscle Soreness." *Journal of Strength and Conditioning Research* 17 (January 2003): 197–208.

Fredericson, M., and C. Wolf. "Iliotibial Band Syndrome in Runners: Innovations in Treatment." *Sports Medicine* 35 (May 2005): 451–459.

Gross, M. T., and J. L. Foxworth. "The Role of Foot Orthoses as an Intervention for Patellofemoral Pain." *Journal of Orthopedic and Sports Physical Therapy* 33 (November 2003): 661–670.

Hoffman, Jay. "Resistance Training and Injury Prevention." *American College of Sports Medicine Current Comment* (May 2002): 1–2.

Jacob, T., et al. "Physical Activities and Low Back Pain: A Community-Based Study." *Medicine & Science in Sports & Exercise* 36 (January 2004): 9–15.

Kersch, T. J. "Overuse ABCs." *The Physician and Sports Medicine* 30 (July 2002): 50.

Khaund, R., and S. H. Flynn. "Iliotibial Band Syndrome: A Common Source of Knee Pain." *American Family Physician* 71 (April 2005): 1545–1550.

Magee, L. M. "Return to Play: A Common Sense Guide for Coaches." American College of Sports Medicine, August 2005. www.acsm.org

Margo, K., et al. "Evaluation and Management of Hip Pain: An Algorithmic Approach." *The Journal of Family Practice* 52 (August 2003): 1–14.

Mayo Clinic. "PRICE Is the Right Treatment." *Mayo Clinic Health Letter* 20 (September 2000): 7.

Mayo Clinic. "Sciatica." *Mayo Clinic Health Letter* 21 (February 2003): 1–3.

Mayo Clinic. "Shoulder Pain." *Mayo Clinic Health Letter* 18 (March 2002): 4–5.

Mayo Clinic. "Sports-Related Injuries and How to Avoid Them." *Mayo Clinic Health Letter* 28 (June 2002): 1–2.

Mazzone, M. F., and T. McCue. "Common Conditions of the Achilles Tendon." *American Family Physician* 65 (May 2002): 1805–1810.

McKinley Health Center. "Achilles Tendinitis." University of Illinois, September 2002. www.mckinley.uiuc.edu

McKinley Health Center. "Plantar Fasciitis." University of Illinois, August 2005. www.mckinley.uiuc.edu

McKinley Health Center. "Shin Splints." University of Illinois, September 2002. www.mckinley.uiuc.edu

Miller, L. "Sprains & Strains: What They Are, and What to Do About Them." American College of Sports Medicine, August 2005. www.acsm.org

Nash, C. E., et al. "Resting Injured Limbs Delays Recovery: A Systematic Review." *The Journal of Family Practice* 53 (September 2004): 1–10.

O'Kane, J. W. "Coping with Upper Respiratory Infections." *The Physician and Sports Medicine* 30 (September 2002): 49–50.

Osborne, M. D., and T. D. Rizzo. "Prevention and Treatment of Ankle Sprain in Athletes." *Sports Medicine* 33 (July 2003): 1145–1150

Thacker, S. B. "The Prevention of Shin Splints in Sports: A Systematic Review of Literature." *Medicine & Science in Sports & Exercise* 34 (January 2002): 32–40.

Thompson, C., et al. "Heat or Ice for Acute Ankle Sprain?" *The Journal of Family Practice* 52 (August 2003): 642–643.

Verbunt, J. A., et al. "Disuse and Deconditioning in Chronic Low Back Pain: Concepts and Hypotheses on Contributing Mechanisms." *European Journal of Pain* 7 (January 2003): 9–21.

Wilder, R. P., and S. Sethi. "Overuse Injuries: Tendinopathies, Stress Fractures, Compartment Syndrome and Shin Splints." *Clinical Sports Medicine* 23 (January 2004): 55–81.

Williams, T. M., et al. "Intrinsic Risk Factors for Inversion Ankle Sprains in Male Subjects: A Prospective Study." *American Journal of Sports Medicine* 33 (March 2005): 45–423.

Wittke, R. "Chronic Knee Joint Discomfort." *MMW Fortschritte der Medizin* 147 (June 2005): 28–29, 31–32.

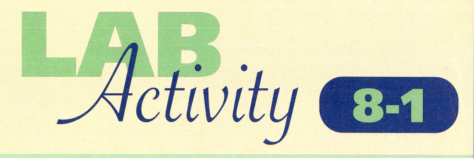

Name _____ **Class/Activity Section** _____ **Date** _____

Phil A. Case Study

Phil is 20 years old and is a student at State College. He has kept himself in good shape and has been running road races for the last 4 years. This morning, while running on White River Road, he stepped into a chuck hole and sprained his ankle. He was able to limp home. You are one of his best friends, and he has come to you for advice. He asks, "Should I go to a doctor?"

1. List five questions you would ask Phil to determine whether you should recommend a doctor:

    a.

    b.

    c.

    d.

    e.

2. Phil answers no to your questions. He asks, "What do you think I should do to keep it from swelling?" List and describe five treatments you would prescribe for Phil's injury:

    a.

    b.

c.

d.

e.

3. Phil wants to keep in shape and plans to start running again as soon as possible. He asks, "Do you think I should try to run tomorrow?" List three steps in the progression of getting back into action. Also, tell him how he might keep in shape while his injury heals:

a.

b.

c.

d.

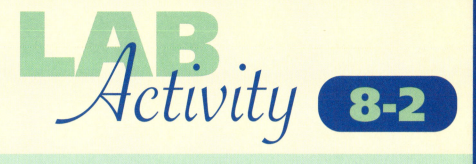

Action Plan for the Back

BACK EXERCISES

Complete the series of back exercises described in Figure 8-3.

1. Describe how your lower back area felt at the completion of the exercise session.

2. Explain how you will fit this exercise regimen into your daily schedule.

BACK CARE

Explain how you will perform the following tasks using proper body mechanics/alignment:

1. Lifting a garage door to open it:

2. Lifting a heavy box to put in the back of a station wagon:

3. Sitting several hours at a desk studying:

4. Driving a car for 5 hours:

5. Standing/working at a checkout counter for 5 hours:

6. Sleeping:

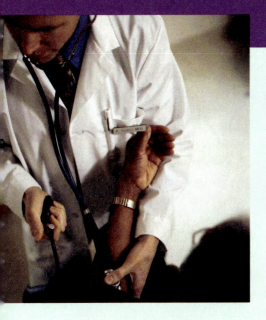

Maximizing Heart Health

9

Chapter 9

"Do it! Move it! No one ever sat their way to success."
—H. Jackson Brown, Jr., ed.,
Dad, a Father's Book of Wisdom

Objectives

After reading this chapter, you will be able to:

1. Identify the six primary cardiovascular disease (CVD) risk factors.
2. Identify the six secondary CVD risk factors.
3. Identify the controllable and uncontrollable risk factors for CVD.
4. Define *arteriosclerosis, atherosclerosis, angina pectoris, myocardial infarction,* and *stroke.*
5. Understand the differences between cardiovascular disease (CVD) and coronary heart disease (CHD).
6. Identify the symptoms of a heart attack and a stroke.
7. Explain the roles of HDL and LDL in heart health.
8. Explain why smoking cigarettes increases heart disease risk.
9. Identify prehypertension, normal blood pressure range, and the blood pressure reading that indicates hypertension.
10. Identify the cholesterol reading that indicates high blood cholesterol.
11. Recognize the CVD risk factors that are positively affected by exercise and identify the two trends that will affect cardiovascular disease in the future.
12. Explain the emerging risk factors for cardiovascular disease (metabolic syndrome, C-reactive protein, and homocysteine).
13. Understand the importance of lifestyle for cardiovascular disease and the mind/body connection.

Terms

- angina pectoris
- arteriosclerosis
- atherosclerosis
- cardiovascular disease
- cholesterol
- collateral circulation
- C-reactive protein
- diabetes mellitus
- diastolic pressure
- high-density lipoprotein (HDL)
- homocysteine
- hot reactors
- hypercholesterolemia
- hypertension
- LDL cholesterol receptors
- low-density lipoprotein (LDL)
- metabolic syndrome
- myocardial infarction (MI)
- plaque
- prediabetes
- prehypertension
- primary risk factors
- risk factors
- secondary hypertension
- secondary risk factors
- stroke
- systolic pressure
- triglycerides
- type A, B, C, and D personality

A Fit and Well Way of Life Online Learning Center www.mhhe.com/robbinsfitwell1e
Go to the Online Learning Center for chapter quizzes, outlines, flashcards, and additional lab activities.

The number one killer in America is not cancer, accidents, or AIDS. It is cardiovascular disease (CVD) (Figure 9-1). Make no mistake: cancer and other diseases are real threats, but cardiovascular diseases kill almost twice as many victims as do all the other leading causes of death. If all major forms of CVD were eliminated, U.S. life expectancy would rise almost 7 years. The tragedy is compounded because cardiovascular diseases are often inaccurately perceived as diseases of the elderly. On the contrary, based on data from the Framingham Heart Study (Chapter 1), approximately 45 percent of heart attack victims are under age 65 and 5 percent are under age 40. Young adults are not exempt from the grim heart disease picture either. It has been revealed that most teenagers already have two or more risk factors for heart disease. The American Heart Association stated that one in six teenagers and one in three people in their 20s showed evidence of atherosclerosis. This information was obtained from autopsies of young accident victims. This is alarming information and confirms that the disease process starts early in life. "Heart disease is a man's disease" is another myth. The fact is that CVD claims the lives of as many women as men, or more, and the gap continues to widen. These diseases demand attention because they are killing too many Americans in the prime of life. Don't become complacent! The way you are living your life now determines your future heart health. Many cardiovascular disease deaths are preventable. You can reduce your chances of developing CVD by assessing your current level of risk and learning ways to reduce those identified risk factors. We realize that education and behavior change are the keys.

The importance of lifestyle and knowledge for the heart health picture is emphasized by the remarks of the world-renowned CVD expert Dr. Jeremiah Stamler. He was asked, "Are diet and exercise enough to cut CVD risk?" He responded, "Yes, along with not smoking. Americans are pushed to solve problems with pills—for cholesterol, for diabetes, for blood pressure. But pills often fail to lower risk to optimum levels. They are costly and have side effects. They ameliorate but don't cure the underlying problem. *Heart disease is caused by adverse lifestyles. If you want to get rid of the disease, get rid of these lifestyles.*"

Are you at risk for heart disease? Would you know what to do if you were? Read the Top 10 List "Ways to Protect Your Heart." This chapter will provide you with valuable information about each of those items and guide you toward maximizing your heart health.

IMPACT OF CARDIOVASCULAR DISEASE

Cardiovascular disease accounts for nearly 38 percent of deaths in the United States, according to American Heart Association (AHA) statistics. In other words, 1 in 2.7 Americans who die each year does so from CVD. How do the death rates from cancer and other causes compare to that from CVD? See Figure 9-1. **Cardiovascular disease** (from *cardio* meaning "heart" and *vascular* meaning "blood vessels") refers to diseases of the heart and blood vessels. Common forms of CVD include coronary heart disease (i.e., heart attack, angina pectoris, atherosclerosis in the heart's blood vessels), congestive heart failure, rheumatic heart disease, congenital heart disease, stroke, high blood pressure, pulmonary (lung) disease, diseases of the arteries and veins, and renal disease. More than one in three Americans suffers from some form of CVD. See Figure 9-2 to see the toll taken by these various forms of CVD. Which type

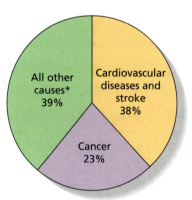

*Includes accidents, diabetes, chronic respiratory diseases, and other diseases and conditions.

FIGURE 9-1 Cardiovascular disease is still the number 1 cause of death in the United States. SOURCE: Centers for Disease Control and Prevention. Causes of death for all Americans in the United States, 2003 Final Data.

TOP 10 LIST

Ways to Protect Your Heart

1. Exercise regularly. Aim for 20 to 60 minutes most days of the week. Performing aerobic exercise regularly helps protect coronary arteries by reducing heart rate, blood pressure, cholesterol level, and body fat.

2. Maintain blood pressure level within normal limits.

3. Maintain blood cholesterol levels within acceptable limits.

4. Don't smoke.

5. Keep your weight within reasonable limits. Weighing too much (especially if you carry the extra pounds in your waistline) raises the risk of a heart attack.

6. Keep blood sugar (glucose) level close to normal.

7. Don't let your triglyceride level exceed 150 mg/dl (or 100 mg/dl if you have other coronary risk factors).

8. Control stress and hostility. Learn and practice stress management strategies and know how to diffuse anger/hostile behaviors.

9. Know the early warning symptoms of angina pectoris and the symptoms of a heart attack and a stroke.

10. Be aware of your genes. If one or more close blood relatives have had a heart attack before age 60, your risk rises substantially. Accordingly, the need to control the primary risk factors for cardiovascular disease is heightened.

Note: In addition to the "Top 10 Ways to Protect Your Heart," eat healthy. This will provide added protection against CVD. Recommendations include reducing homocysteine levels by eating five servings of fruits and vegetables and six servings of grains per day. Also, consuming foods high in antioxidants (vitamins C and E and beta carotene) helps prevent heart attacks by preventing LDL oxidation (which increases clotting and plaque rupture).

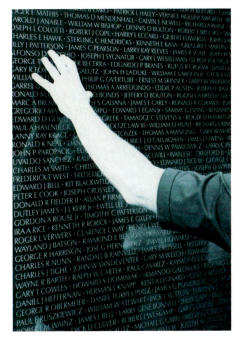

More Americans die each year from cardiovascular disease than would have been killed in 10 Vietnam wars.

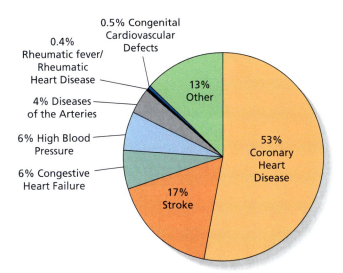

0.5% Congenital Cardiovascular Defects

0.4% Rheumatic fever/ Rheumatic Heart Disease

4% Diseases of the Arteries

6% High Blood Pressure

6% Congestive Heart Failure

13% Other

53% Coronary Heart Disease

17% Stroke

FIGURE 9-2 Percentage breakdown of deaths from cardiovascular diseases; 71.3 million Americans have some form of CVD. United States, 2002. SOURCE: CDC/NCHS.

of CVD claims the most American lives? Studies show that lower educational levels are directly associated with increased incidence of death from CVD.

Coronary heart disease, the most prevalent form of CVD, is still the single largest killer of American men and women (about one of every five deaths). The cost of all CVD in 2006 was estimated by the AHA at $403.1 billion. This figure includes the costs of physician and nursing services, hospital and nursing home services, medications, and lost productivity resulting from disability. While costs for treatment of CVD are spiraling upward, the death rate for these diseases appears to be declining. Advances in medical treatment and education and healthy lifestyle changes can be credited for the declining death rate. However, don't become too complacent about these facts. We still have a long way to go. Cardiovascular disease is the *number one* health concern in the United States. It is a killer. Someone still dies every 35 seconds; more than 2,600 Americans die each day of CVD.

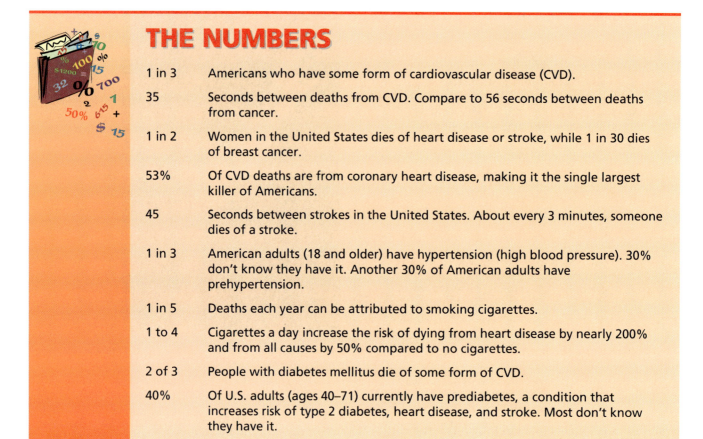

THE NUMBERS

1 in 3	Americans who have some form of cardiovascular disease (CVD).
35	Seconds between deaths from CVD. Compare to 56 seconds between deaths from cancer.
1 in 2	Women in the United States dies of heart disease or stroke, while 1 in 30 dies of breast cancer.
53%	Of CVD deaths are from coronary heart disease, making it the single largest killer of Americans.
45	Seconds between strokes in the United States. About every 3 minutes, someone dies of a stroke.
1 in 3	American adults (18 and older) have hypertension (high blood pressure). 30% don't know they have it. Another 30% of American adults have prehypertension.
1 in 5	Deaths each year can be attributed to smoking cigarettes.
1 to 4	Cigarettes a day increase the risk of dying from heart disease by nearly 200% and from all causes by 50% compared to no cigarettes.
2 of 3	People with diabetes mellitus die of some form of CVD.
40%	Of U.S. adults (ages 40–71) currently have prediabetes, a condition that increases risk of type 2 diabetes, heart disease, and stroke. Most don't know they have it.

Coronary Heart Disease (CHD)

Coronary heart disease includes angina pectoris, myocardial infarction, and the atherosclerotic process in the heart's blood vessels. CHD accounts for more than half of all cases of CVD in men and women. See Figure 9-2. About every 26 seconds an American will suffer a coronary event, and about every minute someone will die from one.

The heart is a muscle (a little larger than a fist) that works all the time. It never stops beating. Each day, the average heart beats 100,000 times and pumps about 2,000 gallons of blood. The heart pumps blood continuously through the circulatory system, which includes the lungs and blood vessels (i.e., arteries and veins). The arteries, arterioles (small arteries), and capillaries (very tiny blood vessels) carry oxygen-and-nutrient-rich blood to all parts of the body. Veins and venules (small veins) carry oxygen-and-nutrient-depleted blood back to the heart and lungs. If all the vessels were laid end to end, they would extend for about 60,000 miles. That's enough to encircle the earth more than twice.

Besides providing oxygen and other nutrients to all tissues of the body, the heart must supply itself with oxygen. This is accomplished by a separate circulatory system, which nourishes only the heart muscle. The two coronary arteries (the right coronary artery and the left coronary artery) branch off the aorta and then divide into many smaller arteries that lie in the heart muscle and feed the heart. See Figure 9-3. The most important factor in your heart's health is the efficiency of your coronary arteries in transporting blood to your heart. The heart requires a steady supply of oxygen-rich blood to function properly. The most common barrier to that supply is coronary artery disease, in which the arteries become blocked or narrowed. Coronary heart disease is most commonly the result of atherosclerosis.

You supply the ingredients for what damages or protects the blood vessels of the heart through what you eat, how you exercise, and how you react to stress. You have the power to make your heart stronger.

Atherosclerosis

What is commonly known as "hardening of the arteries" is **arteriosclerosis,** a general term for the thickening and hardening of arteries. Some hardening of arteries normally occurs as we age. **Atherosclerosis** (*athero* from the Greek work for "paste" and *sclerosis* for "hardness") is a type of arteriosclerosis. It is a progressive condition in which deposits of cholesterol and other lipids, along with cellular waste products, accumulate on the inner walls of coronary arteries or arteries in other places in the body. This buildup is called **plaque.**

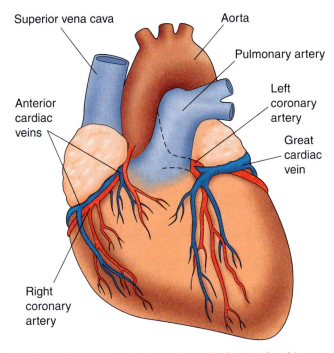

Superior vena cava

Aorta

Pulmonary artery

Left coronary artery

Great cardiac vein

Anterior cardiac veins

Right coronary artery

Smooth muscle

Endothelial cell

Lumen

FIGURE 9-3   Blood supply to the heart. Blood is supplied to the heart from the right and left coronary arteries, which branch off the aorta. If a coronary artery is blocked by plaque buildup or a blood clot, a heart attack occurs; part of the heart muscle may die due to lack of oxygen. Source: David J. Anspaugh, Michael H. Hamrick, and Frank D. Rosato. *Wellness: Concepts and Applications*, 5th ed. New York: McGraw-Hill, 2003, p. 35.

Many scientists think the atherosclerotic process begins with damage to the innermost layer of the artery wall. This layer is called *endothelium* (or *endothelial cell layer*). When these delicate cells are injured, they pull away from each other and form a gap. This "nick" or injury has to be

closed quickly to protect the blood vessel lining. The body tries to repair the "nicks" by covering them with cholesterol (especially the "bad" type) and other substances. Inflammation develops at the site. To counter, the body's immune system sends in white cell protectors to attack the plaque buildup. The resulting plaque gets irritated and unstable and encourages a clot to form.

As the condition progresses, the inner walls of blood vessels become more and more inelastic and clogged and may become hardened and blocked. The real danger comes when the plaque bursts or cracks, causing clotting material to be released and a blood clot to form inside the vessel. A heart attack or stroke may result (see Figure 9-4).

What injures the lining of our arteries, especially the coronary arteries and leads to atherosclerosis? There are many contributing factors that you can largely control: high blood pressure, smoking, high blood cholesterol (the "bad" type and triglycerides), diabetes, high blood levels of some compounds like homocysteine, chronic imflammation from things as diverse as gum (periodontal) disease or sexually transmitted diseases, your reaction to perceived emotional stress, and anger. All of these factors are influenced by lifestyle. Atherosclerosis, a major cause of CVD and coronary heart disease, does not suddenly develop at age 65. It is a long, progressive process beginning in childhood.

Angina Pectoris

Atherosclerosis may lead to **angina pectoris**, or chest pain/discomfort due to CHD. This pain/discomfort occurs when a coronary artery becomes partially blocked, causing an oxygen debt in the heart muscle. Often, angina pectoris is brought on by sudden exertion or vigorous

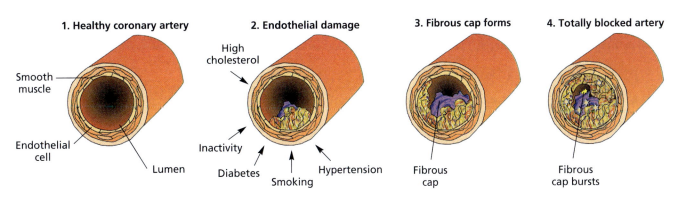

1. Healthy coronary artery   **2. Endothelial damage**   **3. Fibrous cap forms**   **4. Totally blocked artery**

High cholesterol

Smooth muscle

Endothelial cell

Lumen

Inactivity

Diabetes

Smoking

Hypertension

Fibrous cap

Fibrous cap bursts

Progression of atherosclerosis.

FIGURE 9-4

1. **Healthy coronary artery.** The lumen is not narrowed by atherosclerotic plaque, so blood can flow easily through the artery.
2. **Beginning stage of atherosclerosis.** Plaque builds up when the endothelial cells, which line the arteries, are damaged by an unhealthy lifestyle. Circulating platelets and other particles in the blood begin collecting at the injured area.
3. **Advanced atherosclerosis leads to diminished blood flow.** Due to the damage and platelet buildup, plaque continues to accumulate, and then a fibrous cap forms over the plaque.
4. **Totally blocked artery.** The body interprets plaque as an injury to the blood vessel wall. The immune system sends white blood cells to attack the plaque, and eventually inflammation develops. The inflamed plaque may result in the fibrous cap bursting, creating a blood clot that can block the lumen and lead to a heart attack or stroke.

exercise, emotional stress, or even extreme temperatures when the blood flow to the heart is insufficient to meet its oxygen demands. Typical angina is uncomfortable pressure, fullness, and squeezing or pain in the center of the chest. The discomfort may also be felt in the neck, jaw, shoulder, back, or arm. Many types of chest discomfort are not related to angina, such as that caused by acid reflux (heartburn) and lung infection. Angina is a sign that someone is at higher risk of heart attack. The AHA estimates that over 6 million people suffer from angina pectoris, with 350,000 new cases occurring each year.

Myocardial Infarction (MI)

Myocardial infarction (MI), or heart attack, results when one or more of the coronary arteries is partially blocked by atherosclerotic deposits called plaque. When one of the deposits suddenly breaks open, a blood clot (thrombus) forms and chokes off the supply of blood to the heart muscle.

The portion of heart muscle beyond the blockage is deprived of oxygen, resulting in injury or death of that portion. If a damaged area is large enough or in a vital area of the heart, the individual will die. However, many people do survive a heart attack and are capable of living productive lives. See the box "Warning Signs of a Heart Attack."

A number of studies have shown that in some damaged hearts, new blood vessels develop to nourish the area that is being starved of oxygen and other nutrients. This is called **collateral circulation.** Everyone has collateral blood vessels, which are microscopic and are closed under normal conditions. However, in some people with coronary heart disease, these vessels seem to enlarge and form a detour around the blockage to provide alternative routes for the blood. *Exercise* appears to be

one practical way to increase myocardial oxygen demand, which in turn may stimulate the development of collateral vessels. In some cases, coronary angiography (X ray) has revealed increased collateralization after exercise training.

Stroke (Brain Attack)

A **stroke** occurs when blood flow to the brain is interrupted either by a blockage (ischemic stroke) or by a burst blood vessel (cerebral hemorrhage). The brain needs a continuous supply of oxygen-rich blood to function. When a blood clot interrupts the flow of oxygen, the brain does not receive the nourishment it needs, and brain cells die. Stroke, primarily caused by atherosclerosis, is the *third* leading killer of Americans (behind heart attack and cancer). About 700,000 Americans will have a stroke this year—that's someone every 45 seconds. See the box "Most Common Warning Signs of Stroke." It is the chief cause of serious disability and a major contributor to dementia later in life. A stroke can result in paralysis of one side of the body, loss of ability to speak or understand the speech of others, loss of memory, and behavioral change. Because brain cells can't heal, modification of risk factors is important in the prevention of this disease that kills about 160,000 Americans every year. It is not solely a disease of the elderly; more than 28 percent of stroke victims are under age 65. Your risk of stroke increases with these factors:

✔ *Hypertension:* If you have high blood pressure, you are two to four times more likely to have a stroke than is someone with normal blood pressure. It is the most important risk factor for stroke.
✔ *Heart disease:* Sometimes blood clots forming in the heart can move up to the brain and block blood flow.
✔ *Gender:* More than 60 percent of stroke deaths occur in women.
✔ *Diabetes:* Those with diabetes have almost double the risk of stroke.
✔ *Age:* The incidence more than doubles in each decade after age 55.

Warning Signs of a Heart Attack

"Classic" or More Common Signs

- Uncomfortable pressure, fullness, squeezing, or pain in the center of the chest that lasts more than a few minutes or that goes away and comes back
- Pain or discomfort in other areas of the body: shoulder, neck, jaw, back, or stomach, one or both arms

Less Common Signs

- Atypical chest pain, stomach or abdominal pain
- Nausea or dizziness
- Shortness of breath and difficulty breathing
- Unexplained anxiety, weakness, or fatigue
- Palpitations, cold sweat, or paleness

Not all of these signs occur in every heart attack. If some of these symptoms do occur, don't wait. Get help immediately! Call 911.

Most Common Warning Signs of Stroke

- Sudden numbness or weakness of face, arm, or leg, especially on one side of the body
- Sudden confusion, trouble speaking or understanding
- Sudden trouble seeing in one or both eyes
- Sudden trouble walking, dizziness, loss of balance or coordination
- Sudden severe headaches with no known cause

Not all warning signs occur in every stroke. If any or some start to occur, get help immediately. Call 911.

✔ *Race:* African Americans have nearly twice as many fatal strokes as whites and more than twice as many as other minorities. Hypertension and diabetes are the suspected causes. American Indians, Alaska natives, and Mexican Americans have a higher than average risk.

✔ *Lifestyle:* These factors can be controlled: high-fat, high-cholesterol diet; alcohol or cocaine abuse; smoking; and sedentary lifestyle.

✔ Recent studies indicate that the risk of stroke may be higher in women during pregnancy and the 6 weeks following childbirth.

To reduce your risk of stroke:

✔ Exercise regularly.
✔ Keep blood pressure at optimal or normal level.
✔ Do not smoke.
✔ Keep diabetes under control if you have diabetes.
✔ Be evaluated by a sleep specialist if you have sleep apnea.
✔ Keep homocysteine levels at optimal levels by consuming plenty of produce and grains.
✔ Keep infection and inflammation down. Be tested for C-reactive protein, a marker for inflammation in the blood.
✔ Reduce chronic stress, anger, and hostility. Exercise and meditation (or other stress management techniques) are good ways.

RISK FACTORS

Risk factors are the conditions, situations, and behaviors that increase the likelihood that an undesirable outcome (injury, illness, or death) will occur. The risk is established by multiple scientific studies. A risk factor does not cause the undesirable outcome 100 percent of the time, but among those people who engage in the behavior (or experience the condition), a certain number will experience the undesired outcome. The stronger the risk factor's link with a negative outcome, the more likely an individual is to experience the undesired result.

Cardiovascular disease researchers have identified several risk factors that may lead to the development of atherosclerosis. The more risk factors you possess, the greater your chances are of developing CVD. While no one can accurately predict whether you will have a heart attack, you can estimate your odds by evaluating your risk factors. Take the *Are You at Risk for Heart Disease?* test in Lab Activity 9-1 to determine your risk and how to reduce it.

Primary risk factors are linked directly to the development of CVD; they increase the possibility of having a heart attack. *Nearly all primary risk factors are controllable.* Only type 1 diabetes is considered uncon-

trollable due to its genetic link. Type 2 diabetes can be prevented for many years by a healthy lifestyle (i.e., regular exercise, diet, and weight management).

Primary
Controllable Factors
1. Inactivity
2. High blood pressure
3. High blood lipid level
4. Cigarette smoking
5. Obesity
6. Diabetes mellitus (type 1 and type 2)

The **secondary risk factors** contribute to the development of CVD, but not as directly as the primary risk factors do.

Secondary	
Controllable Factors	**Uncontrollable Factors**
1. Stress	3. Age
2. Emotional behavior	4. Male gender
	5. Race
	6. Positive family history

Notice that 8 of the 12 total risk factors are *controllable*. Only 4 risk factors are uncontrollable. The choices you make and the way you live have a profound impact in reducing your total number of risk factors. If you possess several uncontrollable risk factors, it is imperative that you adopt a healthy lifestyle as soon as possible.

Primary Risk Factors

1. Inactivity

Countless studies have linked inactivity to CVD. The surgeon general's report confirmed that physical inactivity is a major health problem in the United States. The report warns couch potatoes, "Beware, sitting around is hazardous to your health." Additionally, the Centers for Disease Control and Prevention (CDC) in Atlanta has named physical inactivity as our nation's most common cardiac threat. Why? Because only 25 percent of Americans engage in physical activity at intensity levels recommended for fitness and health benefits. This leaves close to 75 percent of our population either entirely sedentary or not active enough to reap health benefits. Consequently, it is not surprising to learn that approximately 250,000 deaths (12 percent of deaths) every year in the United States can be attributed to lack

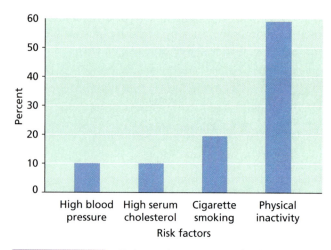

Estimated percentage of U.S. population having selected risk factors for CVD. More Americans are at risk for heart disease because of physical inactivity than because of any other manageable risk factor.

of exercise. Remember, the heart is a muscle and muscles have to be used or they will atrophy. Many experts believe that today's best buy in the prevention of CVD is *exercise* (Figure 9-5).

In yet another ongoing inquiry into the relationship between physical activity and mortality, the Harvard Alumni Study continues to produce results that have led its director, Dr. Ralph S. Paffenbarger, to conclude, "There's no doubt whatever that insufficient activity will shorten your life." Even exercise of moderate intensity (brisk walking or gardening) is beneficial in improving health and well-being. It is vigorous exercise (using the FITT prescription), however, that produces the greatest health benefits and is linked to increased longevity.

The American lifestyle is sedentary. We no longer have to hunt and grow our food, build our homes, or walk to school and work. Our ancestors did not have to build physical activity into their daily lives; it was a part of their lifestyle. Modern conveniences and technology have eliminated physical activity from our lives. The culprits are the automobile, television (with remote control), elevators, escalators, riding lawn mowers, cell phones, and computers and computer games. You can probably add to this list.

University of Tennessee researchers examined the lifestyle of an Old Order Amish community in Canada who still live like most Americans did years ago (i.e., no modern conveniences like electricity, telephone, automobile, etc.). They found that the men accumulated approximately 18,000 steps per day, and the women about 14,000 steps per day. This is far and above the 2,000- to 4,000-step average that is typical of most Americans today. The recommended step goal is around 10,000 steps in a day, which is approximately 5 miles. The lifestyle of the Amish

definitely reaches this goal and more. Refer to Chapter 4 for more information on the 10,000-step lifestyle goal. Do you know how many steps you take in a day?

Vigorous physical exercise is essential to a healthy cardiorespiratory system. Equally important, however, is overall lifestyle and how long you have been exercising. News from the U.S. surgeon general's report provides strong support for physical activity in the prevention of heart disease, high blood pressure, high cholesterol, diabetes, obesity, and cancer. This 1996 government report recommended 30 minutes of moderate-intensity physical activity on most days of the week. It was backed by research documenting that physical activity enhances health by reducing risk of chronic disease. However, in 2002, the Institute of Medicine (IOM) issued a report recommending that Americans spend at least 60 minutes doing moderately intense physical activity, such as brisk walking, every day of the week. This is more than double the daily minimum goal of 30 minutes of physical activity recommended by the surgeon general in 1996. The IOM evidence revealed that it takes more than 30 minutes of activity to maintain ideal weight. The later report reflected the fact that people in the United States are consuming more calories and getting heavier.

A third recommendation entered the picture when the government's new dietary guidelines were released. For the first time ever they included physical activity recommendations. These new guidelines, released in 2005, urge people to get 60 to 90 minutes of physical activity for weight management purposes.

Americans are confused. They are asking, "Should I exercise 30, 60, or 90 minutes a day?" "What about the FITT prescription?" The answer is, it depends on you: how fit you are, whether you are overweight, and what your goals are. Here's how to figure out what is right for you:

✔ *For aerobic fitness,* follow the FITT prescription. Work out for 20–60 minutes at moderate to vigorous intensity (60–80% HRR), three to five

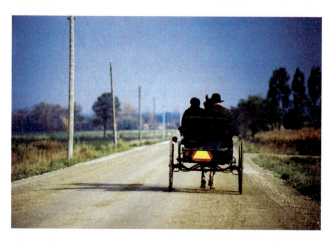

The Amish have no trouble accumulating 10,000 steps a day.

days per week. This will not only promote aerobic fitness but deliver heart and weight management benefits, too. Jog at 5 mph (12-minute mile), walk at 4.5 mph (13–14-minute mile), or bike at 10 mph (6-minute mile). Swimming, heavy yard work (such as chopping wood, shoveling snow), and playing basketball count, also.

✔ *For health benefits,* (to ward off chronic disease), get a minimum of 30 minutes of moderate-intensity exercise (40–60% HRR) *most* days of the week. It should be aerobic activity such as brisk walking at 3.5 to 4 miles per hour (15–17-minute mile). Vigorous work such as raking and bagging leaves can also serve the purpose.

✔ *For weight loss,* get 60 minutes of moderate-intensity exercise (40–60% HRR) most days of the week.

✔ *For weight loss maintenance* (in previously overweight people), get 60–90 minutes of moderate-intensity exercise (40–60% HRR) most days of the week.

✔ It is not necessary to accumulate the total number of minutes of activity all in one bout. The cumulative effect of your activity throughout the day is what counts, including all types of activity, not just doing aerobics or going for a jog. Pulse activity in throughout the day whenever you can.

The old saying "Use it or lose it!" is true. You don't have to run marathons to be physically active. Small increases in daily activity can significantly burn up excess calories, make the heart muscle a stronger and more efficient pump, lower blood pressure, alleviate stress, increase HDL levels, and build self-confidence.

The American Heart Association reports that regular vigorous exercise protects against coronary heart disease and even improves the survival rate after a heart

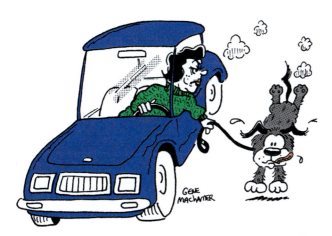

Americans are ingenious at avoiding activity. Dr. Steven Blair compares the dangers of sedentary living to smoking one pack of cigarettes a day. "Improving low fitness seems to be as important as stopping smoking in terms of reducing the risk of dying," he said.

attack. That is life insurance that money cannot buy. The most important thing you can do to improve your health and well-being is to *exercise.*

Exercise is so important for several reasons. It

✔ lowers both systolic and diastolic blood pressure
✔ lowers LDL (the "bad") cholesterol
✔ raises HDL (the "good") cholesterol
✔ decreases inflammation
✔ helps in weight management
✔ reduces stress
✔ reduces risk of type 2 diabetes

The message is this: 30 minutes of moderately intense exercise provides you with significant health benefits. Exercising for 20 to 60 minutes a day at a higher intensity level provides a higher level of fitness benefits and achieves the IOM and government guidelines, too. The point is that to get to 60 minutes, you have to get to 30 minutes first. Get moving!

Ride your bike, walk to school, play tennis instead of watching others doing these activities. Park at the back of the parking lot instead of right next to the building. Get a step pedometer and try to accumulate 10,000 steps in a day. There are many ways to add activity to your daily life. Remember, it doesn't have to be exhausting!

2. High Blood Pressure (Hypertension)

Blood pressure is the force exerted by the heart while pumping blood through the body. It is also the pressure of blood against the arterial walls.

There are two blood pressure levels, recorded as two separate numbers in fraction form (for example, 120/80). When the heart contracts and pumps blood into the arteries, the pressure increases. This is the **systolic,** or pumping, **pressure,** recorded as the upper number. The **diastolic,** or resting, **pressure** is the force of the blood against the arteries when the heart relaxes between beats. It is recorded as the lower number. Both the systolic and diastolic numbers are important. High levels of either or both mean greater risk for heart attack and stroke.

Normal blood pressure is less than 120/80. However, *many experts contend that the new gold standard or "optimal" blood pressure should be 117/75 because damage to the arteries from the pressure of blood pounding through them begins to increase at this point.* This means your risk of CVD increases! **Prehypertension** is acknowledged as blood pressure between 120/80 and 139/89, which until 2003 was considered normal but now is considered to be in the "danger zone" before full-blown hypertension develops. This unsafe condition calls for lifestyle changes and monitoring. **Hypertension,** or high blood pressure, measures 140/90 or more and requires medical treatment. Look at the stages of hypertension listed in Table 9-1.

High blood pressure causes the heart to overwork. Over a period of time, the overworked heart weakens,

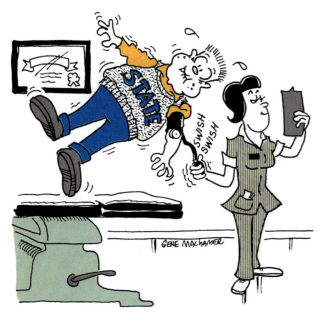

Have your blood pressure checked regularly. High blood pressure causes injuries ("nicks") to the delicate blood vessel lining and leads to atherosclerosis.

enlarges, and has a difficult time keeping up with the demands of the body. High blood pressure also causes blood vessels to become inelastic, severely reducing the amount of blood flow to the body's vital organs. Decreased levels of oxygen and other nutrients can produce heart, brain, and kidney damage. Remember, high blood pressure also leads to heart attacks and strokes.

One in three American adults has high blood pressure, and about 28 percent have prehypertension. In 90 percent of the cases there is no known cause. However, factors that can increase your chances of developing high blood pressure are heredity, cigarette smoking, male gender, age, being an African American, obesity, sensitivity to sodium, heavy alcohol consumption, use of oral contraceptives, and a sedentary lifestyle. In a

small number of cases, hypertension is caused by a specific condition, such as kidney disease, a tumor of the adrenal gland, or a defect in the aorta. This is called **secondary hypertension.** The cause of secondary hypertension can be identified and treated successfully.

How do you know if your blood pressure is too high? The only way of knowing is to have it checked. You cannot feel high blood pressure—and usually there are no symptoms until complications develop. That is why hypertension is called the "silent killer." You can be hypertensive for years and be unaware of the damage occurring. Even warning signs associated with advanced hypertension may go unnoticed but may include headaches, sweating, rapid pulse, shortness of breath, dizziness, nosebleeds, and visual disturbances. It is imperative that you know your blood pressure, because high blood pressure, while it cannot be cured, can be controlled or prevented through specific lifestyle changes. See the Top 10 List "Nondrug Approaches for Reducing Blood Pressure."

3. High Blood Lipid Profile (Cholesterol and Triglycerides)

Research has firmly linked high levels of cholesterol and other blood fats to the development of arterial plaque, a major cause of atherosclerosis and CVD. About half of all Americans have elevated cholesterol levels. Only 35 percent of those with high levels are aware of it, and only 12 percent are being treated for it.

Cholesterol is not a true fat but a waxy substance found in the bloodstream. Because it is soluble in fats rather than in water, it is classified as a lipid, as fats are. About 80 percent of total body cholesterol is manufactured in the liver, while 20 percent comes from dietary sources—mainly from foods of animal origin.

From all the bad press cholesterol gets, you would think cholesterol is our body's enemy. Not true. It is vital for our existence. Cholesterol is necessary for healthy cell membranes, brain cells, digestion, and adrenal

TABLE 9-1	Blood Pressure Stages (Adults 18 or More Years Old)		
Blood Pressure Classification	**Systolic Blood Pressure (mmHg)**	**Diastolic Blood Pressure (mmHg)**	**Recommendation**
Normal	Less than 120	Less than 80	Encourage or maintain lifestyle modifications (healthy diet, maintain healthy weight)
Prehypertension	120–139	80–89	Begin lifestyle modifications (weight reduction, healthy diet such as DASH, increase activity, limit alcohol) and monitoring and possibly treatment
Stage 1 hypertension	140–159	90–99	Lifestyle modifications, medical evaluation, and possibly drug treatment
Stage 2 hypertension	>160	>100	Lifestyle modifications, medical evaluation, and drug treatment

What was once considered normal blood pressure (120/80) is now labeled prehypertension, and treatment is recommended. The higher the blood pressure the greater the chance of a heart attack, heart failure, stroke, and kidney disease.

TOP 10 LIST

Nondrug Approaches for Reducing Blood Pressure

1. *Maintain a healthy weight.* Losing even 5 or 10 pounds, if you are overweight, can reduce blood pressure.

2. *Exercise regularly.* Exercise helps you lose weight and keep it off.

3. *Do not smoke.* Smoking does not cause hypertension but does promote CVD. A hypertensive who smokes is at serious risk.

4. *Keep your sodium intake low (below 2,400 milligrams daily—about 1 teaspoon).* Many people are salt-sensitive, meaning that salt (sodium chloride) elevates their blood pressure.

5. *Avoid alcohol; if you drink alcohol, do so in moderation.* Have no more than one drink daily if you are a woman or two if you are a man.

6. *Eat a well-balanced diet rich in fruits, grains, and vegetables.* This will help you cut back on the consumption of fats and high-calorie foods and lose some excess weight. Reduce caffeine intake. See the DASH eating plan described in Chapter 11.

7. *Increase your calcium intake.* Calcium has been linked to reduction in blood pressure. Daily consumption of 800–1,500 milligrams is recommended. (One glass of milk has approximately 300 mg.)

8. *Increase your intake of potassium.* Studies have documented a blood-pressure-lowering effect of increased potassium intake in people with mild hypertension. Do not exceed 6,000 mg per day. (Bananas are high in potassium.)

9. *Increase fiber intake.* Plant fiber has been observed to lower blood pressure in hypertensive individuals by an average of four to eight points.

10. *Practice a stress management technique such as meditation* or one of those discussed in Chapter 10. Harvard Medical School studies have confirmed the value of stress management in the reduction of high blood pressure.

glands. The problem with cholesterol is that your body makes most of what it needs, and the normal American diet adds much more. Health experts recommend that we keep dietary cholesterol consumption to less than 300 milligrams per day (less than 200 if you have high blood cholesterol). **Hypercholesterolemia** is the term for high cholesterol levels in the blood. See the Diversity Issues box "Who Has High Cholesterol?"

Ninety-five percent of the fats in the body are in the form of triglycerides, a true fat stored in the fat cells and found in the blood. Both high cholesterol and triglycerides increase the risk of developing atherosclerosis.

When evaluating your blood lipid profile for risk of CVD, there are two factors to consider: (1) the total amount of cholesterol/triglycerides found in the blood and (2) the way cholesterol/triglycerides are transported in the bloodstream.

Total Amount of Lipids Knowing your total cholesterol level provides you with a *rough* estimate of your heart disease risk. Blood cholesterol is measured by analyzing a small blood sample in a laboratory. Total cholesterol level includes the amount of cholesterol carried by high-density lipoprotein, low-density lipoprotein, and very low-density lipoprotein. The National Heart, Lung, and Blood Institute relates blood cholesterol level to CVD risk, as illustrated in Table 9-2.

Transportation of Lipids An amazing system is in place to assure cholesterol is circulated wherever it is needed. The action begins in the liver where cholesterol is packaged for delivery. Think of the liver as the cholesterol warehouse.

Like oil and water, cholesterol and blood (because it is mainly water) do not mix. Cholesterol must attach to a protein molecule to be carried through the bloodstream. This combination is called a *lipoprotein*. A lipoprotein analysis gives a more accurate picture of your CVD risk than does total cholesterol alone. A lipoprotein analysis breaks down the total cholesterol into its components, or lipoproteins, of which there are two main types. The first, termed **low-density lipoprotein (LDL)** cholesterol, is damaging to the arteries and carries cholesterol away from the liver out to the body. The second, termed **high-density lipoprotein (HDL)** cholesterol, is protective to the arteries and carries cholesterol back to the liver where it is broken down for removal from the body or sent out again as needed. Problems occur when there is too much LDL cholesterol for the HDLs to pick up promptly, or if there are not enough HDLs to do the job. Additional information about LDLs and HDLs follows:

1. **Low-density lipoprotein (LDL).** LDLs are considered "bad" because they carry a large amount of cholesterol. The lower density of the lipoprotein allows it to attach easily to the inner wall of the blood vessel, thus accelerating the atherosclerotic process. A *high* LDL cholesterol level increases your risk for CVD and stroke (Table 9-2). It is recommended that LDL levels be kept below 130 mg/dl. How can you lower LDLs?
   ✔ Don't smoke.
   ✔ Manage stress.
   ✔ Reduce consumption of saturated and trans fats.
   ✔ Lose weight, if necessary.
   ✔ Consume more fiber and omega-3 fats.

Very low-density lipoproteins (VLDL) are even more dangerous.

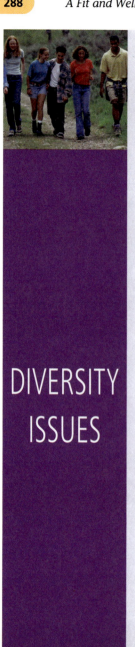

DIVERSITY ISSUES

Risk Factors for Cardiovascular Disease

Who Uses Tobacco Products?

White	32.0%
African American	28.8%
American Indian/Alaska Native	44.3%
Native Hawaiian/Pacific Islander	28.8%
Hispanic/Latino	25.2%
Asian	18.6%

Studies show that smoking prevalence is several times higher among those with less than 12 years of education than it is among those with more than 16 years of education.

Who Has High Blood Pressure (HBP)?

- Men have a greater risk of HBP than do women until age 45. Beyond that age, the percentage of women is higher.
- African Americans, Puerto Ricans, and Cuban and Mexican Americans are more likely to suffer from HBP than are whites.
- The prevalence of hypertension in African Americans in the United States is among the highest in the world.
- 41.8% of African American males and 45.4% of African American females have HBP.
- 30.6% of white males and 31% of white females have HBP.
- 27.8% of Mexican American males and 28.7% of Mexican American females have HBP.

Who Is Physically Inactive?

- People with lower incomes and less than a 12th-grade education are more likely to be sedentary.
- Men (64.2%) are more likely than women (59%) to engage in at least some leisure-time activity.
- Adults with a graduate degree are about twice as likely (80.6%) as adults with less than a high school diploma (41%) to engage in at least some leisure-time activity.

- Prevalence of physical activity:
  - White males — 33.4%
  - White females — 31.8%
  - Black males — 29.5%
  - Black females — 19.6%
  - Mexican American males — 24.9%
  - Mexican American females — 21.8%

Who Is Overweight or Obese?

	Prevalence of Overweight and Obesity (%)	Prevalence of Obesity (%)
White males	69.4	28.2
White females	57.2	30.7
Black males	62.9	27.9
Black females	77.2	49.0
Mexican American males	73.1	27.3
Mexican American females	71	38.4
Hispanic/Latinos (men & women)	38.9	24.7
American Indian/Alaska Native males	76.6	
American Indian/Alaska Native females	61.1	

Overweight in adults is BMI = 25.0 to 29.9. Obesity in adults is BMI = 30.0 or higher.

Who Has Metabolic Syndrome?

- Mexican Americans — 31.9%
- Whites — 23.8%
- African Americans — 21.6%
- Other — 20.3%
- Among African Americans, women had a 57% higher prevalence than did men.
- Among Mexican Americans, women had a 26% higher prevalence than did men.

SOURCE: American Heart Association, 2006 *Heart and Stroke Facts Statistical Update* (National Center, 7272 Greenville Ave., Dallas, TX 75231–4596).

2. **High-density lipoprotein (HDL).** HDL is considered the "good" cholesterol because of the dense structure of the lipoprotein. It is thought that HDL acts as a garbage collector in clearing away plaque and other debris as it flows through the bloodstream to the liver to be excreted from the body. The higher your HDL cholesterol level is, the better and the more protection from CVD it provides. See Table 9-2. HDL levels above 40 mg/dl are recommended. How can you increase your level of HDL?

- ✔ Exercise regularly.
- ✔ Don't smoke.
- ✔ Reduce weight and/or maintain a normal weight.

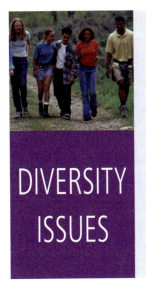

DIVERSITY ISSUES

Who Has High Cholesterol?

	Total Cholesterol 200 mg/dl or Higher	Total Cholesterol 240 mg/dl or Higher	LDL Cholesterol 130 mg/dl or Higher	HDL Cholesterol Less Than 40 mg/dl
Total	49.8%	17.3%	39.5%	22.6%
White males	48.9%	16.5%	43.8%	34.5%
White females	52.1%	18.4%	36.9%	12.4%
Black males	41.6%	12.2%	36.0%	22.7%
Black females	46.8%	17.4%	34.5%	11.3%
Mexican American males	51.9%	16.7%	43.7%	34.4%
Mexican American females	44.8%	13.6%	31.3%	15.4%

SOURCE: 2006 *Heart Disease and Stroke Statistics,* American Heart Association.

TABLE 9-2 *Interpreting the Numbers: Cholesterol Guidelines*

Total Cholesterol	Risk Category
Below 200 mg/dl	Desirable
200–239 mg/dl	Borderline high
240 mg/dl and above	High

LDL Cholesterol	
Below 100 mg/dl*	Optimal
100–129 mg/dl	Near optimal
130–159 mg/dl	Borderline high
160–189 mg/dl	High
190 mg/dL and above	Very high

HDL Cholesterol	
Below 40 mg/dl	Bad
40–59 mg/dl	Better
60 mg/dL and above	Best

Triglycerides	
Below 150 mg/dl	Desirable
150–199 mg/dl	Borderline high
200–499 mg/dl	High
500 mg/dl or above	Very high

*Achieving a goal of less than 170 is recommended if there is a high risk for CVD. SOURCE: National Heart, Lung, and Blood Institute. Cholesterol levels are measured in milligrams (mg) of cholesterol per deciliter (dl) of blood.

✔ High-fiber and low-fat diets may also increase the HDL cholesterol level.
✔ Use monounsaturated fats (e.g., olive oil, canola oil, sunflower oil) as primary fat while keeping total fat intake low.

Alcohol consumption, especially that of red wine, has received attention as a protective factor against heart attack because it is thought to raise HDL cholesterol in the blood and might help prevent clotting that leads to plaque buildup inside arteries. *Moderate* consumption of alcohol (one drink for women per day and two drinks for men per day) is the amount associated with a reduction in the rate of heart attacks. The following amounts are examples of one drink:

✔ 1½ oz. of bourbon, scotch, vodka, gin
✔ 4 oz. wine
✔ 12 oz. beer

If you don't drink, don't start. Recent evidence indicates that similar benefits can be obtained from grape juice *or* red wine, suggesting that the benefit may come from substances (phenols) in the grape skin, not from the alcohol.

Consuming more than two drinks a day is known to damage the heart. A protective effect of alcohol consumption has not been proven, but many adverse effects are well documented. Besides causing automobile accidents and social disruption, excess intake of alcohol can raise blood pressure and triglyceride levels and cause diseases of the liver, pancreas, and nervous system. Even though alcohol consumption above moderate levels adversely affects blood pressure and triglycerides and can damage the heart, alcohol is still NOT considered a primary or secondary heart disease risk factor. To put the benefit of moderate drinking in perspective, the reduction in heart disease risk is comparable to what you might achieve by exercising regularly or by cutting blood cholesterol levels through a low-fat diet.

What causes LDL and HDL to get out of balance in some people? There is genetic variability in how efficiently (or inefficiently) a person metabolizes dietary saturated fat and cholesterol. Some people can eat almost

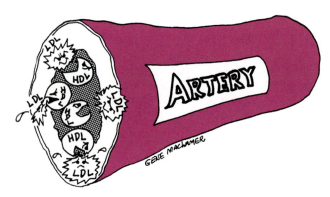

HDL cholesterol clearing away plaque in arteries.

anything and their blood cholesterol levels remain stable. Others find that even a small amount of dietary fat makes their blood cholesterol levels increase. Most of us are somewhere in between on this spectrum.

Drs. Michael Brown and Joseph Goldstein won the Nobel Prize in Medicine in 1985 for their discovery of **LDL cholesterol receptors.** Located primarily in liver cells, these receptors bind and remove cholesterol from the blood. The more cholesterol receptors you have, the more efficiently you can remove cholesterol from the blood. The number of cholesterol receptors is in part genetically determined. Lifestyle factors also influence the number. A diet high in saturated fat and cholesterol produces what Brown and Goldstein termed "double trouble." It not only saturates the receptors, it also decreases their number—a bad combination. Only about 5 percent of the population has genetically high cholesterol levels that remain elevated regardless of lifestyle.

Total Cholesterol/HDL Ratio   Scientists believe that the ratio of total cholesterol to HDL cholesterol is a better indicator of risk for cardiovascular disease than is the total value alone. To determine your ratio, take a laboratory blood test that will reveal your total cholesterol and HDL cholesterol levels. Next, divide the total cholesterol level by the HDL cholesterol level to find the ratio. For example, if the total cholesterol were measured to be 160 and the HDL cholesterol 40, your ratio would be four to one (4:1) (160 ÷ 40 = 4). This would place you in the near optimal category as you can see in Table 9-3. Everyone should strive for a ratio that is 4:1 or lower. The lower this ratio is the lower is the risk for CVD. A ratio above 4:1 increases your CVD risk.

TABLE 9-3	*Ratio of Total Cholesterol to HDL Cholesterol*
Optimal ratio (very low risk)	3.5:1
Near optimal ratio (low risk)	4:1

Average HDL levels in adult Americans are about 45 to 65 mg/dl, with women averaging higher values than men. The female sex hormone estrogen tends to raise HDL levels, which may explain why premenopausal women are usually protected from heart disease. Studies suggest that HDL levels above 70 may protect against heart disease, while those below 35 signal coronary risk.

Triglycerides   **Triglycerides** are manufactured in the body to store excess fats. They are also known as *free fatty acids*, and in combination with cholesterol, they accelerate the formation of plaque. Triglycerides are carried in the bloodstream by very low-density lipoprotein (VLDL). These fatty acids are found in poultry skin, lunch meats, and shellfish. However, they are mainly manufactured in the liver from alcohol, starches, and refined sugars (honey included). Alcohol, starches, and sugars are not fats, but the body can convert them into fats and then dump those fats into the bloodstream. Ways to lower triglycerides include:

✔ Decrease consumption of alcohol, sugar, and refined carbohydrates.
✔ Reduce weight if overweight.
✔ Reduce consumption of animal fats in the diet (poultry skin, lunch meats, shellfish).
✔ Get regular aerobic exercise.
✔ If necessary, take prescribed medications.

As a general rule, you should keep your triglyceride level below 150 mg/dl of blood. However, some reports indicate that triglyceride levels over 100 should be cause for concern. See Table 9-2.

You should know your cholesterol level and have it checked annually, especially if you have a positive family history of CVD. The best way to do this is to have a 12-hour fasting blood test that is analyzed by a reputable laboratory. Over-the-counter tests that don't require fasting are not as reliable. Since cholesterol levels are greatly influenced by diet and lifestyle, follow these guidelines to reduce high levels:

✔ A diet rich in cholesterol—or, worse, one rich in saturated fat (saturated fat is highest in vegetable oils such as tropical and palm, in meat, and in high-fat dairy products) and trans fats (hydrogenated oils in many crackers, cookies, cakes, pies, and pastries)—can increase your blood cholesterol level. Keep total fat less than 30 percent of total calories per day and dietary cholesterol below 300 mg per day. This small modification in dietary fat can reduce cholesterol levels by 10 to 15 percent. (See Chapter 11 for other dietary strategies that affect heart health.)
✔ Reduce body weight if overweight. Weight reduction alone can lower cholesterol and triglyceride levels.

✔ Lowering your stress level also helps offset high cholesterol. See Chapter 10.
✔ Increase daily aerobic exercise. Try to walk more, use escalators and cars less, and be a participant rather than a spectator.
✔ Reduce alcohol, sugar, and caffeine consumption.
✔ Increase consumption of fiber-rich foods such as oatmeal, dried beans and peas, whole-grain breads and cereals, raw fruits and vegetables.
✔ Take your medication, if prescribed.

4. Cigarette Smoking

Cigarette smoking is a primary risk factor. Nicotine increases heart rate and blood pressure and constricts blood vessels. Carbon monoxide also creates cardiovascular stress by impairing the transport of oxygen in the blood. Smoking kills more than 400,000 Americans a year, and 35 percent of those deaths are CVD-related. About one in five deaths from CVD is attributable to smoking. Some health professionals are calling tobacco use a "weapon of mass destruction." Every cigarette package is required by law to carry a consumer warning. One such warning is "Cigarette Smoking Can Kill You."

Even Ann Landers, the nationally syndicated columnist, gave a warning: "Beware, cigarettes are killers that travel in packs." Numerous studies have proved that cigarette smoking causes oral cancer, lung cancer, and emphysema, and in women it is linked to cervical cancer, early menopause, and damage to the fetus during pregnancy. It also leads to the development of wrinkles in men and women. The number of Americans killed each year from smoking is greater than the number killed during World War II and the Vietnam War combined. No level of smoking is safe!

The AHA reports that smokers have more than twice the risk of heart attack of nonsmokers. Even limited smoking (four to five cigarettes per day) increases CVD risk. Also, smoking increases the risk of developing peripheral vascular disease (narrowing blood vessels in the arms and legs), which may lead to the development of gangrene and eventually amputation.

Passive smoke, synonymous with secondhand smoke, is the cigarette smoke inhaled by nonsmokers from environmental air. The U.S. Surgeon General's new report provides conclusive evidence of the alarming public health threat posed by secondhand smoke. It declares smoking bans are the only way to protect nonsmokers. The research reveals that secondhand smoke is remarkably effective in damaging the cardiovascular system:

1. Nonsmokers may be *more* susceptible to heart and vascular damage from secondhand smoke than smokers are even though they absorb much smaller doses of the smoke's toxins. That is because smokers develop compensatory responses

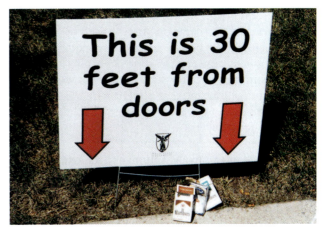

The science is clear: secondhand smoke is not mere annoyance—it's lethal. Smoking bans are heading outdoors, with challenges to the rights of smokers who "puff" outside buildings and on sidewalks. Some states are banning smoking outdoors—within 15 to 30 feet of all public buildings. They are even posting signs to indicate the specific distances. Others are even banning smoking on beaches and in parks.

to some of the adverse cardiovascular effects of cigarette smoke–but nonsmokers do not get the "benefit" of these adaptive responses.

2. Carbon monoxide, a substance in secondhand smoke (and in inhaled cigarette smoke), damages (causes injuries or "nicks") the smooth inner lining of blood vessel walls. This accelerates the atherosclerotic buildup. Carbon monoxide, higher in the blood of smokers but also found in nonsmokers, decreases the amount of oxygen carried in the blood. It also reduces the heart's ability to use the oxygen it does receive.

3. Even low levels of secondhand smoke increase the stickiness of blood platelets in nonsmokers, making it more likely that a clot will form in the narrowed arteries, which can ultimately lead to a heart attack or stroke.

4. Secondhand smoke increases atherosclerosis by lowering HDL cholesterol and increasing LDL cholesterol buildup.

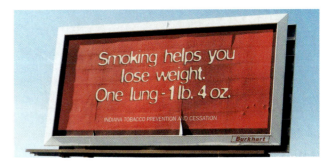

Cigarette smokers are two to four times more likely to develop CVD than nonsmokers.

5. It increases chronic inflammation.

6. It increases cell-damaging free radicals.

7. It decreases the body's levels of antioxidants, which help protect against free radicals.

8. Nonsmokers who live with smokers or work where environmental smoke is present have a 58 to 91 percent higher risk of dying from CVD than do other nonsmokers.

9. It increases insulin resistance.

10. Secondhand smoke is a human carcinogen, killing about 3,000 nonsmokers a year through lung cancer. Smoking is everyone's business!

11. The population burden associated with passive smoking and CVD is estimated to be 65,000 deaths annually in the United States. The simplest and most cost-effective control measure to reduce cost is to *mandate* smoke-free workplaces, schools, and public places.

While studies show that smoking has declined by more than 47 percent since 1965, this downward trend appears to be leveling off. There are still 4,000 new smokers every day. About 80 percent of people who use tobacco begin before age 18 (see Figure 9-6). A non-smoker should not begin to smoke. Smokers should stop *now*. Don't hesitate, do it! Ninety percent of smokers who quit do so on their own!

5. Obesity

Obesity has escalated to epidemic proportions in the United States and is continuing to increase at an alarming rate. See the first Diversity Issues box, "Risk Factors for Cardiovascular Disease." Obesity is uncomfortable; increases the burden on the vital organs, especially the heart; and is directly linked to CVD. Obesity is expensive, too. Annual medical costs for an obese person are 37.7 percent more than those for someone of normal weight.

It is especially risky to have excess body fat in the waist and abdominal area. The distance around the waist and body mass index (BMI) are recommended ways to es-

timate one's body fat. A high-risk waistline is 35 inches or more for women, 40 inches or more for men. See Chapters 3 and 12 for instructions on how to measure your waist and BMI. Skinfold calipers (discussed in Chapter 3) more accurately measure percent of body fat. The CDC considers anyone above 30 pounds over target weight to be obese.

More than 65 percent of the U.S. population is now obese or overweight. In 1980 the number was only 46 percent, up steadily from the 1970s. Child-hood obesity rates have more than tripled since the late 1970s. Ninety percent of people with type 2 diabetes are overweight. Obesity, considered a chronic disease, causes more than 300,000 premature, preventable deaths per year.

In addition, obesity puts women in particular at increased risk of CVD. A study conducted by the Harvard Medical School of 115,000 women ages 30 to 55 found

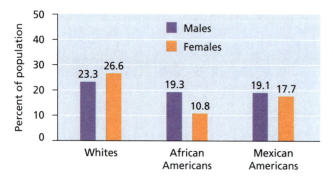

FIGURE 9-6 Prevalence of high school students using any tobacco product by race/ethnicity and sex: United States, 2003.
SOURCE: CDC/NCHS.

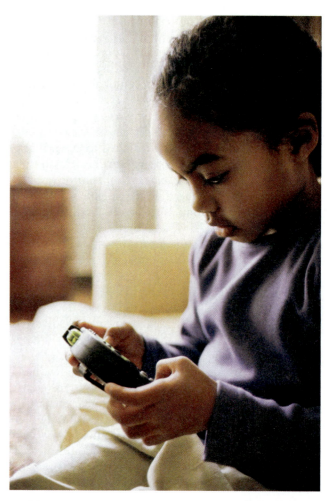

Health experts recommend that school-age children get at least 60 minutes of exercise daily. But, today, too many children spend their time in nonphysical activities such as playing video games. Former President Bill Clinton states, "Our children may grow up to be the first generation with shorter life spans than we had."

that of all the women in the 8-year study who developed CVD, 40 percent had no other risk factors except being 20 percent or more over their ideal weight. Women who had been slim at age 18 and gained weight in adulthood seemed to be at increased risk. The first step in medical treatment for these conditions is usually weight reduction. Obesity is controllable and can be reversed. You can eliminate the obesity risk factor by maintaining a reasonable weight (see Chapter 12). Even modest weight reduction (5 to 10 percent of body weight) can help reduce your risk of CVD and stroke.

Physical inactivity is a major factor in the development of obesity in men, women, and children. Watching too much television is one of the main culprits. The number of television hours watched per person in this country averages about 4 per day. Americans should limit TV viewing to about 1 hour or less a day to prevent physical and mental inactivity. Of course, consuming more calories than are used in daily activity also contributes to obesity. NOTE: Accumulating 10,000 steps expends approximately 500 calories!

6. Diabetes Mellitus (Type 1 and Type 2)

What do blindness, gangrene, kidney failure, heart attack, and stroke have in common? They can all result from diabetes, which eventually strikes one in three people in the United States.

Diabetes mellitus (which includes both type 1 and type 2) is a disease that affects how the body uses *glucose*, a sugar that is the body's main source of fuel. This chronic disease is characterized by the body's inability to produce enough of the hormone *insulin* or use it properly. In the normal digestive process, the food you eat is changed to glucose. Insulin (which is produced in the pancreas) carries the glucose in the blood to the body's cells so that your body gets the energy it needs. In diabetes, this normal process is interrupted. When glucose doesn't reach the cells, it accumulates in the blood and the underfueled cells are starved for energy. This surplus glucose is eliminated by the kidneys, which pass it off in the urine. Too much sugar in the urine and in the blood is a classic sign of diabetes. Diabetes is found in two forms, type 1 and type 2. It is primarily a genetic disease, especially type 1. Type 2 is heavily influenced by obesity. Scientists believe that a genetic predisposition for type 2 can be warded off, even prevented, by lifestyle interventions of weight management and exercise.

In insulin-dependent diabetes, also known as type 1 or juvenile onset, the pancreas makes little or no insulin. The diabetic must receive insulin injections every day to stay alive and must carefully watch his or her diet and exercise regularly. It occurs most often in children or young adults. Symptoms develop rapidly, usually within a period of months or even weeks. Approximately one million Americans have type 1 diabetes.

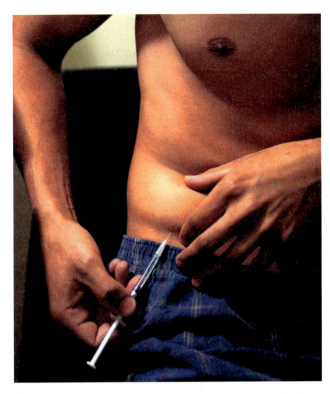

Diabetes has increased at an alarming rate in the United States in the last decade. Health experts are blaming the wired-up, couch potato culture of the 1990s.

More common (90 to 95 percent of diabetics) is non-insulin-dependent diabetes, once known as adult-onset, or type 2, in which the pancreas makes insulin but either the amount is insufficiently released or the body cannot properly use what is available. This type of diabetes can often be controlled without insulin injections through other medications, diet, and weight management. This form of the disease usually occurs in people over 40 years old and is associated with aging and obesity. New data, however, show a dramatic rise of type 2 in children and young adults, making the term "adult-onset diabetes" obsolete. Because the onset of type 2 is gradual, the disease may go undetected for years. Diabetes seriously increases the risk of developing cardiovascular disease. About 75 percent of people with diabetes die of some form of heart, stroke, or blood vessel disease. Part of the reason for this is that diabetes affects cholesterol and triglyceride levels by producing a different kind of LDL that is even worse for the arteries than is ordinary LDL. This accelerates atherosclerosis. Even so, type 2 diabetes can be delayed or averted by weight management and physical activity. One condition shared almost universally by type 2 diabetics is obesity. Not all obese people become diabetic, but *90 percent of people with type 2 diabetes are overweight or obese.*

The surge in youth obesity in this country has paralleled a rise in childhood type 2 diabetes. At one time type 2 diabetes was almost unheard of in children. They almost always had type 1. A new advisory from the American Academy of Pediatrics and the American Diabetes Association calls for diabetes testing of overweight children with any two other risk factors starting at age 10 or at puberty, if it comes earlier. See the projected diabetes rates for those born in 2003 in Figure 9-7.

Many people know their blood pressure and cholesterol levels, but few know their glucose level. A substantially elevated glucose level is the chief diagnostic sign of diabetes. Unfortunately, far too few people are properly tested. As a result, researchers say that nearly half the estimated 17 million people who have type 2 diabetes don't know it.

Now we have identified a condition called **prediabetes** (or insulin resistance), which is a precursor to diabetes. It is defined as a fasting blood glucose between 100 and 125 mg/dl. Millions of Americans have this metabolic condition where the blood-glucose level is only slightly elevated. People with prediabetes can be protected from developing full-blown diabetes—and its life-threatening complications—by losing weight and, if necessary, taking medications to lower their blood sugar.

The main reason why public health experts are urging wider glucose testing is that it is the only way to catch diabetes early. The disease usually causes no symptoms for a decade or more even though it is silently festering the entire time. That's 10 to 12 years during which diabetes quietly eats away at your vision, injures your kidneys and nerves, and sets the stage for CVD. This is damage that would be preventable if only people learned sooner that they have type 2 diabetes.

According to the new American Diabetes Association (ADA) guidelines, all people age 45 and older should have their fasting blood-glucose level tested at least every 3 years. Several groups of people are at greater risk and should be checking for diabetes at least once a year. Get tested, starting at age 35, if you:

✔ Are overweight, especially with extra belly fat
✔ Have a brother, sister, or parent with diabetes
✔ Are nonwhite (i.e., African American, Hispanic, and Native American, especially the Pima tribe of Arizona)
✔ Had a baby weighing more than 9 pounds or had gestational diabetes (diabetes during pregnancy)
✔ Have an HDL cholesterol of 35 or less or a triglyceride level of 250 or more
✔ Have hypertension or take antihypertension drugs
✔ Had a minimally elevated glucose level on a previous test

Two readings of *126 mg/dl or more* on a fasting blood-glucose test taken on different days means you have diabetes. Less elevated reading, from *100 to 125*, indicate impaired fasting glucose, which means you have prediabetes or are insulin resistant and face a sharply increased risk of diabetes (see Table 9-4). Regardless of your glucose level, you are probably prediabetic if you have low HDL, high triglycerides, high blood pressure, or excessive abdominal fat (i.e., a waist measurement of more than 35 inches for a woman and 40 inches for a man).

The following lifestyle changes can improve insulin resistance:

✔ Regular moderate exercise
✔ Losing weight (5 to 7 percent of body weight)
✔ Stopping smoking
✔ Eating a high-fiber diet
✔ Eating a diet low in simple carbohydrates (sugar and other sweets) and alcohol or following the DASH diet

They may also help improve the associated HDL, triglyceride, and blood pressure problems. Those steps can also help people who have type 2 diabetes (and sometimes even those with type 1) control their glucose level.

Two symptoms that occur in many people with diabetes are increased *thirst* and *frequent urination*. That's because excess glucose circulating in your body draws water from your tissues, making you feel dehydrated. To

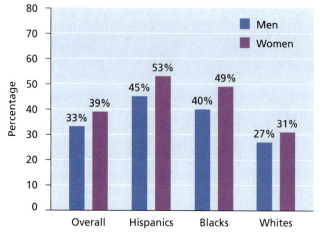

FIGURE 9-7 *Children born in 2003: Who will have type 2 diabetes?* A third of the people born in the United States in 2003 will develop diabetes. The chances of developing diabetes are highest among women and minorities. Minorities have a combination of genetic predisposition and higher obesity rates that puts them at risk.

TABLE 9-4	*Blood-Glucose Levels*
Normal	65 to less than 100 mg/dl
Prediabetes:	100–125 mg/dl
Impaired fasting glucose or insulin resistance	
Diabetes	126 mg/dl or more

quench your thirst, you drink a lot of water and other beverages, and that leads to more frequent urination. Other signs and symptoms of type 2 diabetes are:

- ✔ Flu-like symptoms (since glucose is not reaching your cells you may feel tired and weak)
- ✔ Weight loss or weight gain
- ✔ Blurred vision
- ✔ Frequent hunger
- ✔ Dry skin
- ✔ Slowly healing wounds
- ✔ Itching, tingling, or numbness in the extremities
- ✔ Frequent vaginal or skin infections
- ✔ Combinations of these symptoms

Unless detected and controlled, diabetes can ultimately lead to stroke, heart disease, kidney failure, blindness, amputation of limbs from gangrene, and death. See Table 9-5. According to the ADA, the disease is a leading cause of death in this country, and diabetics are two to four times as prone to heart attack and stroke as are nondiabetics. Assess your risk of developing diabetes by completing Lab Activity 9-4, *Are You at Risk for Diabetes?*

Secondary Risk Factors

These factors are associated with increased risk of CVD, though not as directly as the primary risk factors.

1. Stress

Stress is unavoidable. It includes happy, wonderful, and positive events as well as sad, destructive, and negative ones. For example, the death of a family member and the birth of a child, while perceived differently, are stressors that produce the same physiological response in the body. Job stress may be particularly unhealthy. High blood pressure is three times more common among people who have jobs with high demands but little control (assembly line worker, waitress), or people who are unrecognized for their efforts. Stress has been found to cause a rise in heart rate, blood pressure, and blood cholesterol, and it can lead to excessive smoking or eating–all linked to CVD. The type of stress is not that important. Indianapolis 500 race car drivers have higher cholesterol levels after they race than before. Tax accountants have increased cholesterol around April 15. Students have higher cholesterol levels during exams. Stress causes chemical wear and tear on the body by releasing stress hormones into the bloodstream. Large amounts of stress hormones are found in the bloodstreams of people who react to stressful situations with hostile and angry behavior. However, low levels of stress hormones are found in the bloodstreams of people who react normally to stressful events. How you react to stress seems to be the critical factor. You should recognize stress in your life (the positive and the negative) and

---

TABLE 9-5   *Complications of Diabetes*

Over time, untreated or poorly controlled diabetes can cause debilitating and even life-threatening complications.

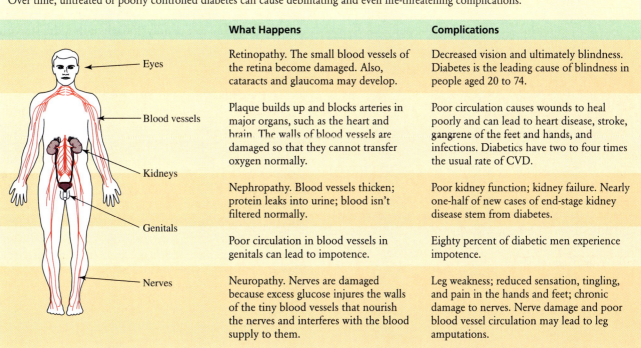

		What Happens	Complications
	Eyes	Retinopathy. The small blood vessels of the retina become damaged. Also, cataracts and glaucoma may develop.	Decreased vision and ultimately blindness. Diabetes is the leading cause of blindness in people aged 20 to 74.
	Blood vessels	Plaque builds up and blocks arteries in major organs, such as the heart and brain. The walls of blood vessels are damaged so that they cannot transfer oxygen normally.	Poor circulation causes wounds to heal poorly and can lead to heart disease, stroke, gangrene of the feet and hands, and infections. Diabetics have two to four times the usual rate of CVD.
	Kidneys	Nephropathy. Blood vessels thicken; protein leaks into urine; blood isn't filtered normally.	Poor kidney function; kidney failure. Nearly one-half of new cases of end-stage kidney disease stem from diabetes.
	Genitals	Poor circulation in blood vessels in genitals can lead to impotence.	Eighty percent of diabetic men experience impotence.
	Nerves	Neuropathy. Nerves are damaged because excess glucose injures the walls of the tiny blood vessels that nourish the nerves and interferes with the blood supply to them.	Leg weakness; reduced sensation, tingling, and pain in the hands and feet; chronic damage to nerves. Nerve damage and poor blood vessel circulation may lead to leg amputations.

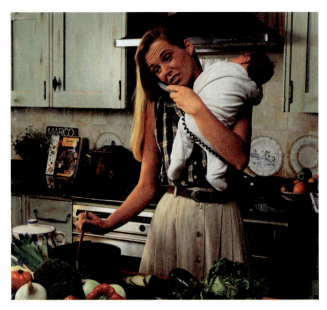

Performing several tasks at the same time is an excellent example of how hectic life in the 21st century has become.

learn to handle the stressful situations in a healthful manner. Coping with stress successfully is vital in today's hectic, in-the-fast-lane lifestyle. Exercise, relaxation techniques, and behavioral modification are excellent methods for reducing stress. Research shows that one of the most important resources for dealing with stress is a good social support system (i.e., family and friends). We need to change the way we look at or perceive stressful situations. Problems are to be solved, not worried about. Read more about ways to reduce stress in Chapter 10.

2. Emotional Behavior

Several studies have linked emotional behavior to increased risk of heart disease. Until recently there were just three emotional behavior patterns or **personality types—Types A, B,** and **C.** Now a newly coined personality type, **Type D** (which stands for "distressed"), has been identified and may be the type with a dangerous risk for CVD. The Type A individual exhibits aggressiveness, competitiveness, and impatience and is a workaholic. Type As demonstrate a high degree of time urgency—a tendency to do two or three things at the same time. The Type B individual is more relaxed, noncompetitive, patient, and slow to anger. Type Cs are actually classified as Type As but learn to cope with emotional stress by using the five Cs: control, commitment, challenge, choices in lifestyle, and connectedness. Such people welcome change, considering it a challenge. They are committed to goals, gaining confidence as a result (see Chapter 10). Type Cs are called *"hardy"* stress resisters.

Early studies identified Type A people as the ones at greater risk of having heart attacks. However, more recent research indicates that it is only when a Type A person exhibits the behaviors of *hostility* and *anger* that a serious risk is apparent. These behaviors arouse the fight-or-flight response, significantly elevate blood pressure, overstimulate the production of stress hormones, and have been documented to increase coronary artery atherosclerosis. Some studies have found that hostility levels are a more accurate predictor of heart disease than high cholesterol, hypertension, smoking, or obesity. The other Type A behaviors do not seem to be as significant but may eventually lead to hostile, angry reactions to stress. That's why Type A behavior should be recognized. Type Bs with these negative behaviors will also suffer adverse health consequences.

Type D people possess negative emotions and tend to be depressed, anxious, irritable, insecure, and distant. They have a joint tendency toward "negative effectivity" (worry, irritability, gloom) and "social inhibition" (discomfort in social interactions, reticence, and a lack of social poise). Some scientists believe that the social and emotional problems associated with Type D personality can increase the chances of developing cardiovascular disease. Hypertension and CHD have been linked to those identified as Type Ds. They seem to have more inflammation throughout the body and exaggerated blood pressure and other negative reactions to stress. Among people who already have heart conditions, those with Type D personalities are less responsive to treatment, have poorer quality of life, and also are more likely to die prematurely.

Twenty percent of apparently healthy people experience extreme surges in blood pressure when confronted with the challenges of everyday life. They are called **hot reactors** because their systolic blood pressure can rise from 120 to a deadly 300 when they are stressed. They often go untreated until felled by a stress-induced heart attack or stroke. Hot reactors can be found in all emotional behavior types.

We are not born with hot reacting, angry, and hostile behaviors. These behaviors are learned, and for the sake of our health, we can unlearn them. Learning to modify Type A and D behaviors, especially hostility, anger, and hot reacting, is not difficult and may add years to your life. How does a "hostile heart" become less angry and cynical—and become a "trusting heart"?

Carry a notebook and record every time you feel angry and/or hostile. Once you have done this for a while, you will start to recognize the situations that provoke these reactions and be able to head off the troublesome behavior. Other suggestions follow:

1. *Stop angry, cynical thoughts.* Every time you have a cynical thought, think to yourself, "STOP!" This is called *thought stopping* and is an effective behavior modification technique when practiced regularly.

Prescription for Action

Date: *Do one more today*

✔ Write down the top two reasons your last fitness program didn't work. Then, write down what you'll do this time to avoid those same pitfalls.

Reasons failed: Strategies to counter:
- •
- •

✔ Get your blood pressure checked.
✔ Do two of the following to maintain a healthy blood pressure or reduce hypertension:
- • Have a high-fiber snack (something with at least 5 or more grams of fiber).
- • If you smoke, cut in half the number of cigarettes smoked today.
- • Avoid alcohol.
- • Reduce caffeine.

✔ Measure your waist.
✔ Calculate your BMI.
✔ Read food labels and avoid all trans fats (anything hydrogenated or partially hydrogenated).
✔ Get 30 minutes of exercise today.
✔ Reflect on the meaningful people in your life. Connect with two of them today via e-mail, telephone, or letter.

Prescribed by: *YOU*

2. *Practice laughing at yourself.* Once you realize how silly your anger is in many situations, laughing at yourself will quickly replace fuming.
3. *Be empathetic.* Put yourself in the other person's shoes. Often the other individual is a victim of circumstances, too.
4. *Reason and understand your anger.* There will be times when anyone would be angry in the same situation, but you must say, "I have this trait, and it is bad for my health." Decide if the situation warrants your attention and if you have an effective response. If not, take a "time out" from the situation.
5. *Learn to relax.* Practice the excellent "stress busters" (such as exercise, meditation, etc.) in Chapter 10.
6. *Practice patience and trust.* Instead of getting irritated while standing in a line, concentrate on a relaxing word (such as "quiet") until your anger subsides. Trust that others are not out to cheat you.

7. *Become a good listener.* Pay attention to what others are saying and do not interrupt. This may help you understand the situation better *before* you jump to an angry response.
8. *Live as if you had a serious disease.* You will soon see that the little problems that once riled you up aren't really so important.
9. *Learn to forgive.* Compassion is the strongest medicine for anger. Blame leads to anger; forgiveness heals.

3. Age

Being older has some advantages (wisdom and experience), but protection from CVD is not one of them. As you age, your risk for developing heart disease increases. This does not mean that coronary heart disease is *only* a disease of the old. You don't suddenly drop dead one day at age 45 from a "heart attack." At any age and certainly at age 18, you have atherosclerotic plaque in your arteries. It accumulates over time, and by the time you've gained "age," you've also increased the private stash of cholesterol in your arteries. There is little that can be done to stop the calendar. Adopting a healthy lifestyle early in life may add years to your life and life to your years.

4. Male Gender

Although CVD is the leading cause of death for both men and women, males have a higher risk of heart attack, especially earlier in life. The gender factor exists because men have heart attacks 10 years earlier than women. Until age 55, men also have greater risk for hypertension than women do. The incidence of stroke is higher for males than females under age 65. The increased male risk is not clearly understood. Some credit the increased risk to the male sex hormone testosterone, which triggers the production of low-density lipoproteins, thereby clogging blood vessels. Others say a male's lifestyle may be the culprit. We do know that a female's hormonal makeup is protective until menopause. Female hormones signal the liver to produce more "good" cholesterol (HDL) and make blood vessels more elastic than a male's blood vessels, especially during childbearing years. Once women reach menopause (usually in their early to middle 50s), their rates of heart-related problems equal or surpass those of men.

It is imperative that males modify other risk factors to protect their cardiovascular systems (i.e., increase physical activity, maintain a healthy weight, don't smoke, keep blood pressure and cholesterol levels at recommended levels, manage stress, and modify emotional behaviors).

5. Race

According to the AHA, African Americans have the greatest risk of all races for heart attack and stroke. High blood pressure develops earlier in life in blacks than in

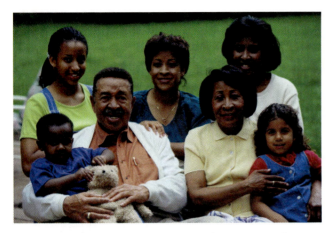

African Americans have increased risk for heart attack, stroke, and diabetes.

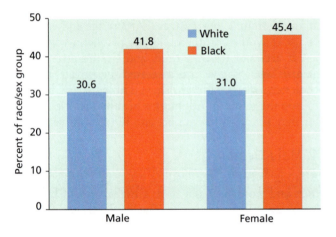

FIGURE 9-8 Estimated percentage of population with hypertension by race and sex among U.S. adults. Hypertensives are defined as persons with a systolic level ≥140 and/or a diastolic level ≥90 or those who reported using antihypertensive medication.

whites and is generally more severe (see Figure 9-8). One explanation for this higher incidence is that many African Americans share a mutation in a gene that helps control blood pressure. A hereditary intolerance to sodium may also account for the danger. African Americans' and Mexican Americans' risk of diabetes and obesity is twice that of any other ethnic groups in the United States (see Figure 9-7). Social and economic stresses may also contribute to increased cardiovascular disease risk. It is paramount that early heart health intervention and education programs be supported for African American populations. Also, being aware of these risks, African Americans should adopt a healthy lifestyle early. See the first Diversity Issues box for additional population information.

Heart disease and stroke risks are high among Mexican Americans, American Indians, and native Hawaiians also. Again, this increased risk is due to higher rates of obesity and diabetes.

6. Positive Family History

A family history of heart disease in brothers, sisters, parents, or grandparents increases your risk of developing CVD. Tendencies toward high blood pressure, stroke, peripheral blood vessel disease, rheumatic fever, high blood lipid levels, obesity, and early heart attack appear to be somewhat hereditary. This is why your physician is so interested in your family history. A family's lifestyle also may contribute to heart disease and stroke. For example, family members may be overweight, smoke, eat large amounts of cholesterol and saturated fat, or be physically inactive. You should find out as much as possible about your family's medical history. You can be alerted early to a possible risk and take preventive measures.

The Emerging Risk Factors

Metabolic Syndrome

Also known as syndrome X, insulin-resistance syndrome, and prediabetes syndrome, **metabolic syndrome** is a dangerous cluster of symptoms that raise the risk of heart disease, stroke, diabetes, and some cancers. It is defined as having three or more of the following:

✔ Elevated blood pressure: blood pressure higher than 130/85
✔ Elevated glucose: fasting blood sugar of at least 100 mg/dl (a sign of insulin resistance)
✔ High triglycerides: triglycerides of 150 or higher
✔ Low HDL ("good") cholesterol: HDL cholesterol less than 40 for men and 50 for women
✔ Obesity: a waist measurement of more than 35 inches for women and 40 inches for men

Do you have metabolic syndrome? It is a silent disease that affects approximately 25 percent of white Americans and even more African Americans, Mexican Americans, and Native Americans. Scientists know a lot about the components that make up metabolic syndrome, but they know less about the overall syndrome. The key element seems to be insulin resistance, but that is largely a result of obesity and lack of exercise. Thus, the root cause is hard to determine.

The best treatment for metabolic syndrome is a healthy diet, regular exercise, and weight loss, even if you don't lose much. See the first Diversity Issues box.

Homocysteine

Homocysteine is an amino acid in the blood and a natural by-product of protein metabolism. The consumption of protein from meat or vegetable sources (such as soy) starts a series of biochemical reactions that ultimately leads to the production of homocysteine. Normally homocysteine is converted into nondamaging amino acids by folacin (often called folate or folic acid) and vitamins B_6 and B_{12}. However, in some individuals these processes are impaired, and homocysteine accumulates in greater quantities than it would normally. Studies have shown that too much homocysteine in the blood is related to a higher risk of CHD, stroke, peripheral vascular disease, and cognitive decline (or dementia). Further, it is known that homocysteine causes injuries (or "nicks") and inflammation in cells lining the arteries, makes the blood more prone to clotting, and promotes the oxidation of low-density lipoprotein, which makes it more likely that cholesterol will be deposited as plaque in the blood vessels. A high homocysteine level is considered to be a risk factor for CVD, much like a high level of cholesterol.

Homocysteine levels in the blood are strongly influenced by diet as well as genetic factors. The dietary components with the greatest positive effects are folic acid and vitamins B_6 and B_{12}. Folic acid and the B vitamins help break down homocysteine and thus lower concentrations in the blood. Also, studies reveal that low blood levels of folic acid are linked with a higher risk of fatal CHD and stroke.

Along with diets high in protein and low in B vitamins, heavy smoking has been linked to high homocysteine levels. Heavy smokers have up to 50 percent higher homocysteine levels than nonsmokers. Homocysteine levels above 15.8 micromoles/liter have a threefold greater risk of heart attack than do lower levels. You should aim for a level of 9 mg/dl or less.

Although evidence for the benefit of lowering homocysteine levels is lacking, people with high risk should be strongly advised to get enough folic acid and vitamins B_6 and B_{12} in their diets. Foods high in these nutrients include:

- ✔ Folacin: leafy greens, broccoli, wheat germ, beans, whole grains, fortified oatmeal
- ✔ Vitamin B_6: whole grains, bananas, potatoes, beans, fish, meat, poultry
- ✔ Vitamin B_{12}: meat, poultry, liver, eggs, dairy, fish, fortified cereals, soy products

It has been suggested that laboratory testing for homocysteine levels can improve the assessment of CHD risk. It may be particularly useful in people who have a personal or family history of CVD but in whom the well-established risk factors (inactivity, smoking, high blood pressure, obesity) do not exist.

C-Reactive Protein (CRP)

It is true that the primary and secondary risk factors increase the risk for heart disease, but scientists have known for some time that they are not the only culprits. Inflammation of the blood vessels can also trigger heart attacks and strokes by causing plaque buildup in the arteries to rupture, creating a blood clot that induces a heart attack or stroke. The process begins when the body interprets plaque in the arteries of the heart as an injury to the blood vessel wall. The immune system attacks the plaque, resulting in inflammation. Inflammation can be measured with a blood test that checks for a substance called **C-reactive protein,** a marker for this inflammation. CRP is produced by the liver in response to inflammation somewhere in the body and is now recognized as an important factor in heart disease. Elevated levels of CRP are linked to an increased risk for heart attack and stroke. A person can have no outward signs of inflammation but still have subtle inflammation and hence elevated CRP.

Twenty-five percent of Americans who have heart attacks have no identifiable risk factors. That is why scientists have been searching persistently for another piece of the puzzle; CRP looks to be one of the missing pieces.

Doctors are not recommending universal blood testing for CRP because even something as simple as the common cold (or minor injuries) can boost it. What causes the inflammation?

- ✔ Bacterial infections (such as chlamydia or other sexually transmitted disease)
- ✔ Obesity (fat cells release proteins that cause low-level inflammation)
- ✔ High LDL and low HDL
- ✔ High blood pressure and smoking (both damage the lining of blood vessel walls)
- ✔ Lingering infections (anything from chronic gum disease or sinus infections to urinary-tract infections).

What can be done?

- ✔ Regular exercise: physically fit people have lower CRP levels.
- ✔ Cholesterol-lowering drugs called statins also reduce CRP, as do aspirin and some other medications. Low doses of aspirin (e.g., "baby" aspirin) are recommended for patients with coronary disease who are not taking other anticoagulants and do not have contraindications to aspirin. Also, antibiotics work.
- ✔ Not smoking: smoking harms the entire cardiovascular system.
- ✔ Diet: people who eat a diet with a high-glycemic load have higher CRP. See Chapter 11 for information on a high-glycemic diet. Also, eat foods rich in omega-3 fatty acids (salmon, tuna, sardines, flax seed).
- ✔ Brush your teeth thoroughly and get dental checkups.

TREATMENT FOR BLOCKED CORONARY ARTERIES

As you have discovered, most of the risk factors linked to coronary heart disease can be controlled. The way you live, the choices you make, can have a profound impact

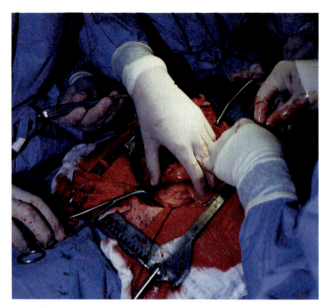

The cost of cardiovascular diseases and stroke was an estimated $403.1 billion. This figure includes health-care expenditures and lost productivity for the year 2006. Each year these costs increase.

on the health of your cardiorespiratory system. When coronary arteries become blocked, usually the first treatments prescribed are diet modification (low fat) and exercise therapy. These are two major areas of one's life that, if maximized, can have positive results. When these methods are unsuccessful, the following procedures may be required.

Drug Therapy

This involves drug treatment affecting the supply of oxygen to the heart muscle or the heart's demand for oxygen. Some drugs (coronary vasodilators) cause the blood vessels to relax, enlarging the opening inside them. Blood flow then improves, and more oxygen reaches the heart. Nitroglycerine is the most commonly used drug in this category. Another category of drugs (beta blockers) slows down the heart rate or reduces blood pressure, thus decreasing the heart's need for oxygen, reducing its workload. There are many other classifications of drugs used to treat CVD as well (e.g., the statins).

Angioplasty (or Balloon Angioplasty)

The AHA describes this treatment as a nonsurgical procedure that improves the blood supply to the heart by dilating a narrowed coronary artery. The blocked part of the coronary artery must be identified before this technique is performed. During this process (cardiac catheterization), a doctor guides a thin plastic tube (catheter) through an artery in the arm or leg into the coronary arteries. A liquid dye, visible in X rays, is in-

jected into the catheter, and X ray movies are taken as the dye flows through the arteries. Doctors can identify obstructions in the arteries by tracing the flow of the dye. Once obstructions are identified, a catheter with a balloon tip is inserted inside the first catheter; the balloon tip is inflated at the obstruction site. This compresses the plaque and enlarges the opening of the blood vessel. The balloon is deflated, and both catheters are removed. The process injures the vessel wall, causing the area to grow new cells. Some people grow too many cells, reclogging the artery. About 20 percent of people who have this treatment have narrowed arteries within 6 months. The introduction of stints (cylinders that prop the arteries open) has substantially reduced the risk of arteries reclosing. However, the reclosure risk is still 10 to 20 percent within the first year.

Coronary Bypass Surgery

This is a surgical technique in which doctors take a blood vessel from another part of the body (usually the leg) and use it to detour around a blockage in the coronary artery. Blood flow to the heart is restored.

 # THE FUTURE . . . FOCUS ON LIFESTYLE

The cost of treating cardiovascular diseases in this country is staggering. Many scientists believe we will be more successful if we focus on prevention rather than rely on expensive, high-tech treatments. "An ounce of prevention is worth a pound of cure" will in all likelihood be the slogan of the 21st century. Heart disease prevention in our future will focus primarily on lifestyle changes and approaches that involve "mind and body" concepts. Many scientists are already substantiating these trends in their research and medical practices.

One example is Dr. Dean Ornish, cardiologist, clinical professor of medicine at the University of California at San Francisco, and pioneer in the treatment of CVD. He found that after treating his patients with the current, recommended medical procedures—medication, angioplasty, (balloon technique), and coronary bypass surgery, all expensive and dangerous—most did not stay well. Despite the procedures, some died and many returned for further treatment. He began to question the wisdom of such dramatic medical care for heart disease. He found it interesting that lifestyle factors could trigger all mechanisms known to cause CVD. The lifestyle choices we make each day, such as what we eat, how we respond to stress, how much we exercise, and whether we use tobacco, have a profound impact on the heart's health. With this concept in mind, he developed a plan that focuses on lifestyle. His program, "Reversing Heart Disease," is having significant success in reducing atherosclerosis without medication or surgical procedures. The program involves the following lifestyle changes:

1. A special diet is recommended. The Reversal Diet is 10 percent fat, 70 to 75 percent carbohydrate, 15 to 20 percent protein, and 5 milligrams of cholesterol per day. In comparison, the typical American diet is 40 to 45 percent fat, 25 to 35 percent carbohydrate, 25 percent protein, and 400 to 500 milligrams of cholesterol per day. The Reversal Diet allows, but does not encourage, moderate alcohol consumption (less than 2 oz. per day). It excludes caffeine, allows moderate use of salt and sugar, and is not restricted in calories.
2. Smoking is prohibited.
3. Thirty minutes a day or 1 hour every other day of moderate exercise is prescribed.
4. Stress management methods are prescribed every day. These include yoga stretches, progressive relaxation, abdominal breathing, meditation, and imagery.
5. Psychological support should be enhanced. This involves increased time spent talking about feelings with friends and family and participating in spiritual and religious activities.

Mind and Body Connection

The traditional risk factors explain only a portion of the known causes of heart disease. Why do some people develop heart disease while others do not? Clearly, all the risk factors are important, but could there be something more? Are there common psychological—and perhaps even spiritual—factors that lead to or prevent coronary heart disease? Is there an unconscious connection between mind, body, and spirit that would explain the unknown causes of heart disease?

Scientists are examining these questions: Is laughter good for you? Can prayer bring down blood pressure? Does a bad marriage or a divorce suppress your immune system? Does listening to others lower blood pressure? Is a cynic more likely to have heart trouble? To each of these questions there is a scientist able to answer "YES!" and provide data to back it up. There is a whole field of mind/body research tapping into the interaction between our immune systems and our bodies, minds, moods, and spirit. Just as we learned the importance of exercise and nutrition to our health, we are discovering ways to go deeper into inner wellness. Ponder these studies that support the mind/body concept:

✔ Norman Cousins (now deceased), author, philosopher, and former professor at the Department of Psychiatry and Bio-behavioral Sciences at UCLA Medical School, found that laughter heals because it replaces fear and stress with serenity and homeostasis. He taught others never to underestimate the capacity of the human mind and body to regenerate, even when the prospects seem most dismal. His research confirmed that positive emotions boost health.

✔ Larry Scherwitz, professor of psychology at the University of California, found that people who overuse the self-centered pronouns "I," "me," and "mine" are twice as likely to have heart attacks. These people are hostile, have a low level of trust in others, and put their self-centered interests and pleasures ahead of others.

✔ Redford Williams of Duke University found that cynics, being full of contempt for other people, and angry hostile people have more than their share of heart trouble.

✔ Many scientists have developed psychological tests to measure levels of anger that bring on heart attacks. Studies linking social support (i.e., loving family, happy marriage, one or two close friends, support groups) to vitality, longevity, lowered blood pressure, and healthier immune systems confirm that emotions may regulate health. These head and heart factors are powerful medicine.

✔ Dean Ornish, M.D., is convinced that one cause of blocked coronary arteries stems from three kinds of loneliness (or isolation): (1) we feel isolated from ourselves, (2) we lack "connectedness" and intimate relationships with others, and (3) we have a cosmic loneliness of the spirit (or higher part of ourselves). He feels that isolation leads to chronic stress and to illnesses such as heart disease and that real intimacy and feelings of connectedness with others can be healing. He argues that the ability to be intimate with ourselves, with others, and with a higher spirit—within ourselves—is the key to emotional health and essential to the health of our hearts as well.

✔ Mind/body connection authority Jon Kabat-Zinn, author of *Full Catastrophe Living*, advocates meditation as a technique to bridge the gap between the mind and the heart to improve health, ease pain, and reduce stress.

✔ Another authority on the mind/body connection, Bill Moyers, author of *Healing and the Mind*, explored the latest research in the field of medicine known as psychoneuroimmunology. He found evidence supporting the ways in which thoughts, feelings, and emotions influence our health. Moyers documents the importance of mind/body interactions in the prevention and treatment of illness.

Frequently Asked Questions

Q. The United States is such a diverse nation with many different ethnic populations. Are the leading causes of death the same for each?

A. Look at Figure 9-1. You can see at a glance that CVD disease is by far the number one killer of all people in the United States, regardless of ethnicity. Far down the list is cancer, followed by accidents. Every 34 seconds someone in this country dies of CVD, whereas every 56 seconds someone dies of cancer.

Q. I recently had my cholesterol tested. Why didn't the figures for LDL and HDL cholesterol add up to the total cholesterol number?

A. Because the total includes several other substances. About 10 to 15 percent of the total consists of other particles, notably very low-density (VLDL) and intermediate-density lipoprotein (IDL). While these also contribute to clogged arteries, there hasn't been enough research to correlate specific VLDL and IDL numbers with heart risk, so doctors generally don't consider them. As you know, more important than total cholesterol, since it is a hodgepodge of different substances, are the HDL and LDL numbers. The isolated LDL and HDL numbers, with diametrically different effects on the heart, are the best indicators of coronary risk. Ask your doctor for those scores, available on a blood test called total lipid profile.

Q. My friend, who just had a full body scan, suggested that I should get one, too. Is a full body scan recommended? What are the pros and cons?

A. Full body scans are CT (computed tomography) examinations of the entire body that are being offered to healthy people to look for early signs of disease. Diagnostic CT scanning to examine specific parts of the body when there is a problem has been used for decades. But scanning almost the entire body for screening is a new concept.

Full-body CT screening is controversial. The potential benefit is the early detection of significant disease, such as tumors or plaque in the coronary arteries. The risk is that of radiation exposure. X rays can cause damage to cells in your body. Even at low doses there is a risk of causing cancer. That's too high a risk for a test that is not medically necessary, especially if you have one every few years.

Another downside is the likelihood that the scan will reveal some abnormality in the body that is benign or inconsequential. But because the abnormality has been "seen" on the scan, you may have to have additional anxiety-provoking tests. The exam also has its limitations—it can't detect every abnormality, so it does not absolutely rule out the possibility of cancer or other disease.

Cost is a factor, too. These scans are not cheap, and they are not covered by health insurance. The American College of Radiology does not sanction full body scans for screening healthy people.

Q. Is it really OK to eat eggs two or three times a week even though I'm on medication to keep my cholesterol down?

A. Yes, it is. Research shows that two or three eggs weekly are not apt to raise blood cholesterol. The real villain is saturated animal fat, found in whole milk, fatty meat, cheese, and butter. A Harvard study of 120,000 men and women found that a daily egg did not boost the risk of heart disease or stroke. Eggs are rich in choline, needed for proper brain functioning, and the antioxidant lutein, believed to help protect eyes from macular degeneration.

Q. Why does exercise prevent heart disease?

A. Here's at least part of the answer. In addition to lowering blood pressure, cholesterol, and body fat, certain components in the bloodstream called cytokines act either to promote atherosclerosis (atherogenic) or to prevent it (atheroprotective). Research published in the *Journal of the American Medical Association* studied the effect of long-term exercise on those blood factors. The participants worked out for an average of 2½ hours per week for 6 months. After the exercise program, production of the atherogenic blood factors fell by 58.3 percent and the level of atheroprotective factors rose by 35 percent. In any individual, the amount of change was proportional to the level of activity. In other words, the participants who exercised more enjoyed more of the beneficial effects in their blood levels. Those who exercised less had a smaller response. It appears that with every extra minute you exercise, your body is producing more protection and undergoing less destruction of your arteries. Although there is likely an upper limit (or point of diminishing returns), this study gives you one more reason to exercise.

Q. Don't more women die from breast cancer than heart disease?

A. No. Across nearly all racial and ethnic groups, heart disease is the number one killer of women just as it is the number one killer of men.

Q. How often should I have my blood cholesterol measured?

A. Adults should be screened at *least* once every 5 years, but more frequently if the total cholesterol is elevated, HDL is low, and/or they have other cardiac risk factors.

Q. How many people in the United States adhere to a lifestyle that reduces the risk of coronary heart disease?

A. It is somewhat difficult to pinpoint the exact number, but findings from the Nurse's Health Study (involving more than 80,000 women) may give us some insight. The study revealed that women in this low-risk category make up only *3 percent of the population*, a pitifully low number. That means 97 percent of the U.S. population does not! The study confirmed that the risk of heart disease can almost be eliminated if we follow a few rules. The heart-healthy lifestyle defined in this study involves:

- Engaging in moderate to vigorous physical activity for at least half an hour per day.
- Not smoking.
- Eating healthy and consuming a diet:
  - Low in saturated fat (found in animal products) and trans fat (found in cookies, crackers, pies, cakes, donuts, candy, margarine)
  - High in fiber
  - High in folate (found in green leafy vegetables, orange juice, fortified cereals, legumes, and whole grains)
  - High in omega-3 fatty acids (found in fish)
  - Low in glycemic foods (sweets, etc., which raise glucose levels)
  - Averaging at least half a drink of an alcoholic beverage a day
- Not being overweight

Q. How long do most people have diabetes before it is diagnosed?

A. It often depends on what type of diabetes they have. Millions of American adults and children have diabetes and don't know it, many of them for years. Early detection is important because diabetes can cause more complications the longer it goes untreated. Type 1 diabetes is probably hard to overlook because it often begins with sudden and severe signs and symptoms, such as nausea, vomiting, and stomach pain. Thus, it is diagnosed soon after it starts, usually within a few weeks to a few months. People with type 2 diabetes, in contrast, often don't have noticeable symptoms for a long time. On average, people have diabetes for 8 years before it is diagnosed. Regular visits to your doctor and regular fasting blood-sugar tests can help detect the disease early (see Tables 9-4 and 9-5).

Q. I can find all kinds of information on high blood pressure but not much on low blood pressure. How low is too low?

A. Within limits, the lower your blood pressure the better. For most people, blood pressure is not too low unless it causes signs and symptoms such as light-headedness or fainting. Normal blood pressure is less than 120/80 millimeters of mercury (mmHg). Unusually low blood pressure should be evaluated by a physician. Unlike high blood pressure, there are no clear-cut standards for the diagnosis of low blood pressure. Low blood pressure is not a specific disease. It is usually a sign of an underlying problem.

Summary

Heart disease is the number one killer in the United States. Extensive studies have identified 12 factors that increase the risk of developing coronary heart disease. These factors lead to the development of atherosclerosis. The most significant factors are inactivity, high blood pressure, a high blood lipid profile, cigarette smoking, obesity, and diabetes. These six are labeled *primary* and can be controlled (except type 1 diabetes). Only type 1 diabetes is linked to heredity. Type 2 is influenced by genetics but can be prevented by a healthy lifestyle (involving weight management and exercise). There are seven additional factors labeled *secondary*. The first two of these are controllable. They are stress and emotional behavior (especially negative emotional behaviors such as hostility and anger). The other four secondary risk factors, which cannot be controlled, are age, male gender, race, and positive family history. Recently identified contributors to CVD are metabolic syndrome, C-reactive protein, and homocysteine. The more risk factors you have and the longer they are present, the greater the chance you have of developing heart disease. By age 20, you already have fatty deposits present in your coronary arteries. If your risk of CVD is low, keep up the good work by maintaining a healthy lifestyle. However, if your coronary risk is high, now is the time to act. You can't do anything about your race, heredity, sex (gender), or age. However, you can choose to act on those risk factors under your control.

If the coronary arteries become blocked due to advanced atherosclerosis, there are several treatments available. These include exercise and diet modification, drug therapy, angioplasty, and coronary bypass surgery. The cost of treating CVD continues to spiral upward every year. To counter this trend, many scientists are convinced that preventing CVD through lifestyle change is the key to maximizing heart health.

Adopting a healthy lifestyle early in life can add years to your life and life to your years. In addition, great discoveries await us as the field of mind and body research gains wider acceptance in the quest for increased well-being.

Let the words of Don Ardell inspire you to maximize your potential to be the best you can be: "Excellence ain't easy. If it were, everyone would be doing it and it would be ordinary. Know that in lots of ways, the deck is stacked against anyone who wants to excel. Do it anyway."

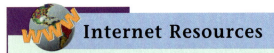

Internet Resources

America On the Move
www.americaonthemove.org
Help to add 2,000 steps a day and reduce calories by 100 calories a day.

American Diabetes Association
www.diabetes.org
National nonprofit organization providing diabetes research, information, and advocacy.

American Heart Association
www.americanheart.org
Includes statistics and information on heart disease and stroke risk.

American Stroke Association
www.strokeassociation.org
Provides information on strokes.

Centers for Disease Control and Prevention
www.cdc.gov
Provides links to health and disease information. Lead federal agency for enhancing and promoting disease prevention and health education. Can find information about how the U.S. is doing on *Healthy People 2010* goals.

Cooper Institute for Aerobics Research
www.cooperinst.org
Has exercise and health research information.

DASH: Dietary Approaches to Stop Hypertension
www.nhlbi.nitt.gov/health/public/heart/hbp/dash
Provides dietary information to lower high blood pressure.

Diabetes Personal Health Decisions
www.diabetes.org/diabetesphd
Online risk profile tool for diabetes.

Harvard Medical School Health Publications
www.healthharvard.edu
Consumer-friendly site features a Heart Letter, Mental Health Letter, Women's Health Letter, Men's Health Letter, and special health reports.

Health A to Z
www.healthatoz.com
You can search for information on general health topics.

Healthfinder, U.S. Government
www.healthfinder.gov
Lists government health resources and offers links to over 500 consumer health sites.

Healthy People 2010
www.healthypeople.gov
Provides information on the goals, objectives, leading health indicators, and priority areas in the federal government's publication *Healthy People 2010*.

Healthy People 2020
www.health.gov/healthypeople
Has information and guidelines for a healthy America.

Journal of the American Medical Association
www.ama.assn.org
Provides abstracts and news update summaries of latest *JAMA* reports.

Mayo Clinic
www.mayohealth.org
You can search by major health/disease subject area.

MedlinePlus
www.nim.nih.gov/medlineplus
National library of medicine.

National Heart, Lung, and Blood Institute
www.nhlbi.noh.gov/index.html
Gives information and statistics about heart and lung disease.

National Institutes of Health
www.nih.gov
Has links to a vast number of health sites and provides up-to-date research about disease prevention and treatment. Part of the U.S. Department of Health and Human Services.

National Library of Medicine
www.nim.nih.gov
You can search for published scientific medical literature.

Shape Up America
www.shapeup.org
Dr. Koop (former U.S. surgeon general) provides information on exercise and diet.

Smoke Clinic
www.smokeclinic.com
Helps people stop smoking. Provides a structured program similar to those used in real-world smoking clinics.

U.S. Surgeon General
www.surgeongeneral.gov/topics/obesity
Provides information on weight management.

Web MD
www.webmd.com
Has news items, advice, and articles on health.

Your Disease Risk
www.yourdiseaserisk.harvard.edu
An interactive site to assess your disease risk factors.

Bibliography

ACSM's Resource Manual for Guidelines for Exercise Testing and Prescription, 5th ed. Leonard A. Kaminsky, ed. Philadelphia: Lippincott Williams & Wilkins, 2006.

American Heart Association. "Heart Disease and Stroke Statistics–2006 Update." National Center, 7272 Greenville Avenue, Dallas, TX 75231-4596. 2006.

Blair, S. N., and T. S. Church. "The Fitness, Obesity, and Health Equation." *Journal of the American Medical Association* 292 no. 10 (September 8, 2004): 1232–1234.

Case, P. E., et al. "Stemming the Tide: Are You Prepared for the Diabetes Epidemic?" *ACSM's Health & Fitness Journal* 10, no. 1 (January/February 2006): 7–13.

Center for Disease Control. "New Data Show Obesity and Diabetes Still on the Rise." National Center for Chronic Disease Prevention and Health Promotion, December 30, 2002.

Christou, D. D., C. L. Gentile, et al. "Fatness Is a Better Predictor of Cardiovascular Disease Risk Factor Profile Than Aerobic Fitness in Healthy Men." *Circulation* 11 (April 18, 2005): 1904–1914.

Danesh, M. B., et al. "C-Reactive Protein and Other Circulation Markers of Inflammation in the Prediction of Coronary Heart Disease." *New England Journal of Medicine* 350, no. 14 (April 1, 2004): 1387–1397.

Denollet, J. "DS14: Standard Assessment of Negative Affectivity, Social Inhibition, and Type D Personality." *Psychosomatic Medicine* 67 (2005): 89–97.

Dietz, W. H., and T. N. Robinson. "Overweight Children and Adolescents." *New England Journal of Medicine* 352, no. 20 (May 19, 2005): 2100–2109.

Flegal, K. M., et al., "Excess Deaths Associated with Underweight, Overweight, and Obesity." *Journal of the American Medical Association* 293, no. 15 (April 20, 2005): 1861–1867.

Glantz, S. A., and W. W. Parmley. "Anger Proneness Predicts Coronary Heart Risk." *Circulation* 101 (March 2000): 20–34.

Greenland, P., M. D. Knoll, et al. "Major Risk Factors as Antecedents of Fatal and Nonfatal Coronary Heart Disease Events." *Journal of the American Medical Association* 290, no. 7 (August 20, 2003): 891–902.

Guloti, M., H. P. Black, et al. "The Prognostic Value of a Nomogram for Exercise Capacity in Women." *New England Journal of Medicine* 353, no. 5 (August 4, 2005): 346–475.

Hansson, G. K. "Inflammation, Atherosclerosis, and Coronary Artery Disease." *New England Journal of Medicine* 352, no. 16 (April 21, 2005): 1685–1695.

Hittel, D. S., W. E. Kraus, et al. "Exercise in Muscles of Overweight Men and Women with Metabolic Syndrome." *Journal of Applied Physiology* 98 (January 2005): 168–179.

Hu, F. B., et al., "Adiposity and Physical Activity as Predictors of Mortality." *New England Journal of Medicine* 352, no. 13 (March 31, 2005): 1381–1384.

Keys, A. "Coronary Heart Disease in Seven Countries." *Circulation* 41 (Suppl. 1, 1970): 1.

Krause, W. E., and P. S. Douglas. "Where Does Fitness Fit In?" *New England Journal of Medicine* 353, no. 5 (August 4, 2005): 517–519.

Manson, J. E., et al. "Walking Compared with Vigorous Exercise for the Prevention of Cardiovascular Events in Women." *New England Journal of Medicine* 347, no. 10 (September 5, 2002): 716–725.

Miller, G. E., K. E. Freedland, et al. "Cynical Hostility, Depressive Symptoms, and the Expression of Inflammatory Risk Markers for Heart Disease." *Journal of Behavioral Medicine* 26, no. 6 (December 2003): 501–515.

Mitka, M. "Diabetes Management Remains Suboptimal." *Journal of the American Medical Association* 293, no. 15 (April 20, 2005): 1845–1846.

National Heart, Lung, and Blood Institute (NHLBI). "Seventh Report of the Joint National Committee on Prevention, Detection, Evaluation, and Treatment of High Blood Pressure (JNC 7) Express. 2003."

Preston, S. "Deadweight?–The Influence of Obesity on Longevity." *New England Journal of Medicine* 352, no. 13 (March 31, 2005): 1135–1137.

Ribisl, P. "Exercise–The New Penicillin: Inflammation and Chronic Disease." *ACSM's Health and Fitness Journal* 7, no. 4 (July/August, 2003): 28–30.

Ridker, P. M., J. E. Buring, et al. "C-Reactive Protein, the Metabolic Syndrome and Risk of Incident Cardiovascular Events: An 8-Year Follow-up of 14719 Initially Healthy American Women." *Circulation* 107, no. 3 (2003): 391–397.

Roberts, C. K., and J. R. Barnard. "Effects of Exercise and Diet on Chronic Disease." *Journal of Applied Physiology* 98 (January 2005): 3–30.

Schum, J. L., R. S. Jorgensen, et al. "Trait Anger, Anger Expression, and Ambulatory Blood Pressure: A Meta-Analytic Review." *Journal of Behavioral Medicine* 26, no. 5 (October 2003): 395–415.

Stephenson, J. "Reducing Diabetes Deaths." *Journal of the American Medical Association* 291, no. 21 (June 2, 2004): 2534–2540.

Toole, J. F., and M. R. Malinow. "Lowering Homocysteine in Patients with Ischemic Stroke to Prevent Recurrent Stroke, Myocardial Infarction, and Death." *Journal of the American Medical Association* 291, no. 5 (February 4, 2004): 565–755.

Walters, P. H. "Childhood Obesity: Causes and Treatment." *ACSM's Health and Fitness Journal* 7, no. 1 (January/February 2003): 17–22.

Weiss, R. J., J. Dziura, et al. "Obesity and the Metabolic Syndrome in Children and Adolescents." *New England Journal of Medicine* 350, no. 23 (June 3, 2004): 2362–2374.

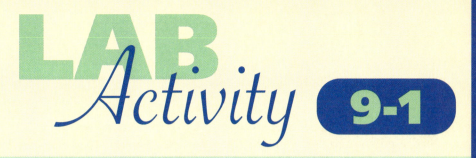

Name _____ **Class/Activity Section** _____ **Date** _____

Are You at Risk for Heart Disease?

Your chances of developing CVD depend on a variety of habits and risk factors. Smoking, physical activity, stress management, blood pressure, and cholesterol are important prognosticators for heart disease. Read each question and circle the most appropriate response as it relates to your lifestyle. Finally, add the points associated with your response to obtain your total score and risk of developing heart disease.

1. Do you smoke cigarettes?	Yes	12
	No	0
2. Do you use other tobacco products (pipe, cigars, chewing, snuff)?	Yes	3
	No	0
3. Do you usually exercise vigorously at least three times a week for 20 to 60 minutes?	Yes	0
	No	10
4. How would you describe your lifestyle?	Sedentary (inactive)	6
	Somewhat active	2
	Very active	0
5. What is your blood pressure?	High 140/90 +	9
	Normal	0
	Don't know	2
6. What is your total cholesterol	High 240 mg/dl+	9
	Desirable	0
	Don't know	2
7. Has anyone in your family ever been told he or she had any form of heart disease (parents or siblings <55 years)?	Yes	5
	No	0
8. Have you ever had any of the following?		
a. Pain or discomfort in chest and surrounding areas?	Yes	2
	No	0
b. Unaccustomed shortness of breath with mild exertion?	Yes	2
	No	0

9. What is your gender?	Female	0
	Male	4
10. Have you ever been told you have diabetes?	Yes	4
	No	0
11. Have you suffered a personal loss or misfortune in the past year that had a serious impact on your life? (e.g., job loss, disability, separation/ divorce, jail term, or the death of someone close to you)?	No	0
	Yes, 1 serious loss or misfortune	1
	Yes, 2 or more	2
12. Do you feel you handle everyday stress well?	Yes	0
	No	2
13. Would you describe yourself as a type D or an angry/hostile person (i.e., aggressive, competitive, time-conscious)?	Yes	4
	No	2
14. If you are male, what is your age?	Under 40	1
	40+	3
If you are female, what is your age?	Under 50	0
	50+	3
15. What is your race?	White	0
	African American	3
	Hispanic	1
	Other	1
16. How would you describe your weight?	Normal/below	0
	Normal to +30 lb.	1
	+30 lb. or more	2
17. Do you consume meat, eggs, cheese, butter, whole milk, and fried foods?	0 to 5 times/week	0
	5 to 10 times/week	2
	2 to 3 servings/day	3
	Over 3 servings/day	6
	Your Total Score	_____

SCORING

Scores of 0 to 16
Your risk is **low** for developing heart disease at this time. Evaluate your risk every year, since risk factors such as blood pressure, cholesterol levels, and age change from year to year. If you have any uncontrollable risk factors, you would be wise to modify other risk factors to protect your cardiorespiratory system.

Scores of 17 to 29
Your risk is **average** or moderate. Your score indicates there is room for improvement on some risk factors. If you have any uncontrollable risk factors, it is imperative to modify other risk factors to protect your cardiorespiratory system.

Scores of 30+
You have a **high** risk of developing heart disease. You should take action **immediately** to modify all controllable risk factors.

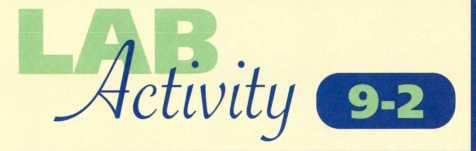

Name _____ **Class/Activity Section** _____ **Date** _____

Evaluation of "Are You at Risk for Heart Disease?"

After completing the *Are You at Risk for Heart Disease?* assessment, answer the following questions:

1. List the factors you identified that contribute to your risk of coronary heart disease.

2. List at least five personal lifestyle changes you can make to lower your risk for heart disease. Be specific; don't say, "Eat better," for example.

3. Take the *Are You at Risk for Heart Disease?* assessment for a parent or friend. What is his or her score? What advice would you give to help to lower his or her score?

4. List **your** personal controllable risk factors. How can you make changes in each one to become more heart healthy?

5. List **your** personal *uncontrollable* risk factors.

6. What if some physicians refused to treat people when they discover that they smoke or don't exercise or have diets high in fat? Discuss how you feel about this decision.

7. "You've got to die of something, so why worry about a healthy lifestyle?" Argue against.

8. "My grandmother lived to be 90 years old and never thought about a healthy lifestyle. So I won't either." Why is this *not* such a good idea?

9. "I don't smoke cigarettes, so cigarettes don't affect me." Respond and explain your response.

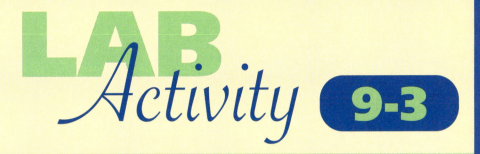

LAB Activity 9-3

Name _____ **Class/Activity Section** _____ **Date** _____

How to Mend a Broken Heart

Read the opening scenario concerning Rob in Chapter 1 of your text. You were the physician on call when he was brought in. Complete a medical history on this patient and answer his wife's questions.

1. List Rob's four primary risk factors for heart disease given in the scenario.

2. List Rob's two secondary risk factors for heart disease.

3. What three or four lifestyle changes will you tell Rob to make to reduce his heart disease risk?

Rob's wife has read the chart. She is distraught and has several questions for you. Please respond.

4. "Doctor, I really don't understand some of the words used on the chart. What is angina? Myocardial infarction? What is atherosclerosis, and will it ever go away?"

5. "I saw that his cholesterol was 280, his HDL level was 28, and his LDL level was 174. His cholesterol and HDL ratio was 10, and his triglycerides were 325. What do each of these mean? What is normal or desirable for each?"

   a.

   b.

   c.

   d.

   e.

6. "Rob doesn't want to quit smoking—he's smoked for 20 years. Why is smoking bad for his heart?"

7. "A nurse said Rob needs a special exercise program to aid in recovery. Won't exercise strain his heart? What good will it do?" (Give three benefits.)

8. "Rob enjoys having an occasional glass of wine. Will he have to give this up?"

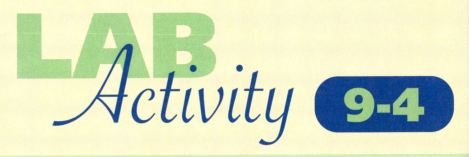

LAB Activity 9-4

Are You at Risk for Diabetes?

Answer the questions in Part I to evaluate your risk for developing diabetes. Complete Part II to learn more about diabetes and the connection it has to heart disease.

PART I

Yes	No	
____	____	1. I am overweight (body mass index greater than 27; to calculate your BMI, multiply your weight in pounds by 705, divide the result by your height in inches, then divide that result by your height in inches again). What is your BMI? _____.
____	____	2. I get little or no exercise.
____	____	3. I have a parent with diabetes.
____	____	4. I am African American, Hispanic American, or Native American.
____	____	5. I am over 40 years of age (counts as one "yes" answer; if over 65 years of age, counts as two "yes" answers).
____	____	6. I am a woman who had diabetes during pregnancy or delivered a baby weighing more than 9 pounds.
____	____	7. I have a brother, sister, or parent with diabetes.
____	____	8. I have high blood pressure and/or high cholesterol.
____	____	9. I had a minimally elevated glucose level on a previous test (100–125 mg/dl).

Scoring: Each "yes" answer increases your risk of developing diabetes.

PART II

1. How many "yes" answers did you have? _____

2. Discuss your potential risk for developing diabetes. _____

_____

_____

_____

3. List the warning symptoms of type 1 and type 2 diabetes. _____

_____

_____

_____

_____

4. Discuss the difference between type 1 and type 2 diabetes. _____

_____

_____

_____

_____

5. What can you do to prevent or reduce your risk of developing diabetes? _____

_____

_____

_____

_____

6. Why is diabetes such a serious disease? _____

_____

_____

_____

_____

7. Why does diabetes increase the risk for heart disease? _____

_____

_____

_____

_____

8. What segments of the U.S. population are at increased risk of diabetes? _____

_____

_____

_____

_____

9. How does diabetes affect the eyes, blood vessels, kidneys, genitals, and nerves? _____

_____

_____

_____

_____

_____

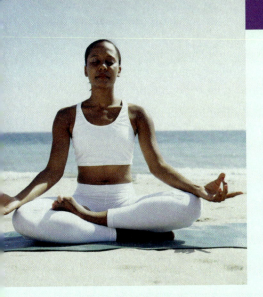

Chapter 10

Coping with Stress 10

Happiness is an inside job.
—H. Jackson Brown, Jr., ed.
Dad, a Father's Book of Wisdom

Objectives

After reading this chapter, you will be able to:

1. Define the terms *stress, stressor,* and *stress response.*
2. Explain the three stages of the stress response.
3. Define and give examples of eustress, distress, optimal stress, acute stress, and chronic stress.
4. Explain how perception and control are involved in stress.
5. On the Life Event Stress Test, measure the number of life changes you have encountered this year and be able to predict your susceptibility to a stress-related illness.
6. Explain the difference between daily hassles and daily uplifts and know how each affects overall health.
7. Describe six harmful effects of too much stress.
8. Contrast Type A, Type B, Type C, and Type D personalities.
9. Describe a hot reactor's behavior and the health consequences of this behavior.
10. List angry/hostile behavior modification techniques.
11. List the strategies for managing stress.
12. Define and list the benefits of the relaxation response.

Terms

- acute stress
- autogenic training and imagery
- biofeedback training
- chronic stress
- daily hassles
- daily uplifts
- distress
- eustress
- faulty perception
- fight-or-flight response (Alarm Reaction Stage)
- General Adaptation Syndrome (GAS)
- hardiness
- Hatha yoga
- hot reactors
- meditation
- mindfulness meditation
- optimal stress
- progressive relaxation
- psychoneuroimmunology
- psychosomatic disease
- reframing
- relaxation response
- stage of exhaustion
- stage of resistance
- stress
- Stress Response
- stressors
- transcendental meditation (TM)
- Type A personality
- Type B personality
- Type C personality
- Type D personality

A Fit and Well Way of Life Online Learning Center www.mhhe.com/robbinsfitwell1e
Go to the Online Learning Center for chapter quizzes, outlines, flashcards, and additional lab activities.

Lisa was the oldest child of three and the first in her family to go to college. Living on campus was wonderful—it meant new friends, open visitation in the residence hall, and no curfew. But by the end of the school year, her life had changed for the worse.

Her GPA was barely above a C average, which was far below her high school performance. There never seemed to be enough hours in the day to keep up with all the reading. Also, she felt exhausted most of the time and had trouble waking up for early classes. It was no wonder: The "action" never settled down on her hall before 12:30 or 1:00 A.M. The parties on the weekends were awesome. There were so many, she couldn't decide which one to go to, and so she went to them all. She would stay out partying until 6 A.M., grab a bite, and then sleep all day. With all the partying, fast food, and beer, her waistline also began to slip, 15 pounds worth! Then, just before final exams, her parents announced that they were getting a divorce. Had her college expenses created a financial burden on the family budget and contributed to the divorce? She felt guilty and partially responsible for her parents' problems. Now she would have to move back home and work full-time at the local discount store to help pay for college. Would it be possible to finish the nursing degree by taking night classes? Antonio, her boyfriend, was pressuring her to drop out of school so that they could get married. He complained that she devoted too much time to schoolwork and not enough to him. Her mother would now have to go back to work and would expect Lisa to help take care of her younger brothers and assist with the household chores. Feeling fatigued and stressed out, she wondered, with work and family obligations, when she would study. Would she have any time for herself? Was she the only one in college with such problems? How complicated her life had become.

This scene just described is not that uncommon on the typical college campus. The many challenges faced by college students are stressful and can cause feelings of anxiety. Stiff competition for grades, career choices, selection of classes, test anxiety, sense of loss of family and home, balancing work and school, peer pressure, inadequate sleep, poor nutritional habits, low physical fitness levels, and increased social involvement contribute to high levels of stress. Clearly, college is a stressful environment that makes demands on you physically, socially, intellectually, and emotionally. It's no wonder that you sometimes feel anxious, irritable, and stressed out.

Contrary to what many college students believe, stress does not "evaporate" after graduation. The amount of time the average person spends at work has increased rather than decreased in the last 2 decades. Many people have second jobs or work extended hours in demanding professional jobs. Also, nearly three times as many married women with children work full-time now as did in 1960. Experts call today's young adults the "overworked Americans." A great majority of adults have enough time for work, chores, and sleep but not enough time for friends, self, spouse, and children.

The pace of life seems to be accelerating. Federal Express overnight service is no longer quick enough—the letter needs to be faxed immediately. Receiving one telephone call at a time is not enough; now, with call waiting, two or more can be received at once. Even the traditional places of refuge in the 21st century—the car and the home—are being transformed into offices away from offices: with fax machines and computers in the home and cell phones, Blackberries, fax machines, and the Internet in the car, work stress never ends. We often do not have time to recover from one stressful situation before we face another one.

No one is exempt from stress. This is good because a certain amount is beneficial for an optimal level of health and achievement and because it helps us cope with emergency situations. Figure 10-1 illustrates how the "right" amount of stress improves health and performance but how our health and well-being can be adversely affected by excessive stress. Too much stress (chronic stress) ultimately exhausts the body's ability to adapt; vital organs wear out, and various illnesses may appear. This is especially true when stress is perceived to be negative or harmful. Stress is a normal part of life, so why do so few people understand it or know how to manage it? Improvement in the quality of life is dependent on *balancing* the demands made on you and developing effective ways to *manage* stress. Look back at *Assessing Your Wellness,* Lab Activity 1-2. How balanced was your wellness wheel? Balance in the seven dimensions of wellness has implications for how well you cope with the demands of life.

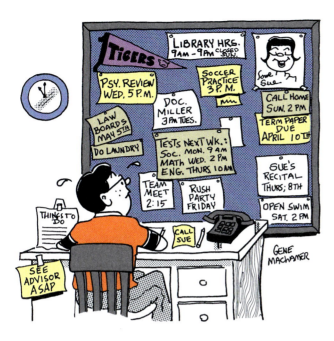

College students have many demands on their time and must plan wisely.

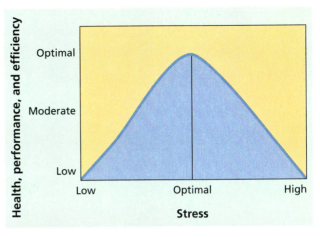

FIGURE 10-1   Optimal stress and the relationship to health and performance. Everyone has a point at which the "right" amount of stress improves performance, health, and efficiency.

WHAT IS STRESS?

Dr. Hans Selye, the foremost stress authority of the 20th century, defined **stress** as the "nonspecific response of the body to any demand made upon it." It is the response of the body to any type of change and to any new, threatening, or exciting situation. *Nonspecific* means that the body reacts the same way regardless of the cause. Stress comes in two forms: *acute* and *chronic*. **Acute stress** is the body's response to imminent danger. (See Fight-or-Flight [Alarm Reaction].) **Chronic stress** is caused by prolonged stress, more than an individual can cope with or control. (See Harmful Effects of Stress.) **Stressors,** factors causing stress, can be pleasant or unpleasant, real or imagined, and can be of different types. All cause the body to adapt. For example, *physical* stressors include illness, accidents, injury, lack of sleep, heat, cold, and noise. *Psychological* or *emotional* stressors involve pressures and deadlines with work or school, problems with loved ones, the need to pay bills, getting ready for the holidays (or vacation), parenting, final exams, rejection, depression, divorce, and marriage. Less obvious sources include crowds, traffic, even starting a new job.

Dr. Selye described the ways in which we react to stress as either *eustress* (good) or *distress* (bad). In both cases the physiological response is the same. In the case of **eustress,** which refers to happy, pleasant events (holidays, getting married, etc.), health and performance improve even as stress increases. In contrast, **distress** refers to unpleasant or harmful stress (flunking an exam, breakup of a relationship, etc.) under which health and performance begin to decline. **Optimal stress** is a point at which eustress and distress are intense enough to motivate and physically prepare us to perform optimally yet not intense enough to cause the body to overreact or sustain harmful effects. Figure 10-1 illustrates this concept. Optimal stress gives athletes the competitive edge and public speakers the enthusiasm to project with charisma. Overstress results in poor performance and produces overreaction, poor concentration, test anxiety, and health problems. When experiencing positive stress, individuals feel in control. Negative stress causes out-of-control feelings.

Regardless of the cause, the adaptation (or reaction) to stress is both psychological and physiological and leads to what Dr. Selye called the **General Adaptation Syndrome (GAS).** Today, the GAS is called the **Stress Response.**

THE STRESS RESPONSE: A THREE-STAGE PROCESS

Hans Selye summarized the Stress Response in a three-stage process:

1. **Fight-or-flight response (Alarm Reaction Stage):** The body prepares to cope with a stressor. The response is a warning signal that a stressor is present. Physiological and psychological responses appear. This is a primitive survival mechanism and a response to imminent danger (to acute stress). It gave early humans the energy to fight aggressors or run from predators (e.g., the caveman or woman could escape the jaws of a hungry lion [stressor] by swiftly running [fight-or-flight]). Stress today is rarely the life-and-death type, but our bodies react as if it is. See Figure 10-2.

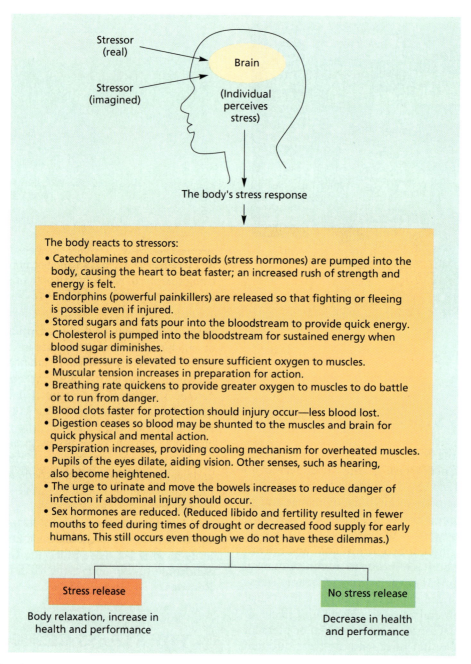

Stressor (real)

Brain

Stressor (imagined)

(Individual perceives stress)

The body's stress response

The body reacts to stressors:

- Catecholamines and corticosteroids (stress hormones) are pumped into the body, causing the heart to beat faster; an increased rush of strength and energy is felt.
- Endorphins (powerful painkillers) are released so that fighting or fleeing is possible even if injured.
- Stored sugars and fats pour into the bloodstream to provide quick energy.
- Cholesterol is pumped into the bloodstream for sustained energy when blood sugar diminishes.
- Blood pressure is elevated to ensure sufficient oxygen to muscles.
- Muscular tension increases in preparation for action.
- Breathing rate quickens to provide greater oxygen to muscles to do battle or to run from danger.
- Blood clots faster for protection should injury occur—less blood lost.
- Digestion ceases so blood may be shunted to the muscles and brain for quick physical and mental action.
- Perspiration increases, providing cooling mechanism for overheated muscles.
- Pupils of the eyes dilate, aiding vision. Other senses, such as hearing, also become heightened.
- The urge to urinate and move the bowels increases to reduce danger of infection if abdominal injury should occur.
- Sex hormones are reduced. (Reduced libido and fertility resulted in fewer mouths to feed during times of drought or decreased food supply for early humans. This still occurs even though we do not have these dilemmas.)

Stress release

Body relaxation, increase in health and performance

No stress release

Decrease in health and performance

FIGURE 10-2   Physical reactions to stressors.

2. **Stage of resistance:** The body actively resists and attempts to cope with the stressor. Eventually the body loses the ability to keep up with the demands that stress puts on it and wears out.

3. **Stage of exhaustion:** Adaptation energy is exhausted, and signs of fight-or-flight reappear. During the exhaustion phase, immunity breaks down. The organ systems of the body malfunction. Disease or even death may occur. For example, high blood pressure (caused by excessive stress) promotes kidney and heart damage, which can kill the individual if allowed to continue.

Fight-or-Flight (Alarm Reaction)

The body responds to stress, whether emotional or physical (real or perceived), by activating a series of mechanisms collectively known as the fight-or-flight response. These fight-or-flight mechanisms work best when the danger is clear, well defined, and short-term (acute, not chronic).

Our stress responses were programmed for life in a primitive state, thousands of years before we became "civilized." No longer are our stresses a simple matter of life-and-death threats; they now involve intricate and complex challenges. When the body is stressed, two main groups of hormones are released into the bloodstream: the catecholamines (i.e., adrenaline, epinephrine, and norepenephrine) and the corticosteroids (i.e., cortisone and cortisol). Both groups have positive and negative effects on the body. The positive effects occur during acute short-term stress (Figure 10-2), and the negative effects occur during chronic stress.

Many examples of the fight-or-flight response can be found even in today's world. Imagine this scenario: You are crossing the street on your way home when suddenly you see a car quickly approaching you. Instinctively, your muscles tense, and you jump back on the curb with such force that you fall back into a newspaper stand and cut your head, which quickly stops bleeding. The fight-or-flight response saved your life (the quick backward jump and the cut that stops bleeding). Other examples of the response, normally described as "superhuman" acts, are in reality the fight-or-flight response in action. Perhaps you can add others to this list:

✔ A person lifts an automobile off an injured individual at an accident scene.
✔ A young hiker amputates his arm to save his life after getting it caught between two boulders in a climbing accident.
✔ After having both arms ripped off by a farm machine, a young farmer manages to telephone for help by dialing 911 with a pencil clenched in his teeth.
✔ A mother knocks down a locked bedroom door to rescue her children from a burning house.
✔ A student outruns a mugger on a dark corner of the campus.

These are only a few examples that have required action to prevent or minimize physical harm. A few minutes after the frightening event (acute stressor), the individuals return to their normal physiological state. Other stressors, the kind you encounter every day, such as noise, arguments, keys locked inside the car, missed deadlines, traffic tickets, or any new situation that causes us to adapt, have the same potential for eliciting the fight-or-flight response. Ironically, the strains and hassles of life in a civilized world have transformed this lifesaving mechanism into a potentially life-threatening one.

We are designed to cope with acute stress much better than with chronic stress. Unfortunately, physical and emotional stress in modern times tends to be chronic rather than acute. The pace of life accelerates every year. Constant hurrying, common in today's lifestyle, is associated with the chronic arousal of the fight-or-flight response. We often do not have time to recover from one stressful situation before we face another one.

Innate physiological stress responses (Figure 10-2) have evolved over the centuries to help us survive danger and prepare us for swift action whether or not it is needed. However, the buildup of unused stress products produces excessive wear and tear on the body and even

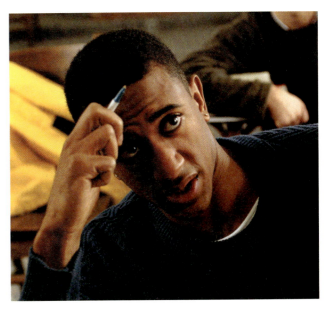

Chronic arousal of the fight-or-flight response causes chemical wear and tear on the body.

increases the rate of aging. When stressors inappropriately provoke the fight-or-flight reaction many times a day, the body repeatedly responds as if experiencing real emergencies. The fight-or-flight response is often appropriate and should not be thought of as always harmful. It is a necessary part of our physiological makeup, a useful reaction to many situations in our current world. However, we need to learn how to avoid triggering the stress response except in real emergencies and develop effective ways to play out the response once it is evoked.

Stage of Resistance

The longer our bodies stay in a chronic "on guard" resistance stage, the more likely we are to experience ill effects. Today we don't have much opportunity to play out the fight-or-flight response physically, which is needed in *acute stress* situations, because today's stress is mostly *chronic*. Though we chronically evoke the fight-or-flight response, modern society does not accept the natural response associated with it. For example, you do not run away from or hit your boss when he or she reprimands you. Our innate reactions have not changed, but society has. The response is turned on, but we do not use it appropriately. As a result, the body remains in the resistance stage for longer periods. Our sedentary lifestyles decrease outlets for fight-or-flight hormones that are pumped into the body. Stress becomes harmful when it is prolonged and/or perceived as negative to the recipient.

Learning stress management skills is important in coping with the stresses of life. People who have learned these skills may still overreact to a stressor but will relax more quickly to the resting physiological state than will people who have not learned these skills.

Stage of Exhaustion

The exhaustion stage of the stress response can ultimately result in death if it is not countered. Thankfully, the final point of this stage is not often reached. If our bodies are successful in resisting stress, exhaustion does not follow. We usually adapt to the stress and make whatever adjustments are necessary to cope whether the stress is physical or psychological. However, the body has its limits. They are different in every person, but when the body reaches its limit, it collapses. Learn and practice regularly one or more of the stress management skills described in this chapter to reduce the unhealthy consequences of stress in your life.

 PERCEPTION AND CONTROL

Your reaction to a specific event (stressor) is different from everyone else's. Things that are distressful for you can be an exhilarating pleasure for others or have little impact either way, as is readily illustrated by observing passengers on a steep roller-coaster ride. Whether a particular stressor causes a negative reaction depends on whether the person *perceives* that stressor as being negative.

Faulty perception occurs when an individual assesses a situation (or stressor) as threatening regardless of its actual threat. It is unnecessarily seeing a situation as hopeless, harmful, or negative. Faulty perception of stress is the real culprit and is the cause of most people's problems. This concept was confirmed by the research of Dr. Richard Lazarus, who found that prolonged unmanaged faulty perception of stress results in negative health consequences. Lazarus's research asserted that we are, after all, thinking, cognitive creatures. We are able to assess the positive and negative consequences of any situation or threat and apply a coping strategy (such as problem-solving) that may provide us with a sense of control (actual or perceived) that may affect our perception of stress. One person may *perceive* a stressor as threatening and as a result experience a full-blown fight-or-flight response. Another may encounter the same event and simply take it in stride. How do you perceive snakes, the announcement of an exam, competition, being cut off in traffic, being called in to see the boss, a doctor's appointment, being called on to contribute to class discussion, and a professor requesting to speak with you after class? These situations do not bother some individuals but are agonizing to others.

Before gearing up to fret, fight, or flee when facing a stressor, ask yourself, "Does a threat really exist? Is the issue important to me? Can I make a difference?" If the answer to any of these questions is no, do not waste your energy. It is not worth it. Some situations are truly threatening and require high-energy stress responses. When the threat you perceive in a situation is real, go ahead and gear up. You can then benefit from the energy generated by your natural stress response by applying it to the situation at hand.

Control is a major factor in the total stress picture. The core cause of much stress is the sense that one is "not in the driver's seat." The *perception (real or unreal) of not having control* is very stressful. The way to turn a stressful incident into something that is not stressful is to gain a sense of control over it. Managing stress means empowering yourself to take control rather than relinquishing the control to events, to other people, to your environment, or to the calendar. People who handle stress best tend to control their lives and look for active solutions to the problems and circumstances of their lives. You are responsible for allowing stressful situations to raise your blood pressure and heart rate. We can all recall events that made us angry one time but did not even faze us the next. Why is this? It is because we *allowed* ourselves to become upset. Perhaps the situation was complicated by nasty weather, lack of sleep, or a buildup of particular events. The bottom line is that this particular time we *allowed* the event to provoke an angry response. Whether to allow stressful events to provoke physiological reactions that may increase vulnerability to illness and disease is your decision. By taking charge, you can decide whether to be an overstressed, nervous wreck or a calm, collected person.

Important ways to gain control over your life include:

✔ Make healthy lifestyle decisions—getting regular exercise and adequate sleep. Not smoking, eating nutritionally, and not overindulging in alcohol allow you to exert control.

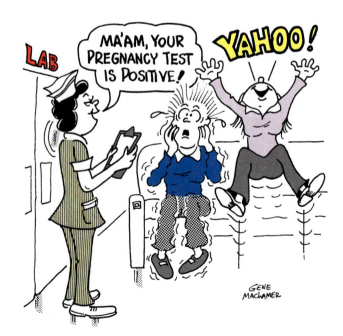

We perceive stressors differently.

THE NUMBERS

75% to 90%	All visits to health-care providers that result from stress-related disorders.
90%	American adults who experience high stress levels one or two times per week; a fourth of all American adults are subject to crushing levels of stress nearly every day.
30%	College freshmen who report feeling overwhelmed a great deal of the time during the beginning of college.
2nd	Rank of suicide as a leading cause of death in the college population. It is often linked to untreated depression and triggered by stressful events, high levels of anger and anxiety, or major life change events.
25%	Students who feel like dropping out of school due to stress at one point or another.
75%	College students who feel "really stressed" at least one day of the week.
54%	People with high blood pressure who are Type Ds. Type Ds are four times more likely to suffer a second heart attack than the non-D types.
30%	Reduction of cardiovascular disease risk that has been linked to the regular practice of meditation.

✔ Learn and implement time management skills. Getting organized helps spread stress out instead of having it pile up. See Strategy 3b and Lab Activity 10-6 in this chapter.

✔ Learn when to say no. Only you know when to take on added duties and assignments and when your "plate is full" and you must say, "No, sorry, not at this time. I have too many irons in the fire." This puts you in charge of your precious time.

✔ Regularly practice relaxation techniques and employ often the other stress-coping strategies found later in this chapter. Commit to restoring a sense of control and reduce symptoms of stress in your life. See Lab Activities 10-2 and 10-4.

Remember, only you can decide if you want to manage your stress. It is your responsibility to exert control over your life. The key to surviving and even thriving on stress is improving cognitive problem-solving skills to better cope with faulty perception. Take charge of *you–for you.*

HARMFUL EFFECTS OF STRESS

Stressors (i.e., all events, emotions, or situations, good or bad) cause you to react and force you to adapt. This adaptation to the stresses of life isn't harmful unless you are overloaded with too much in a short time–too many life change events and hassles, especially the ones perceived as undesirable or uncontrollable. In today's society, stress has increased dramatically. In essence, your fight-or-flight responses stay aroused 24 hours a day, 7 days a week. This is *chronic stress,* and it travels with us daily, everywhere we go. We pay a high price for not dealing with chronic stress. It can lead to a psychosomatic disease.

A **psychosomatic disease** (*psych* refers to the mind; *somatic* refers to the body) is a physical ailment that is mentally induced. The mind and the body are an interrelated whole–what affects one ultimately affects the other. **Psychoneuroimmunology** is a specialized branch of medicine that studies the mind/body connection. Harvard's Dr. Herbert Benson has determined that about 75 to 90 percent of visits to health-care professionals are "in the stress-related, mind body realm."

Chronic stress, resulting in long-term activation of the stress response system, can disrupt almost all your body's processes, increasing your risk of obesity, insomnia, digestive complaints, heart disease, and depression. The following paragraphs summarize the impact it has on the body.

Long-term stress suppresses your *immune system,* making you more susceptible to colds and other infections. In fighting infection, substances that cause inflammation are released. Prolonged stress doesn't allow the body to turn off the inflammatory responses once the infection is cleared. This can lead to high C-reactive protein levels and increase plaque buildup and the risk of cardiovascular disease. In some cases, stress can have the opposite effect, making the immune system overreactive. The result is an increased risk of autoimmune diseases, in which the immune system attacks the body's own cells. It can also worsen the symptoms of autoimmune diseases.

If your fight-or-flight response never shuts off as in chronic stress, the *nervous system* is negatively affected. A wide variety of adverse psychological symptoms may be produced ranging from severe depression, persistent feelings of anxiety and helplessness, to impending doom. Behavioral problems such as sleep disturbances, loss of sex drive, disordered eating, and excessive drinking, along with nervous habits (e.g., nail biting), phobias, and addictions may occur.

The negative effects of chronic stress on the *cardiovascular system* include increased blood pressure and cholesterol and triglyceride levels. These are all linked to heart attacks, strokes, and increased accumulation of abdominal fat—a marker for higher risk of heart disease and diabetes. Chronic stress is linked to the development of insulin resistance—a risk factor for diabetes.

Chronic stress damages other body systems as well. It often affects the *digestive system,* causing countless gastrointestinal problems (e.g., stomachache, diarrhea, and irritable bowel syndrome). Research has shown that among overweight persons, stress leads to overeating, whereas among thin people, it tends to lead to loss of appetite. Migraine headaches, asthma, and many *skin conditions* (e.g., psoriasis, acne, hives, and eczema) are worsened or triggered by chronic stress. Some studies reveal it even promotes *aging, osteoporosis,* and *cancer.* It has been theorized that the inability to cope with stress, rather than the stress itself, may lead to the development of cancer.

Managing stress in our lives means adapting and changing as circumstances demand and learning to *listen.* Listen to our bodies, our feelings, and our relationships and be *aware* of the common signs of stress. See Table 10-1.

Sure, a few weeks in crisis mode won't kill us, but the earlier we learn coping skills and change unhealthy habits, the healthier and more productive we will be throughout our lives. If you live in isolation or without essential social support, you might try to reach out by joining a volunteer, civic, or church group or perhaps seeking counseling. You can learn cognitive skills to change faulty perceptions of the stressful events in your life. If you smoke, try to quit. Eating a healthy diet is another way to confirm that you care about your own well-being. Regular physical exercise fits into the picture, too. See the other stress-coping strategies later in this chapter if you are experiencing many of the symptoms in Table 10-1 (or feel particularly "stressed out") so that you can avoid a serious psychosomatic disease. The sage advice of Eubie Blake, the famous jazz musician who lived to be 100 years old, is applicable here: "If I knew I was going to live this long, I'd have taken better care of myself."

MEASURING YOUR STRESS

In 1967, two psychiatrists at the University of Washington School of Medicine, Thomas H. Holmes, M.D., and Richard H. Rahe, M.D., observed that certain life events coincided with illness. According to those doctors, change, whether for "good" or "bad," causes stress, leaving humans more susceptible to illness. Even simple changes, such as in eating habits, job routine, and extra school work, can increase one's susceptibility to stress-related diseases. After studying the medical histories and personal biographies of patients, the doctors found a curious link between life-changing events and illnesses such as heart disease, gastrointestinal problems, even psychological problems (depression, anxiety, etc.); they developed a list of life changes that range from minor to severe and assigned points to each one based on the amount of stress evoked. The list includes both the positive (eustress), such as a vacation trip or marriage, and the negative (distress), such as trouble with a relationship or, most stressful, the death of a child or spouse. The original test was revised recently to keep pace with the new millennium and to more effectively reflect the stress of college/school. Take a few moments to complete the Life Event Stress Test, identifying the events that have occurred in your life during the last year, in Table 10-2. The

Prescription for Action

Date: *Do one or more today*

✔ Think of an act of kindness and then do it for a stranger.
✔ Get 8 hours of sleep tonight.
✔ Go to a humorous or uplifting movie (or get a video/DVD of one).
✔ Reflect on the meaningful people in your life. Connect with two of them today via e-mail, telephone, or letter.
✔ Watch a sunset tonight and/or a sunrise tomorrow.
✔ Get your study area organized.
✔ Write in a journal. Record the best things that have happened to you this week.
✔ Volunteer your services to a worthy project/group that interests you.

Prescribed by: ___*YOU*___

TABLE 10-1	*Common Signs of Stress*

Check the signs of stress that you have experienced lately. Stress affects many dimensions of your life.

PHYSICAL

_____ Headaches	_____ Allergy flare-up, rashes, hives
_____ Asthma attack	_____ Muscle twitches or eye twitches
_____ Gastrointestinal (constipation and/or diarrhea, indigestion, stomach cramping or bloating, nausea or vomiting)	_____ Heart pounding, racing, or beating erratically
	_____ Restlessness
	_____ Fatigue
_____ Acne flare-up	_____ Stiff or tense muscles
_____ Excessive dryness of hair or skin	_____ Difficulty sleeping (insomnia, sleeping too much, sleeping too little)
_____ Frequent colds, flu, low-grade infections/herpes flare-ups	
_____ Chest pain	_____ Trembling hands
_____ Neck, back, or shoulder pain	_____ Weight gain or loss
_____ Increased perspiration (excess sweating, cold sweaty hands)	_____ Teeth grinding

EMOTIONAL/SOCIAL/BEHAVIORAL

_____ Depression	_____ Loss of appetite or excessive eating
_____ Sadness	_____ Mood swings
_____ Restlessness	_____ Fidgeting
_____ Feeling burned out	_____ Paying less attention to appearance
_____ Inability to relax	_____ Resentment
_____ Difficulty in completing work or school assignments	_____ Impulsive actions
_____ Questioning your personal worth	_____ Loneliness
_____ Feeling sensitive to criticism	_____ Bouts of anger/hostility
_____ Often feeling suspicious	_____ Social withdrawal or need to be with people most or all of the time
_____ Crying spells	
_____ Being accident-prone	_____ Trouble getting along with others
_____ Increased use of alcohol/drugs/tobacco products	_____ Diminished sex drive

MENTAL

_____ Disorganization (losing things, making dumb mistakes)	_____ Negative attitude and/or negative self-talk
_____ Irritability	_____ Confusion
_____ Difficulty making small decisions	_____ Lethargy
_____ Restlessness, poor concentration, boredom	_____ Decreased productivity
_____ Worrying, anxiety, phobias	_____ Depression
_____ Forgetfulness (memory problems)	_____ Loss of sense of humor

SPIRITUAL

_____ Emptiness	_____ Sadness
_____ Loss of meaning	_____ Intolerance
_____ Doubt	_____ Loss of direction
_____ Being unforgiving	_____ Cynicism
_____ Martyrdom	_____ Apathy
_____ Lack of intimacy	

total score on this self-test offers some insight into one's risk for illness as a result of recent life events. Stressful change in itself won't necessarily harm you. That depends, at least in part, on how you perceive the event, and whether you feel in control of the situation; the support you can rely on from family and friends; and your stress coping skills. Lab Activity 10-1 provides an excellent evaluation of your score on this self-test.

The test can be an effective tool when used to anticipate major life events so that you can take *control* of the stress they produce. No one would suggest that we get rid of holidays, vacations, and weddings. But we

should take all life changes, including these positive ones, into account when planning our lives. Realizing there are certain life events you cannot control is equally important in stress reduction. Remember, change is inevitable; that's what living is about. But keep in mind that you can plan ahead for change and regulate the timing of many events (stressors) to prevent them from draining much of your adaptation energy. Spread change over time. When you feel in control, you perceive stressful situations as much less stressful; thus, there is less chance of provoking a stress-related illness. Change in life situations alone may not be enough to

TABLE 10-2 *Life Event Stress Test*

To get a feel for the possible health impact of the recent changes in your life, think back over the last year and circle the "stress points" listed for each of the events you experienced during that time. Then total your points. Your score is termed your life change units (LCU). This is a measure of the amount of significant change in your life to which you have had to adjust. In other words, your LCU is a measure of the stressors you have encountered this year. If an event has occurred more than once, multiply the score for that event by the number of times it has occurred.

LIFE CHANGE EVENT

Home and Family

Event	Points
Death of spouse	119
Death of other family member:	
child	123
brother or sister	102
parent	100
Divorce	96
Separation from spouse:	
due to marital problems	76
due to work	53
Gain of a new family member:	
birth of a child	66
adoption or remarriage	65
a relative moving in with you	46
Change in the marriage status of your parents:	
divorce	59
remarriage	50
Major change in health or behavior of family member	55
Marriage	50
Change in arguments with spouse	50
Change in residence:	
move within the same town or city	25
move to different town, city, or state	47
Major change in living conditions	42
Spouse beginning or ending work	46
Child leaving home:	
to attend college	41
due to marriage	41
for other reasons	45
In-law problems	38

Health

Event	Points
An injury/illness that:	
kept you in bed a week or more or sent you to the hospital	74
was less serious than above	44
Pregnancy	67
Miscarriage or abortion	65
Major change in your usual type and/or amount of recreation	28
Major change in eating habits	27
Major change in sleeping habits	26
Major dental work	26

School/College

Event	Points
Beginning or ending school/college	38
Change of school/college	35
Failing an important course	22
Increase in class workload	20

Event	Points
Lack of enough money	18
Change of major	11
Lower grade(s) than expected	10

Work

Event	Points
Loss of job:	
fired from work	79
laid off from work	68
Retirement	52
Change to a new type of work	51
Change in your responsibilities at work:	
demotion	42
transfer	32
promotion	31
more responsibilities	29
Change in your work hours or conditions	35
Troubles at work:	
with coworkers	35
with persons under your supervision	35
with your boss	29
other work troubles	28
Taking course(s) to help you in your work	18

Financial

Event	Points
Major change in finances:	
decreased income	60
investment and/or credit difficulties (or credit card debt)	54
increased income	38
Foreclosure on a mortage or loan	58
Loss or damage of personal property	43
Major purchase (over $10,000), mortgage, loan(s), car	37
Moderate purchase (under $10,000)	20

Personal and Social

Event	Points
Being held in jail	75
Death of a close friend	70
Major decision regarding your immediate future	51
An accident	48
"Falling out" of a close personal relationship	47
Engagement to marry	45
Sexual difficulties	44
Girlfriend/boyfriend problems	39
New, close personal relationship	37
Major personal achivement	36
Change in religious beliefs	29
Change in social activities	27
Change in personal habits	26
Change in political beliefs	24
Vacation	24
Minor violation of the law	20

Total Score _____

Score	Rating	Implication for Illness
≤249	Low Stress	37% chance of getting a stress-related illness in the next year or two. Consider yourself fortunate.
250–500	Moderate Stress	51% chance of getting a stress-related illness in the next year.
≥501	High Stress	80% chance of getting a stress-related illness in the next year.

Note: These predictions are not absolute. Your final score is influenced by individual perception of these events, your coping/stress management skills, and the social support of family and friends. Adapted from T. E. Holmes and R. H. Rahe, "The Social Readjustment Scale." *Journal of Psychosomatic Reasearch* 11 (1967): 213–219.

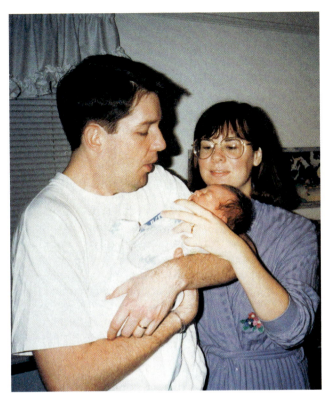

Even happy life events add to our total stress picture.

cause illness. When these changes are perceived as distressing and result in prolonged emotional and physiological wear and tear, your risk of illness increases. Some people are more vulnerable to certain types of stress than others are. If you would like to find out what type of stress you are most susceptible to and how well you cope with stress, complete *Measuring Your Stress and Coping Skills* (Lab Activity 10-5). This test also measures coping skills for dealing with stress.

Establishing coping strategies such as the ones discussed later in this chapter is a positive way to block the development of a stress illness. Well-timed social support is one of the best coping mechanism we have. When you are experiencing many life changes but have family and friends with whom you can discuss your problems, you probably will avoid a stress illness. An individual experiencing fewer life changes but with less support may become ill.

DAILY HASSLES AND UPLIFTS

Studies by Richard Lazarus and colleagues suggest that it is not only the major "life events" that have a negative impact on health but also other factors called *daily hassles*, and these may be even more harmful. **Daily hassles** are the events or interactions in your daily life that you find bothersome, annoying, or negative in some way. These irritating demands include common problems

such as losing things, chronic car problems (or running out of gas on the way to work/school), time demands/deadlines, exams (i.e., preparing for, taking), traffic jams, arguments, and family concerns. Various studies show that hassles are strongly related to episodes of illness, even when there are no major life events to consider. Having too many things to do, roommate problems, not enough sleep, parking problems on campus, and money difficulties were the most frequently reported hassles of students at Ball State University. Examine the Top 10 List "Hassles/Uplifts of College Students" to see how the hassles in your life compare.

Everyday hassles can be the "straw that broke the camel's back" if they are added to your life at a time when it is already overloaded with stressful events. The average person is as likely to be "nibbled to death" by everyday hassles as to be overwhelmed by tragedies. The way you handle daily hassles depends to a large degree on your score on the Life Event Stress Test. When scores are high (i.e., you are overstressed), you are more likely to react to daily hassles with less tolerance and a shorter fuse. For example, after Akiko's mother died of cancer, she had to leave college in her first year and enroll at the local community college in her hometown because she was needed at home to care for her younger brothers. On top of this, she lost her billfold (with driver's license and credit cards) on the first day of classes at the new school. The hassles of too many things to do, losing the billfold, caring for the home and her brothers, and keeping up at school were overwhelming. Frustration boiled over into stress and anger, and she soon became ill. As with any stressor, the way you perceive it is critical. What constitutes a hassle or an uplift varies greatly from person to person. Concern about weight may not be a hassle to you but may be a real problem to a person for whom physical appearance is a top priority.

The counterpart to daily hassles are **daily uplifts.** These are positive events that make us feel good. Fridays, payday, going shopping, and having a date were

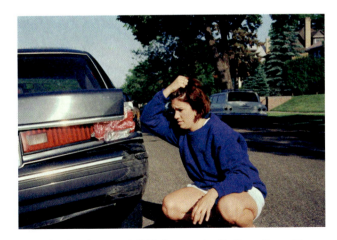

Everyday hassles can "nibble" us to death. Sometimes it's not the mountain in front of you but the grain of sand in your shoe that brings you to your knees.

TOP 10 LIST

Hassles/Uplifts of College Students

Hassles

1. Misplacing or losing things
2. Troubling thoughts about your future
3. Not getting enough sleep
4. Money problems
5. Social obligations
6. Concerns about weight and physical appearance
7. Too many things to do (registration for classes, exams, getting low grades, extracurricular groups, everyday chores, chronic car problems)
8. Concerns about meeting high standards (not living up to expectations, getting low grades)
9. Being lonely (relationship issues)
10. Child care problems

Uplifts

1. Being visited, e-mailed, phoned, or sent a letter
2. Visiting, phoning, or writing someone
3. Having fun (socializing, partying, being with friends)
4. Completing a task
5. Recreation (sports, games, etc.)
6. Hugging and/or kissing (relating well with spouse or lover)
7. Getting enough sleep
8. Being complimented
9. Having someone to listen to you
10. Eating out

the uplifts most often listed by students at Ball State. Research has shown that these little daily uplifts can reverse the negative effects of daily hassles. An appropriate balance between hassles and uplifts may be the important ingredient in your overall health and well-being. These daily uplifts may protect you from stress-related illnesses.

List the events in your everyday life that you find bothersome. How many of them can you eliminate? How many will you have to deal with in some manner? List the daily uplifts you find enjoyable. Can you find ways to add to this list? How does your list compare to the Top 10 list of hassles and uplifts?

TYPE A, B, AND D PERSONALITIES AND STRESS

We all know people who have the "hurry-up-itis" syndrome. They always are rushed, never have enough time, usually need more than 8 hours a day to complete a day's work, could not survive without a cell phone or laptop computer, and appear to be doing four or five things at one time. The woman who impatiently pushes ahead of you in line at the grocery, the young man who honks the horn of his automobile indicating that you should hurry up, and the friend who constantly looks at his or her watch all exhibit Type A behavior.

The **Type A personality** is described as competitive, ambitious, driven, impatient, workaholic, and *always* rushed. Type As put big demands on themselves to accomplish more in less time. They have little time for or interest in hobbies or leisure pursuits and have few intimate friends. The key problem with Type A behavior is stress. Type As put themselves under constant pressure, and their bodies react by producing extra amounts of stress hormones.

The **Type B personality** is the opposite—relaxed, casual, unaggressive, and patient. Most Type Bs build time into the day for absorbing activities such as exercise, hobbies, and friendship. They speak more softly, are less obsessed with success, and tend to deal more effectively with stressful situations.

Research led many to believe that the individual who exhibits Type A behavior is prone to developing coronary heart disease, with increased risk of suffering a heart attack. However, newer research indicates that the personality behaviors of *hostility, cynicism, and anger are the major culprits that increase the risk of heart disease and not the Type A personality itself.* People exhibiting hostility, cynicism, and anger in response to stress produce greater amounts of hormones that damage the cardiorespiratory system. These traits are also related to atherosclerosis, higher diastolic blood pressure and cholesterol levels, and increased clotting potential, and they can alter heart rhythms. Some studies have found that hostility levels are a more accurate predictor of heart disease than high cholesterol, hypertension, smoking, or obesity. The problem is that the components of Type A behavior can be harmful if they lead to the development of hostile, angry behavior. This is especially true in the case of chronic hurrying, a hallmark characteristic of Type A behavior. Chronic hurrying, synonymous with Type A behavior and life in the 21st century, is especially stressful when we want to hurry but are stuck in situations where all we can do is wait, such as heavy traffic and long lines. The frustration boils over into stress and *anger*. It is now clearly understood that Type Bs exhibiting angry, cynical, and hostile behaviors suffer the same negative effects as do Type As.

✔ Do you become enraged when a car in front of you cuts you off?
✔ Do you find it intolerable to wait in lines?
✔ Do you lash out with gestures, raised voice, and increased heart rate when someone does something that seems incompetent, messy, selfish, or inconsiderate to you?

✔ Do you often instigate arguments with others?

✔ Do you have a tendency to feel defensive?

✔ Do you frequently feel other people aren't doing their part to solve a problem?

People with a hostile personality trait that leads to a heightened risk of heart disease typically can answer "yes" to these questions.

The latest research strengthens the dangers of truly harmful emotions and has led to the identification of a new personality called **Type D.** Type D increases risk of cardiovascular disease and is potentially lethal to those who have already suffered a heart attack or stroke. Type D (for "distressed" personality) people possess negative emotions and tend to be depressed, anxious, insecure, and distant. A newly developed 14-question personality test defines overall distress in terms of two emotional states: "negative affectivity (worry, irritability, gloom)" and "social inhibition (discomfort in social interactions, reticence, and a lack of social poise)." "Yes" or "no" responses to questions like the following (a brief version of the 14-question test) might reveal if you are a Type D personality with negative affectivity and social inhibition:

✔ I make contact easily when I meet people.

✔ I often talk to strangers.

✔ I am often unhappy.

✔ I am often irritated.

✔ I take a gloomy view of things.

✔ I find it hard to start a conversation.

✔ I would rather keep people at a distance.

✔ I often find myself worrying about something.

✔ When socializing, I don't find the right things to talk about.

Don't panic if you think you might be a Type D. Type D personality is not a mental illness. It is a collection of normal human traits. There are many Type D individuals who are living healthy lives and functioning quite well. Even the most distress-prone person can learn to cope with stress and beat back anxious thoughts. If you feel you may be distress-prone, you can take practical steps to make it less toxic. Exercise, a wholesome diet, and relaxation techniques such as meditation will reduce almost everyone's risk of cardiovascular disease. And lifestyle changes that protect your heart can improve your emotional state as well.

The Hot Reactor

Another example of how the combination of angry behavior and stress can be lethal has been discovered by Robert S. Eliot. He has found that many apparently healthy individuals are prime candidates for stress-related heart attacks or strokes because of the extreme reactions they demonstrate in response to daily stress. He labeled these people **hot reactors** because when stressed, they produce astronomical amounts of powerful hormones

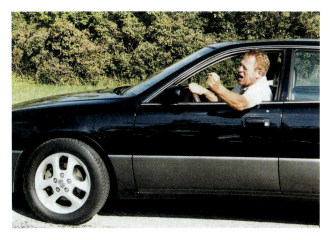

Being a "hot reactor," as in road rage, can be deadly.

called catecholamines (adrenaline and norepinephrine) that damage the cardiovascular system and disrupt the electrical rhythm of the heart. Abnormally high blood pressure and dangerous heart muscle lesions are the results of the massive doses of these stress hormones being released into the bloodstream. (Systolic readings can rise from 120 to a deadly 300.) Additionally, anger can trigger an acute myocardial infarction (heart attack) when atherosclerotic plaque ruptures and the resulting clot blocks an artery. Thus, venting anger by "blowing off steam," losing your cool, and lashing out can be dangerous to your health. Many people ask, "Isn't it better to express anger—to let it out rather than bottle it up inside?" Now you know that the answer is NO! It is healthier to diffuse these harmful feelings by using the techniques described in Chapter 9.

Hot reactors are guilty of faulty perception. They perceive nearly every stressor as a life-and-death issue and constantly perceive a loss of control in their daily lives. Daily challenges at work or school (deadlines, friendly competition, dealing with the kids, disagreement with a neighbor) trigger an overblown fight-or-flight reaction. The fight-or-flight reaction is a human response meant to be used only in real life-and-death situations. Squandering doses of these powerful hormones on mundane situations (e.g., missing a green light, standing in a checkout line, and running out of dental floss) is a characteristic of a hot reactor. Hot reactors may be either hard-driving Type As, more placid Type Bs, or the distressed Type D.

Constant stress causes many people to bristle with aggressiveness, hostility, cynicism, and anger. Our increasingly complex world fosters the development of the Type A and D personalities. We reward the student who excels in the classroom, the winning athlete, the "superwoman" (with career and family), the youngest-ever CEO, the secretary who never takes a break, the executives who talk business over lunch, and the college student who works, carries a full load of classes, is an A student, and volunteers at church.

Life-threatening overreaction to stress is neither innate nor inevitable. People are not born with this trait. They learn it, and they can unlearn it. Reframing is an excellent way to calm hot, angry reactions to stress. Read more about reframing later in this chapter. Take a few minutes now to read the Top 10 "Stress Reduction Tips." Learn and use one or more of the strategies for managing the stress in your life found in this chapter. You can take charge and be in control of your life. Ask yourself, "Is this situation worth dying for?" Stop sweating the small stuff and remember, it is all small stuff! Assess your reaction to stress by taking the behavior quiz in Table 10-3.

ANGRY/HOSTILE BEHAVIOR MODIFICATION

Okay, so you have angry/hostile tendencies. What can you do about it? We know that many angry/hostile behaviors are learned and become habits. You can learn to modify your behavior and control hot, angry, and hostile reactions to stress in more healthful ways. Try these behavior modification suggestions:

1. Every day find "me time." It recharges your batteries. Everyone can spare 15 minutes or so a day to calm down and reflect on happy memories. Watch a sunset or listen to your favorite music.

TABLE 10-3   *Quiz to Identify Your Type A, Angry/Hostile, Hot Reactor Behavior*

Answer **yes** or **no** to the following statements:

PART I: ARE YOU A TYPE A?

Yes	No	
____	____	1. I hate to wait for anyone or anything.
____	____	2. I often interrupt others when they are speaking.
____	____	3. I am usually rushed. There's never enough time in the day.
____	____	4. I feel guilty when I have nothing to do or when I play.
____	____	5. I get impatient when others perform tasks incompetently.
____	____	6. I eat faster than most of my friends do.
____	____	7. I feel stretched to my limits at the end of the day.
____	____	8. I think about other things during conversations.

Scoring

Part I: Statements in this section demonstrate Type A behavior. If you said yes to *three* or more of these statements, you probably fall into the Type A category.

PART II: ARE YOU TOO ANGRY?

Yes	No	
____	____	1. I am quick-tempered.
____	____	2. When driving, I get irritated at drivers who cut me off or drive too slowly. I frequently blow my horn, tailgate, and try to pass them.
____	____	3. I have been so mad that I have thrown things or slammed a door.
____	____	4. I remember irritating incidents and get mad again.
____	____	5. I am annoyed when others are incompetent at their jobs.
____	____	6. I get angry when I am affected by others' mistakes.
____	____	7. I think salespeople are trying to cheat me.
____	____	8. I feel my anger is justified. I feel an urge to punish people–to get back at them.
____	____	9. I frequently feel irritated when I stand in line or drive in heavy traffic.
____	____	10. I like to have the last word in an argument.
____	____	11. In a checkout express line, if the person in front of me has more items than the limit, I get annoyed.
____	____	12. I feel upset when I am not given recognition for doing good work.
____	____	13. When I am angry, I keep things inside, pout, and sulk.
____	____	14. When I get angry, I say nasty things.

Scoring

Part II: Statements in this section demonstrate angry/hostile/cynical/hot reactor behavior. Even one yes response to any of these statements is too many and may be raising your risk of heart disease. Have a friend or loved one who knows you also check the statements for you. Was there a change in any of the answers to the statements?

TOP (10) LIST

Stress Reduction Tips

(After Implementing the Five Stress Management Strategies Outlined in This Chapter)

1. Learn to lighten your load. Simplify. Remind yourself that you are not the general manager of the universe. Someone else has that job and doesn't need any help.
2. Live within your budget and don't use credit cards for ordinary purchases.
3. Simplify and unclutter your life. Start with cleaning out your wallet or purse, then your desk or study area, then a drawer or closet.
4. Allow extra time to do things and get places.
5. Listen to relaxing music while driving, working, or thinking.
6. Do something for the kid in you every day. Set aside time to play and laugh.
7. Worry constructively and only about things you can control. Don't sweat the small stuff. It's all small stuff.
8. Weed out trivia. Write down important things and forget unimportant details. Don't overburden your memory.
9. Live in the present. Clear your mind of unpleasant experiences and emotions. Let it go!
10. Every night, think of one thing for which you are grateful and record it in your journal.

SLOW DOWN!

---

2. Develop a game plan for what you want to accomplish in life (both long-term and short-term) and set priorities. Let some things go. Sometimes we need to step back from leadership roles to create time—to exercise, to eat right, etc. Keep things in balance, Don't let your long-term goals lose out to your short-term pressures.
3. Practice relaxation techniques daily, especially meditation.
4. Develop a sense of humor about life. *He or she who laughs lasts.*
5. Laugh more.
6. Spend more time with friends and make those friendships more intimate.
7. Anticipate stresses and regulate their number and timing when possible.
8. Maintain a flexible schedule. Don't schedule appointments and activities unnecessarily.
9. Learn to say no and to protect your precious time.
10. Delegate more.
11. Listen to others without interrupting.

12. Avoid irritating, competitive people.
13. Allow extra time to do things and to get places.
14. Carry a paperback with you to read while waiting in lines or for appointments.
15. Develop a caring attitude (most people are doing the best they can).
16. Learn to savor food instead of grabbing fast food and eating "on the run."
17. Purposely choose the longest line in which to do your business (at the bank, at the checkout in the grocery store, in a fast-food restaurant, or in a discount department store).
18. Discontinue polyphasic behavior (doing two or more things at once).
19. Build a time each day for exercise or another absorbing activity.
20. Read a good book.
21. Spend an entire afternoon in a museum or art gallery.

THE STRESS-RESISTANT HARDY PERSON

Have you ever imagined what George Washington or any of our other founding fathers would think about our modern, high-tech, fast-paced world? They might be surprised by computers, fax machines, television with 24-hour global news, heart transplants, overcrowded calendars, never-ending deadlines, and chronic shortages of time. Certainly they would agree that we have just cause to feel overwhelmed by our daily schedules and would be glad not to be participating in the 21st

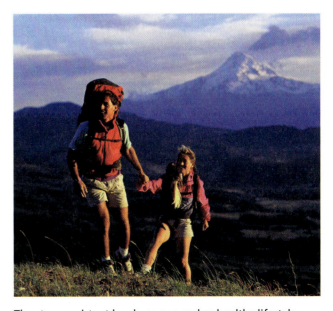

The stress-resistant hardy person makes healthy lifestyle choices and has a sense of connectedness to others.

century with us. Yet we all know some people who, in spite of it all, seem relatively insulated from the potential negative effects of their hectic pace. Their lives are as full as ours, but they seem to carry on, taking "everything in stride"—often with a sense of enjoyment and fun. Who are these effective copers? Are they born this way, or are they bred—learning strategies for coping with stress that protect them from being overwhelmed and feeling stressed-out?

Two psychologists, Dr. R. Flannery of Harvard University Medical School and Dr. S. Kobasa, independently researching these questions, discovered that even when highly stressed, many individuals have a lower incidence of physical illness, lower amounts of anxiety and depression, and increased longevity. These stress-resistant individuals were labeled "hardy." "**Hardiness**" is an ability to resist the ill effects of stress. The hardy have strong immune systems and are optimists. The same study found that people lacking "hardiness" were more prone to illness in the face of stress. They are pessimists with weak immune systems. A hardy soul is a Type A who has been relabeled a **Type C personality** because of the five unique personality traits he or she possesses for adapting to life stress. We call the Type C traits the *Five Cs:*

✔ *Control:* Control is the opposite of helplessness. The hardy person has a sense of internal control (influence) over life events and their outcomes. These people take daily hassles in stride. They think ahead, plan, and make lists of what needs to be done. They seek active solutions to problems. Do you feel "in control" of your life? If not, what plan can you implement that will help you gain more control?

✔ *Commitment:* Commitment is the opposite of alienation and is typified by meaningful involvement in life (i.e., with one's family, job, and community). The hardy person has a sense of purpose in life and sets short- and long-term goals. Rearing one's children, having friends, participating in community projects, having religious values (or spirituality in some form), reaching career goals, and working to complete your degree are examples of personal commitments that help us unstress. List one or two goals to which you have made a commitment.

✔ *Challenge:* The hardy person perceives life change as a potential opportunity and a challenge rather than a threat. These people continue to learn from positive and negative experiences. Hardy people are highly confident in their ability to do their work. They accept setbacks as a part of life and as an opportunity for growth. They are positive thinkers and view bad situations as temporary and changeable.

✔ *Choices in lifestyle:* Hardy individuals make lifestyle choices that enhance health and reduce stress. They reduce their use of caffeine, nicotine,

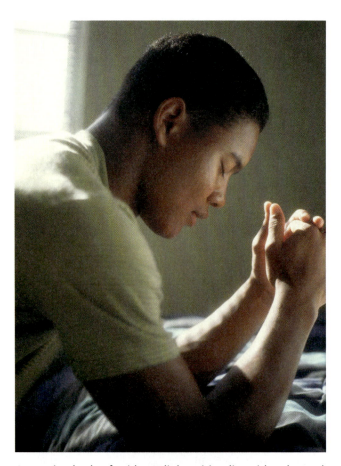

A growing body of evidence links spirituality with enhanced health—including cardiovascular and immune function. Spirituality has been found to reduce the risk of disease, increase the rate of recovery from surgery, and lower the overall death rate.

alcohol, and sugar and incorporate aerobic exercise and relaxation activities into their lives. How much caffeine do you consume every day? Do you practice any of the relaxation techniques in this chapter? Sydney J. Harris said it best: "The time to relax is when you don't have time for it."

✔ *Connectedness:* Hardy people develop a network of social support that includes helping and being helped by others. They have developed a sense of "connectedness" to others. They are actively involved with others. Studies show that social interaction is important. It may lower the pulse rate and blood pressure, enhance the immune system, and boost the production of endorphins. When you're in a caring relationship with another person, these health benefits accrue. Do you have one or more close friends to whom you feel "connected" (i.e., sharing troubles, ambitions, and desires) or whom you can count on for emotional support?

Research on the hardy, stress-resistant Type C personality has made it clear that the five interrelated traits of control, commitment, challenge, lifestyle choices (personal health practices), and connectedness are important factors that buffer us from the ravages of our modern lifestyles and help us adapt and even flourish in the face of them. How many of these hardiness traits do you possess? Lab Activity 10-3, *Becoming Stress-Resistant and Hardy,* will help you strengthen these traits in your life. Can you think of two ways you can apply the knowledge of these five traits to your life, bolstering your "hardiness" rating?

BUILDING SKILLS FOR STRESS MANAGEMENT

Relaxation training is being recommended, in combination with medication, nutrition, and exercise, not only to reduce stress but to treat chronic pain and illness, such as heart disease, high blood pressure, diabetes, infertility, and cancer. Relaxation is also being used in easing depression, painful AIDS symptoms, headaches, and back pain. The concept of relaxation as "good medicine," once dismissed by scientists, is accepted now, thanks to the work of several pioneers in the mind/body field.

As you have learned, when an individual is stressed, the body responds with an outpouring of hormones to prepare him or her to either fight or take flight (the stress response). Performance and work decline when you feel stressed out. When you are relaxed and feeling in control, the mind and body function efficiently and effectively. Dr. Herbert Benson of the Harvard Medical School, the founder of the Mind/Body Medical Institute at New England Deaconness Hospital in Boston, discovered that with effort and training in the use of meditation, we can learn to quiet down and summon at will the healing changes in body chemistry called the **relaxation response.** Benson found that the relaxation response is the body's built-in defense mechanism against the harmful effects of the inappropriate elicitation of the fight-or-flight response caused by everyday living.

The innate physiological changes produced by the relaxation response, which we can elicit to counteract stress, include the following:

✔ Decreased oxygen consumption and metabolic rate, lessening strain on the body's energy resources
✔ Increased intensity and frequency of alpha brain waves associated with deep relaxation
✔ Reduced blood lactates (substances in the blood associated with anxiety)
✔ Decreased anxiety, fears, and phobias and increased positive mental health (i.e., less anxiety and greater feeling of control)

✔ Significant decreases in blood pressure in hypertensive individuals (which remained lowered throughout the day)
✔ Reduced heart rate and slower respiration
✔ Decreased muscle tension
✔ Increased blood flow to the arms and legs
✔ Improved quality of sleep

Dr. Redford Williams, director of the Behavioral Medical Research Center at Duke University, found that distressed, angry, hostile people suffered more heart disease than did calm ones. Williams, like Benson, believes relaxation and other stress-management techniques are critical ways to reduce negative emotions.

Dr. Jon Kabat-Zinn, another stress pioneer, is known for using stress-reduction programs, especially mind/body interactions and mindfulness meditation, at the University of Massachusetts Medical Center to help patients suffering from chronic pain and stress-related disorders. While traditional meditation involves training the mind on a single point of focus, such as a word or phrase, **mindfulness meditation** (i.e., non-mantra meditation) involves nonjudgmental awareness of whatever a person happens to be experiencing at the time—and learning to experience it calmly, whether it is pleasant or unpleasant. Kabat-Zinn describes *mindfulness* as waking up and living in harmony with oneself and the world. He encourages his patients to cultivate some appreciation for the fullness of each moment they are alive. He asserts that it is important to be "in touch" with each moment so that we may live our lives with greater satisfaction, harmony, and wisdom. What he's talking about is conscious attention to behavior. Mindfulness meditation is not an attempt to escape from problems or difficulties. On the contrary, it is a willingness to go nose to nose with pain, confusion, and loss. For example, people using mindfulness meditation to cope with chronic pain would not try to distract themselves from the pain but would experience the pain without fear or anxiety (emotions that make the pain more intense). Those who practice mindfulness meditation, focusing only on what is going on at the present—for 20 minutes a day—can produce the relaxation response and benefit from all of its antistress effects. It has been successfully used for many medical conditions including asthma, cancer, coronary artery disease, fibromyalgia, HIV/AIDS, rheumatoid arthritis, stomach ulcers, and chronic pain.

You can't change the complexities of life, but you can develop strategies that enable you to cope more effectively. You can learn to relax, to quiet down the mind and body (so you can get "in touch" or "connected to" your inner thoughts, feelings, goals, and values), and successfully manage the stress in your life. Review behavior change in Chapter 2 and Table 10-4 to assess your current stage of behavior change relative to stress management.

TABLE 10-4   *Tips for Behavior Change—Managing Stress*

STAGES OF CHANGE: IN WHAT STAGE ARE YOU?

1. Precontemplation: "Stress is no problem for me."
2. Contemplation: "I wish I could get control of my stress level."
3. Preparation: "I am going to start working on managing my stress."
4. Action: "I am actively taking steps to control my stress."
5. Maintenance: "I have been able to control my stress level for this entire year."

PROCESS OF CHANGE

After identifying your current stage, try using some of the following selected processes and behavior strategies that are appropriate for your particular stage to facilitate your transition into the next stage:

- Consciousness raising: Assess your level of stress (Table 10-2, Life Event Stress Test)
- Social liberation: Identify stress management self-help groups/workshops on campus
- Emotional arousal: Read about the long-term ill effects of stress on the body
- Self-liberation: Keep a diary of daily stressors, reactions, and coping skills used
- Countering: Do deep breathing exercises when feeling stressed
- Helping relationships: Use stress-management support group in your residence hall

By following one or more of the six stress management strategies in this chapter every day, you will be well on your way to becoming a stress-hardy person. Enjoy!

The six stress management strategies described here include:

1. Exercise
2. Relaxation techniques
3. Lifestyle change
4. Reframing
5. Laughter and humor
6. Create a memory bank

STRATEGY #1: EXERCISE

Get physical. An avalanche of research reveals that aerobic exercise promotes health and energy and is a powerful antidote for stress, anxiety, and even moderate depression. Many physicians recommend exercise to their "stressed" patients instead of medications such as tranquilizers. Exercise allows us to play out the inappropriate fight-or-flight response, use the muscles that are tensed for action, and reduce the adrenaline being pumped into the bloodstream. A number of studies suggest that exercise reduces the intensity of the stress response, shortens the time it takes to recover from stress, and helps ward off illness in people experiencing stress. While stress increases blood pressure and platelet stickiness (the factor that increases clotting), exercise reduces them. Regular exercise also helps reduce abdominal obesity, improves insulin sensitivity, and slows the progression of artery disease.

Exercise is a natural way to relax and renew energy. When hassles and problems begin to pile up in the office or at school, change into your workout clothes and take a vigorous run, a swim, or a brisk walk. The effect is amazing. Headaches, tension, anxiety, aggressiveness, and irritability are diminished. Vigorous exercise increases the release of endorphins, brain chemicals that may alleviate the harmful effects of stressors by producing a more relaxed state. Besides better stress management, the psychological benefits of exercise, documented by research, are increased self-esteem, increased alertness, and decreased depression and anxiety.

Although aerobic vigorous exercise is best, even a 30-minute walk can do wonders to relieve tension. What is the number one reason people give for not exercising? "I don't have the time to exercise." Anyone can squeeze in 20 minutes, the minimum amount of time recommended for an aerobic workout! (The FITT prescription is 20–60 minutes of moderate to vigorous aerobic exercise. See Chapter 4.) For basic health benefits, 30 minutes of moderate-intensity exercise is recommended. Play tennis or racquetball, golf, dance, bowl, swim, rake leaves, garden, bike, or do whatever. Enjoy physical activity. It is the healthiest thing you can do for yourself, and it's inexpensive.

STRATEGY #2: RELAXATION TECHNIQUES

Practice the following relaxation techniques to find the ones that you feel most comfortable using and that work for you. For best results, set aside some time every day for relaxation. The seven relaxation techniques described here are meditation, autogenic training and imagery, Jacobson's progressive relaxation, abdominal breathing, hatha yoga, massage, and biofeedback training.

2a. Meditation

Meditation is a mental exercise that affects body processes, producing physical benefits. The purpose of meditation is to gain control over your attention—to internally quiet down, allowing *you* to choose what to focus on and block out distracting thoughts.

Meditation actually dates back to biblical times, but the type practiced in the Eastern cultures of India and Tibet was exported to the Western world by the Maharishi Mahesh Yogi. The Maharishi popularized the **transcendental meditation (TM)** method. In recent years, TM and meditation in general have been subjected to a battery of scientific studies. Especially revealing and conclusive were the experiments conducted at the Harvard School of Medicine by Dr. Herbert Benson and at the School of Medicine, University of California, San Francisco, by Dr. Dean Ornish. They found that meditation in general was a simple yet powerful, easy-to-learn, nonchemical stress reducer that produced the relaxation response. They call meditation the "universal stress antidote" and assert that it is compatible with modern medicine. Other experts agree that meditation is now mainstream. They feel that a proficient meditator develops a sense of wholeness and is able to face stress, pain, and illness with equanimity and triumph over his or her problems. Meditation is merely a discipline for training the mind to focus, for developing greater calm, relief, and understanding. This, in turn, leads to a greater sense of control and happiness.

To bring the relaxation response benefits into your everyday life, learn to meditate. Meditation, recognized as one of the most powerful antidotes for stress, should be practiced for 10 to 20 minutes, twice a day. Soon you will be enjoying the relaxing periods of stillness and quietness of the mind that meditation produces. (Use Lab Activity 10-2 for additional practice.) Meditation involves the following four essential elements:

1. *A quiet, comfortable environment.* A place where you will not be disturbed is essential. However, once you become experienced, you will be able to meditate almost anywhere.
2. *A comfortable position.* A position that will allow you to remain in the same posture for approximately 20 minutes is necessary to avoid any undue muscular tension. Lying down or sitting in an overstuffed chair may cause you to lose your focus and fall asleep.
3. *Focusing your attention on something repetitive or unchanging such as a mantra, a mental device, or the breath.* For starters, you can keep it simple by focusing on your breathing, feeling the air as it moves in and out. Use your breath as an anchor to bring you back when your attention is disrupted. A mantra can also be used. A mantra is a silently repeated word, phrase, sound, or thought such as *one, love, peace,* or *omh.* The mantra should be easy to pronounce and short enough to repeat silently as you exhale. Or use a mental device, an unchanging object such as an object in the room where you meditate. Gaze at the object fixedly. Select any one of the three methods to help you maintain your focus, shut out outside stimuli, and keep you calm. The method may vary but the relaxation benefits do not.
4. *A calm, relaxed attitude.* Relax. Try not to try. Let it happen. The harder you try, the more tense you

get. Disregard outside noise and thoughts. When distracting thoughts and noise intrude—it is normal that they will occasionally—calmly return your focus to the slow, steady repetition of the mantra or to the mental device.

2b. Autogenic Training and Imagery

Autogenic means "self-generating" or "self-induced." The **autogenic training and imagery** technique uses mental concentration exercises to bring about sensations of warmth and heaviness in the limbs and torso and then uses relaxing images to expand the relaxed state. Both meditation and autogenic training lead to the relaxation response. Many who find meditation too easy and boring enjoy autogenic training because of the switches of focus from one part of the body to another and the use of imagery. Autogenic training has been successful in the treatment of chronic and lower back pain. Otherwise, the physiological and psychological benefits are similar to those of meditation.

Autogenic training should be done with the eyes closed while you are lying down or in a seated position. Whatever position you choose, be sure that you are relaxed and comfortable. Eliminate muscle tension in any part of the body by changing position slightly. Practice for 10 to 30 minutes, one or two times a day, to become skillful at this technique.

The six steps to autogenic training follow:

1. Concentrate on heaviness of arms and legs, beginning with dominant side.
2. Concentrate on warmth of arms and legs, beginning with dominant side.
3. Concentrate on warmth and heaviness of heart and chest.
4. Concentrate on breathing rhythm.
5. Concentrate on warmth of abdominal area.
6. Concentrate on coolness of forehead.

After the six stages of autogenic training have been mastered, transfer body relaxation to mind relaxation by using images of relaxing scenes, such as the following:

- ✔ Sinking into a mattress
- ✔ A sack of sugar melting away in the rain
- ✔ Floating out to sea
- ✔ A feather floating in the sky
- ✔ A soaring bird
- ✔ Clouds drifting by
- ✔ Ocean surf splashing on the sand
- ✔ A warm, relaxing fire burning in the fireplace
- ✔ A sailboat drifting on a calm lake

Use images you find relaxing. They may be different from those used by your friends.

2c. Jacobson's Progressive Relaxation

Edmund Jacobson, a physician, designed for his tense patients a series of exercises called **progressive relaxation** that emphasizes the relaxation of voluntary skeletal muscles—that is, the muscles over which you have control. He taught his patients to contract a muscle group and then relax it, progressing from one muscle group to another until the entire body was relaxed. The idea was to learn to recognize tenseness and be able to relax consciously whenever it was needed. This method of relaxation, named after its developer, does not produce the relaxation response. However, if practiced regularly, it is beneficial in helping people relax. It has been used in the treatment of insomnia and psychological conditions such as poor self-concept, depression, and anxiety.

There are many routines of contract-relax exercises for progressive relaxation. Try the progressive relaxation routine in this chapter (Table 10-5), which begins at the head and ends at the feet, or develop your own routine. With practice, you will be able to eliminate the contraction phase and focus on relaxation.

TABLE 10-5	*Progressive Relaxation Routine*

1. Lie on your back on the floor in a quiet place with the lights dimmed. Remove shoes. Let feet relax and rotate outward. Arms should be beside body, palms turned upward.
2. Proceed slowly over the body, tensing a muscle group and then relaxing it. Stop if cramping or pain develops.
3. Face: Squint eyes, wrinkle nose, make a face, and then relax. Open mouth wide and stick out tongue. Close mouth and clench teeth. Now relax.
4. Neck: Nod head downward to touch chin to chest. Relax.
5. Head: Try to touch right ear to right shoulder and left ear to left shoulder. Relax and center head over torso.
6. Shoulders: One at a time, shrug shoulder up toward ear; pull shoulder down from ear; press hard against floor. Relax.
7. Hands and arms: Squeeze fingers together, making a fist. Relax. Raise right arm, bending at elbow, and "make a muscle" with biceps. Relax. Repeat with left arm. Relax. With arms on floor, stiffen both arms, make fists. Relax.
8. Back: Try to squeeze shoulder blades together. Relax. Press lower back area into floor. Relax.
9. Abdomen: Suck in abdominal muscles. Relax.
10. Buttocks: Contract buttock muscles. Relax.
11. Thighs: Contract thigh muscles, one at a time and then both at the same time. Relax.
12. Calves: Flex toes back toward head and then extend or point toes away from head, using right leg and then left leg. Relax.
13. Toes: Curl toes under, first right foot and then left foot. Relax.
14. Be aware of relaxed state of body.

TABLE 10-6	*Abdominal Breathing*

1. Inhale and exhale fully through the mouth.
2. Inhale slowly and push out your abdomen (stomach) as though it were a balloon inflating. Move your chest as little as possible.
3. Exhale *slowly* and allow stomach to flatten.
4. Repeat the pattern. On each "in" breath, let belly balloon, and on each "out" breath, let it flatten.
5. Each "out" breath is an opportunity to rid the body of tension.

2d. Abdominal Breathing

Most of us breathe in short shallow breaths, expanding only the chest, especially when we're under stress. This is called *thoracic breathing* and is not the proper way to breathe. It does not allow the lungs to fill and empty completely, and it can increase muscle tension.

During stressful situations, it is even more important to breathe from the abdomen. This method allows more oxygen to enter the body and relaxes the muscles. You can practice the steps described in this chapter at almost any time or in any place, even on the telephone, in class, or at a meeting. Practice at least once a day so that it becomes natural when you use it in stressful or fatiguing situations. This procedure has produced excellent results for many (Table 10-6).

2e. Hatha Yoga

The most familiar form of yoga is **Hatha yoga,** or physical yoga. It is a discipline that involves the use of various exercises or postures (called *asanas*) in combination with proper breathing rhythm to remove tension and inflexibility in the body. It also improves muscular strength, muscular endurance, and body alignment. Hatha yoga

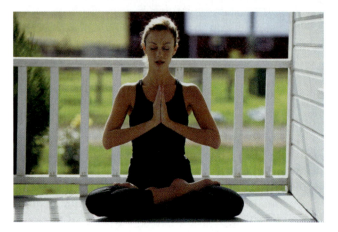

Yoga is a relaxing form of exercise. See Lab Activity 5-2 in Chapter 5 for a sample yoga routine. The Sun Salutation is one of the most practiced yoga routines.

should not be associated with religious or spiritual groups. The physiological and psychological benefits of Hatha yoga received thorough research, confirming it to be an excellent form of exercise and an aid to improving the health and well-being of those who practice it.

2f. Massage

When you are bombarded with too much stress, the muscles in the neck, shoulders, and back can become tight and stiff to the point of pain. Without relaxation, these muscles can become chronically tight and can cause much distress. One of the most enjoyable ways to relieve this condition is to have a massage.

There are several popular forms of massage:

1. *Swedish massage,* the most familiar form, involves kneading and stroking the muscles to decrease tension and increase circulation.
2. *Shiatsu,* originating in Japan and China, is a technique that is a form of acupressure. Pressure is applied with the thumbs or fingers along acupuncture meridians. The idea is to restore balance so that the chi (vital energy believed to be linked to the life force) flows freely and in a balanced manner.
3. *Sports massage* combines Swedish strokes and stretching to help prevent injuries and facilitate flexibility.
4. *Deep tissue massage* uses slow strokes and deep finger pressure to reach deeper layers of muscle to relieve painful areas.
5. *Hot stone massage* involves placing heated stones on different areas of the body to relax the muscles and prepare them for massage.

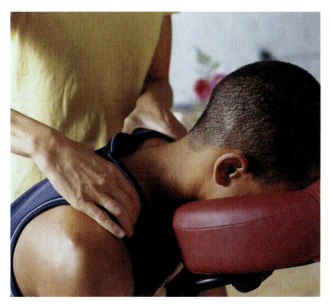

Massage is one of the most enjoyable stress relievers.

Massage given by a spouse or friend can be just as pleasant. You can even massage yourself when tight neck and shoulder muscles are tense. Put on your favorite music and enjoy.

2g. Biofeedback Training

Biofeedback training is a technique in which machines measure certain physiological processes of the body. The machines then convert this information to an understandable form and feed it back to the individual. This process gives a person access to biological information not usually available to one's consciousness. Proponents of biofeedback believe that by mentally recognizing involuntary biological responses such as heart rates, you can control them. With feedback training, stressors are not removed but the response to them is controlled. Control of physiological arousal is an important step in stress management. A major drawback of biofeedback is the cost and availability of the machines and the lack of trained professionals to operate them.

STRATEGY #3: LIFESTYLE CHANGE

Seven important elements are involved in helping us successfully cope with the daily stresses of our hectic, fast-paced lives. They are the impact of diet; time management; alcohol, drugs, cigarettes; plenty of restful sleep; developing satisfying relationships; learning when to seek the help and support of others; and scheduling "me time" and listening to music. This is an area that you control . . . take charge!

3a. The Impact of Diet

Proper diet is an important part of your stress management program and an area in which you can definitely exert *control.* A nutritious diet will help you look and feel good, plus it will strengthen your immune system. Many feel that poor diet can increase susceptibility to stress by causing fatigue and irritability. This is especially true for individuals who are eating too many meals away from home, missing meals, or eating on the run. Unfortunately, there are no miracle foods to boost energy and reduce stress. The best advice for surviving the stress of modern life is to eat three nutritious meals a day and follow these guidelines to help keep you from feeling irritable and uptight:

1. Reduce (below 250 milligrams per day) or eliminate the caffeine in your diet. Caffeine is a stimulant and magnifies the effects of stress. Also, avoid or minimize the use of stimulating drugs (diet pills and oral decongestants) that may cause added agitation.

2. Limit foods containing sugar, especially if you have been skipping meals. It robs the body of B-complex vitamins and may induce anxiety and failure to cope with stressful situations.

3. Limit your intake of sodium because excessive fluid buildup leads to discomfort and increased stress. Too much sodium (salt) can also increase blood pressure due to the fluid buildup. Keep salt consumption below 2,400 milligrams a day—about one teaspoon.

4. Limit alcoholic beverage consumption. Alcohol makes people feel relaxed and less stressed while they're drinking it but leaves them feeling more tired the next day.

3b. Time Management

Insufficient time appears to be the plague of the 21st century. College students frequently complain about the lack of this precious commodity. How well you manage your time plays a large role in how much pressure you feel. You should manage your time as if your life depended on it, because it does. The goal of time management should not be the elimination of leisure time (relaxation, etc.); rather, it should be the elimination of life's real time wasters. Use *Time Management*, Lab Activity 10-6, to practice this important stress management lifestyle strategy. Also, review the Top 10 "Tips on How to Reduce College Stress by Improving Studying and Test-Taking Skills." Time management experts suggest these time-saving tips:

TOP 10 LIST

Tips on How to Reduce College Stress by Improving Studying and Test-Taking Skills

1. Choose a quiet place—no friends, stereo, telephone, TV, and so on.
2. Learn to manage your time. Follow a daily schedule that includes time for classes, completing reading and writing assignments, exam preparation, meals, exercise, job, "me time," and so on.
3. Plan on doing 2 hours of studying for each hour you spend in class.
4. Take short breaks after each hour of studying.
5. Don't skip classes.
6. Don't give in to peer pressure to join midweek get-togethers.
7. Don't rely on cramming.
8. Master test-taking skills:
   - Read all directions carefully.
   - Survey the test. Will certain sections take more time, count more?
   - Outline answers for essays.
   - Work on one question at a time.
   - Mark difficult items and return to them later.
9. Don't hesitate to seek help if you are having difficulty with a course.
10. Encourage yourself with positive thinking ("I can do well in this course").

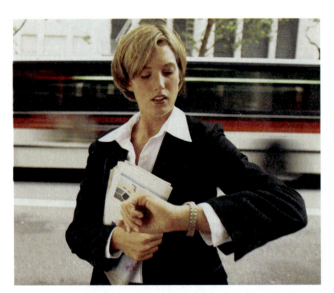

How well do you manage your time? Those who always feel rushed are less likely to be happy than those who almost never feel rushed. "Chronic" stress may be a trigger for depression. Depressed people have higher levels of the stress hormone cortisol, and long-term exposure is unhealthy.

1. Analyze how you spend time and then evaluate that use of time. Keep a diary. You may find you are wasting too much time.

2. Learn to set short- and long-range goals. Write them down. This helps you plan for today and for the future.

3. Learn how to set priorities. Not everything you do is number one on your list of important things. With goals in mind, you will know how to prioritize your activities. Items on the "Do" list must get done; items on the "Maybe" list are those you would like to take care of today, if possible; and those on the "If Possible" list are those you would like to do once the activities on the first and second lists are completed.

4. Use a planner calendar to schedule your priorities into your day, week, and year. This will help you organize and simplify your life by keeping track of important dates, appointments, and meetings. A planner calendar is productive. By systematically planning your day, you can see more clearly what needs to be done. Minor tasks need no longer

overshadow major ones. A few minutes of planning can control hours of chaos. A planned day allows you to schedule stress-reducing breaks and rest periods and to have time for family, friends, personal development, and hobbies. Gaining control over your life reduces stress.

5. Take 5 to 10 minutes at the end of the day to evaluate how well you managed your time. How many of your goals did you check off today? Good time managers use this technique daily to assess time wasted, reprioritize goals (even dumping some), and maintain progress in achieving their short- and long-range goals.

6. Adopt the following time-saving strategies:
   - Learn how to stop being inefficient. This is an art that anyone can learn. Go through mail one time only. Start a task with the intention of completing it now. Don't look it over and put it aside for later. You will have wasted time looking it over the first time.
   - Learn to say no to nonessential tasks! Know your limits. Don't allow too many demands to be made "on your time." Learn to delegate certain activities to others when possible.
   - Practice quick relaxation tricks frequently throughout the day. Get up and go for a drink of water. Give yourself a massage on the neck, shoulders, and forehead. This energizes you to complete tasks more efficiently.

3c. Alcohol, Drugs, and Cigarettes

Alcohol is a powerful depressant drug that temporarily masks but doesn't solve your problems. It can increase stress by creating new problems—hangovers, arrests, traffic violations, fights, and accidents. Taking illegal drugs can only increase stress. Why risk ruining your physical and mental health and experiencing the stress of being arrested? Do not smoke cigarettes or use other tobacco products (snuff, chewing tobacco). Nicotine is a stimulant that increases stress.

3d. Get Plenty of Restful Sleep

Take care of yourself. Most people need 7 to 9 hours of restful sleep each night. Getting enough sleep can make you more alert, less irritable, and better able to cope with stressful situations. Cumulative sleep loss has debilitating and even fatal effects. Poor judgment and other declines in cognitive performance lead to increased risks of accident and injury when sleep is shortchanged. Driving while sleep-deprived (getting 6 hours of sleep or less the night before), according to researchers, is nearly as risky as driving while intoxicated! Quality of life decreases dramatically if fatigue dominates the day. When short on sleep people tend to overeat and underexercise. Tired people are less productive at work and in the classroom, less patient with others, and less interactive in relationships. Good sleep is as important as regular exercise and good nutrition to coping with life's stresses and keeping yourself in top form physically, mentally, and spiritually. You know you are getting enough sleep if you wake up in the morning before the alarm goes off, feel refreshed and rested, and are alert throughout the day. If you have any of the following signs and symptoms, you may not be getting enough sleep:

✔ You routinely ignore the alarm clock or snatch a few extra minutes to snooze before getting up.
✔ You look forward to catching up on your sleep on the weekend.
✔ You have to fight to stay awake during class, during long meetings, in overheated rooms, or after a heavy meal.

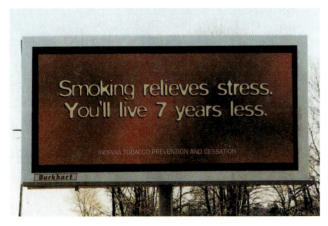

Some individuals use smoking as a way to cope with everyday stress.

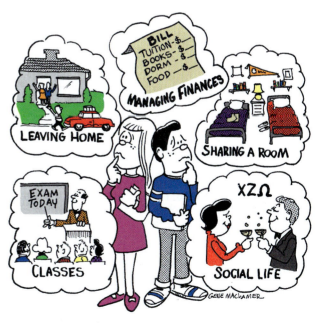

College students face many stresses.

✔ You're irritable with friends, family members, or coworkers.
✔ You have difficulty concentrating or remembering.
✔ It takes you more than 30 minutes to fall asleep at night.
✔ You wake repeatedly throughout the night.
✔ You wake up groggy and not well rested.
✔ Your roommate, spouse, or partner complains about your snoring or fitful sleeping.

Review the guidelines in Table 10-7 if you have concerns about the quality of your sleep.

3e. Develop Satisfying Relationships

Having close friends with whom to share the joys and sorrows of living is a huge asset in protecting your health. Recent research confirms that loneliness is bad for your heart. It is linked to blood vessel problems that may lead to high blood pressure in younger adults and greatly increases blood pressure in men and women over 50 years of age. Club membership, religious or civic activities, and volunteer work have been shown to protect against the physical effects of stress. Unhappiness, de-

pression, and feelings of isolation can be caused by lack of close emotional bonds with friends, a spouse, or family members. Intimate relationships and social support can become a powerful life-support system when internal resources have fallen short. Social support can provide direct reinforcement for healthy behaviors and indirectly buffer disappointments that would otherwise lead to excessive stress. Friends are not just nice, they are a necessity. You have to *be a friend to have a friend*. Make the effort. It's good health and happiness insurance.

3f. Learn When to Seek the Help and Support of Others

There will be stressful situations you will not be able to deal with alone. Don't be embarrassed about seeking professional help. Developing a variety of support groups such as family, friends, coaches, counselors, or physicians can be helpful. Talking to someone gives you a different perspective on worries and concerns.

3g. Schedule "Me Time" and Listen to Music

Schedule a regular time for yourself and make that time inviolate. It is your special time. Let nothing else interfere. This is an excellent way to balance the stresses of work or school. "Me time" can include learning to do nothing (loafing) at times and feeling okay about it. This time does not have to be a long period; it can be as brief as 15 minutes a day. Many people enjoy listening to their favorite music during their "me time." Music has been found to be therapeutic, relaxing, and an excellent way to calm the mind. According to a study at the Cornell Center for Complementary and Integrative Medicine, music can lower stress hormones by as much as 25 percent when you listen for 15 minutes or more a day.

TABLE 10-7	*Improve Your Quality of Sleep*

To improve your quality of sleep, implement the following helpful guidelines:

- Stick to a regular schedule for sleeping and waking. Try to stick to that schedule even on weekends. Consistency helps your body know when it's time to go to sleep and wake up.
- Don't eat or drink a lot before bedtime.
- Sleep primarily at night. Avoid frequent daytime naps—they may disrupt sleep at night.
- Develop a soothing bedtime routine. A warm bath or shower before bedtime relaxes tense muscles.
- Create a dark, quiet, and comfortable place to sleep. A slightly cool room is ideal.
- Get adequate exposure to bright light each day. Get outside as much as possible, especially at midday during short winter days.
- Exercise regularly—but not within a few hours of bedtime. Don't overtrain, though; this has the opposite effect on sleep.
- Check your medications. Many contain ingredients (such as caffeine) that can cause insomnia (e.g., pain relievers, decongestants, asthma/cold/antihistamine medications, exercise and diet aids).
- Acknowledge the sources of stress in your life and devise a plan to eliminate the ones you can.
- Practice relaxation techniques.
- Modify your lifestyle. Reduce or eliminate caffeine, tobacco, and alcohol, especially before bedtime. While alcohol may help people fall asleep, it usually produces a light restless sleep, often causing the individual to awaken suddenly during the night, unable to sleep again.

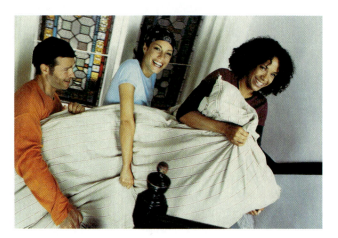

Having friends you can rely on (like helping on moving day) can enhance the immune system. Social support is a key factor in reducing the stress in our hectic lives.

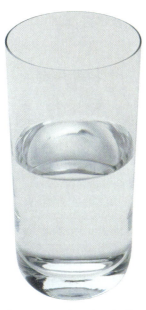

Reframing: Is the glass half empty or half full?

STRATEGY #4: REFRAMING

Reframing means consciously reinterpreting a situation in a more positive light. It is a way of looking at life in a positive manner. This makes you better able to deal with problems when they come. Is the glass half empty or half full? Viewing yourself as a sick person because you have asthma is different, for example, from perceiving yourself as a healthy person who also happens to have asthma. In the case of the driver who cuts you off in traffic, you might tell yourself, "Maybe she had some emergency." This is an excellent way to diffuse anger and negativism. See if you can learn to "reframe" life's stumbling blocks into challenges. Look at the bright side of each situation. Take control of your reactions to events. Learn to be an optimist. Good things happen to people who expect them. Positive emotions and laughter play an important role in keeping well and fit. Optimists have higher hardiness scores (and stronger immune systems), whereas pessimists are more likely to resort to anger and hostility.

STRATEGY #5: LAUGHTER AND HUMOR

Laughter and its subtle companion humor can provide psychological relief from tension, anxiety, anger, hostility, and emotional pain. Laughing is like "internal jogging"—it causes endorphins (pain-relieving chemicals) to be released in the brain. Laughter is a natural tranquilizer with no negative side effects. It helps relax the blood vessels and boosts blood circulation. In one study, laughter increased blood flow 22 percent; under stress, blood flow decreased 35 percent. Laughter and humor reduce anger

and anxiety, increase joy, provide a greater sense of control, lower production of stress hormones, and improve immune function.

Make an effort (and practice it, too) to see the humor in everyday situations. Don't be afraid to laugh at yourself whenever you make a silly mistake. After all, we are only human. Scientific evidence is beginning to support the biblical axiom that "a merry heart doeth good like a medicine." Bob Hope, a Hollywood comedian who lived to be 100 years old, is a good example of this axiom. When asked about his life's work he answered: "I have seen what a laugh can do. It can transform almost unbearable tears into something bearable, even hopeful."

STRATEGY #6: CREATE A MEMORY BANK

Happiness comes from noticing and enjoying the little things in life. Take 5 minutes of your day, every day, to savor the special experiences of your life. Store them in your memory bank. Journaling will help you remember them. When you look back over your day (and your life), what special memories do you fondly recall: roasting marshmallows over a campfire, watching the sunset, smelling a rose, the glow after a satisfying workout, birds singing early in the morning, a beautiful morning sunrise, newborn animals, a hug that said "I care"? What can you do today to increase your store of pleasant memories?

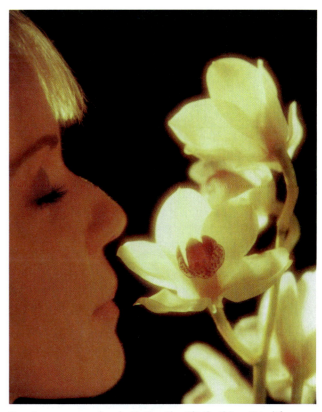

Create a memory bank. Notice the "little things" in life.

Frequently Asked Questions

Q. Can spirituality uplift one's health?

A. Modern medicine, with its high-tech wizardry, can do wonders for the body but little for the soul. And until recently medical research avoided spirituality.

In the last decade a growing number of researchers have put spirituality and religion under the microscope. The research so far suggests that having a spiritual dimension in your life may help you get healthy when you are sick and stay healthy when you are well.

There are several plausible explanations for a faith-health link: Religion and spirituality may encourage healthy habits and help reduce stress, perhaps by promoting social support; an optimistic outlook; and deep relaxation during prayer, meditation, or another relaxation technique.

Q. I think my boyfriend might be depressed. How large a problem is depression (more than just "the blues") among college students? What are the symptoms of depression?

A. Combine the academic pressures of college life with the fact that the age of onset for mental disorders is often 18–25, and it is not a surprise that students are especially vulnerable. The following can be symptoms of depression:
- a persistent feeling of sadness, anxiety, or "emptiness"
- feelings of hopelessness and worthlessness
- loss of interest in activities
- fatigue or lack of energy
- trouble concentrating
- insomnia, early morning awakening, or oversleeping
- thoughts of suicide

Seek professional help immediately if you, a loved one, or a friend exhibit signs of depression.

Q. I sleep 5 to 6 hours a night and don't feel tired during the day. Am I getting enough sleep?

A. Probably not. Roughly 5 percent of people claim that's all the sleep they need to function well during the day. But getting so little slumber may harm your health even if it doesn't impair your performance. Without enough sleep:
- You may notice a decline in your ability to learn; your problem-solving, speaking, and writing skills; your reaction time; and your stamina.
- You are more likely to become tense and moody and to have trouble getting along with others.
- The body's immune system may weaken. People who report daytime sleepiness have worse overall health and higher mortality rates than do well-rested people.
- The risk of developing insulin resistance increases. This may predispose people to diabetes, high

blood pressure, coronary heart disease, stroke, and possibly cancer.
- Weight gain and reductions in muscle mass may occur due to inhibited nocturnal surges of growth hormone.

Q. Last year I thought it was a good idea to attend a college in another state. Now that I am four states away from home, I'm not so sure. I don't know anyone in my residence hall much less on campus. All my friends went to in-state schools. Last week I felt like I was getting sick. Can loneliness affect my health?

A. It sure can. Researchers at Carnegie Mellon University studied college freshmen coping with their first semester away from home. They found that freshmen who felt the loneliest and most socially isolated had the weakest immune response to the flu virus. Their studies show that loneliness and social isolation can have an impact and that the first semester of college can be "really stressful." College students aren't the only ones whose health may suffer with those feelings. Loneliness and social isolation have previously been associated with immune detriments in other age groups.

Q. Can stress really cause premature aging?

A. Yes! Just look at any U.S. President after a few years in office. A groundbreaking study at the University of California found that chronic stress appears to accelerate the aging process by shortening the life span of the immune system cells. The cells of people under lots of stress aged the equivalent of 9 to 17 years more than the cells of people under little stress. What's more, it wasn't just the stress itself but the perception of stress (or how the person perceives the stress) that can lead to faster aging. The researchers suspect that stress hormones such as cortisol are to blame. They also believe it may be more or equally important how you view your life and cope with demands, and what kind of support you have. The meaning is clear: people at risk for high stress can slow down cell aging through exercise, meditation, prayer, or other stress-reducing strategies. Health can indeed be an example of "mind over matter."

Q. I heard on TV that stress can make you fat. Is this true?

A. Yes! The fight-or-flight reaction, which is triggered on an almost continuous basis in some people, causes a release of stress hormones. One of them is cortisol. High cortisol levels are associated with overeating, craving high-caloric fatty and sugary foods, and relocating fat from the circulation and storage depots to the deep internal abdominal area. Research has demonstrated that moderate to vigorous exercise and stress management activities can offset the negative effects of cortisol and reduce the health risks associated with stress-induced obesity.

Q. What is Tai Chi? Is it a beneficial form of exercise?

A. Tai Chi is an ancient Chinese exercise form that combines relaxed, slow movement with a calm, alert mental state. The practitioner keeps his or her body relaxed and upright, focusing throughout the exercise sequence on natural diaphragmatic breathing. The Chinese have long touted Tai Chi's medical benefits, practicing it for health, vitality, relaxation, and self-defense. Medical research has begun to confirm that Tai Chi practice has a positive effect on health by:

- Reducing diastolic and systolic blood pressure.
- Improving strength and balance.
- Improving emotional health (i.e., reduced tension, depression, anger, improved general mood).
- Possibly positively affecting the immune system.

Q. The nation seems to be in the middle of an anger epidemic. Why is this?

A. Bad tempers are everywhere. The media report incidents of road rage, airplane rage, cell phone rage, grocery store rage, parking lot rage, and youth sports activities rage. Leading social scientists confirm that the nation is in the middle of an unsettling and deadly anger trend. This all-too-frequent display of rage is described as a fuming, unrelenting sense of anger, hostility, and alienation that simmers for months, even years, without relief. Eventually, all it takes is a triggering incident, usually minor, for a hostile person to go ballistic. Why?

- Stress is a hallmark of the anger epidemic, and the major contributing factors are lack of time and intrusive technology. Cell phones, pagers, and so on allow us to be interrupted anywhere, at any time. This constant accessibility and compulsive use of technology fragments what little time we have, adding to our sense of urgency and overload.
- Multitasking. People feel the need to do several things at the same time (e.g., drive and talk on the phone).
- High expectations and sense of entitlement, pressure to achieve more and live the "good life." People feel they are entitled to fulfillment at any cost because of materialism and consumerism.
- Lack of manners. Rude and selfish behavior has increased, and so has anger at the bad behavior of others.
- Lack of connection. Families are not doing things together the way they used to. Social support also has diminished.
- Media. Television programs (talk shows such as *The Jerry Springer Show,* crime shows, shows such as *Dateline* and *20/20,* and the evening news) continually show examples of rage outbursts, almost convincing the viewing public that it's okay or at least normal.
- We feel it's normal. We are exposed to more violence, which makes it mainstream.

Summary

Stress is unavoidable. Optimal levels of stress improve health and performance, but excess levels, especially when chronic and perceived as negative, can be hazardous to your health. Major life events—death of a spouse, marriage, and divorce, for example—are significant stressors. Other, more common stressors are daily hassles (missed sleep, rush-hour traffic, losing things). We learn to cope with major life events and daily hassles in a variety of ways. Some are healthy; some are not. Healthy stress management strategies include exercise, relaxation techniques, lifestyle changes, reframing, laughter and humor, and creating a memory bank. Hassles can be countered with the giving and receiving of daily uplifts (compliments, hugs, and getting enough sleep).

Four stress-coping behavior types—Types A, B, C, and D—have been identified. Type As are described as rushed, competitive, and impatient. These behaviors often lead to angry, hostile, and cynical reactions when the individual is stressed, which are, in turn, the lethal risk factors for coronary heart disease. Type Bs are more relaxed than Type As, but if they demonstrate anger and hostility, they also will develop negative health consequences. Hot reactors perceive every stressor as a life-and-death situation and may be either Type A or Type B. Type Ds are "distressed" and exhibit two emotional states: negative affectivity (worry, irritability, gloom) and social inhibition (discomfort in social interactions, reticence, and a lack of social poise). Type Ds are especially at risk for cardiovascular disease. Type Cs are often referred to as "hardy." Type Cs possess the Five Cs: They accept challenges, feel they are in control of their lives, have a strong commitment or purpose in life, make healthy lifestyle choices, and have a strong sense of connectedness to others.

Your wellness is dependent on how well you balance the stress in your life, how well you can modify your angry and hostile behavior, and how successfully you take charge of your life. As one wise person said, "If you can't fight and you can't flee, flow."

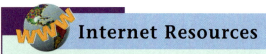

Internet Resources

American Foundation for Suicide Prevention
www.afsp.org
Provides information about depression and suicide.

American Institute of Stress
www.stress.org
Dedicated to advancing our understanding of the role of stress in health and illness, the nature and importance of mind/body relationships, and the inherent and immense potential for self-healing.

American Massage Therapy Association
www.amtamassage.org
Provides a list of certified massage therapists in your area.

American Psychological Association
www.apa.org
This scientific organization's site provides studies of the mind and behavior.

American Yoga Association
www.americanyogaassociation.org
Gives information on how to start practicing yoga and how to choose a yoga teacher. Has an online store for books, DVDs, videos, etc.

Ask Dr. Weil
www.drweil.com
Offers information about alternative health topics.

Association for Applied Psychophysiology and Biofeedback
www.aapb.org
Provides information about biofeedback and mind/body interactions.

Center for Anxiety and Stress Treatment
www.stressrelease.com
Provides resources to help manage and regain control of your life.

Health Behavior News Services
www.hbns.org
Resource for most recent research about how people can change their behaviors to improve their health. Topics include stress, diet, exercise, cardiovascular health, diabetes, HIV/AIDS, and addictions.

Healthfinder
www.healthfinder.gov
Consolidates official government health resources and offers links to over 500 consumer health sites.

The Humor Project
www.humorproject.com
Provides articles, speakers' bureau, discussion boards, and publications on utilizing humor for the release of stress.

Mayo Clinic
www.mayoclinic.com
Provides reliable health and wellness information, including information on stress.

Meditation Center
www.meditationcenter.com
Provides simple instructions and information about a variety of meditation techniques.

Mind/Body Medical Institute
www.mbmi.org
Harvard's Dr. Herbert Benson provides the latest information about mind/body stress reduction.

National Institute of Mental Health (NIMH)
www.nimh.nih.gov
Part of the National Institutes of Health (U.S. Department of Health and Human Services). Provides up-to-date research and information pertaining to a wide variety of wellness topics.

Stress Busters
www.stressrelease.com/strssbus.html
Site dedicated to reducing workplace stress. Includes stress-building beliefs and stress-busting techniques.

Stress, Depression, Anxiety, Sleep Problems, and Drug Use
www.teachhealth.com
Provides information on recognizing stress and the biological bases of stress, a stress test, and stress management techniques.

Stress Less
www.stressless.com
Provides sources for over 1,421 stress-reducing products.

Transcendental Meditation
www.tm.org
Provides information on TM.

Web MD
www.webmd.com
Provides valuable health information and tools for managing health.

Yoga Basics
www.yogabasics.com
Provides information on newsletters and articles, has a yoga products section.

Yoga Journal
www.yogajournal.com
Provides video demonstration of the Sun Salutation and other postures. Gives information on yoga conferences, yoga products, videos, etc.

Bibliography

Barnes, V. A., et al. "Impact of Meditation on Resting and Ambulatory Blood Pressure and Heart Rate in Youth." *Psychosomatic Medicine* 66, no. 6 (November/December 2004): 909–914.

Benson, H. *The Relaxation Response.* New York: Avon Books, 1976.

Birkel, D. *Hatha Yoga: Developing the Body, Mind and Inner Self.* Dubuque, IA: Eddie Bowers, 1999.

Bluementhal, J. A., et al. "Effects of Exercise and Stress Management Training on Markers of Cardiovascular Risk in Patients with Ischemic Heart Disease." *Journal of American Medical Association* 293, no. 13 (April 13, 2005): 1626–1634.

Crady, T. "College of the Overwhelmed: The Campus Mental Health Crisis and What to Do About It." *Journal of College Student Development* 46, no. 5 (September/October 2005): 556–558.

Davidson, R. J., J. Kabat-Zinn, et al. "Alterations in Brain and Immune Function Produced by Mindfulness Meditation." *Pychosomatic Medicine* 65 (2003): 564–570.

Denollet, J. "DS14: Standard Assessment of Negative Affectivity, Social Inhibition and Type D Personality." *Psychosomatic Medicine* 67, no. 1 (2005): 89–97.

Frey, B. B., T. P. Daaleman, et al. "Measuring a Dimension of Spirituality for Health Research: Validity of the Spirituality Index of Well-Being." *Research on Aging* 27, no. 5 (September 1, 2005): 556–577.

Galper, D. I., et al. "Inverse Association Between Physical Inactivity and Mental Health in Men and Women." *Medicine and Science in Sports & Exercise* 38, no. 1 (January 2006): 173–178.

Grossman, P., et al. "Mindfulness-Based Stress Reduction and Health Benefits, a Meta-Analysis." *Journal of Psychosomatic Research* 57 (2004): 35–43.

Hampton, T. "Stress and Memory Loss." *Journal of the American Medical Association* 292, no. 23 (December 22, 2004): 2963.

Holmes, T. E., and R. H. Rahe. "The Social Readjustment Rating Scale." *Journal of Psychosomatic Research* 11 (1967): 213–219.

Hummer, R. A. "Commentary: Understanding Religious Involvements and Mortality Risk in the United States." *International Journal of Epidemiology* 34, no. 2 (April 1, 2005): 452–453.

Kabat-Zinn, John. *Wherever You Go You Are There.* New York: Hyperion, 1994.

Kobasa, S. C. "The Hardy Personality: Toward a Social Psychology of Stress and Health." In Sanders, R. S., and J. Suls, eds., *Social Psychology of Health and Illness.* Hillsdale, NJ: Erlbaum, 1982.

Kong, K., D. Birkle, et al. "p38MAP Kinase Inhibitor Reverses Stress-Induced Myocyte Dysfunction." *Journal of Applied Physiology* 98 (January 2005): 77–84.

La Forge, R. "Aligning Mind and Body: Exploring the Disciplines of Mindful Exercise." *ACSM's Health & Fitness Journal* 9, no. 5 (September/October 2005): 7–14.

Largo-Wright, E., et al. "Perceived Problem Solving, Stress, and Health Among College Students." *American Journal of Health Behavior* 29, no. 4 (July/August 2005): 360–370.

Lepore, S. J., et al. "It's Not That Bad: Challenges to Emotional Disclosure Enhance Adjustment to Stress." *Anxiety, Stress, and Coping* 17, no. 4 (December 2004): 341–361.

Lett, Robin M. "A Multidimensional Investigation of the Relationships Among Spiritual Maturity, Spiritual Experience, and Health Promoting Behaviors." Ph.D. dissertation, Ball State University, Muncie, IN, March 2002.

Maglione-Garves, C. A., et al. "Cortisol Connection: Tips on Managing Stress and Weight." *ACSM's Health & Fitness Journal* 9, no. 5 (September/October 2005): 20–23.

Miller, G. E., K. E. Freedland, et al. "Cynical Hostility, Depressive Symptoms, and the Expression of Inflammatory Risk Markers for Coronary Heart Disease." *Journal of Behavioral Medicine* 26, no. 6 (December 2003): 501–515.

Peterson, J. "Ten (Lame) Reasons People Commonly Give for Not Exercising." *ACSM's Health & Fitness Journal* 10, no. 1 (January/February): 44.

Rosch, P. J., editor-in-chief. "Can Laughter and Humor Help You Live Longer?" *Health and Stress, The Newsletter of the American Institute of Stress* (November 2005): 1–13.

Rosenthal, R. "Stressed Out: An Examination of College Students' Reactions to Stress." *Journal of College and Character,* October 12, 2000. www.collegevalues.org

Schum. J. L., R. S. Jorgensen, et al. "Trait Anger, Anger Expression, and Ambulatory Blood Pressure: A Meta-Analytic Review." *Journal of Behavioral Medicine* 26, no. 5 (October 2003): 395–415.

Scott, S. "Combating Depression with Exercise." *ACSM's Health & Fitness Journal* 9, no. 4 (July/August 2005) 3–33.

Seeman, T. E., et al. "Religiosity/Spirituality and Health, A Cristic Review of the Evidence for Biological Pathways." *American Psychology* 58, no. 1 (January 2003): 53–63.

Selye, Hans. *Stress Without Distress.* New York: Lippincott, 1984.

Tacon, A. M, et al. "Mindfulness Meditation, Anxiety Reduction, and Heart Disease: A Pilot Study." *Family and Community Health* 26, no. 1 (January 2003): 25–33.

Voelker, R. "Stress, Sleep Loss, and Substance Abuse Create Potent Recipe for College Depression." *Journal of the American Medical Association* 291, no. 18 (May 12, 2004): 2177–2179.

Wilson, G., and M. Prithard. "Comparing Sources of Stress in College Student Athletes and Non-Athletes." *Athletic Insight, The Online Journal of Sport Psychology* 7, no. 1 (March 2005).

Winterowd, C. "The Relationship of Spiritual Beliefs and Involvement With the Experience of Anger and Stress in College Students." *Journal of College Student Development* 46, no. 5 (September/October 2005): 515–529.

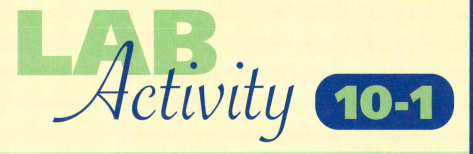

LAB Activity 10-1

Evaluation of the Life Event Stress Test

After completing the Life Event Stress Test (Table 10-2) in this chapter, answer the following questions:

1. What was your score? _____

2. What was your rating? _____

3. Discuss the results of this test in terms of its implication for your having a stress illness this year. List at least four or five factors that influence this implication.

4. Describe one of the relaxation techniques (Strategy #2) you would enjoy practicing on a regular basis. Why did you select this one?

5. List and discuss *three* stress management strategies you could incorporate into your current lifestyle. How will you do so? Be specific.

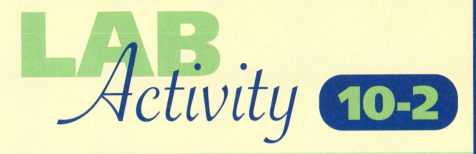

Name _____ **Class/Activity Section** _____ **Date** _____

How to Meditate and Experience the Relaxation Response

Meditation is recognized as a valuable antidote for stress. This powerful mind/body approach is a natural, nonchemical, inexpensive method to help you calm down and gain greater control over your life. Meditation relieves stress by lowering the level of the powerful stress hormones that inhibit immune function and interfere with our natural healing processes. Meditation increases body/mind relaxation by calming feelings of depression, panic, fear, and pain. Learning to meditate is a do-it-yourself self-help project. You do not need a guru, special lessons, an expensive club membership, or an expert to help you learn how to meditate. You can't simply wish to be a more relaxed person; meditation is a skill that takes commitment and practice. For meditation to be helpful, plan now to incorporate meditation into your daily schedule so that you too may profit from its numerous benefits.

Read the following helpful meditation guidelines before you begin:

1. The best times to meditate are before breakfast and before dinner. Do not meditate directly after a meal. After eating, the blood is diverted toward the stomach area, aiding the digestive process. This diversion inhibits complete relaxation.

2. Find a quiet room and sit in a comfortable chair. A straight-back chair is best because you do not want to be so comfortable that you fall asleep. Rest your arms on the arms of the chair or in your lap.

3. Wear nonrestrictive clothing while meditating or loosen your clothes.

4. Relax all your muscles as best you can without forcing it. Focus on your breathing.

5. The goal is to meditate for 20 minutes, but don't worry about meditating for a full 20 minutes at first. As you become more comfortable with the process, you will be able to progress to 20 minutes or more, twice a day.

6. Do not smoke cigarettes or drink coffee, tea, or colas before meditating. These substances are stimulants and will not promote relaxation.

7. It is helpful to disconnect the telephone. Also, *do not* set the alarm clock for 20 minutes.

8. Relax and enjoy this time. Your problems will be there when you're finished. However, they will seem less distressing after meditation if you commit yourself to the time necessary to do it.

9. Don't come out of the meditative state too abruptly.

10. Practice regularly. It takes practice to learn to sit still, meditate, relax, and calm the mind. Be patient. You won't discover the benefits unless you practice every day.

The four guidelines involved in learning how to meditate are as follows:

1. *Find a quiet environment.* Find a quiet room and sit in a comfortable chair. A straight-back chair is best because you don't want to be so comfortable that you fall asleep.
2. *Choose a comfortable position.* It is best to close your eyes (unless you are using a mental device). There should be no tension in your forehead or eyes. Breathe easily and naturally through your nose. Rest your arms on the arms of the chair or in your lap.
3. *Focus your attention on something repetitive or unchanging, such as a single word, phrase, sound, thought, or prayer (called mantras).* A fixed gazing at an unchanging object or image may also be used. For starters, though, you can keep it simple by focusing on just your breathing, feeling the air as it moves in and out. Use the breath as an anchor to bring you back when your attention is disrupted. As you gain experience, you may wish to select and use a mantra that you can focus on silently. The mantra should be easy to pronounce and short enough to repeat silently as you exhale. Focusing your attention on your breath, on a mantra, or on an unchanging object helps block out distracting thoughts and sounds that will interfere with the meditative process. Relax all your muscles as best you can without forcing it. Focus on your breathing. Now silently repeat the mantra very, very slowly without a break on every exhale. Many meditators like to use as a mantra a word, such as *one, love, calm,* or *peace,* as they slowly exhale. Use whatever feels comfortable to you.
4. *Maintain a calm, relaxed attitude.* Do not force yourself to relax or watch yourself relax; the rhythm of the mantra (or the fixed gazing) will be interrupted, and so will your relaxation period. It is normal for distracting thoughts to occur; do not worry about them–let them pass when this happens. Return your focus to the repetition of the mantra, mental device, or breathing rhythm.

Continue to meditate for approximately 20 minutes. It is recommended that you meditate twice a day for 20 minutes each time.

When you stop meditating, give your body time to adjust. Keep your eyes closed for 1 minute and let regular thoughts return. Next, open your eyes and focus on the objects in the room. Take several deep breaths. Stretch while seated. When you feel ready, stand and stretch.

MEDITATION LOG SHEET

Practice meditating for 1 week. Use the following log to record the time of day, the location, the length of time, and comments about the meditative session. Make copies of this log form as needed.

Day	Time of Day	Location	Length of Meditation	Comments
Sunday				
Monday				
Tuesday				
Wednesday				
Thursday				
Friday				
Saturday				

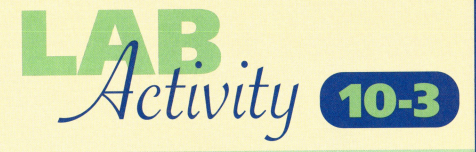

Becoming Stress-Resistant and Hardy

List two ways your "hardiness" can be strengthened in each of the following categories:

1. *Control:* Do you feel you are in control of your life? List at least two ways you can gain more control. (Example: Plot out the courses you need to complete your degree, semester by semester.)

2. *Commitment (task involvement):* How can you build commitment in your life (e.g., family, friends, studies, work, community)? List at least two ways to improve commitment. (Example: I will complete my nursing degree by 20_.)

3. *Challenge:* Do you see changes and/or setbacks as challenges instead of stumbling blocks? Give at least two examples that have occurred recently or list two strategies you can use in the future. (Example: So I didn't do well on this anatomy pop quiz. . . . Now I know that I need to study daily, go for tutoring, and/or go to study sessions for this course.)

4. *Choices in lifestyle:* How healthy is your current lifestyle? List at least two improvements you can make in your lifestyle. (Example: I will get at least 8 hours of sleep every night for 2 weeks.)

5. *Connectedness:* Do you have anyone you can count on for emotional support? Do you feel *connected* with at least one other person or group? Do you have close friends and family members? List at least two ways to improve connectedness. (Example: Twice a week I will either e-mail, telephone, or write a note to keep in touch with friends I rarely get to see.)

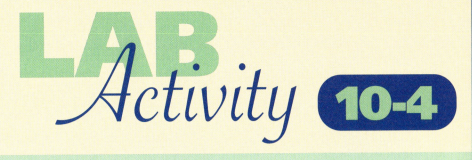

LAB Activity 10-4

Relaxation

There are many ways to relax—meditation, progressive relaxation, autogenic training, and imagery. Hatha yoga, massage, and abdominal breathing are excellent tension relievers too. You cannot simply wish to become a more relaxed person. Becoming relaxed is a *skill* that takes *commitment* and *practice*. Make the commitment now!

Choose any relaxation technique in Strategy #2 in Chapter 10 and practice it for 20 minutes every day for 1 week. Then respond to the following questions. Before you begin, rate your current ability to relax. How good are you at relaxing? Mark the line where you would rate your current relaxation skill:

Very Poor	Poor	Average	Good	Excellent

1. How often do you practice relaxation now? Circle one: never, once in a while, every day. Explain (i.e., why don't you practice relaxation, what method do you use, how often do you practice?):

2. Do you believe you could benefit by improving your ability to relax? Explain your response.

3. Which relaxation technique did you choose to practice? Why did you select this technique? Describe your experience with this technique (i.e., how you felt before and after).

4. Did this technique help you feel relaxed? Why or why not?

5. Is this a skill you feel you can use to manage the stress in your daily life? Explain.

6. Would you like to try any of the other techniques? If so, which ones and why?

7. Do you think relaxation is important in the management of your stress? Why or why not?

8. Take the Life Event Stress Test (Table 10-2). What was your score? _____ What was your implication for illness? Discuss why and give two ways you can more effectively manage the stress in your life.

9. What role does diet play in the total stress picture in your life? List three ways you can improve the diet-stress connection in your everyday life.

10. List the top two daily hassles and top two daily uplifts in your life.

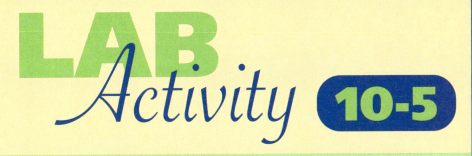

LAB Activity 10-5

Measuring Your Stress and Coping Skills

This is a four-part test. The first three parts are designed to give you an indication of how vulnerable you might be to certain types of stress and make you aware of how they might affect you. The last part of the test will provide you with information on how to cope with stressful situations.

Part I

Choose the most appropriate answer for each of the 10 questions.

	a. Almost always true	b. Usually true	c. Usually false	d. Almost always false
1. When I can't do something my way, I simply adjust and do it the easiest way.	—	—	—	—
2. I get upset when someone in front of me drives slowly.	—	—	—	—
3. It bothers me when my plans are dependent on others.	—	—	—	—
4. Whenever possible, I tend to avoid large crowds.	—	—	—	—
5. I am uncomfortable when I have to stand in long lines.	—	—	—	—
6. Arguments upset me.	—	—	—	—
7. When my plans don't flow smoothly, I become anxious.	—	—	—	—
8. I require a lot of space in which to live and work.	—	—	—	—
9. When I am busy at a task, I hate to be disturbed.	—	—	—	—
10. I believe that it is worth waiting for all good things.	—			—
Total score				—

SCORING

For 1 and 10, a = 1, b = 2, c = 3, d = 4; for 2 through 9, a = 4, b = 3, c = 2, d = 1. This test measures your vulnerability to stress from being frustrated or inhibited. Scores in excess of 25 seem to suggest some vulnerability to this source of stress.

Part II

Check or mark the letter of the response that best answers the following 10 questions. How often do you

	a. Almost always	b. Very often	c. Seldom	d. Never
1. Find yourself with insufficient time to complete your work?	—	—	—	—
2. Find yourself becoming confused and unable to think clearly because too many things are happening at once?	—	—	—	—
3. Wish you had help to get everything done?				
4. Feel your boss/professor expects too much from you?	—	—	—	—
5. Feel your family and friends expect too much from you?	—	—	—	—
6. Find your work/school infringing on your leisure hours?	—	—	—	—
7. Find yourself doing extra work to set an example to those around you?	—	—	—	—
8. Find yourself doing extra work to impress your superiors?	—	—	—	—
9. Have to skip a meal so that you can get work completed?	—	—	—	—
10. Feel that you have too much responsibility?	—	—	—	—
Total score				—

SCORING

a = 4, b = 3, c = 2, d = 1. This test measures your vulnerability to overload, that is, to having too much to do. Scores in excess of 25 seem to indicate vulnerability to this source of stress.

Part III

Answer each question as it is generally true for you.

	a. Almost always true	b. Usually true	c. Usually false	d. Almost always false
1. I hate to wait in lines.				
2. I often find myself racing against the clock to save time.	—	—	—	—
3. I become upset if I think something is taking too long.	—	—	—	—
4. When under pressure I tend to lose my temper.	—	—	—	—
5. My friends tell me that I tend to get irritated easily.	—	—	—	—
6. I seldom like to do anything unless I can make it competitive.	—	—	—	—
7. When something must be done, I'm the first to begin even though the details may still need to be worked out.	—	—	—	—
8. When I make a mistake, it is usually because I've rushed into something without giving it enough thought and planning.	—	—	—	—
9. Whenever possible, I try to do two things at once, such as eating while working or planning while driving or bathing.	—	—	—	—
10. When I go on a vacation, I usually take along some work to do just in case I get a chance.	—	—	—	—
Total score				—

SCORING

a = 4, b = 3, c = 2, d = 1. This test measures the presence of compulsive, time-urgent, and excessively aggressive behavioral traits. Scores in excess of 25 suggest the presence of one or more of these traits.

Part IV

This scale was created largely on the basis of results compiled by clinicians and researchers who sought to identify how individuals cope with stress. This scale is an educational tool, not a clinical instrument. Its purpose therefore is to inform you of ways in which you can effectively and healthfully cope with the stress in your life. At the same time, through a point system, it will give you some indication of the relative desirability of the coping strategies you are using. Simply follow the instructions given for each of the 14 items listed. Total your points when you have completed all the items.

1. Give yourself 10 points if you feel that you have a supportive family. _____

2. Give yourself 10 points if you actively pursue a hobby. _____

3. Give yourself 10 points if you belong to a social or activity group (other than your family) that meets at least once a month. _____

4. Give yourself 15 points if you are within 5 pounds of your ideal body weight, considering your height and bone structure. _____

5. Give yourself 15 points if you practice some form of deep relaxation at least three times a week. Deep relaxation exercises include meditation, imagery, and yoga. _____

6. Give yourself 5 points for each time you exercise 30 minutes or longer during an average week. _____

7. Give yourself 5 points for each day you consume at least five servings of fruits and vegetables during an average week. _____

8. Give yourself 5 points if you do something just for yourself that you really enjoy during an average week. _____

9. Give yourself 10 points if you have a place in your home/department/residence hall you can go to in order to relax and/or be alone. _____

10. Give yourself 10 points if you practice time management techniques in your daily life. _____

11. Subtract 10 points for each pack of cigarettes you smoke during an average day. _____

12. Subtract 5 points for each evening during an average week that you take any form of medication or chemical (including alcohol) to help you sleep. _____

13. Subtract 10 points for each day during an average week that you consume any form of medication or chemical substance (including alcohol) to reduce your anxiety or calm you down. _____

14. Subtract 5 points for each evening during an average week that you bring work home—work that was meant to be done at your place of employment. (This does not include schoolwork.) _____

Total score _____

SCORING

Now calculate your total score. A perfect score would be 115 points or more. If you scored in the range of 50 to 60, you probably have an adequate collection of coping strategies for most common sources of stress. You should keep in mind, however, that the higher your score, the greater your ability to cope with stress in an effective and healthful manner.

Source: Daniel Girdano and George S. Everly, *Controlling Stress and Tension: A Holistic Approach*, © 1979, pp. 62, 67, 108–109. Adapted by permission of Prentice-Hall, Englewood Cliffs, New Jersey.

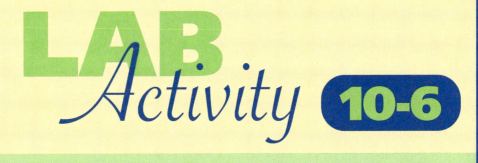

LAB *Activity* 10-6

Time Management

I. LIFETIME AND YEARLY GOALS

Read the time management strategies in Chapter 10 (Strategy 3b). Complete sections A and B before proceeding to parts II and III.

A. *Setting lifetime goals.* List three to five goals you wish to accomplish in your lifetime. Next, prioritize them by numbering them from 1 to 5:

-
-
-
-
-

B. *Setting yearly goals.* List three to five goals you wish to accomplish this year. Next, prioritize them by numbering them from 1 to 5:

-
-
-
-

Keep Part I to review at a later date.

II. DAILY TIME STUDY LOG (Make copies of this form as needed.)

Analyze how you spend your time by keeping a daily log for 1 week. Record at half-hour intervals the activities you do. At the end of each day, use a highlighter to identify the times of the day you feel were wasted. Then plan for tomorrow in regard to how to correct the wasted time and how to be more productive.

7:00 A.M.	7:00 P.M.
7:30 A.M.	7:30 P.M.
8:00 A.M.	8:00 P.M.
8:30 A.M.	8:30 P.M.
9:00 A.M.	9:00 P.M.
9:30 A.M.	9:30 P.M.
10:00 A.M.	10:00 P.M.
10:30 A.M.	10:30 P.M.
11:00 A.M.	11:00 P.M.
11:30 A.M.	11:30 P.M.
Noon	Midnight
12:30 P.M.	12:30 A.M.
1:00 P.M.	1:00 A.M.
1:30 P.M.	1:30 A.M.
2:00 P.M.	2:00 A.M.
2:30 P.M.	2:30 A.M.
3:00 P.M.	3:00 A.M.
3:30 P.M.	3:30 A.M.
4:00 P.M.	4:00 A.M.
4:30 P.M.	4:30 A.M.
5:00 P.M.	5:00 A.M.
5:30 P.M.	5:30 A.M.
6:00 P.M.	6:00 A.M.
6:30 P.M.	6:30 A.M.

III. WEEKLY GOALS

A. *Set goals:* Think through the entire week and list the specific goals you wish to accomplish (or tasks you wish to complete) this week. Schedule into the week your appointments, obligations, and other responsibilities. Be sure to leave time for work projects, schoolwork, exercise, time with family and friends, and play/recreation time for you (watching TV, socializing).

-

-

-

-

-

B. *Prioritize:* To beat the negative effects of stress, you have to learn to prioritize. Not everything on your list can be number one. Prioritize the week's tasks now by numbering them from 1 to 5.

C. *Complete a weekly evaluation:* After completing the Daily Time Study Log in Part II, evaluate how successfully you managed your time this week. Explain in a few sentences how you did. What goals/tasks did not get completed? Should they be eliminated or reestablished on next week's list? Explain.

IV. DAILY PLANNING

The goal of time management is not to eliminate leisure time (time for self, family, friends, etc.); it is to eliminate life's real time wasters and redundancies.

A. *Analyze your time and set goals.* After completing a week of the Daily Time Study Log in Part II (analyzing how you spend your time) and establishing Weekly Goals in Part III, you are ready to begin daily planning. Look over the goals and tasks you have prioritized for the week. Include any of them you want to check off today. Write the goals/tasks that must get done today on the "Must do" list (no more than five items on this list). This way you are more likely to get all the things done and will feel a greater sense of accomplishment and control. The ones you would like to take care of today put on the "Maybe" list, and those you would like to complete if all items are completed on the first and second lists put on the "If possible" list. Be sure to schedule into the day appointments, meetings, study time, exercise, recreation (and/or time to do nothing), and errands. Make extra copies of this form as needed.

B. *Prioritize and schedule priorities into your day.*

Must do:

-
-
-
-
-

Maybe:

-
-
-
-
-

If possible:

-
-
-
-

C. *Evaluation.* A good time manager takes 5 to 10 minutes each day to evaluate how he or she did.

1. How did you do today? Explain in a few sentences.

2. Did you check off everything on the "Must do" list? List what did not get checked off. Will it be added to tomorrow's list?

3. How did you do on the "Maybe" and "If possible" lists?

4. How many hours today did you feel were unproductive or wasted? Why? Explain in a few sentences.

5. Were you able to say no or delegate any chores that would have made too great a demand on your time? Describe.

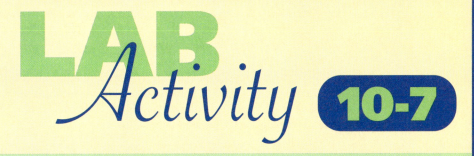

Changing Behavior Using the Transtheoretical Model

Using a highlighter, trace a path on the algorithm as you answer each question. Highlight your stage of change. Continue the activity on the back of this sheet.

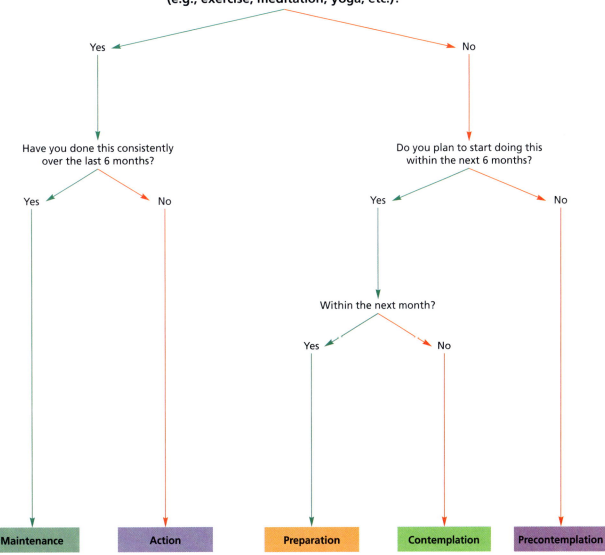

Do you use specific stress management strategies most days of the week (e.g., exercise, meditation, yoga, etc.)?

Yes

No

Have you done this consistently over the last 6 months?

Do you plan to start doing this within the next 6 months?

Yes   No

Yes   No

Within the next month?

Yes   No

Maintenance   Action   Preparation   Contemplation   Precontemplation

Once you've identified which stage of change you are in, it is important to use the processes that are most useful in progressing to the next stage or remaining in maintenance.

In the box, write your stage of change. Then list the processes that are most useful in that stage (see Figure 2-2 in Chapter 2). Use only the processes that apply to your stage of behavior change. You may not need to use all six. Under each process that you use, give two specific behavior strategies (see Table 2-1 in Chapter 2) that could help you progress to the next stage or maintain if you're in the maintenance stage.

The stage I am in =

Process 1. _____

    Behavior strategy -a.

    Behavior strategy -b.

Process 2. _____

    Behavior strategy -a.

    Behavior strategy -b.

Process 3. _____

    Behavior strategy -a.

    Behavior strategy -b.

Process 4. _____

    Behavior strategy -a.

    Behavior strategy -b.

Process 5. _____

    Behavior strategy -a.

    Behavior strategy -b.

Process 6. _____

    Behavior strategy -a.

    Behavior strategy -b.

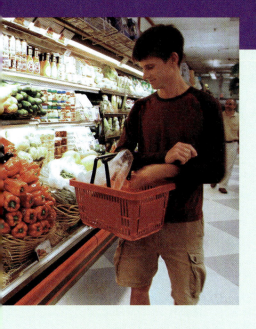

Eating for Wellness

*Let your food be your medicine,
and your medicine be your food.*
—Hippocrates

Objectives

After reading this chapter, you will be able to:
1. List the nine *2005 Dietary Guidelines for Americans*.
2. List the six major nutrients and describe their main function in the body.
3. Identify the percentages of calories recommended in the diet for carbohydrates, proteins, and fats.
4. Identify the health benefits of fiber and list good food sources of fiber.
5. Differentiate between complex and simple carbohydrates.
6. Identify the correct descriptions of cholesterol, saturated fats, monounsaturated fats, polyunsaturated fats, and trans fats and state the recommended daily limits of each.
7. Calculate fat gram allowances for specific daily calorie intakes.
8. Describe the role phytochemicals and antioxidants play in nutritional health, and identify foods high in these compounds.
9. Identify four preventive factors relating to osteoporosis.
10. Describe the USDA's MyPyramid food guidance system.
11. Give 10 specific examples of small changes that can be incorporated into daily food selections and preparations that could make a significant change in your nutritional wellness.
12. Look at a food label and identify the largest ingredient; calculate the percentage of calories that come from fat, carbohydrates, and protein; identify the sources of fat.
13. Identify three ways to eat nutritiously in a fast-food restaurant.

Terms

- antioxidants
- carbohydrates
- cholesterol
- complex carbohydrates
- fat
- fat soluble vitamins
- fiber
- free radicals
- glycemic index (GI)
- glycogen
- hydrogenation
- insoluble fiber
- ketone bodies
- lactovegetarian
- macrominerals
- minerals
- monounsaturated fat
- nutrient density
- omega-3
- osteopenia
- osteoporosis
- ovo-lactovegetarian
- phytochemicals
- phytoestrogens
- polyunsaturated fat
- protein
- saturated fat
- semivegetarian
- simple carbohydrates
- soluble fiber
- strict vegetarian (or vegan)
- trace minerals
- trans-fatty acids (trans fats)
- vitamins
- water soluble vitamins

 A Fit and Well Way of Life Online Learning Center www.mhhe.com/robbinsfitwell1e
Go to the Online Learning Center for chapter quizzes, outlines, flashcards, and additional lab activities.

*I*n a world where so many things seem out of our hands, taking control of what you eat is an important personal way to affect how you feel. Fundamental knowledge about nutrition can make a tremendous contribution to your level of wellness. It can help you make food choices that will enhance your health and vitality. This knowledge can also help you decipher social influences and messages related to eating. This is another step toward assuming self-responsibility for your well-being and health. Learning about nutrition can be exciting. Eating is a daily activity, and so you have many opportunities to affect your wellness in a positive way. Food not only sustains life but also has a clear link to *disease prevention.* Scientists are finding that certain foods (especially fruits, vegetables, and whole grains) are directly associated with the prevention of cardiovascular disease and certain cancers—the leading causes of death in our country. We are fortunate to live in a country where food is plentiful; we have wide and varied choices. We must learn, however, to make healthy choices because we live in an environment where unhealthy choices are also plentiful.

We tend to see diet as affecting only the physical dimension of wellness. Food, however, can be associated with all the dimensions. Much of our social life revolves around food. Providing food is an important sign of caring. Eating and being fed are intimately connected with our deepest feelings. Table 11-1 gives examples of how food relates to all seven dimensions of wellness. Perhaps you can think of other connections.

After reading this chapter, you should be able to make responsible food choices in your pursuit of high-level wellness. You have heard it before, but it is remarkably true: You are what you eat.

CHANGING TIMES

In the agricultural lifestyle of the past, most people grew and prepared their food. Foods were fresh and simple. Early Americans consumed much greater amounts of fresh fruits, vegetables, and grains and lesser amounts of salt, fats, refined sugars, and processed foods than Americans do today. Today's fast-paced technological society has contributed to drastic changes in the way we eat.

TABLE 11-1	*Food Is Associated with Every Dimension of Wellness*
Dimension	**How Food Is Associated**
Physical	Food is required for physiological nourishment, genetic growth, and survival.
Emotional	Food is often used as a reward, to please, to soothe feelings, and to ease depression or stress.
Social	Food is often at the heart of social events, celebrations, and family interactions.
Intellectual	Having a healthy relationship with food requires informed consumerism, knowledge about the science of nutrition and sound dietary principles, and the ability to read food labels.
Spiritual	Food is used in rituals and is part of spiritual cleansing. Abstention from eating or eating particular foods often accompanies spiritual growth experiences. Food is used in many death rituals throughout the world.
Environmental	The human need for food demands food and crop quality and protection from contamination, protection of the food chain, and strategies for combating world hunger.
Occupational	Food is often a part of business meetings and social gatherings and breaks at work. Also, the income generated by our occupations determines our food choices. Institutional food preparation is big business. The business of "food" provides a lot of jobs.

Dual-career and single-parent families are commonplace. As parents juggle careers, child care, social and professional meetings, education, and recreation, meals are often skipped, eaten on the run, or thrown together quickly. More than ever, meals are consumed behind the wheel of a car in what food industry experts call "dashboard dining." Even most gas stations have become mini-marts. As a result, the food preparers are often fast-food restaurants or manufacturers of frozen, processed, or snack foods. In the last 30 years our daily intake of food has dramatically shifted from at-home sit-down meals to snacking, with chips, sodas, hamburgers, french fries, and pizza leading the charge. Food preparation and advertising are big business, and the purpose of mass advertising is to sell products, not necessarily to enhance our nutrition. Supermarket shelves are lined with packaged food products bearing little resemblance to the original farm product. Most are highly processed, often

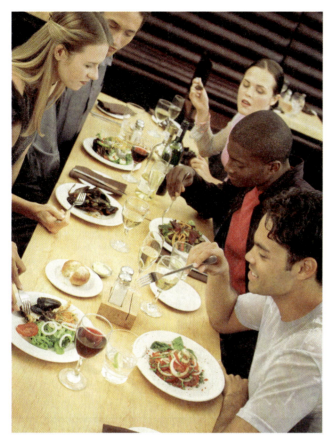

Eating is one of life's pleasures, and the choices we make can have a dramatic impact on our present and future well-being.

stripped of key nutrients. The result is a new form of malnutrition. Rather than a lack of food, we find ourselves eating too much of the wrong foods. As we have progressed from eating wheat and berries to consuming tacos and french fries, the incidence of heart disease, obesity, type 2 diabetes, and cancer has increased. This progression has also cost us our vitality and seriously compromised our immune systems.

Poor diet is said to contribute to 4 of the top 10 leading causes of death in our country. Studies repeatedly identify six shortfalls in our eating habits:

1. Too few fruits and vegetables
2. Too little fiber
3. Too much fat
4. Too many refined sugars
5. Too much food overall
6. Inadequate water intake

Take a serious look at these habits. How many of them relate to you?

A U.S. Department of Agriculture survey revealed some interesting facts about nutrition knowledge and behavior in this country. Although public awareness of the importance of nutrition continues to grow with the help of all types of media and educational materials, only 23 percent of Americans declare an interest in improving their diet. The majority know that their diet is poor but feel that healthful eating is too complicated or that they'll have to give up their favorite foods. According to government statistics, only 10 percent of the population can be classified as having a "good" diet. Television contributes to the problem by presenting mixed messages about diet and nutrition. We are exposed to hundreds of commercials for sugary, high-fat snacks, often featuring enchanting music, jingles, and appealing characters. In prime-time programming, nutrition is anything but balanced—grabbing a snack is the norm.

In college, you are faced with the perhaps new responsibility of buying and preparing your meals or making daily cafeteria or food court selections. Unfortunately, many college students are unaware of or apathetic about the implications of poor dietary habits on the future development of chronic diseases. Many young adults have been raised in the "happy meal" world of snacks and fast foods. Studies have shown that a majority of college students do not consume the recommended five to nine servings of fruits and vegetables a day, do not eat enough fiber, and eat too much saturated fat. In one study, 59 percent of students said they know their diet is worse since they started college. Unfortunately, many of these habits often continue into later adulthood. Since maintaining healthy dietary habits is essential to lifelong wellness, the college years can be a crucial time to develop healthy practices.

Healthful eating *can* be enjoyable and is easier to sustain than most people think. The underlying approach for dietary choices should be to combine basic nutrition *knowledge* with positive and practical *action*. Small, gradual changes can collectively produce substantial and sustainable dietary improvements. The purpose of this chapter is to help you begin adopting these improvements.

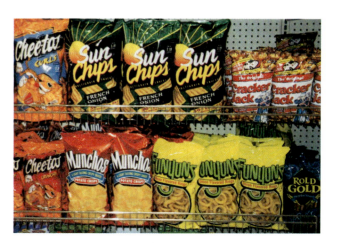

We have become a "snack food nation," consuming over $50 billion in snacks each year.

TABLE 11-2	2005 Dietary Guidelines for Americans*

1. Balance nutrients with calories.
Many people are eating too many calories yet failing to eat enough nutrient-dense foods. Limit the intake of saturated and trans fats, cholesterol, added sugars, and salt. Choose foods high in vitamins, minerals, and fiber. The USDA's MyPyramid and the DASH eating plan are good plans that translate nutrient recommendations into food choices. (Both plans are covered later in this chapter.)
2. Manage weight.
With overweight and obesity becoming a major public health problem in the United States, most Americans need to reduce the number of calories they consume. By making small daily decreases in food intake and increasing activity, gradual weight gain over time can be avoided.
3. Be physically active.
To prevent chronic diseases, engage in moderate-intensity physical activity at least 30 minutes on most days. To prevent weight gain, engage in approximately 60 minutes of moderate-intensity activity. For sustained weight loss, aim for 60–90 minutes daily of moderate-intensity activity. You can do the activity all at once or spread it out in shorter bouts throughout the day.
4. Food groups to encourage.
Eat 5–9 servings of fruits and vegetables every day. Each week aim to get a variety from all vegetable subgroups (dark green, orange, legumes, starchy vegetables, etc.). Make half of all grains eaten whole grains. Consume 3 cups of low-fat dairy per day.
5. Eat the right fats.
Consume less than 10 percent of calories of saturated fats and less than 300 mg/day of cholesterol. Keep total fat intake between 20–30 percent of calories with most coming from sources of polyunsaturated and monounsaturated fatty acids, such as fish, nuts, and vegetable oils. Limit intake of trans fats.
6. Make your carbohydrates count.
Choose fiber-rich fruits, vegetables, and whole grains often. Choose foods with less added sugars and artificial sweeteners.
7. Get less sodium and more potassium.
Consume less than 2,300 mg of sodium (approximately 1 teaspoon of salt) per day. Choose and prepare foods with little salt. At the same time, consume potassium-rich foods such as fruits and vegetables.
8. Go easy on alcoholic beverages.
If you drink, do so in moderation (no more than one drink a day for women, two for men).
9. Keep food safe to eat.
Wash hands and surfaces; keep raw and cooked foods separate; chill and defrost foods properly; avoid raw or undercooked foods.

*Recommended for healthy Americans age 2 and over.

SOURCE: U.S. Department of Health and Human Services, U.S. Department of Agriculture. *Dietary Guidelines for Americans 2005*. January 2005. www.healthierus.gov/dietaryguidelines

Dietary Guidelines for Americans

As a service to the American people, the U.S. Department of Health and Human Services publishes the *Dietary Guidelines for Americans*. Revised every 5 years, these guidelines (Table 11-2) help answer the question "What should we eat to stay healthy and prevent chronic diseases?" The guidelines reflect the newest research on diet and health relationships, with the purpose of giving *practical* suggestions on how to make healthy diet adjustments. It is impossible to specify the perfect diet for every individual. However, these guidelines point out positive directions for everyday food selections that can help you maintain optimal health. The newest guidelines also recognize the value of physical activity and the importance of weight management by giving specific guidelines for exercise and calories. In 2002, the Institute of Medicine (the scientific advisory group to the National Academy of Sciences) identified specific guidelines for us to follow. These guidelines are listed in Table 11-3.

In regard to these guidelines, nutritionists concur that the main challenge no longer is solely determining what eating patterns to recommend. It has become obvious that simply issuing and disseminating recommen-

TABLE 11-3	Daily Diet Recommendations
Cholesterol	Less than 300 mg
Carbohydrate	45–65% of calories
Protein	10–35% of calories
Total fat	20–35% of calories
Saturated fats/trans fats	Less than 10% of calories
Fiber	25 grams for women, 38 grams for men
Added sugars	Less than 25% of calories

SOURCE: National Academy of Sciences, Institute of Medicine. "Dietary Reference Intakes for Energy, Carbohydrates, Fiber, Fat, Fatty Acids, Cholesterol, Protein and Amino Acids." September 5, 2002.

dations is insufficient to produce change in most people's eating behavior. As in making most lifestyle changes, you need:

- ✔ *Knowledge* (to identify problem diet behaviors and how to improve them)
- ✔ *Motivation* (to make healthy changes)
- ✔ *A supportive environment* (to maintain changes in restaurants, supermarkets, worksite and school food services, nutrition labeling, and nutrition education in the schools)

For many, the dietary guidelines seem difficult to attain in this fast-food, grab-it-and-go world. Rather than viewing them as impossible and unrealistic, let them inspire you, not intimidate you! Remember that these are *goals*. Look for ways to shift from wherever you are now, up a few notches. For example, add an extra serving of fruit to your day; try a new vegetable at dinner; substitute low-fat yogurt for cake as a dessert; walk an extra 15 minutes after classes.

So, where are the trans fats? What constitutes a "serving" of vegetables? What qualifies as a "whole" grain? Where are the "good" fats? How do you eat out healthfully? These questions are addressed in the following sections, and we will give practical suggestions for making daily food choices that will enhance your nutritional wellness and get you closer to reaching the goals in the *Dietary Guidelines*.

NUTRITION BASICS

Your body is a priceless machine that needs fuel. This fuel should be composed of six major nutrients: carbohydrates, proteins, fats, vitamins, minerals, and water. These nutrients fulfill three main functions in the body:

1. Provide energy
2. Build and repair body tissues
3. Regulate body processes

Only the carbohydrates, fats, and proteins contribute energy or calories (kcal) to your diet. To function at optimal efficiency, you need a balance of all six of the essential nutrient groups.

Carbohydrates

Carbohydrates are the major source of energy for the body. They are the body's preferred form of energy. In fact, some cells, like brain cells, use only carbohydrates for fuel. Carbohydrates are stored in the liver and in muscles in the form of **glycogen.** It is recommended that our daily caloric intake be 45 to 65 percent carbohydrate. Carbohydrates have mistakenly earned the reputation of being fattening even though they provide only 4 calories per gram. Of course, any calories consumed in excess of body energy needs are stored as body fat. If we analyze the two types of carbohydrates, this unearned reputation can be understood. Carbohydrates, with the exception of milk sugar, come from plants. The two types are **simple carbohydrates** (sugars) and **complex carbohydrates** (starches).

Simple Carbohydrates (Sugars)

When you see the suffix *-ose* as an ingredient on a package label (as in sucrose, fructose, dextrose, and maltose)

or see *corn sweetener, corn syrup, molasses, sorbitol,* or *honey*, think *sugar*. The presence of these refined and processed sugars in our diet accounts for carbohydrates' "fattening" reputation. Instead of consuming the natural simple sugars found in fruits and milk, we consume too much of these hidden processed sugars.

The major sources of added sugars in Americans' diets are:

1. Soft drinks
2. Cakes, cookies, pies
3. Fruit ades and drinks such as fruit punch and lemonade
4. Dairy desserts such as ice cream
5. Candy

These refined sugars have been extracted from their natural sources and have little nutritional value other than the calories they contain—hence the name "empty calories." Excess sugar throws the entire body chemistry off balance, causes fatigue, and dramatically weakens the immune system for up to 6 hours after ingestion. Even if you profess not to eat sweets, you probably consume more sugar than you realize because it is hidden in so many processed foods, such as chocolate milk, ketchup, barbecue sauce, cereals, and juice drinks. Proclaimed "low-fat" foods are often loaded with added sugars. One average 12-ounce cola drink contains 10 teaspoons of sugar. Eight ounces of low-fat fruit yogurt contain 7 teaspoons of sugar. Jell-O is 83 percent sugar. Check your breakfast cereal. Some are nothing more than "candy" fortified with vitamins. Look for cereals with no more than 5 or 6 grams of added sugar per serving.

Complex Carbohydrates (Starches)

The starches are potatoes, rice, whole grains, beans, and vegetables. These foods are low in calories. They are nutritionally dense, a rich source of vitamins and minerals

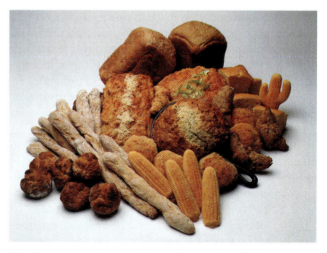

Whole-grain products are better for your health than refined flours.

that provides a steady amount of energy for many hours. What *is* fattening are the calorie-rich additives we often add to these foods (butter, sour cream, jams, gravies, sauces). Complex carbohydrates should constitute 35 to 55 percent of our total caloric intake, while simple sugars should be limited to only 10 percent. Carbohydrates supply many vital nutrients, such as vitamins, minerals, and water. In addition, they supply an important non-nutrient: dietary fiber. **Fiber** is the part of plant food that is not digested in the small intestine, where most other foods are digested and absorbed into the bloodstream. Fiber is not a single substance but a large group of widely different compounds with varied effects on the body. Formerly called *roughage* or *bulk*, fiber once was thought of primarily as a filler—it takes up room, leaving less space for high-fat, high-calorie items. That is still one of fiber's potential benefits. Even though fiber does not provide vitamins or minerals, foods that are high in fiber are often rich in vitamins and minerals. Researchers recognize that fiber plays a role in reducing the risk of heart disease, cancer, and diabetes. Look at the Top 10 "Reasons to Eat More Fiber." As you can see, a high-fiber diet contributes to health in a multitude of ways. There are two types of fiber: insoluble and soluble. Both play important roles in your nutritional health.

Insoluble fiber comes from the cell walls of plants and is not digested by the body. Insoluble fiber absorbs water as it passes through the digestive tract, increasing fecal bulk. It quickens the passage of food through the system, helping to prevent constipation. This type of fiber acts as a deterrent to digestive disorders, including cancer of the colon and rectum, because it decreases the time your system is exposed to toxic substances in waste materials. Whole-wheat bran is the richest source of insoluble fiber. This valuable bran is lost when whole-wheat flour is refined to produce white flour and wheat flour (used in most breads, crackers, and cereals). Lentils, skins of fruits and root vegetables, and leafy greens are other good sources of insoluble fiber.

Soluble fiber travels through the digestive tract in a gel-like form, pacing the absorption of carbohydrates. This prevents dramatic shifts in blood sugar levels and can help control diabetes. A diet rich in soluble fiber has also been shown to reduce blood cholesterol levels, especially LDL, thus reducing the risk of cardiovascular diseases. However, this effect occurs primarily when fiber is coupled with a diet low in saturated fats. Oat bran, beans, vegetables, and fruits are rich sources of soluble fiber, though most plant foods contain both types of fiber. Animal foods never contain fiber.

According to the American Cancer Society, approximately one-third of cancer deaths are related to what we eat. Eating between 25 and 38 grams of fiber daily is recommended (about double the amount in the current American diet). Not enough is known about how each kind of fiber (soluble and insoluble) works, and so there is no set recommended dietary ratio for ei-

TOP 10 LIST

Reasons to Eat More Fiber

1. It curbs overeating. Because fiber-filled foods take up more room in your stomach than other foods, you feel full faster.

2. It decreases your hunger. Fiber is slower to digest, and so it keeps hunger at bay longer.

3. It whisks away calories. Because most fiber leaves the body undigested, the calories in fiber-rich foods are less accessible to the body. For each gram of fiber you consume, you absorb about 7 fewer calories from food.

4. It reduces the risk for heart disease, hypertension, and high cholesterol.

5. It cuts the fat. Fiber-rich foods are naturally low in fat.

6. It may reduce the risk for type 2 diabetes. Eating fiber while reducing sugar in the diet has been linked to a more stable blood sugar and insulin control.

7. It helps keeps you regular. Fiber is called the body's "broom" because the insoluble fiber binds with water to usher waste out of the body.

8. Its sources are nutrient-dense. Fruits, vegetables, and fortified high-fiber breads and cereals are filled with tons of vitamins, minerals, and antioxidants.

9. It may protect against breast cancer. Fiber binds to estrogen—an important breast-cancer risk factor—reducing blood levels of this hormone.

10. It may protect against colon cancer. Fiber binds with and removes carcinogens from the body and speeds movement through the digestive tract.

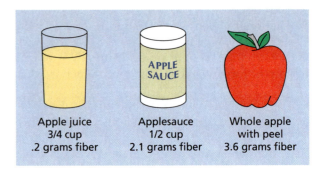

Apple juice
3/4 cup
.2 grams fiber

Applesauce
1/2 cup
2.1 grams fiber

Whole apple
with peel
3.6 grams fiber

A fiber profile.

ther type. How much is 30 grams of fiber? If you were to eat 1 cup of bran cereal, ½ cup of carrots, ½ cup of beans, a medium-size apple, and a medium-size pear in one day, you would have consumed 30 grams of fiber. Table 11-4 shows the fiber content of some common foods.

For busy students and adults, breakfast is one of the best meals to get a jump start on fiber consumption for

TABLE 11-4	*Fiber in Selected Foods*
Food	**Fiber (grams)**
Bran cereal (1/2 c.)	10
Beans, lentils, peas (1/2 c.)	6–9
Spaghetti, whole wheat (1 c.)	6
Mini-wheat cereal (1 c.)	5
Chex cereal (1 c.)	5
Cauliflower (1/2 c. cooked)	5
Pear (1 med.)	5
Sweet potato (1 med.)	5
Peas, frozen (1/2 c.)	4.5
Quick oatmeal (1/2 c. dry)	4
Popcorn (6 c.)	4
Potato, baked (1 med.)	4
Brown rice (1/2 c. cooked)	4
Berries (1/2 c.)	4
Pork and beans (1/2 c.)	4
Almonds (1/4 c.)	3.9
Apple (1 med.)	3.5
Whole wheat bread (1 slice)	3
Broccoli (1/2 c. cooked)	3
Orange (1 med.)	3
Triscuit crackers (7 crackers)	3
Spinach, canned (1/2 c.)	3
Banana (1 med.)	3
Cheerios (1 c.)	2
Corn, canned (1/2 c.)	2
White bread (1 slice)	.6
Iceberg lettuce (1 c.)	.5
Cornflakes (1 c.)	.5

the day. Check the labels of various breakfast cereals. Many have 5 or more grams of fiber per serving. Add some fresh fruit and you have a great start toward those 25 to 38 grams.

Whole Grains Versus Refined Flours

Whole grain consists of three parts: bran (outer layer), endosperm (middle layer), and germ (core). When grains are refined through processing, the bran and germ are removed. This takes away most of the nutrients and fiber. These refined flours are then used to make white bread, rolls, pasta, rice, bread sticks, pizza crusts, crackers, cereals, cookies, pretzels, etc. As a result, not all grains are created equal. Whole-grain products are nutritional powerhouses, whereas refined flours have little nutritional value. Many experts believe that Americans' overconsumption of refined flours is contributing to the explosion of obesity and type 2 diabetes, since these refined products play havoc with our insulin levels. Unfortunately, fiber has been eliminated from most snack and fast foods.

Since the *Dietary Guidelines* emphasize increased consumption of whole grains, look for whole-grain breads, bagels, pasta, cereal, crackers, and rice. Even though the outer package of a product may say "multi-grain," "seven-grain," "made with whole grain," or even "wheat," carefully check the ingredient list. Look for the words "whole grain," "whole wheat," "whole oats," "wheat bran," "oat bran," "bulgur," or "oatmeal" as the first ingredient. These are whole grains! Wheat flour, enriched wheat flour, unbleached flour, and oat flour *are not* whole grains. Enriched wheat flour is a refined grain to which the manufacturer has added back some of the vitamins that were lost during the refinement. The term "enriched," however, does not mean that fiber or other nutrients were restored. Don't be fooled by the color, also. Dark-colored breads are not always whole wheat. Manufacturers often add food coloring to refined flours to make the product darker. This does not mean refined flours are bad for you. Simply put, whole grains are a far healthier choice.

Glycemic Index

One of the newest topics in nutrition is the glycemic index. The **glycemic index (GI)** is a scale that measures the extent to which a food affects blood-glucose (sugar) levels. A food that quickly raises blood-glucose levels is said to have a *high*-GI (e.g., white bread). In the long run, a diet with a lot of high-GI foods can cause obesity, type 2 diabetes, an increased chance of some cancers, and heart disease. *Low*-GI foods (e.g., brown rice) result in a small rise in blood sugar and can help reduce fat storage and the chance of type 2 diabetes as well as raise the levels of good HDL cholesterol in some people. Whereas high-GI foods can increase your appetite, low-GI foods create more of a feeling of fullness. Common sense would suggest that all complex carbohydrates are low-GI and all simple carbohydrates are high-GI. The fact is, the distinction between simple and complex carbohydrates does not always hold true for the glycemic index level. For example, look at the following examples of high- and low-GI foods:

High GI	**Low GI**
White potato	Sweet potato
White bread or bagel	Sourdough or whole wheat bread
Instant white rice	Spaghetti
Rice cake	Beans
Pretzels	Peanuts
Total cereal	All-Bran cereal
Banana	Apple
Pop-Tart	Yogurt

If you have ever felt hungry or felt a sudden drop in blood sugar 1½ hours after eating pancakes, you've experienced the impact of eating a high-GI food. Not all nutrition experts have embraced the glycemic index as a calculator of "good" and "bad" foods. To people who suffer from fluctuations in their blood-sugar levels, however, the glycemic index may be helpful in selecting foods. For a more comprehensive list of the glycemic index of foods, log on to www.mendosa.com/gi.htm or www.glycemicindex.com or look at *The New Glucose Revolution* (see the bibliography at the end of this chapter).

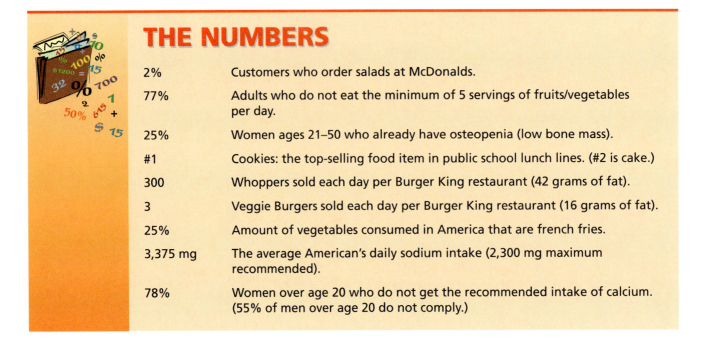

THE NUMBERS

2%	Customers who order salads at McDonalds.
77%	Adults who do not eat the minimum of 5 servings of fruits/vegetables per day.
25%	Women ages 21–50 who already have osteopenia (low bone mass).
#1	Cookies: the top-selling food item in public school lunch lines. (#2 is cake.)
300	Whoppers sold each day per Burger King restaurant (42 grams of fat).
3	Veggie Burgers sold each day per Burger King restaurant (16 grams of fat).
25%	Amount of vegetables consumed in America that are french fries.
3,375 mg	The average American's daily sodium intake (2,300 mg maximum recommended).
78%	Women over age 20 who do not get the recommended intake of calcium. (55% of men over age 20 do not comply.)

Proteins

Hundreds of different kinds of proteins make up the cells of the body. **Protein** is the major substance used to build and repair tissue, maintain chemical balance, and regulate the formation of hormones, antibodies, and enzymes. Protein can also be used as a source of energy, but only if there are not enough carbohydrates or fats available. It is not an efficient source of energy, however. When protein is broken down, the nitrogen part of the protein molecule is left. The kidneys are overworked trying to excrete this excess nitrogen. Also, if your body must rely on protein for energy, the protein is not available for building and repairing tissue—its real function.

Each gram of protein provides 4 calories of energy. We need protein daily, and most of us consume more than enough. The Institute of Medicine recommends that the amount of protein adults eat for good health can be 10–35 percent of total daily calories. Protein needs vary throughout the life cycle due to different growth stages. Growing children need more protein per body weight than adults do. Pregnant or lactating women, competitive athletes, and people over age 55 may need a little extra protein. Persons age 19 and older can approximate their daily protein need in grams by multiplying their weight (in pounds) by 0.36.

Example: 130-lb. person × 0.36 = 46.8 or 47 grams of protein daily
To give you an idea of how little food this is, 47 grams of protein would be:
4 oz. of meat (a piece roughly the size of your palm)
2 cups of skim milk

Example: 180-lb. person × 0.36 = 64.8 or 65 grams of protein daily
65 grams of protein could be fulfilled with:
1 cup oatmeal
1½ cups macaroni and cheese
1½ cups skim milk
1 large bowl of chili with beans

Most Americans meet or exceed the amount of protein needed. (Average consumption is about 100 grams per day.) Excessive protein (especially excessive red meat consumption) has been linked to kidney disease and some cancers.

Good sources of protein are found in animal and plant foods. Meat, poultry, fish, eggs, and milk products are good sources of animal protein. Many of these sources also contain high amounts of fat and cholesterol, and so you are wise to select some plant sources of protein: legumes (beans and peas), whole grains, pastas, rice, and seeds. These plant proteins are also a great source of fiber.

Fats

Fat is the most concentrated form of food energy, providing 9 calories per gram, more than twice the energy provided by carbohydrates and proteins. Fat adds texture and flavor to food. It helps satisfy the appetite because it is digested more slowly. Also known as *lipids*, fats are necessary for growth and healthy skin and for transporting fat soluble vitamins in the body. Fats are also linked to hormone regulation. Because of their concentrated form, fats are an efficient way to store energy. Like

TABLE 11-5		*Comparison of Fats*	
		CHARACTERISTICS	EXAMPLES
LIMIT IN THE DIET	SATURATED	Raises total cholesterol. Raises "bad" LDL cholesterol. Increases risk of heart disease. Increases risk of some cancers.	Red meats; poultry skin; coconut and palm oils; butter; cheese; luncheon meats; whole milk; hot dogs; chocolate; bacon; lard
LIMIT IN THE DIET	TRANS	Raises total cholesterol. Raises "bad" LDL cholesterol. Lowers "good" HDL cholesterol. Increases risk of heart disease. Increases risk of some cancers.	French fries and other deep-fried foods; many fast foods; stick margarine; shortenings; cookies; crackers; doughnuts; candy; pies and cakes; dips; some boxed foods such as ramen noodles
USE ONLY SMALL AMOUNTS	POLYUNSATURATED	Lowers total cholesterol. Lowers "bad" LDL cholesterol. May reduce risk of heart disease.	Corn, soybean, safflower, and sunflower oils; tub margarines; mayonnaise; salad dressings
PREFERRED CHOICES, BUT USE IN MODERATION	MONOUNSATURATED	Lowers total cholesterol. Lowers "bad" LDL cholesterol. May raise "good" HDL cholesterol. May reduce risk for heart disease. May reduce risk for some cancers.	Olive, peanut, and canola oils; avocado; olives; most nuts; peanut butter (without added hydrogenated oils)
PREFERRED CHOICES	OMEGA-3 (considered a special type of polyunsaturated fat)	Lowers total cholesterol. Lowers risk for heart disease and stroke. Inhibits atherosclerosis and inflammation in blood vessels. May lower blood pressure. Reduces blood clots. Can reduce occurrence of cancerous tumors.	Cold-water fish (salmon, tuna, halibut, mackerel, sardines, herring); lesser amounts in walnuts, flaxseed and flaxseed oil, green leafy vegetables, canola oil, wheat germ, soybeans

protein, however, fats are not a good *single* source of energy. Fats burned for energy in the absence of carbohydrates produce a toxic waste product called *ketone bodies*. *Ketosis*, a buildup of poisonous **ketone bodies,** causes fatigue and nausea and overtaxes the kidneys. Extreme cases can cause brain damage. Fat is burned more completely in the presence of carbohydrates, another reason to have a diet high in complex carbohydrates (and to avoid weight-loss diets that promote very low carbohydrate and calorie intake).

An important distinction should be made among the three types of fatty acids. Dietary fats comprise a combination of three forms—saturated, monounsaturated, and polyunsaturated. Even though they are complex mixtures, they are classified simplistically by their overall saturation and chemical structure. Canola oil, for example, is classified primarily as a monounsaturated fat, even though it is also made up partially of polyunsaturated fatty acids. Table 11-5 identifies and compares types of fats according to their primary fatty acid structure.

An easy observation shows that with a few exceptions, **saturated fats** are primarily in foods of animal origin (e.g., red meats, cheese, whole milk, hot dogs, luncheon meats), whereas most vegetable fats are unsaturated. Additionally, all animal fats contain cholesterol. (Vegetable foods have no natural presence of cholesterol.) Diets high in saturated fat have a strong link to heart disease and stroke. They elevate blood cholesterol levels, which in turn can lead to clogged arteries (atherosclerosis). **Polyunsaturated fats** come mostly from plant foods and are a healthier fat to consume. **Monounsaturated fats** also come from plant foods. When "mono" fats replace saturated fats in the diet, they not only decrease total and LDL cholesterol but also appear to raise HDLs—an added benefit.

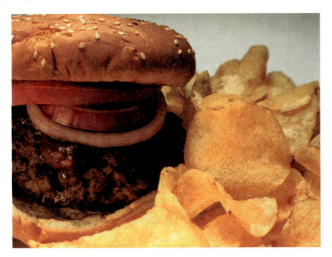

Our love for fats contributes to heart attacks, strokes, and some cancers.

Regardless of the types of fats, we need to be more discriminating in our selections. We have a tendency to eat too much total fat, saturated fat, and trans fats. Most nutritionists recommend that our daily calories consist of only 20–35 percent fat, keeping saturated and trans fats under 10 percent of our calories. The excessive fat in our diet is the main reason Americans have so many heart disease deaths. Thirty to 40 percent of cancers in men and 60 percent of cancers in women have been attributed to diet, with excessive saturated and trans fats being prime culprits. The amount and type of dietary fat eaten—not the amount of cholesterol consumed—have the greatest impact on the blood cholesterol level. Dietary cholesterol also affects the level of blood cholesterol but to a lesser and more variable extent than does the fat content of the diet.

Monounsaturated fat and polyunsaturated oils are often turned into solid unhealthy saturated fats by a manufacturing process called **hydrogenation.** This technique adds hydrogen atoms to these fats as a way to prolong the shelf life of a product and improve the texture of some foods (e.g., pastries, pie crusts, cookies). Avoid completely and partially hydrogenated oils! Like saturated fats, they elevate the blood cholesterol level. During the process of hydrogenation, some fatty acid molecules become rearranged and convert to a **transfatty acid** (sometimes called **trans fats**). Trans fats are linked to coronary artery disease and some cancers. Scientists now believe that trans fats may be more harmful than saturated fats to artery health because they raise "bad" LDL cholesterol and lower "good" HDL cholesterol in the blood—the worst possible combination! In studies at the Harvard School of Public Health, researchers discovered that persons who consumed the most trans-fatty acids had a 50 percent greater risk for heart attacks than those who consumed the least. Trans fats were also linked to increased waist size—another risk factor for heart disease. Regardless of the number of

calories consumed, trans fats appear to affect the body in a specific way to increase this harmful abdominal fat. Foods typically high in trans fats include margarine, crackers, cookies, doughnuts, pies, french fries, chips, cakes, taco shells, frostings, peanut butter, some cereals, and candy. And because foods can still be called "cholesterol-free," implying a certain healthfulness, this is misleading if they contain hydrogenated oils and trans-fatty acids. Because trans-fatty acids are present in so many manufactured foods, the U.S. Food and Drug Administration mandated that a food's level of trans fats be listed on its label beginning in 2006. The Institute of Medicine has not established a safe or recommended level of trans fat intake. However, people are urged to eat as little as possible. Many manufacturers have already begun eliminating heart-hazardous trans fats from their products as evidenced by the margarines, snacks, and baked goods that advertise on their labels "zero trans fats."

Be a wise consumer and watch out for "hidden" fats in commercially prepared foods. Whereas it is obvious that butter, oils, and the visible fat on meats have a high fat content, the fat in crackers, peanut butter, pastries, dips, sauces, and deep-fried fast foods is less obvious. It is important to be able to decipher food labels and understand where the fats are in our heavily processed food supply. Remember, "completely" or "partially hydrogenated oils" equals trans-fatty acids.

Newly developed fat substitutes (such as Olestra and Simplesse) are being used in many commercially prepared foods. These substitutes are made from soybeans or various milk and egg proteins with the purpose of duplicating the taste and texture of fat—without the caloric fat content. Read the food labels for any side effects or contraindications from these substitutes. Some can cause abdominal distress.

Regardless of the source, it is important to moderate your overall fat intake because all fats are high in calories. If a little oil is needed in food preparation, choose small amounts of olive oil or canola oil. Choose fish over red meat. And remember that a small handful of nuts can supply health benefits. Table 11-6 shows you how to figure your daily fat allowance to adhere to recommended fat-calorie guidelines.

With so much emphasis on low-fat eating, some people may try to cut their fat grams to almost zero. Remember that a little dietary fat is necessary for basic metabolic functions, especially for the absorption of fat soluble vitamins. A minimum of 10 to 20 grams per day should satisfy these requirements.

Fish Oils

Studies of the diets of Eskimos and Asian fishers have revealed interesting information about fats. Their diets provide 40 percent of daily calories from fats. Yet Eskimos are listed among the people with the lowest rates of

TABLE 11-6 *Determining Your Fat Gram Allowance*

It is recommended that we consume no more than 35 percent of our daily calories from fat. For better artery health and weight loss, 20 to 30 percent consumption is preferred. If you know your approximate daily caloric intake, it is easy to calculate your desired fat grams.

Example: Terry consumes 2,000 calories per day. He wishes to stay at a 30 percent fat-calorie guideline.

30% × 2,000 calories = 600 fat calories
600 calories ÷ 9 (calories per gram of fat) = 66.6 or 67 grams of fat

An easy way to estimate your fat gram limit per day is to divide your ideal weight in half. Keep your number of fat grams per day under this number. (If your ideal weight is 140 lb., your fat gram limit should be 70 g per day.) For people with higher weight this estimate is not quite as accurate (e.g., someone whose ideal weight is 220 lb. should probably *not* be eating 110 grams of fat each day).

FAT GRAMS PER DAY FOR SPECIFIC CALORIE INTAKES AND PERCENTAGES

Daily Calories	20%	25%	30%	35%
1,200	27g	33g	40g	47g
1,400	31g	39g	47g	54g
1,600	36g	44g	53g	62g
1,800	40g	50g	60g	70g
2,000	44g	56g	67g	78g
2,200	49g	61g	73g	86g
2,500	56g	69g	83g	97g
2,800	62g	78g	93g	109g

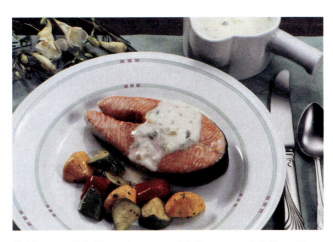

Cold-water fish like salmon are rich in omega-3 fatty acids.

heart disease in the world. Why? They eat lots of fish, and fish are rich in **omega-3** fatty acids. A diet rich in omega-3 fatty acids inhibits atherosclerosis in coronary arteries and can reduce the blood cholesterol level. Populations in countries that consume high amounts of omega-3 fatty acids from fish have lower incidences of breast, prostate, and colon cancer than people in countries that consume less omega-3s. The American Heart Association recommends eating fish twice a week to get heart-healthy omega-3 fatty acids. The best omega-3 sources are salmon, mackerel, herring, tuna, and sardines. Omega-3s are also available from plant sources such as flaxseed and walnuts.

Cholesterol

Cholesterol is not a true fat. It is a fatlike waxy substance found in animal tissue. It plays a vital role in the body's functioning. Your liver manufactures all the cholesterol that you physically need. However, most of us consume more cholesterol by eating animal products (meat, egg yolks, cheese, dairy products, shrimp, liver). A diet high in fats and cholesterol has been linked to atherosclerosis; therefore, you are prudent to limit animal products in your diet. It is recommended that you restrict cholesterol consumption to 300 mg per day. (One egg yolk equals approximately 213 mg cholesterol; a hamburger patty or chicken breast has approximately 80 mg.) Remember, vegetable foods contain no cholesterol unless it is added in processing or food preparation.

Vitamins

Vitamins are the organic catalysts necessary to initiate the body's complex metabolic functions. Although these chemical substances are vital to life, they are required in only minute amounts. Because of our adequate food supply, symptoms of vitamin deficiencies are rare. However, some factors may alter one's requirements (aging, illness, stress, pregnancy, smoking, dieting). Vitamins fall into two categories: fat soluble and water soluble. Vitamins A, D, E, and K are **fat soluble vitamins**, which means they are transported and stored by the body's fat cells and liver. They are stored in the body for relatively long periods (many months). Vitamin C and the B complexes are **water soluble vitamins.** They remain in various body tissues for a short time (usually only a few weeks). Excesses are excreted.

Minerals

Minerals are inorganic substances that are critical to many enzyme functions in the body. Two groups of minerals are necessary to the diet: macrominerals and trace minerals. **Macrominerals** are needed in large doses (more than 100 mg daily). Examples are calcium, phosphorus, magnesium, potassium, and sodium. **Trace minerals** are needed in much smaller amounts. Examples are iron, zinc, copper, iodine, fluoride, and selenium. Table 11-7 lists vitamins and minerals, their functions, good food sources of each, and adult recommendations.

Three minerals deserve special attention: calcium, iron, and sodium.

TABLE 11-7	Vitamins and Minerals			
Vitamins	**Functions**	**Sources**	**Daily Value (DV)***	**Upper Level (UL)†**
Fat Soluble				
A (retinol)	Promotes growth and repair of body tissues; keeps skin cells moist; builds resistance to infection; promotes bone and tooth development; aids in vision	Green leafy vegetables, yellow fruits and vegetables, eggs, butter, margarine, cheese, milk, liver	5,000 IU‡ or 1,500 mcg	10,000 IU
D	Regulates absorption of calcium and phosphorus; promotes normal growth of bone and teeth	Vitamin D–fortified milk products, fish, eggs, fortified margarines, sunlight (absorbed through the skin)	400 IU	2,000 IU
E (alpha-tocopherol)	Essential in preventing oxidation of other vitamins and fatty acids; maintains cell structure	Vegetable oil, green and leafy vegetables, whole grains, egg yolks, nuts, wheat germ	30 IU	1,100 IU (synthetic) 1,500 IU (natural)
K (phylloquinone)	Aids in blood clotting	Cabbage, cauliflower, spinach, green vegetables, liver, cereals	80 mcg	30,000 mcg
Water Soluble				
C (ascorbic acid)	Builds resistance to infection; aids in tissue repair and healing; involved in tooth and bone formation	Citrus fruits, strawberries, tomatoes, potatoes, melons, broccoli, peppers, cabbage	60 mg	2,000 mg
B_1 (thiamine)	Needed to convert carbohydrates into energy; promotes normal function of nervous system	Whole grains, fortified grain products, milk, pork, legumes, nuts, meats	1.5 mg	50 mg
B_2 (riboflavin)	Combines with proteins to make enzymes that affect function of eyes, skin, nervous system, and stomach	Meat, dairy products, whole grains, green leafy vegetables	1.7 mg	200 mg
B_3 (niacin)	Aids in energy production from fats and carbohydrates	Meat, poultry, fish, liver, nuts, whole grains, legumes	20 mg	35 mg
B_6 (pyridoxine)	Aids in protein metabolism and red blood cell formation	Whole grains, meat, fish, poultry, legumes, milk, green leafy vegetables	2.0 mg	100 mg
Folic acid (folacin)	Aids in red blood cell formation; aids in synthesizing genetic material	Meat, poultry, fish, eggs, broccoli, asparagus, legumes	400 mcg	1,000 mcg
B_{12} (cobalamin)	Aids in function of body cells and nervous system	Animal foods only; meat, poultry, fish, eggs, dairy products	6 mg	3,000 mcg

Calcium

Calcium is the body's most abundant mineral and is critical to many body functions. If the calcium supply in the blood is too low, the body withdraws calcium from the bones. This inadequate supply of calcium is a major factor contributing to **osteoporosis**, an age-related condition of insufficient bone mass. Healthy bone is living tissue that is continuously being replenished. Most of the adult skeleton is replaced about every 10 years. In osteoporosis, the formation of bone fails to keep pace with lost bone tissue. The result is porous, brittle bones susceptible to fracture. Women are more susceptible to os-

teoporosis because they have smaller, less dense bones. However, men are also at risk. In fact, one in four men over age 50 will break a bone as a result of osteoporosis.

According to a report from the U.S. surgeon general, roughly 10 million Americans over age 50 have osteoporosis (brittle bones). Another 34 million have **osteopenia**—a bone density that is lower than normal. "The bone health status of Americans appears to be in jeopardy, and left unchecked it is only going to get worse as the population ages," says the surgeon general. By 2020, it is predicted that half of all Americans over age 50 will be at risk for fractures from weakened bones. Os-

| TABLE 11-7 | Vitamins and Minerals (continued) | | | |

Minerals	Functions	Sources	Daily Value (DV)*	Upper Level (UL)†
Macrominerals				
Calcium	Aids in bone and tooth formation; aids in use of phosphorus, helps muscle contraction and heart function	Dairy products, green leafy vegetables, broccoli, fish	1,000 mg	2,500 mg
Phosphorus	Aids in metabolism and energy production	Dairy products, eggs, meat, fish, poultry, legumes, whole grains	1,000 mg	4,000 mg
Magnesium	Activates important enzyme reactions	Whole grains, nuts, legumes, green vegetables	400 mg	350 mg from supplements only
Potassium	Regulates body fluids and the transfer of nutrients across cell walls	Citrus fruits, juices, bananas, potatoes, spinach	4,700 mg	None
Sodium	Regulates fluid balance in cells; aids in muscle contraction	Table salt, milk, seafood (abundant in most foods except fruits)	1,500 mg	2,300 mg
Trace				
Iron	Essential for oxygen transport in the blood	Liver, meat, poultry, fish, dried fruit, whole grains, legumes, green vegetables	18 mg	45 mg
Zinc	Aids in metabolism and growth of tissue	Seafood, poultry, eggs, whole grains, vegetables	15 mg	40 mg
Copper	Involved with iron in the formation of red blood cells, affecting overall metabolism	Liver, nuts, shellfish, meat, poultry, vegetables	2 mg	10 mg
Iodine	Forms thyroid hormone	Iodized salt, seafood	150 mcg	1,100 mcg
Selenium	Necessary for normal growth and development, and for use of iodine in thyroid function; has antioxidant properties	Seafood, meat, liver, grains	70 mcg	400 mcg
Chromium	Works with insulin to help the body use blood sugar	Whole grains, bran cereals, meat, poultry, seafood	120 mcg	1,000 mcg

*Daily Value (DV): These levels, also called U.S. Recommended Daily Allowances (USRDAs), appear on food and supplement labels. There is only one DV for everyone over age 4.

†Upper level (UL): These levels are the highest levels that pose no risk. As intake increases above the UL, so does the risk of adverse effects.

‡IU = International Units.

SOURCE: National Academy of Sciences, 2002, 2004.

teoporosis is a "silent" condition because many are unaware that their bones are thinning until one breaks. Some bone loss is normal with aging in both males and females. However, osteoporosis is *not* part of normal aging. Therefore, it is vitally important that you build strong bones during young adulthood. In actuality, strong bones begin in childhood. With good nutrition and physical activity, bones can remain strong throughout a lifetime. Consumption of adequate dietary calcium from preadolescence through young adulthood is one critical factor in building bone mass. Current calcium consumption is dangerously low. It's estimated that most Americans consume only 500 to 800 milligrams of calcium daily.

Your present habits determine your bone density later in life. Up to about age 25, as calcium is added to the diet, the rate at which bone is replaced is greater than the rate at which it breaks down. By age 25 to 30, you've reached your peak bone mass—the point at which your bones are as dense and strong as they'll ever be. Forty to 60 percent of this peak bone mass is built during the teenage years. By age 40, bone mass begins to decline slowly in both men and women. After menopause, women lose bone mass rapidly due to a drop in the estrogen level. Osteoporosis cannot be cured—it can only be prevented, or its progression delayed. That is why it is critical that teens and young adults take action to build as much bone mass as possible while they are

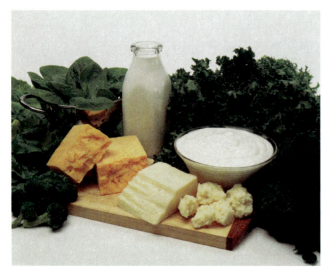

Dairy products are not the only sources of calcium in the diet.

young to slow the rate of bone loss later in life. The number of cases of osteoporosis will continue to sky-rocket if today's young adults don't adjust their diets and exercise habits. See Table 11-8 for the recommended calcium intake for various age groups. A negative balance of only 50–100 mg of calcium per day over a long period of time is sufficient to produce osteoporosis.

TABLE 11-8	Optimal Calcium Requirements (Recommendations of the National Institutes of Health)

Age	Calcium (mg/day)
1–3	500
4–8	800
9–18	1,300
19–50	1,000
51 and older (men)	1,200
51 and older (women)	1,500

For your information:

1 cup yogurt = 300 mg	1 cup cottage cheese = 150 mg
1 cup milk = 300 mg	1½ oz. hard cheese = 350 mg
1 cup cooked broccoli = 90 mg	3 oz. sardines = 370 mg
1/2 cup ice cream or frozen yogurt = 100 mg	4 oz. tofu = 145 mg
	1 slice whole-wheat bread = 25 mg
1/2 cup spinach = 100 mg	
8 oz. orange juice with calcium = 350 mg	1 packet instant oatmeal = 150 mg
1/3 cup nonfat dry milk = 300 mg	1 cup kale = 180 mg
3/4 cup Total cereal = 1,000 mg	1 Viactiv soft chew = 500 mg

Note: Your body absorbs only 500 mg of calcium at a time, so spread your intake throughout the day.

Food labels list calcium content as "% Daily Value." To convert to milligrams (mg) of calcium, add a zero. For example, if one serving has 15% DV for calcium, it has 150 mg.

Recent studies show that calcium isn't the only factor in creating strong bones. Other dietary and lifestyle habits contribute to bone health. To keep your bone "banks" filled, check out the Top 10 List below.

TOP 10 LIST

Ways to Keep Your Bone "Banks" Filled

1. Eat calcium-rich foods every day—low-fat dairy products, spinach, hard cheeses, broccoli, fish with edible bones (salmon, sardines). Sprinkle nonfat dry milk into casseroles, soups, meat loaf, and sauces.

2. Get regular vigorous exercise. Exercises that create muscular contraction and gravitational pull on the long bones or create weight-bearing impact are the best (jogging, aerobics, weight training, tennis, jumping rope).

3. Ingesting an adequate amount of vitamin D is necessary for bones to absorb calcium. Getting 400 IU/daily of vitamin D is critical for bone health. Older people should probably get more, especially if they get little sun exposure.

4. Do not smoke. Smoking reduces the production of estrogen and negatively affects calcium absorption.

5. Avoid excesses of alcohol and sodium. Both increase urinary loss of calcium.

6. Watch your protein intake. Eating excessive protein can cause urinary calcium excretion if calcium and vitamin D intake is low. Because of this, the popular high-protein, low-carbohydrate diets can contribute to dissolution of bone if inadequate amounts of calcium and vitamin D are consumed.

7. Limit consumption of soft drinks. Today's young adults have tripled their consumption of soft drinks and cut their consumption of milk by more than 40 percent, robbing them of bone-building calcium during this critical stage of bone formation. The risk? More bone fractures and a future of osteoporosis.

8. If you have lactose intolerance (trouble digesting dairy products), lactose-free products are available at some stores. Or experiment with dairy foods lowest in lactose: ricotta, mozzarella, parmesan, American, and cheddar cheeses; tofu; some yogurts; sherbet; 1 percent low-fat cottage cheese.

9. Look for calcium-fortified foods such as orange juice and cereals.

10. Consider a calcium supplement—ideally in the form of calcium citrate, the most readily absorbed form.

Iron

Iron deficiency is a nutritional problem for some people, particularly women, teenagers, and endurance athletes. Due to menstruation, women need to ingest more iron than men do. Iron deficiency may cause chronic fatigue and listlessness. To increase your iron intake, take the following steps:

1. Eat foods rich in iron (lean meats, poultry, fish, fortified cereals and grains, green vegetables, beans, peas, and nuts).
2. Consume iron-rich foods with foods high in vitamin C to triple iron absorption (a hamburger and tomato, cereal and orange juice).
3. Keep consumption of tea and coffee under 3 cups per day (caffeine reduces the absorption of iron).
4. Use cast-iron cookware (iron is absorbed into the food in a form readily assimilated into the body).

Iron supplementation should not be done indiscriminately. Prolonged consumption of large amounts can cause a disturbance in iron metabolism for some people, contributing to atherosclerosis and heart attacks. This excessive iron buildup is more prevalent in men than in women, because women lose blood through menstruation each month. Individuals concerned about their iron level should consult a physician.

Sodium

Many people can reduce their chances of developing high blood pressure by consuming less salt. The American Heart Association and the National Academy of Sciences recommend no more than 1,500 mg of sodium per day for healthy adults. (One teaspoon of table salt contains 2,400 mg of sodium.) Most Americans consume much more than that daily, some up to 8,000 mg! We consume sodium most commonly in the form of table salt and in the processed foods we eat. Even if you never salt your food, 90 percent of processed foods contain sodium—even milk does. In this way, sodium becomes "hidden" in our diet. Boxed rice dishes, pizza, soups, frozen dinners, luncheon meats, and many snacks are loaded with salt. Sodium is also present in other popular condiments, such as monosodium glutamate (MSG), meat tenderizer, ketchup, salsa, soy sauce, mustard, barbecue sauce, and salad dressings. It is even present in many medications—antacids, for instance. Fast-food restaurants are "salt mines." Eating a breakfast biscuit with egg and sausage adds up to 1,200 mg of sodium. Excess sodium consumption has been one factor linked to hypertension in some sodium-sensitive individuals. Excesses of sodium also increase calcium loss in urine, which is detrimental to bone density. Therefore, be conscious of your sodium intake and try to keep it within the recommended range.

Water

Water is often called the forgotten nutrient. However, it is *the most important* nutrient because it serves as the medium in which the other nutrients are transported. Almost all the body's metabolic reactions occur in this medium. Water also helps rid the body of wastes, aids in metabolizing stored fat, and helps control body temperature. Water composes approximately two-thirds of your body weight. Your exact percentage of water weight varies depending on your body composition. Lean tissue contains more water than does fat tissue. Lean muscle tissue is about 73 percent water; fat tissue is only 20 percent water. Being dehydrated can result in feelings of fatigue, stress, headaches, constipation, and hunger. You should drink before you feel thirsty, because thirst is a sign that you're already dehydrated. One's water needs vary, dependent on body size, activity level, and climate. Drinking water is important, but also remember that water is a component of many foods (apples, lettuce, melons, potatoes, soups, tomatoes, fruit juices, etc.). Caffeinated beverages such as coffee, tea, and colas have a slight diuretic effect but also count. Alcohol, however, dehydrates you because your body uses up water to metabolize it. Are you getting enough water? If so, your urine is clear, almost colorless. (See Chapter 7 for more information on water consumption.)

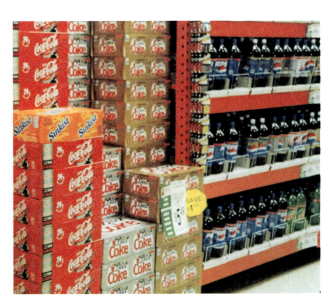

The average teenager consumes three cans of carbonated soft drinks every day. Twice as much soda as milk is consumed today; 20 years ago the reverse was true. The result? Fat teens and brittle bones.

PHYTOCHEMICALS AND ANTIOXIDANTS: DISEASE FIGHTERS

Research is exploding in a new area of dietary study: examining the power of specific food components to ward off chronic diseases. These food components, known as **phytochemicals** (meaning "plant chemicals"), are present in foods such as fruits, vegetables, grains, legumes, and seeds. Phytochemicals are also in garlic, licorice, soy, and green tea. Phytochemicals have been associated with the prevention and treatment of at least four of the leading causes of death in the United States: cancer, cardiovascular diseases, diabetes, and hypertension.

There are hundreds of helpful phytochemicals. These plant pigments and enzymes interact with hormone receptors, suppress malignant changes in cells, enhance immune function, and reduce cholesterol levels. Excitement is building in this new area of nutrition research as scientists continue to uncover the relationship between these plant chemicals and disease prevention. Phytochemicals, with peculiar names such as carotenoids, pectins, lignins, flavonoids, indoles, lycopene, quercetin, and lutein, translate into a cornucopia of fruits and vegetables. Eating a wide variety of colorful fruits and vegetables gives you a full range of these powerful internal bodyguards that help fight off everything from cataracts to cancer to arthritis.

One particular group of phytochemicals, called **phytoestrogens** (plant estrogens), have a structure similar to that of the body's own hormones. Found particularly in soy products (soy milk, soy nuts, tofu, etc.), they may reduce the long-term harmful effects of the body's own hormones, commonly associated with breast, colon, and prostate cancers. Soy products may also be linked to the reduction of blood cholesterol.

Phytochemicals, along with certain vitamins (A, C, E) and selenium, are known as antioxidants. **Antioxidants** are compounds that come to the aid of every cell in the body that faces an ongoing barrage of damage because of the normal aging and oxygenation process (living and breathing), environmental pollution, chemicals and pesticides, additives in processed foods, stress, and sun radiation. As aging and exposure occur, our bodies create **free radicals**, singlet oxygen molecules that damage our cells and tissues. This free radical assault on the body contributes to a number of chronic diseases, such as atherosclerosis, arthritis, cancer, cataracts, heart disease, stroke, and an array of other degenerative diseases. Antioxidants (phytochemicals, carotenoids, vitamins C and E, etc.) that are plentiful in fruits and vegetables neutralize these free radical chemical reactions, thereby suppressing cell deterioration and slowing the aging process.

Realizing the power of these substances, Americans need to take action by eating a wide variety of fruits and vegetables—at least five servings per day. Check out these antioxidant "all-stars":

- ✔ apples
- ✔ broccoli
- ✔ green and red peppers
- ✔ cantaloupe
- ✔ spinach
- ✔ carrots
- ✔ tomatoes
- ✔ raspberries
- ✔ onions
- ✔ grapes
- ✔ strawberries
- ✔ kale
- ✔ Brussels sprouts
- ✔ blueberries
- ✔ sweet potatoes
- ✔ cabbage
- ✔ raisins and grapes
- ✔ oranges

How many of these have you eaten in the last 3 days? Remember, an apple a day may indeed keep the doctor away!

Nutritional Supplements

Are vitamin supplements necessary? Vitamins do not contain energy or calories. Therefore, extra vitamins will not provide more energy or power. Eating a variety of foods is a preferred way to maintain an adequate intake

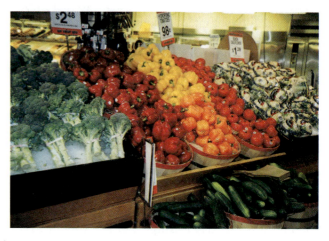

Fruits and vegetables are true "disease fighters." Yet a majority of adults admit to eating only one or two servings per day.

of vitamins, minerals, fiber, and other nutrients. However, with today's lifestyle, most people are not consuming a varied and balanced diet. Manufacturers' processing and preserving, food irradiation and chemical pollution, nutrient-depleted soil, and shipping and storage practices have significantly reduced the nutritional value of foods. Other lifestyle factors, such as smoking, consuming alcohol, stress, and using drugs such as aspirin and oral contraceptives, may increase the need for vitamin or mineral supplementation. Most medical authorities have been reluctant to recommend supplements on a broad scale for healthy people who eat healthy diets. After all, the benefits from food are more complex than merely delivering so many milligrams of this or that nutrient. However, the accumulation of research in recent years has shown that extra amounts of certain vitamins (especially the antioxidants) may play a significant role in preventing chronic diseases such as heart disease and cancer. Also, because most Americans aren't eating enough fruits, vegetables, and whole grains, supplements of vitamin B_{12}, vitamin D, folic acid, vitamin E, and calcium are most common. And frankly, some of these nutrients are hard to get in sufficent quantities from food alone. Anyone with irregular diet patterns, those on a weight-reduction regimen, pregnant or lactating women, strict vegetarians, and elderly people should consider a nutritional supplement or multivitamin. This could offer some nutritional insurance.

In fact, the *Journal of the American Medical Association* issued a report based on a review of more than 30 years of scientific studies that acknowledged that all adults should take a daily multivitamin. This statement is a startling reversal of the medical community's past denial of the need for dietary supplements. However, it is also important to realize that not all supplements are created equal. Not only are people taking vitamin and mineral supplements, but herbs, enzymes, amino acids, human growth hormones, energy and sexual enhancers, and diet pills are flying off drugstore shelves. In the United States, supplements are not considered "drugs," thereby escaping the scrutiny of the U.S. Food and Drug Administration (FDA). However, a 2003 ruling by the FDA forces manufacturers to label their products accurately to ensure that what's written on the label is what's actually contained in the product. In the past, approximately 15 percent of supplements contained either too much or too little of the stated ingredients or contained contaminants. Companies are also now prohibited from making disease claims in their advertising or on their labels such as "cures cancer" and "lowers cholesterol." More regulations are pending in Congress because illnesses and deaths have occurred as a result of people misusing supplements. Remember that dietary supplements are not a substitute for a healthy diet. Nutrient and nutrient-food interactions are so complex that merely relying on pills to fill in all the gaps would be a

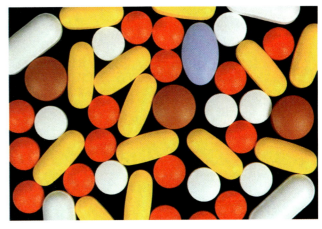

Taking supplements cannot replace a balanced diet but can fill some specific nutritional gaps for some people.

mistake. Therefore, consider the following suggestions if you choose to take a supplement:

1. Look for the seal from the United States Pharmacopoeia (USP) that sets safety and purity standards.
2. Buy from an established company rather than from a late-night infomercial provider.
3. Check the label for a company website or telephone number. Does the company have a Current Good Manufacturing Practices (CGMP) certification and/or a National Nutrition Foods Association (NNFA) rating?
4. Educate yourself about the supplements you take (see Internet Resources at the end of this chapter).
5. Talk to your physician, since some supplements may interact with the prescription medicines you are taking.

THE WELL-BALANCED DIET

Eating healthy is exciting. Nutritious eating does not doom you to "nutrition martyrdom"—eating flavorless foods, counting grams, or passing up favorite desserts. Eating right means having a wide variety of foods, some in moderation, throughout the week. There are no "forbidden" or "bad" foods—only bad eating habits. If you have a high-fat snack one day, make sure to balance it with low-fat foods at other meals. Eating should remain one of life's pleasures. Americans are fortunate to have food choices that are varied, plentiful, and safe to eat. Nutritionists often refer to three words when attempting to simplify the principles of good nutrition: *variety, moderation,* and *balance.* Do you eat the same thing for breakfast every day? For lunch? For snacks? Despite our access to diverse foods, we have a tendency to consume relatively few types of foods and often become locked into standard meals that often are culturally influenced. Why

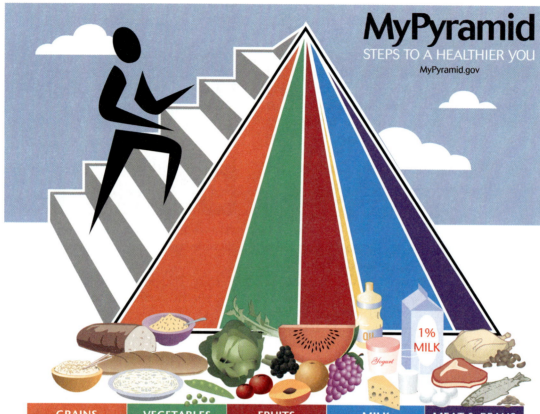

MyPyramid
STEPS TO A HEALTHIER YOU
MyPyramid.gov

GRAINS	VEGETABLES	FRUITS	MILK	MEAT & BEANS
Make at least *half* your grains "whole." 1 oz. is equivalent to: 1 slice bread; 1 c. dry cereal; ½ c. cooked rice, cereal, or pasta; ½ bagel, English muffin, or bun; 1 4½" pancake; 3 c. popcorn; 1 6" tortilla; 1 small muffin	Eat a variety of vegetables: dark green; orange; beans, peas, and lentils. A ½ c. equivalent is: ½ c. raw or cooked vegetables; 1 c. raw leafy vegetables; ½ c. vegetable juice	Choose fresh, frozen, canned, or dried fruits rather than fruit juices. A ½ c. equivalent is: 1 small whole fruit; ½ c. canned, frozen, or fresh fruit; ½ c. 100% fruit juice; ¼ c. dried fruit	Choose fat-free or low-fat milk, yogurt, and cottage cheese. Choose lower-fat cheeses. 1½ oz. cheese is equivalent to 1 c. milk	Choose lean meat, poultry, or fish—baked, broiled, or grilled. 1 oz. is equivalent to: 1 oz. cooked meat; 1 T. peanut butter; ¼ c. dry peas, beans, or lentils; 1 egg; ½ oz. nuts
2,000-calorie diet = 6 oz. daily	2½ c. daily	2 c. daily	3 c. daily	5½ oz. daily
2,400-calorie diet = 8 oz. daily	3 c. daily	2 c. daily	3 c. daily	6½ oz. daily
2,800-calorie diet = 10 oz. daily	3½ c. daily	2½ c. daily	3 c. daily	7 oz. daily

Oils:

The USDA recommendation that corresponds to the thin, yellow stripe is that "most of your fat sources come from fish, nuts, and vegetable oils" and that you "limit solid fats like butter, stick margarine, shortening and lard."

Physical activity:

Find your balance between food and physical activity
- Be sure to stay within your daily calorie needs.
- Be physically active for at least 30 minutes most days of the week.
- About 60 minutes a day of physical activity may be needed to prevent weight gain.
- For sustaining weight loss, at least 60 to 90 minutes a day of physical activity may be required.
- Children and teenagers should be physically active for 60 minutes every day, or most days.

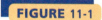

FIGURE 11-1 The USDA MyPyramid. Specific pyramids for 12 different caloric levels are available at www.MyPyramid.gov. Source: U.S. Department of Agriculture, Center for Nutrition Policy and Promotion, April 2005.

not have rice, chili, or pizza for breakfast rather than eggs, bacon, and donuts? The *2005 Dietary Guidelines* provides a sound framework for helping us make food choices.

USDA's MyPyramid

In 2005, the U.S. Department of Agriculture (USDA) introduced a new food guidance system as a graphic companion to the *2005 Dietary Guidelines for Americans*. Called MyPyramid, the graphic replaces the old food guide pyramid. The multicolored stripes that run from the bottom of the pyramid up to its apex represent the spectrum of food choices, with the width of each stripe approximating the quantity of food each of us should consume from each group (e.g., the green "vegetables" stripe is much wider than the purple "meat & beans" stripe). By showing a person climbing the steps at the side of the new pyramid, physical activity is emphasized as an essential link with healthy eating as key components of healthy living. MyPyramid is actually 12 different pyramids. It was designed to be personalized, based on varying ages, genders, and activity levels.

The website, www.MyPyramid.gov, allows you to enter your personal data and then view your customized pyramid. Figure 11-1 shows the USDA MyPyramid with a few example guidelines—based on a 2,000-, 2,400-, and 2,800-calorie diet. In viewing the pyramid, pay attention to the recommended serving sizes. For example, a single restaurant serving of pasta may actually be 5 ounces of grains (2½ cups)! And, if it is made of refined flour, it does not count as a "whole" grain. MyPyramid.gov has many tools to help you plan your diet—lists of foods in each striped category, tracking worksheets, specific serving size guidelines, and more. Visit MyPyramid.gov to learn more about your personalized eating plan. Lab Activity 11-2 allows you to explore your pyramid in depth.

MyPyramid is meant to be not a rigid prescription but a general guide for eating a variety of foods. Fats and sugars are sometimes added to grains, fruits, and vegetables (with sauces, toppings, and preparation methods), making them less healthy choices. For example, having a buttery alfredo sauce on pasta is not as healthy as having a tomato-rich marinara sauce. In the dairy group, a glass of skim milk would be healthier than a milk shake. For fruit, apple pie has more fat and calories than an apple. Also remember that there are "good" fats such as omega-3s and that whole-wheat grains are healthier than white flour grains. Thus, it is up to you to make wise choices within each food group.

As you evaluate your diet, use the Top 10 List on how to add more fruits and vegetables to your day. Also, since most people underestimate the size of their food portions, train your eye to estimate what a cup, an ounce, or a tablespoon is. By using Table 11-9, "Eyeball Your Servings," you can get a quick estimate of what portions should be on your plate without carrying around measuring cups.

TOP 10 LIST

Answers to "How Am I Supposed to Eat All Those Fruits and Vegetables?"

To further promote healthy eating, the National Cancer Institute initiated a national campaign encouraging all Americans to eat five to nine servings of fruits and vegetables every day. Contrary to what most people say, with some planning it is surprisingly easy to do. Here are some suggestions for adding produce to your life:

1. Start your day with a glass of 100 percent fruit juice (not fruit "drink"). Six ounces is a serving.
2. Top your cereal or pancakes with sliced bananas, berries, apples, or raisins.
3. Create a veggie omelette, pizza, pita sandwich, or burrito.
4. Iceberg lettuce is the least nutritious of vegetable greens. Try romaine, spinach, red leaf, chicory—add other veggies.
5. Add chopped fruits to yogurt or pudding and as an ice cream topping; make a fruit smoothie using skim milk and fruit.
6. Add tomatoes, carrots, zucchini, peppers, spinach, or broccoli to pasta and rice salads and pasta sauces. Frozen or canned veggies work fine.
7. Top baked potatoes with assorted cooked veggies or salsa.
8. Fortify stews, soups, and casseroles with extra veggies (e.g., add broccoli, peppers, or peas to your standard macaroni and cheese).
9. Replace chips with raw veggies for dipping.
10. Keep dried fruits, raw veggies, and fresh fruits available for quick snacks.

TABLE 11-9 Eyeball Your Servings

Use these common references for estimating standard serving sizes:
1 cup of pasta = closed fist
3-ounce serving of meat = palm of your hand or a deck of cards
1 ounce cheese = size of your thumb or four dice
1 medium potato = computer mouse
2 tablespoons peanut butter = golf ball
½ cup rice or cooked vegetables = scoop of ice cream
1 standard bagel = hockey puck
1 teaspoon margarine = the tip of your thumb
1 medium orange or apple = baseball
1 muffin or dinner roll = plum
1 small cookie or cracker = poker chip

DASH Eating Plan

Because high blood pressure affects nearly one in three American adults, the National Heart, Lung, and Blood Institute has developed an eating plan that is a slight modification of MyPyramid. Called DASH (Dietary Approaches to Stop Hypertension), this eating plan has received accolades from the medical community for its effectiveness in lowering blood pressure. Since individuals with *normal* blood pressure at age 55 have a 90 percent lifetime risk of developing hypertension, the DASH plan should be considered seriously by everyone. DASH is based on the following principles:

✔ Reduction of overall fat, saturated fat, and cholesterol

TABLE 11-10	*The DASH Eating Plan*

The DASH eating plan is based on 2,000 calories a day. The number of daily servings in a food group may vary from those listed, depending on your caloric needs. Use this chart to help you plan your menus or take it with you when you go to the store.

Food Group	Daily Servings (except as noted)	Serving Sizes	Examples and Notes	Significance of Each Food Group to the DASH Eating Plan
Grains and grain products	7–8	1 slice bread 1 oz. dry cereal* 1/2 cup cooked rice, pasta, or cereal	Whole-wheat bread, English muffin, pita bread, bagel, cereals, grits, oatmeal, crackers, unsalted pretzels and popcorn	Major sources of energy and fiber
Vegetables	4–5	1 cup raw leafy vegetable 1/2 cup cooked vegetable 6 oz. vegetable juice	Tomatoes, potatoes, carrots, green peas, squash, broccoli, turnip greens, collards, kale, spinach, artichokes, green beans, lima beans, sweet potatoes	Rich sources of potassium, magnesium, and fiber
Fruits	4–5	6 oz. fruit juice 1 medium fruit 1/4 cup dried fruit 1/2 cup fresh, frozen, or canned fruit	Apricots, bananas, dates, grapes, oranges, orange juice, grapefruit, grapefruit juice, mangoes, melons, peaches, pineapples, prunes, raisins, strawberries, tangerines	Important sources of potassium, magnesium, and fiber
Low-fat or fat-free dairy foods	2–3	8 oz. milk 1 cup yogurt 1½ oz. cheese	Fat-free (skim) or low-fat (1%) milk, fat-free or low-fat buttermilk, fat-free or low-fat regular or frozen yogurt, low-fat and fat-free cheese	Major sources of calcium and protein
Meats, poultry, and fish	2 or less	3 oz. cooked meat, poultry, or fish	Select only lean; trim away visible fats; broil, roast, or boil instead of frying; remove skin from poultry	Rich sources of protein and magnesium
Nuts, seeds, and dry beans	4–5 per week	1/3 cup or 1½ oz. nuts 2 Tbsp. or 1/2 oz. seeds 1/2 cup cooked dry beans or peas	Almonds, filberts, mixed nuts, peanuts, walnuts, sunflower seeds, kidney beans, lentils	Rich sources of energy, magnesium, potassium, protein, and fiber
Fats and oils†	2–3	1 tsp. soft margarine 1 Tbsp. low-fat mayonnaise 2 Tbsp. light salad dressing 1 tsp. vegetable oil	Soft margarine, low-fat mayonnaise, light salad dressing, vegetable oil (such as olive, corn, canola, or safflower)	DASH has 27 percent of calories as fat, including fat in or added to foods
Sweets	5 per week	1 Tbsp. sugar 1 Tbsp. jelly or jam 1/2 oz. jelly beans 8 oz. lemonade	Maple syrup, sugar, jelly, jam, fruit-flavored gelatin, jelly beans, hard candy, fruit punch, sorbet, ices	Sweets should be low in fat

*Equals 1/2 to 1 1/4 cups, depending on cereal type. Check the product's Nutrition Facts label.

†Fat content changes serving counts for fats and oils. For example, 1 Tbsp. of regular salad dressing equals 1 serving; 1 Tbsp. of a low-fat dressing equals 1/2 serving; 1 Tbsp. of a fat-free dressing equals 0 servings.

SOURCE: U.S. Department of Health and Human Services. National Heart, Lung, and Blood Institute.

✔ Increased fruits, vegetables, and low-fat dairy foods
✔ Increased fiber by including whole grains
✔ Restriction of sodium
✔ Increased magnesium, potassium, and calcium (which help the body excrete excess salt)

Check out Table 11-10, which describes the DASH eating plan. Everyone could benefit by adopting many of the DASH guidelines.

Making Positive Changes

All this information about nutrition can seem confusing and sometimes appear contradictory; for example, how do you consume enough meat for iron yet reduce saturated fat? Eggs are a good source of protein, but how do you make sure daily cholesterol milligrams don't exceed 300? You certainly hear enough about what *not* to eat. We believe in a positive approach to a wellness lifestyle, and Table 11-11 gives many general tips to help you eat more nutritiously in today's fast-paced world. These suggestions are ways to incorporate the dietary guidelines into sensible and simple practices. Significant improvements in your nutritional health can be accomplished with *simple* changes. For example, using Prochaska's transtheoretical model for behavior change (see Chapter 2), participants in a research study were successful in lowering and maintaining their dietary fat intake to below 30 percent of their calories by using five specific action-based techniques:

1. Switching to low-fat or nonfat cheeses and dairy products
2. Eating bread, rolls, pancakes, and muffins without butter or margarine
3. Taking the skin off chicken
4. Using low-cal or nonfat salad dressings
5. Regularly eating fruit or veggies as snacks (grapes, raisins, carrots, bananas, etc.)

You may want to go back and review Prochaska's behavior change theory to help identify your current stage of change in regard to some of your dietary practices. Look at the specific behavior change strategies that could help you make a healthy dietary change. See Table 11-12 for one example.

People eat food, not numbers. So rather than focusing on constant measuring, counting, and weighing, dietary change should involve practical changes that can become lifetime habits. It is not advisable or possible to do a complete overhaul of your diet. It is easier, and usually more lasting, to make small and gradual changes. Realize that no one is perfect or eats perfectly all the time. You do have choices, though. If nothing else, try to select foods high in **nutrient density**. Nutrient-dense foods provide substantial nutrients (vitamins, minerals, phytochemicals, fiber, etc.) with relatively few calories,

---

TABLE 11-11   *20 Tips for Nutritional Wellness*

1. Use fresh, unprocessed foods whenever possible.
2. Remove the skin from poultry (the source of most of the saturated fat).
3. Eat low-fat dairy products.
4. Eat fish once or twice a week (baked or broiled, *not* fried or breaded).
5. Instead of focusing a meal on meat, use a small amount of meat (diced, shaved, chopped, sliced) to mix in with vegetables and rice or pasta.
6. Steam, bake, broil, or roast foods, using a cooking rack to allow fat to drain from the food.
7. Select salad oils, cooking oils, and margarines made with unsaturated fats. Soft, tub margarines with liquid oil listed as the first ingredient are good choices.
8. Use a nonstick vegetable oil spray for sautéing.
9. Use deli luncheon meats such as sliced chicken breast and turkey instead of high-fat bologna, salami, beef, or hot dogs.
10. Use applesauce in place of the oil in brownie, cake, and quick-bread recipes.
11. Use plain low-fat yogurt as a substitute for sour cream in dips and on baked potatoes. Fat-free sour cream and cream cheese are also available. Evaporated skim milk can substitute for cream in recipes.
12. Eat a meatless dinner several nights a week.
13. Use ground turkey or soy-based crumbles in casseroles, chili, spaghetti sauce, tacos, and skillet dinners that normally require ground beef.
14. When making scrambled eggs, separate the eggs, eliminating half the yolks. If a recipe calls for one egg, substitute two egg whites to reduce the cholesterol.
15. Decrease at least by half the margarine or butter called for in preparing packaged rice and pasta mixes (with minimal effect on taste).
16. Take advantage of nonfat chips, dips, snacks, cereals, cookies, and crackers that are appearing on grocery shelves almost daily. (Remember, however, that "no fat" doesn't necessarily mean "no calories.")
17. Try canned fruit with natural juices as a tasty topping for pancakes and french toast, rather than butter and syrup.
18. Top pizzas, baked potatoes, and stuffed burritos with broccoli, mushrooms, zucchini, peppers, salsa, or onions rather than meats.
19. Try powdered "nonbutter" sprinkles or "butterlike" sprays as toppings for vegetables.
20. Use breads and cereals that list 100 percent whole wheat or "whole grain" as the first ingredient.

TABLE 11-12	*Tips for Behavior Change: Eating Five to Nine Servings of Fruits/Vegetables Every Day*

STAGES OF CHANGE: IN WHAT STAGE ARE YOU?

1. Precontemplation: "I don't like fruits and vegetables, and I'm in good health. So why would I want to eat them?"
2. Contemplation: "I realize fruits and vegetables have a lot of nutritional value and could probably cut my risk of future chronic diseases."
3. Preparation: "I've been spending more time in the produce section of the grocery store, learning more about different fruits. I have even started buying and trying some new kinds."
4. Action: "I have been eating five servings every day for about 2 months."
5. Maintenance: "I eat at least seven servings (sometimes more!) every day and have done so for over 6 months. I can't imagine not eating them every day!"

PROCESSES OF CHANGE

After identifying your current stage, try using some of the following selected processes and behavior strategies appropriate for your particular stage to facilitate your transition into the next stage (refer to Figure 2-2).

- Consciousness-raising: Read about health benefits of eating fruits and vegetables.
- Social liberation: Investigate new fruits and vegetables at the grocery store and new recipes.
- Self-reevaluation: Write down pros and cons of making this major dietary change.
- Self-liberation: Map out a plan (e.g., drink a glass of juice and slice a banana onto cereal at breakfast; carry an apple in backpack for a snack; have a green vegetable at dinner every night; snack on grapes, carrot sticks, or other fruits/veggies while studying).
- Reward: Treat yourself to a rich fruit dessert once a week (cobbler, pie, etc.).
- Environment control: Have plenty of fruits/vegetables available in room/apartment.

fat, and sugar. Examples of nutrient-dense foods are fruits, vegetables, legumes, and whole grains. These foods allow you to meet your nutritional needs without overconsuming calories. They fill you up (as opposed to "empty calorie" foods like pastries, chips, sodas, and alcohol that are high in calories and lack many nutrients).

A good way to assess your nutritional habits is to record everything you eat for 3 to 7 days in a log. By observing types and quantities of food consumed, you can best judge if your diet is nutritionally sound—that is, if it conforms to the *Dietary Guidelines* and mimics your Pyramid. Keeping a food log can help you set goals for making positive dietary changes. (There is a sample Food Log form in the Lab Activities section at the end of this chapter.) You may prefer to use one of the many computer programs or websites or the tools that accompany www.MyPyramid.gov for dietary assessment. At the end of this chapter you will find helpful websites with links to information on the nutritive values of foods, even fast foods. It may be tedious to keep records for several days, but this experience creates an awareness of food choices and quantities as well as of where improvements can be made.

Nutrition Labeling

Now that you understand the basics of nutrition, how do you find out the nutritional content of the foods you are eating? You do this by reading labels. Read about what you are eating. Part of self-responsibility is becoming a nutrition-wise consumer. The federal government regulates food labeling and requires processed and packaged foods to have uniform labels. This uniformity can help consumers make healthy choices. Study the sample label in Figure 11-2 to learn how to read a label.

Remember these points when reading labels:

1. Check serving size. You may eat two to three servings if the stated serving size is skimpy.
2. Watch for hidden sugars added to a product: syrup, sucrose, molasses, corn sweetener, dextrose, maltose, honey, and so on.
3. Check fat content. Avoid hydrogenated fats.
4. Some crackers, pastries, cookies, candies, and instant cocoas are made with coconut and palm oil, which is more saturated than beef fat.
5. Select *whole*-wheat bread ("wheat flour" means refined *white* flour—the bran and wheat germ have been removed). All whole-wheat bread is brown, but not all brown bread is whole wheat.
6. Fortified foods contain added vitamins and minerals not originally in the food or present in lower amounts. Breakfast cereals are commonly fortified. Can you name the vitamin with which milk is commonly fortified?

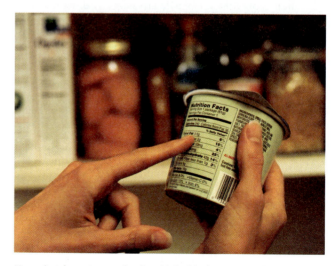

Knowing how to read a food label helps you understand how a particular food fits into your daily allowances.

Serving sizes are standardized to reflect the amounts of food people actually eat. They are also expressed in common household and metric measures. (You should note whether you are consuming more than one serving.)

With only 5g of saturated fat, and 1.5 g of trans fat, where is the rest of the 13 total grams of fat? It could be unsaturated fats, which are not currently required on a label.

This mandatory list of nutrients includes those most important to today's consumers. In the past, the concern was vitamin and mineral deficiencies. Now the worries pertain to fat, cholesterol, sodium, types of carbohydrates, and protein amounts.

This means that in a 2,000-calorie diet 65 grams is equal to 30 percent fat.

This information can help you calculate what percentage of calories of this food comes from fat, carbohydrates, and protein.

CHECK YOURSELF:
What % of calories of this food comes from fat? carbohydrates? protein?
FAT: 13 grams X 9 cal/gram = 117 fat calories. 117/261 = 45 This marcaroni and cheese is 45% fat.
CARBOHYDRATES:
31 grams X 4 cal/gram = 124 carbohydrate calories. 124/261 = .47. This macaroni and cheese is 47% carbohydrate.
PROTEIN: 5 grams x 4 cal/gram = 20 protein calories. 20/261 = .08. This macaroni and cheese is 8% protein.

MACARONI AND CHEESE
Nutrition Facts

Serving Size 1/2 cup (114g)
Servings Per Container 4

Amount Per Serving

Calories 261	Calories from Fat 117

	% Daily Value*
Total Fat 13g	**20%**
Saturated Fat 5g	25%
Trans Fat 1.5g	10%
Cholesterol 30mg	**10%**
Sodium 660mg	**28%**
Total Carbohydrate 31g	**11%**
Sugar 5g	**
Dietary Fiber 1g	4%
Protein 5g	**

Vitamin A 4% • Vitamin C 2% • Calcium 15% • Iron 4%

* Percents (%) of a Daily Value are based on a 2,000-calorie diet. Your Daily Values may vary higher or lower depending on your calorie needs:

	Calories	2,000	2,500
Total Fat	Less than	65g	80g
Sat Fat	Less than	20g	25g
Cholesterol	Less than	300mg	300mg
Sodium	Less than	2,400mg	2,400mg
Total Carbohydrate		300g	375g
Fiber		25g	30g

1g Fat = 9 calories
1g Carbohydrates = 4 calories
1g Protein = 4 calories

** No daily values have been determined for sugars and protein intake.

Ingredients: Enriched wheat flour (contains niacin, reduced iron, vitamin B$_1$, vitamin B$_2$, folic acid), cheddar cheese cultures, partially hydrogenated soybean and/or cottonseed oil, non-fat milk, salt, corn syrup, monosodium glutamate, citric acid, natural and artificial flavors, yellow 5 and 6.

% Daily Value shows how a food fits into the overall daily diet. For each item, it shows the percentage or recommended daily consumption for a person eating 2,000 calories a day (e.g., 5 grams of saturated fat is 25 percent of the *recommended* daily value of 20 grams).

No Daily Value for trans fats has been established. If a product lists 0 grams trans fat, it could still contain up to 0.5 grams per serving (but still be advertised as "trans free").

Percentage of daily requirements for selected vitamins and minerals

Recommended daily amounts of each item for two average diets. (If you eat less than 2,000 calories, you will have to adjust the Daily Values.)

Based on 10 percent consumption

Based on 60 percent consumption

Voluntary components that will be allowed on labels are calories from saturated fat, polyunsaturated fat, monounsaturated fat, potassium, soluble and insoluble fiber, sugar, alcohol, other carbohydrates, and other essential vitamins and minerals.

Ingredients are listed in descending order by weight. The ingredient in the largest quantity is always listed first.

FIGURE 11-2 How to read a food label.

7. Enriched foods have lost nutrients during processing and then have had them replaced by the manufacturers. For instance, when wheat is turned into white flour, it loses at least 50 to 80 percent of many nutrients. Of these, iron, niacin, thiamine, and riboflavin are replaced, but other nutrients lost in the milling process, such as fiber, zinc, and copper, are not restored.

EATING OUT

Eating out has become routine for many of us. One in five Americans eats in a fast-food restaurant each day. Meal preparation time at home has decreased due to changing lifestyles, and it is evident this trend will not reverse. In this fast-paced world, people want food fast. Many fast-food restaurants pride themselves on the ability to have a meal in your hands 90 seconds after you place your order. The fast-food industry is a multi-billion dollar industry, and there is considerable emphasis by food companies in getting the consumer to form an emotional bond with their products. Even though most people know the connections between diet and health, many still rate price, convenience, and taste of food as the main factors affecting their food choices. For every dollar spent by the World Health Organization on preventing the diseases caused by our industrialized, Western diet, more than $500 is spent by the food industry promoting their unhealthy foods! Most fast-food chains supply nutrient information on their food products, on their websites, or in brochures. What has this information revealed about the nutrient value of fast food? Are fast foods "junk" foods? Nutritionists have found that fast-food items do have significant amounts of some nutrients (especially protein), but many tend to be low in fiber and high in calories, sodium, and fat. How often do you rely on these foods? What other foods are you eating during the day? Occasional visits to fast-food restaurants will have little effect on the nutritive value of your total diet. In response to consumer demand, many chains have become diversified and have added many more items to their menus. Many offer healthier items such as salads and fruit. However, it is still up to you to make a wise selection. For many, it is difficult to get ample amounts of fruits, vegetables, and whole grains by eating consistently at fast-food establishments. A fast-food meal can easily total 1,600 calories, 65 grams of fat, and 1,500 milligrams of sodium. Check out the Top 10 List for suggestions on healthy eating at fast-food restaurants.

Restaurant eating in general (not only eating fast foods) has become a way of life for many. Many restaurants offer low-fat, low-calorie choices, often identified on the menu. Some list fat grams and other nutritional

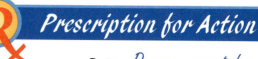

Prescription for Action

Date *Do one or more today*

✔ Eat a whole-grain cereal for breakfast and top it with fruit.
✔ Substitute skim milk, water, or 100 percent fruit juice for a sweetened soft drink.
✔ Make sure your dinner plate has two different-colored vegetables on it.
✔ Try an all-veggie pizza, burrito, wrap, or sandwich.
✔ Choose fruit for dessert or for a snack.

Prescribed by ___*YOU*___

TOP 10 LIST

Fast Tips for Fast Foods

1. At sub shops choose lean meats and avoid tuna salad, bacon, oils, regular mayonnaise, and high-fat cheeses. Try the all-veggie sub.

2. Salad bars are a wise choice for vitamins A and C and fiber; go easy on the dressings, high-fat cheeses, bacon, olives, sour cream, and refried beans. If the bar has pita bread, tacos, or tortillas, why not stuff them with veggies?

3. Potato bars are another good choice if you avoid the heavy cheese and butter-type sauces, bacon, and sour cream.

4. Chicken and fish sound healthy, but many are coated with fat. Select the baked or grilled ones without breading or skin.

5. Pizza is a great choice, especially if the toppings are vegetables; avoid pepperoni, sausage, bacon, and olives.

6. Hamburgers—order the small one instead of the "jumbo" burger. Try the veggie burger.

7. Drink skim milk or juices instead of a shake or soda.

8. When eating Mexican food, emphasize soft corn tortillas, beans, chicken, and vegetables (easy on the cheese).

9. For breakfast, avoid croissants, biscuits, sausage, bacon, butter, and the danish. Better choices are pancakes, English muffins, bagels, bran muffins, and whole-grain cereals.

10. Ask for salad dressings "on the side" and use sparingly. Select nonfat or low-fat dressings.

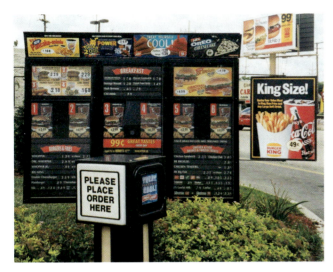

We spend almost 50 percent of our food dollars taking out, driving through, or sitting down for a restaurant meal. In comparison, in 1980 it accounted for only 25 percent of our budgets.

information. Having nutritional knowledge can help you make healthy selections. Ask the server how foods are prepared. Are they baked or fried? Can lower-fat sauces or condiments be substituted? Can the vegetable of the day be substituted for french fries? Salads are not always healthy if loaded with bacon, high-fat cheeses, and full-fat dressings. Check out the à la carte menu. Baked potatoes, salads, vegetables, and soups can often be ordered to make up a meal. Watch portion sizes. Restaurants have a tendency to feed us too much food! Split a meal with a friend or utilize the "doggie bag." When looking at your overall diet, keep your entire day's and week's intakes in perspective. No foods should be totally forbidden. Everyone enjoys an occasional burger and fries, cheesecake, or pepperoni pizza. Try to live by the "80-20 rule": 80 percent of the time eat nutritionally dense, healthy foods; 20 percent of the time indulge! Remember: *variety, moderation,* and *balance.*

SPECIAL NUTRITIONAL CONCERNS

High-level wellness means adjusting to life changes and seeking information for special situations. This section discusses dietary considerations for vegetarians, pregnant women, the elderly, and those engaging in regular, vigorous exercise.

Vegetarian Diet

For a variety of health and moral reasons, many people prefer a vegetarian diet. A vegetarian diet can be nutritious and healthy. From not eating animal foods, vege-

tarians normally have lower body fat, blood cholesterol, blood pressure, and rates of coronary heart disease than do meat eaters. They also have a lower than average risk of various cancers and type 2 diabetes because of their high consumption of beans, fruits, and vegetables. There are different vegetarian diets, however. Careful planning and food selection are important to avoid nutritional deficiencies. All vegetarian diets emphasize the use of vegetables, fruits, and grains as main staples. Some diets exclude all animal products, while some include dairy products and eggs.

Here are the types of vegetarians:

1. **Strict vegetarian** (or **vegan**) consumes only plant foods. (Vitamin B_{12} supplementation is recommended because it is not in any plant foods.)
2. **Lactovegetarian** will consume plant foods and dairy products but no meat or eggs.
3. **Ovo-lactovegetarian** will consume plant foods, dairy products, and eggs.
4. **Semivegetarian** only excludes red meat.

Meat is not essential to your diet, but protein is. Therefore, following a vegetarian diet requires careful planning and food selection to consume sufficient vitamins and minerals (especially the B vitamins, vitamin D, calcium, zinc, and iron). Search for good-quality protein sources such as legumes (beans), nuts, grains, seeds, and soybean products. A thorough knowledge of nutrition is essential. For example, combining a good source of vitamin C with whole grains and legumes will greatly enhance iron absorption from grain and legumes. Drinking fortified soy milk will help you obtain calcium and vitamin B_{12}. Vegetarians can easily adapt MyPyramid by substituting beans, nuts, tofu, peas, and veggie/soy meats in the meat category. For those who do not consume dairy, calcium can be obtained from soy milk, broccoli (and other green leafy vegetables), fortified orange juice, tofu, and almond butter. By also consistently selecting whole grains rather than refined flours, adequate vitamins and minerals can be consumed. With care, the vegetarian diet can be nutritionally complete.

Pregnancy

Many women become more nutritionally aware and eat more wisely during pregnancy. This makes sense. It is an enormous responsibility to be in control of the nutritional well-being of another human. Good nutritional habits before conception give the baby an even healthier start. Good nutrition can improve infant birth weight and reduce infant mortality. It has become recognized that a deficiency in folic acid (a B vitamin) is linked to neural tube birth defects. Therefore, the U.S. Public Health Service has issued a public health recommendation that all women of childbearing age should consume

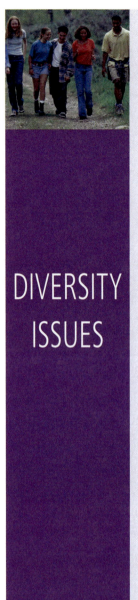

DIVERSITY ISSUES

Ethnic Food Choices

America loves more than burgers and fries. Ethnic foods are popular. Check out these suggestions. (Remember, any food in huge portions can contribute extra fat, calories, and salt.)

	CHOOSE	AVOID
MEXICAN	rice and beans, salsa, soft tacos, chicken or bean burritos, chicken or vegetable fajitas, corn tortillas, grilled chicken or seafood, nonfat or low-fat refried beans, black bean soup	refried beans made with lard, taco chips and shells, cheese sauces, sour cream, guacamole, fried appetizers, chimichangas, nachos, tostadas, fried ice cream, chili con queso
CHINESE	wonton soup, steamed rice, soft noodles (lo mein), chicken, shrimp, stir fries, vegetables, Hunan or Szechuan dishes, steamed spring rolls	breaded and deep-fried meats, fried rice, fried noodles, egg rolls, fried wontons, General Tso's chicken, crab rangoon
ITALIAN	marinara and tomato-based sauces, grilled fish and chicken, minestrone or fagioli (bean) soup, pasta primavera, pasta with red clam sauce, vegetable pizza, steamed clams, marsala or cacciatore dishes	alfredo, carbonara, or other cream sauces, parmigiana dishes, cannelloni, ravioli, manicotti, garlic bread, fried calamari, deep-crust pepperoni pizza, sausage pizza, cannoli
INDIAN	baked breads (chapati), tandoori chicken or fish, yogurt-based curry dishes, dal (lentils), rice pilaf, hummus, kabobs, basmati rice	fried breads (bhatura, poori, paratha), ghee (clarified butter), fried appetizers (pakoras), samosas, korma (meat in cream sauce)
THAI	chicken and seafood dishes (larb, po tak), broiled beef with onions (yum neua), tofu and vegetables, Thai salad	fried fish, chicken or duck, curries, peanut sauces, yum koon chaing (sausage with peppers), crispy noodles, coconut milk curries
GREEK	tabouli (bulgur salad), dolmas (rice wrapped in grape leaves), tzatziki (yogurt and cucumbers), shish kabob, pita bread	moussaka, gyros, baklava, vegetable pies (spanakopita), baba ghanouj (eggplant appetizer), deep-fried falafel

0.4 mg (or 400 mcg) of folic acid per day. The evidence is so clear and the concern so great that the FDA has mandated that folic acid be added to "enriched" grain products.

Pregnancy is not a time to diet. Weight gain and some increased fat deposition are necessary and healthy. Be sure to increase calcium, iron, and protein. Your physician may recommend a vitamin supplement because many vitamin needs are increased. Although some additional vitamins and minerals are needed, only about 300 extra calories per day are necessary for fetal growth and metabolic expenditure. A woman may be "eating for two," but normal energy expenditure is not double. Therefore, it is important to eat nutritionally dense foods. Twinkies, chocolate chip cookies, and potato chips offer few nutrients to a growing baby. Alcohol and caffeine should be limited because they increase nutrient excretion and adversely affect fetal development.

Aging

Many factors may interfere with good nutrition in older adults: economics, isolation, dentures, chronic health disorders, loss of taste, and medications. Nutrient absorption may decrease, especially for calcium and zinc. The widow or widower whose partner had always prepared the meals might start eating fast foods or frozen dinners. The depressed and lonely surviving partner may eat very little. Proper nutrition throughout life and into later life can minimize degenerative changes and help you maintain productivity and wellness. However, your 65-year-old body will not be the same one you fed at age

25. If you decrease activity and your body composition changes (increase in fat, decrease in lean), caloric intake should be decreased. Maintaining an active lifestyle can keep energy requirements from decreasing drastically. Although energy needs may drop as you age, nutrient needs do not diminish significantly. You must make your calories count. Be sure to eat adequate fiber and calcium and fewer fats and refined sugars. In many ways good nutrition (along with proper exercise) can help slow the aging process.

Sports and Fitness

Do you play competitive soccer? Are you training for a half-marathon? Is lap swimming every morning your fitness routine? Nutrition complements physical activity as you pursue a wellness lifestyle. However, the basic nutritional needs of an active person vary little from those of the more sedentary. *Everyone* needs a wide variety of healthy foods. If you are physically active, you burn more calories and have less chance of gaining weight (while eating more). Nevertheless, you do not need a special diet. There are many myths surrounding athletic performance and nutrition. An athlete (even a body builder) does not benefit from consuming massive amounts of protein. The typical American diet contains adequate amounts of protein—even to support an athletic lifestyle. Athletes who train heavily may need a little more. (See Frequently Asked Questions.) These increased protein needs can be satisfied easily through small adjustments in the normal diet—skim milk, yogurt, skinless chicken breast, and beans can provide excellent high-quality protein.

The main fuel for exercising muscles, glycogen, comes from carbohydrates. The best are the complex ones (breads, pastas, cereals, potatoes, rice, fruit), which provide plenty of vitamins and minerals. Persons engaged in fitness activities should consistently follow a 55 to 65 percent carbohydrate diet-proportion guideline. For those engaging in heavy exercise training, a diet with 65 to 70 percent of its calories from carbohydrates may be necessary to refuel glycogen stores. High-sugar snacks consumed before exercising can decrease performance. Carbohydrate loading (that is, manipulating diet and training to increase glycogen stores in the muscles) has not been shown to be effective for athletes participating in events requiring less than 1½ to 2 hours of continuous, noninterrupted effort.

The benefits of vitamin and mineral supplementation is a current area of study in regard to nutrition for competitive athletes. Large doses of the antioxidant vitamins C, E, and beta-carotene have shown promise in minimizing muscle damage and soreness in hardworking athletes. However, there is no evidence that consuming supplements containing vitamins, minerals, herbs, protein, or amino acids will build muscle or improve sports performance. Muscle overload through training, not supplementation, builds muscle. Research is exploding in this area.

Dehydration is a major contributor to poor athletic performance. Athletes, like everyone else, should drink plenty of water every day. They should drink 16 oz. (2 cups) of fluid two hours prior to exercise and a cup more (8 oz.) immediately before the workout. Add another 8 oz. of fluid every 20–30 minutes during exercise to match fluid loss in sweat (more in hot weather or if you sweat a lot). Do not wait until you are thirsty. Thirst is not a reliable indicator of dehydration because it usually does not occur until after 2 to 4 pints of body water are lost. The inclusion of electrolytes in sports drinks has been shown to be beneficial for rehydrating athletes who are exercising for long periods (60 to 90 minutes). (See Chapter 7 for more information on water consumption and sports drinks.) In regard to nutrition, the key to sports and fitness performance is the same as the key to general wellness and vitality: a balanced diet.

Frequently Asked Questions

Q. I work out quite a bit: endurance biking and weight training. Don't I need a lot more protein than a casual exerciser does?

A. Many athletes overestimate the amount of protein they need, thinking that more is better. Some studies indicate that more grams of protein than the normal recommendation (i.e., weight in pounds multiplied by 0.36) may help somewhat, while other studies show no improvement in workload capacity or strength. In the studies that recommend more protein, weight in pounds multiplied by 0.54 to 0.64 is the additional amount sufficient for strength and endurance athletes. If you are typical, you probably eat more than enough protein. For example, if you weigh 180 pounds, your recommended protein intake is approximately 65 grams (180 lb. × 0.36). If you increase to 180 lb. × 0.54 or 180 lb. × 0.64, the result is 97 to 115 total grams of protein. To put this in food perspective, 70 grams of protein would be 8 ounces of skinless chicken breast and 2 cups of skim milk. An addition of 1 cup oatmeal, 1 cup cottage cheese, and 2 tablespoons peanut butter brings the total to 115 grams of protein. As you can see, the typical American diet contains a sufficient amount of protein to support even the most active lifestyle. Remember, more carbohydrates, *not* protein, are needed for energy fuel, and excessive protein does not build muscle faster. Excessive protein intake puts extra strain on the kidneys.

Q. I hate milk and know I don't get enough calcium. Can't I take a calcium supplement? If so, what kind?

A. It is best to get enough calcium in the diet, but like you, many people struggle with this. There are many types of calcium supplements, some more absorbable than others. The most absorbable form of calcium is calcium citrate, and it can be taken without food. Avoid oyster shell calcium, coral calcium, dolomite, and bone meal products due to possible lead contamination. Calcium carbonate (the type found in antacids) is less absorbable than calcium citrate. Also, you absorb more from divided doses (500 mg or less) than from taking a high dose of calcium all at once. In addition to calcium, it is important to get the recommended levels of magnesium, zinc, and vitamin D to enhance the absorption of calcium. Remember, you can also obtain calcium from nondairy foods: calcium-fortified orange juice, sardines, oatmeal, whole grains, broccoli, and tofu.

Q. I keep seeing more foods labeled "organic" in my grocery store. What does that mean?

A. In the past, "organic" was never officially defined. Growers and manufacturers could slap "organic" on any food they wanted and not be breaking any regulations. This has changed. Under the new federal regulations, "organic" indicates that a food has been made with ingredients grown without chemical fertilizers, genetic engineering (scientific tinkering with a plant's DNA), and irradiation (a process that uses low levels of radiation to kill bacteria). "Organic" meat denotes that the animals have not been administered antibiotics, have had access to outdoor land, and have been fed organically grown feed.

Q. Which is better to eat, butter or margarine?

A. It is best to limit consumption of *all* fats, including butter and margarine. Butter is high in saturated fat, which raises "bad" LDL cholesterol. Regular margarine is high in trans-fatty acids (hydrogenated oils), known to increase the "bad" LDL cholesterol *and* decrease the "good" HDL cholesterol. Therefore, if you must use a spread, look for lower-fat or lighter kinds of margarines that say "trans-free" on the label. These are better for you. Both margarine and butter have the same number of calories, approximately 100 calories per tablespoon. You may want to try some of the butter sprinkles, butter-flavored mixes, and butter sprays, which are fat-free.

Q. I don't like many vegetables. Is it okay to get all my phytochemicals strictly from fruit?

A. If you absolutely cannot stand vegetables, eating extra fruit can compensate to some degree, but fruits and vegetables are not nutritionally identical. Both fruits and vegetables contain about the same vitamins and minerals, but vegetables offer a wider array of phytochemicals and carotenoids that help fight cancer, heart disease, and more. How about trying to add some new sauces or spices to vegetables to make them more flavorful? Or add shredded carrots, zucchini, or spinach to pasta sauces or meat loaf. Add steamed broccoli or peas to macaroni and cheese. Throw a handful of veggies into soup. They make great pizza toppings. There are many creative ways to add vegetables to your diet. And you may find you like them!

Q. I love pizza. Is it considered an unhealthy "junk food"?

A. It all depends on the toppings you choose. Ordering a vegetable-topped pizza is generally a pretty healthful choice. Also, a thin crust is better than a thick crust. When you load a pizza with pepperoni, sausage, bacon, or extra cheese, the fat and calories skyrocket. Since an entire large veggie pizza rarely contains even one cup of vegetables, why not add some more on your own? In the 10 minutes you wait for a pizza to be delivered or to preheat the oven, you can sauté some mushrooms, onions, peppers, broccoli, or spinach to add to the pizza. Chopped tomatoes or even canned vegetables will do. Use your imagination!

Q. Are fresh fruits and vegetables more nutritious than frozen, canned, or dried?

A. Not really. Most frozen, canned, and dried fruits or vegetables can be as nutritious as fresh produce. The frozen and canned versions are usually processed quickly using fresh-picked produce. To maximize vitamin content, use little water in preparation. Eating fruits and vegetables in a variety of forms will ensure a balance of important nutrients. When choosing frozen, canned, or dried versions, try to choose products without added sauces, sodium, or sugars.

Q. Since I have classes during mid-day, I never have time for lunch. What healthy and filling items can be packed in a backpack to get me through the day?

A. Many of us are busy or on-the-go during lunchtime. The following items can be packed in a backpack, office drawer, or car to fill an empty stomach: fresh or dried fruits, 100% fruit juices, bagels, carrots or celery sticks, granola or cereal bars, snack-size cereal boxes or crackers, soy nuts, rice cakes, whole-wheat fig bars, almonds, peanut butter–or cheese-filled whole-wheat crackers.

Summary

Although diet is not singled out as a specific risk factor for coronary heart disease, dietary factors are often interrelated with patterns of physical activity as major contributors to heart disease, stroke, obesity, atherosclerosis, osteoporosis, and some types of cancer. While many dietary components are involved in diet and health relationships, a primary factor is our high consumption of fats (especially saturated fats). These fats are often consumed at the expense of fruits, vegetables, and complex carbohydrates that may be more conducive to health.

Like many, you may admit to having some poor nutritional habits. You may rationalize this with some of the following:

- I'll do better after I get out of school and have more time. (Frankly, you will probably be busier after graduation.)
- But I feel fine! (Like smoking, poor eating habits may not noticeably affect your health for years.)

- I don't have any control over what the cafeteria serves. (However, you do have *choices* in the cafeteria and between meals.)
- I don't have enough money to buy the right foods. (On the contrary, milk is cheaper than soft drinks; a bunch of bananas costs less than a bag of potato chips.)
- I'm going to die anyway, so I might as well eat what I like. (Yes, we are all going to die. However, lifetime dietary habits significantly affect the *quality* of the last 10 to 20 years of your life.)

Wellness involves making informed choices rather than rationalizing. Improved eating habits can positively affect your health—now and later in life. Therefore, learn about the foods you are eating. Read food labels. The heart of good nutrition is *nine dietary guidelines*, a *pyramid of choices*, and *three simple words: variety, moderation,* and *balance.*

Internet Resources

3-a-Day of Dairy
   www.3aday.org
Emphasizes the importance of dairy products for healthier bones, weight loss, and overall health. Includes articles, research, recipes, and tips.

5 to 9 a Day
   www.5aday.gov
Emphasizes the importance of fruits and vegetable in the diet for prevention of chronic diseases. Gives research, recipes, and resources.

American Dietetic Association
   www.eatright.org
Provides a vast amount of reliable, objective food and nutrition information, including fact sheets, position papers, and healthy eating tips.

American Heart Association: Delicious Decisions
   www.deliciousdecisions.org
Provides basic information about nutrition, tips for shopping and eating out, and healthy recipes.

Ask the Dietitian
   www.dietitian.com
Thoroughly covers all areas of nutrition, food, weight issues, and fitness in a question-and-answer format.

Center for Nutrition Policy and Promotion
   www.usda.gov/cnpp
Promotes healthy eating and provides dietary guidance that links scientific research to consumer issues: food plans, dietary guidelines, nutrition insights, and up-to-date reports.

Center for Science in the Public Interest
   www.cspinet.org
Features the *Nutrition Action Newsletter*, a watchdog of the fast-food and restaurant industry whose mission is to educate the public on healthy eating.

The Diet Channel
   www.thedietchannel.com
Has over 600 links to reliable nutrition information as well as a vast array of up-to-date articles. Also has a lot of food/fitness/body calculators and tools.

Fast Food Facts
   www.foodfacts.info
Has a database of fast-food restaurants with comparisons and the nutritional content of their foods, sorted by calories, fat, cholesterol, and more.

Harvard School of Public Health
   www.hsph.harvard.edu/nutritionsource
Covers current research on all aspects of nutrition, providing tips on healthy eating and dispelling myths. Addresses everything from fiber to weight management to exercise.

MyPyramid
   www.MyPyramid.gov
A U.S. Department of Agriculture site that helps you choose the foods and amounts that are right for you according to the current *Dietary Guidelines*. Provides tips, tracking sheets, resources, and guidelines for healthy eating.

National Dairy Council
   www.nationaldairycouncil.org
Provides timely and reliable nutrition information on the health benefits of dairy foods.

National Osteoporosis Foundation

www.nof.org

Covers facts, risk factors, information, and news related to fighting osteoporosis and promoting bone health.

Nutrition.gov

www.nutrition.gov

Everything you need to know about nutrition issues, dietary guidelines, weight management, supplements, and food safety. Provides science-based guidance and reliable information for all ages from a multitude of federal agencies.

Office of Dietary Supplements

http://dietary-supplements.info.nih.gov

An office of the National Institutes of Health, this site helps consumers, health-care providers, and educators find credible scientific information on a variety of dietary supplements.

USDA Food and Nutrition Information Center

www.nal.usda.gov/fnic

Covers a wide array of information, including dietary guidelines, food composition tables, dietary supplements, healthy eating tips, and fitness/food/body calculators.

U.S. Food and Drug Administration

www.fda.gov

Provides information about the safety and effectiveness of food, drugs, cosmetics, weight-loss products, and any medical devices intended for human use.

The Vegetarian Resource Group

www.vrg.org

Covers all issues and topics regarding vegetarianism.

The following restaurants have nutritional information for their foods online:

www.arbys.com	www.krispykreme.com
www.blimpie.com	www.longjohnsilvers.com
www.bostonmarket.com	www.mcdonalds.com
www.burgerking.com	www.panerabread.com
www.carlsjr.com	www.papajohns.com
www.chick-fil-a.com	www.popeyes.com
www.churchs.com	www.pizzahut.com
www.dairyqueen.com	www.schlotzskys.com
www.dominos.com	www.sonicdrivein.com
www.dunkindonuts.com	www.steaknshake.com
www.fazolis.com	www.subway.com
www.hardees.com	www.tacobell.com
www.jackinthebox.com	www.whitecastle.com
www.kfc.com	

Bibliography

Brand-Miller, J., et al. *The New Glucose Revolution: The Authoritative Guide to the Glycemic Index.* New York: Marlow and Co., 2003.

Byers, T., and C. Doyle. "Diet, Physical Activity and Cancer . . . What's the Connection?" American Cancer Society, Atlanta, 2003.

Centers for Disease Control and Prevention. National Center for Chronic Disease Prevention and Health Promotion. *Behavioral Risk Factor Surveillance—United States, 2004.* www.cdc.gov/brfss

Fletcher, R. H., and K. M. Fairfield. "Vitamins for Chronic Disease Prevention in Adults." *Journal of the American Medical Association* 287 (June 19, 2002): 3127–3129.

Foster-Powell, K., S. H. A. Holt, and J. C. Brand-Miller. "International Table of Glycemic Index and Glycemic Load." *American Journal of Clinical Nutrition* 76 (July 2002): 5–56.

"How Omega-3 Fats May Protect Against Cancer." *American Institute for Cancer Research Newsletter* 84 (Summer 2004): 1, 3–4.

Kaminsky, L. A., ed. *ACSM's Resource Manual for Guidelines for Exercise Testing and Prescription.* Philadelphia: Lippincott Williams & Wilkins, 2006.

Lang, T., and M. Heasman. *Food Wars: The Global Battle for Mouths, Minds and Markets.* London: Earthscan, 2004.

Lemley, B. "What Does Science Say You Should Eat?" *Discover* 25 (February 2004): 43–49.

Liebman, B. "Breaking Up: Strong Bones Need More Calcium." *Nutrition Action Healthletter* 32 (April 2005): 1, 3–8.

National Academy of Sciences. Institute of Medicine. "Dietary Reference Intakes for Energy, Carbohydrates, Fiber, Fatty Acids, Cholesterol, Protein, and Amino Acids." September 5, 2002.

National Academy of Sciences. Institute of Medicine. "Dietary Reference Intakes for Water, Potassium, Sodium, Chloride, and Sulfate." February 11, 2004.

National Osteoporosis Foundation. *Take Action: Healthy Bones, Build Them for Life!* Washington, D.C., 2004. www.nof.org

"New Labeling Helps You Avoid Trans Fats." *Tufts University Health & Nutrition Letter* 23 (January 2006): 1–2.

"Omega-3s: Beyond the Sea." *UC Berkeley Wellness Letter* 22 (July 2005): 4.

"Phytonutrients: The Hidden Keys to Disease Prevention, Good Health." *Environmental Nutrition* 26 (January 2003): 1, 6.

Roberts, C. K., and R. J. Barnard. "Effects of Exercise and Diet on Chronic Disease." *Journal of Applied Physiology* 98 (January 2005): 3–30.

"The Trouble with Trans Fat." *Harvard Women's Health Watch* 11 (March 2004): 1–3.

"Uncle Sam's Diet Book: Putting the New Dietary Guidelines to Work for You." *Tufts University Health & Nutrition Newsletter* 23 (March 2005): 1, 4–5.

Upton, J. "New Roles for Fiber: Focus on Heart Disease, Diabetes, Blood Pressure." *Environmental Nutrition* 28 (April 2005): 1, 6.

U.S. Department of Agriculture. Center for Nutrition Policy and Promotion. "Beliefs and Attitudes of Americans Toward Their Diet." *Nutrition Insights* 19 (June 2000).

U.S. Department of Agriculture. Center for Nutrition Policy and Promotion. "Grain Consumption by Americans." *Nutrition Insights* 32 (August 2005).

U.S. Department of Agriculture. Center for Nutrition Policy and Promotion. *The Healthy Eating Index.* Washington, D.C., December 2002.

U.S. Department of Agriculture. Center for Nutrition Policy and Promotion. *MyPyramid.* Washington, D.C., April 2005. www.MyPyramid.gov

U.S. Department of Agriculture. Center for Nutrition Policy and Promotion. "Report Card on the Quality of Americans' Diets." *Nutrition Insights* 28 (December 2002).

U.S. Department of Health and Human Services. *A Healthier You.* Washington, D.C., November 2005.

U.S. Department of Health and Human Services. *Bone Health and Osteoporosis: A Report of the Surgeon General.* Washington, D.C., 2004.

U.S. Department of Health and Human Services. National Heart, Lung, and Blood Institute. *The DASH Eating Plan.* May 2003.

U.S. Department of Health and Human Services. *The 2004 Surgeon General's Report on Bone Health and Osteoporosis.* October 2004. www.surgeongeneral.gov

U.S. Department of Health and Human Services. U.S. Department of Agriculture. *Dietary Guidelines for Americans 2005.* January 2005. www.healthierus.gov/dietaryguidelines

U.S. Department of Health and Human Services. U.S. Department of Agriculture. *Finding Your Way to a Healthier You: Based on the Dietary Guidelines for Americans.* Home and Garden Bulletin No. 232-CP. 2005.

"Whole Grains: On a Roll." *American Institute for Cancer Research Newsletter* 89 (Fall 2005): 1, 3, 8.

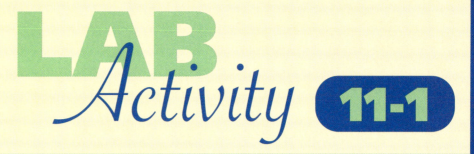

Name _____ **Class/Activity Section** _____ **Date** _____

Food Log

Write down everything you eat and drink for 3 to 5 full days. Make copies of the log as needed. Be sure to note the approximate quantity of food and assess combination foods (e.g., pizza, casseroles, tacos, salads) to list the foods in them. Use the columns at the right to record calories, sodium milligrams, fat grams, cholesterol milligrams, or other information, as desired by you or your instructor.

Date _____
    (12:01 A.M. to 12:00 midnight)

Other possible categories: calories, calcium, cholesterol, fat, sodium, fiber, etc.

Major Food Groups
(list amounts)

	Time	Food	Grains	Vegetables	Fruits	Meat and beans	Milk	Fats, oils, sweets	Fat grams	Calories				
EXAMPLES:	11:45 A.M.	Cheeseburger	2 oz.			4 oz.	1½ oz. cheese	1 Tbsp. mayo	36	490				
	11.45 A.M.	Apple			1 med.				0	80				
	11.45 A.M.	Soda						12 oz.	0	160				
		Totals =												

Vitamin supplements:

Date _____
  (12:01 A.M. to 12:00 midnight)

Other possible categories: calories, calcium,
cholesterol, fat, sodium, fiber, etc.

Major Food Groups
(list amounts)

Time	Food	Grains	Vegetables	Fruits	Meat and beans	Milk	Fats, oils, sweets	Fat grams	Calories				
Totals =													

Vitamin Supplements:

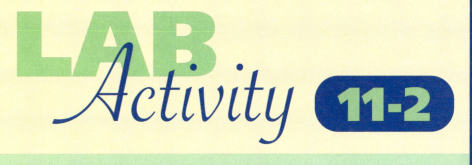

LAB Activity 11-2

Analyze Your Diet

After completing the *Food Log*, analyze your diet as follows.

1. Looking at the *2005 Dietary Guidelines for Americans*, how do you measure up to *each* of the nine guidelines?

   1.   6.

   2.   7.

   3.   8.

   4.   9.

   5.

2. Go to www.MyPyramid.gov and enter your personal data. Print your recommended plan. Compare your average daily diet to what is recommended in MyPyramid. (See Figure 11-1 for serving size equivalencies.)

   Grains: MyPyramid recommendations: _____ My average consumption:_____
   Are half of your grains "whole grains"?_____

   Vegetables: MyPyramid recommendations:_____
   My average consumption:_____

   Fruits: MyPyramid recommendations:_____
   My average consumption:_____

   Milk: MyPyramid recommendations:_____
   My average consumption:_____

   Meat & Beans: MyPyramid recommendations:_____
   My average consumption:_____

   According to MyPyramid, what are your estimated daily calorie needs? _____

   Do you feel you balance your calorie intake with your calorie output most days? _____

3. Identify three positive dietary changes you could implement that would help you come closer to complying with the *Dietary Guidelines* or your Pyramid. Include *what* you could do and a *specific strategy* for how to do it.
    EXAMPLE: *What*? Eat two more servings of fruit every day.
            Strategy? Slice a banana on my cereal every morning; put an apple in my backpack for an afternoon snack each day.

    a.

    b.

    c.

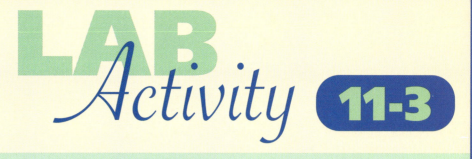

LAB Activity 11-3

How Much Fat?

1. Lisa consumes 2,100 calories per day. To keep her percentage of fat at 30 percent of her calories, figure out how many *grams* of fat she can consume per day. _____ (Show your work.)

   If Lisa wants to eat even *healthier* and limit her fat percentage to 20 percent of her daily calories, how many fat grams can she consume per day? _____ (Show your work.)

2. Robert consumes 2,700 calories per day. To keep his percentage of fat at 30 percent of his calories, how many *grams* of fat can he consume per day? _____ (Show your work.)

   If Robert wants to eat even *healthier* and limit his fat percentage to 25 percent of his daily calories, how many fat grams can he consume per day? _____ (Show your work.)

WHAT ABOUT YOU?

Multiply your body weight by 15 to approximate your caloric intake for a day.

_____ lb. × 15 = _____ calories

Number of daily fat grams at 30 percent of calories = _____ (Show your work.)

Number of daily fat grams at 25 percent of calories = _____ (Show your work.)

Number of daily fat grams at 20 percent of calories = _____ (Show your work.)

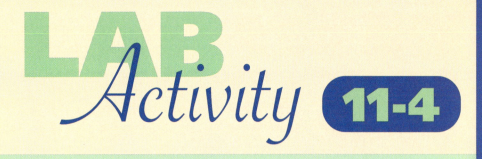

Label Reading Assignment

HONEY WHEAT MUFFIN MIX

<table>
<tr><td>

Directions

Combine mix with:
- 1/3 c. whole milk
- 1 T. oil
- 1 egg

Stir and pour into prepared muffin tin. Bake 15 minutes at 400°.

</td><td>

Nutrition Facts

Serving Size 1 muffin (from 31g mix)
Servings Per Container 6

Amount Per Serving	Mix	Prepared
Calories	123	162
Calories from Fat	27	54

		% Daily Value**	
Total Fat 3g*		**4%**	**10%**
Saturated Fat 0.5g	**3%**		**7%**
Trans Fat 0.5g			
Cholesterol 0mg		**0%**	**12%**
Sodium 210mg		**9%**	**9%**
Potassium 15mg	**<1%**		**1%**
Total Carbohydrate 23g		**8%**	**8%**
Dietary Fiber <1g		**2%**	**2%**
Sugars 12g			
Other Carbohydrate 11g			
Protein 1g			
Calcium		**0%**	**2%**
Iron		**2%**	**2%**

</td><td>

Not a significant source of vitamin A and vitamin C.

*Amount in mix. As prepared, one serving provides 6g fat (1.5g saturated fat; 1.0g trans fat), 35mg cholesterol, 220mg sodium, 45mg potassium, 24g total carbohydrate (12g sugars) and 3g protein.

**Percent Daily Values are based on a 2,000 calorie diet. Your daily values may be higher or lower depending on your calorie needs:

		Calories:	2,000	2,500
Total Fat	Less than		65g	80g
Sat Fat	Less than		20g	25g
Cholesterol	Less than		300mg	300mg
Sodium	Less than		2,400mg	2,400mg
Potassium			3,500mg	3,500mg
Total Carbohydrate			300g	375g
Dietary Fiber			25g	30g

Calories per gram:
Fat 9 • Carbohydrate 4 • Protein 4

Ingredients: Enriched Wheat Flour, Sugar, Hydrogenated Vegetable Oil (Coconut and/or Palm Kernel), Corn Syrup, Salt, Cellulose Gum, Dextrose, Rice Flour, Artificial Flavor.

</td></tr>
</table>

Look at the muffin mix label and respond to the following:

1. What constitutes one serving?

2. Why are there two columns (mix, prepared)?

3. How many grams of total fat are there in two prepared muffins? _____

4. In one prepared muffin, figure out the
   a. percent of calories from fat: _____

   b. percent of calories from carbohydrates: _____

   c. percent of calories from protein: _____

5. Give one source of complex carbohydrate in this product:

6. Give one source of simple carbohydrate in this product:

7. Name the source of cholesterol in this prepared product:

8. Name and comment on the sources of fat in this prepared product:

9. What alternatives or substitutes could be made in preparing these muffins to make them healthier?

10. What is your overall assessment of this food (i.e., nutritional density; sodium, fat, cholesterol content; types of carbohydrates; fiber content)?

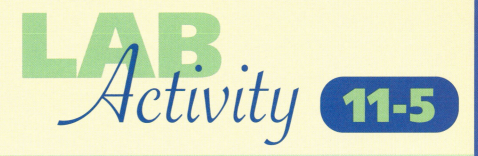

Changing Behavior Using the Transtheoretical Model

Using a highlighter, trace a path on the algorithm as you answer each question. Highlight your stage of change.

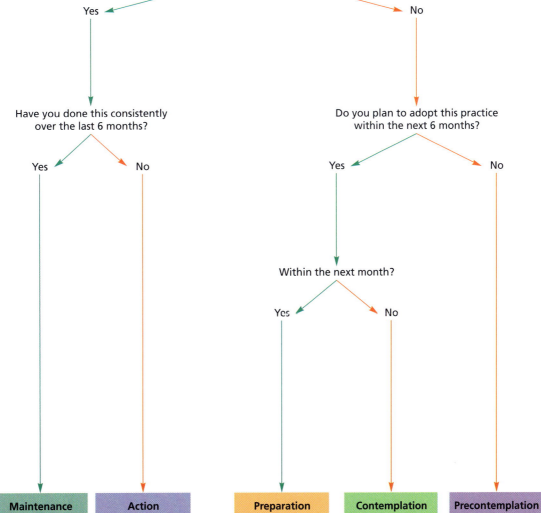

Do you do consume at least five servings of fruits and/or vegetables every day?

Yes — No

Yes → Have you done this consistently over the last 6 months?

Yes — No

No → Do you plan to adopt this practice within the next 6 months?

Yes — No

Yes → Within the next month?

Yes — No

| Maintenance | Action | Preparation | Contemplation | Precontemplation |

Once you've identified which stage of change you are in, it is important to use the processes most useful in progressing to the next stage—*or* remaining in maintenance. In the box, write your stage of change. Then list the processes that are most useful in that stage (see Figure 2-2 in Chapter 2). Use only the number of processes that apply to your stage of behavior change. You may not need to use all six. Under each process, give two specific behavior strategies (see Table 2-1 in Chapter 2) that could help you progress to the next stage—*or* maintain, if you're in the maintenance stage.

The stage I am in = [   ] .

Process 1.   _____

    Behavior strategy –a.

    Behavior strategy –b.

Process 2.   _____

    Behavior strategy –a.

    Behavior strategy –b.

Process 3.   _____

    Behavior strategy –a.

    Behavior strategy –b.

Process 4.   _____

    Behavior strategy –a.

    Behavior strategy –b.

Process 5.   _____

    Behavior strategy –a.

    Behavior strategy –b.

Process 6.   _____

    Behavior strategy –a.

    Behavior strategy –b.

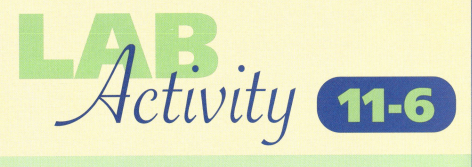

Can You Eat Healthy at a Fast-Food Restaurant?

Using the websites of various fast-food restaurants listed in the Chapter 11 Internet Resources, put together breakfast and lunch/dinner meals that would be typical for many consumers (perhaps one of your "non-health-conscious" friends). Use the nutritional information available on the restaurant's website for each food item selected. Record and total the calories, fat grams, and sodium content for each meal. In step 2, put together "healthy" meals from the same resturant. Record and total the nutritional information. Then answer the discussion questions on the back of this page.

STEP 1   Typical breakfast meal

Choose a restaurant _____

Food item	Calories	Fat grams	Sodium mg.
_____	_____	_____	_____
_____	_____	_____	_____
_____	_____	_____	_____
_____	_____	_____	_____
_____	_____	_____	_____
_____	_____	_____	_____
TOTALS =	☐	☐	☐

Typical lunch/dinner meal

Choose a restaurant _____

Food item	Calories	Fat grams	Sodium mg.
_____	_____	_____	_____
_____	_____	_____	_____
_____	_____	_____	_____
_____	_____	_____	_____
_____	_____	_____	_____
_____	_____	_____	_____
TOTALS =	☐	☐	☐

STEP 2   "Healthy" breakfast meal

(Same restaurant as above)

Food item	Calories	Fat grams	Sodium mg.
_____	_____	_____	_____
_____	_____	_____	_____
_____	_____	_____	_____
_____	_____	_____	_____
_____	_____	_____	_____
TOTALS =	☐	☐	☐

"Healthy" lunch/dinner meal

(Same restaurant as above)

Food item	Calories	Fat grams	Sodium mg.
_____	_____	_____	_____
_____	_____	_____	_____
_____	_____	_____	_____
_____	_____	_____	_____
_____	_____	_____	_____
TOTALS =	☐	☐	☐

LAB Activity ■ CHAPTER 11

1. Comment on the nutritional differences in the meals.
   Calories:

   Fat:

   Sodium:

2. Do you think it is possible to eat healthy (i.e., meet nutritional needs) by eating regularly in fast-food restaurants? Why or why not?

3. What specific tips for food selections would you give someone who must eat in fast-food restaurants regularly?

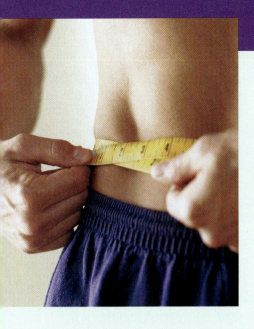

Chapter 12

Achieving a Healthy Weight

12

More die in the United States of too much food than of too little.
—John Kenneth Galbraith

Objectives

After reading this chapter, you will be able to:

1. Differentiate between overweight and obesity.
2. Identify the percentage of adults over age 20 who are overweight and the percentage who are obese.
3. Explain the purpose of the body mass index (BMI) and identify a BMI associated with health problems.
4. List six health conditions associated with obesity.
5. Explain how the location of fat on the body is linked to health risks and calculate waist-to-hip ratios.
6. Identify a risky waist-to-hip ratio and a high-risk waist circumference for both men and women.
7. Describe how each of the following factors contributes to obesity: energy balance, fat cells, set point, heredity, and metabolism.
8. Define the basal metabolic rate (BMR) and identify five factors that affect it.
9. Distinguish a healthy weight-loss program from a fad/diet program.
10. Identify and explain the three major components of effective lifetime weight management.
11. List five ways exercise helps in weight management.
12. Compare and contrast the eating disorders: bulimia nervosa, anorexia nervosa, binge eating disorder, and disordered eating.

Terms

- anorexia nervosa
- basal metabolic rate (BMR)
- behavior modification
- binge eating disorder
- body fat
- body mass index (BMI)
- bulimia nervosa
- calorie (kcal)
- cellulite
- disordered eating
- eating disorder
- essential fat
- fat cells (adipose cells)
- fat-free mass
- glycogen
- lean-body mass (muscle mass)
- liposuction
- obesity
- overweight
- set-point theory
- storage fat
- weight cycling (yo-yo syndrome)

A Fit and Well Way of Life **Online Learning Center** www.mhhe.com/robbinsfitwell1e
Go to the Online Learning Center for chapter quizzes, outlines, flashcards, and additional lab activities.

Americans are preoccupied with weight. It is likely that you know your weight within 5 pounds. Every birth announcement gives the baby's weight to the ounce. Weight scales are commonplace in American bathrooms. This preoccupation has made weight control a multi-billion-dollar business. Americans spend approximately $40 billion yearly on weight-loss products and programs and diet aids. The diet-food industry is the fastest-growing food market.

The craze to lose weight (whether needed or not) is reflected by the millions of Americans who report that they are dieting. Approximately 60 percent of Americans are trying to lose weight on any given day. Bookstore shelves and magazine racks are crammed with diet plans guaranteed to help you lose those extra inches. Television, radio, and newspapers further advertise a multitude of weight-loss options. Advertisements nailed to bulletin boards promise "Lose 30 pounds in 30 days." "Before" and "after" photos touting the benefits of pills, diets, and creams are scattered throughout magazines. In fact, losing weight is so important that 88 percent of dieters say they would give up a job promotion, retirement, or a dream house if they could only reach their target weight! With all this attention and effort, one would predict that the American population would be getting leaner. Paradoxically, obesity rates are climbing in all populations in our country. Overweight and obesity account for over 100,000 U.S. deaths per year, second only to tobacco as the most preventable cause of death. And obesity is increasing in prevalence in both developed and developing countries throughout the world.

The latest national statistics reveal that an alarming 65 percent of American adults age 20 or older are overweight or obese. Among those persons, 31 percent are classified as obese.

The prevalence of obesity among adults has more than doubled in the last 20 years (see Figure 12-1). Consistent with the data for adults, the prevalence of overweight among children ages 6–11 rose from 7 to 16 percent between 1976 and 2002, and more than tripled among adolescents ages 12–19, from 5 to 16 percent during the same time period. The rate is increasing so rapidly that it is predicted that nearly half of all children in North America will be overweight by 2010, and *all* American adults will be overweight by 2030. And the Centers for Disease Control and Prevention estimates that if current obesity trends continue, one-third of all children and one-half of African American and Hispanic children who were born in 2003 will develop type 2 diabetes.

A study of 14 industrialized countries found the highest rates of teenage obesity to be in the United States. This unprecedented epidemic is consistent in all states; in both sexes; and across all age groups, racial and ethnic groups, and educational levels. Because of the substantial increase in the prevalence and severity of obesity, officials predict that the steady rise in life expectancy in the United States during the past two centuries may soon come to an end.

However, there are disparities in overweight and obesity in some segments of the population. For ex-

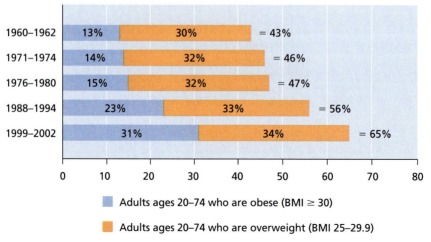

FIGURE 12-1   Americans are getting bigger. SOURCE: Centers for Disease Control and Prevention, National Center for Health Statistics, 2005.

ample, overweight and obesity are particularly common among minority groups (see Diversity Issues).

Because the obesity trend is increasing so rapidly, most health professionals feel that obesity is the most serious health threat to Americans.

Although there is tremendous interest in diets and dieting, many dieters fail to achieve their weight goals, and over 90 percent of those who do lose weight are unable to keep the weight off. At the other extreme, the incidence of eating disorders is at

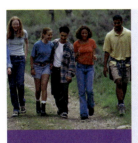

DIVERSITY ISSUES

Weight Differences Among Various Ethnic Groups

- Although overweight and obesity are rising in all age groups, they are substantially more prevalent in women who are members of racial and ethnic minority populations than in non-Hispanic white women.
- Among men, Mexican Americans have a higher prevalence of overweight and obesity than do non-Hispanic whites and or non-Hispanic blacks.
- For non-Hispanic men, the prevalence of overweight and obesity among whites is higher than it is among blacks.
- Among women, non-Hispanic blacks have the highest prevalence of obesity.
- Smaller surveys indicate a higher prevalence of overweight and obesity in American Indians, Alaska Natives, and Pacific Islander Americans and a lower

prevalence in Asian Americans compared with the general population.
- Among all racial and ethnic groups combined, women of lower socioeconomic status are approximately 50 percent more likely to be obese than are women of higher socioeconomic status.
- African American women of all ages report participating less in regular exercise than do white women.
- African American men age 45 and older report less regular exercise than do white women.
- Cultural factors related to dietary choices, physical activity, and acceptance of excess weight among African Americans and other racial-ethnic groups appear to play a role in interfering with weight loss.

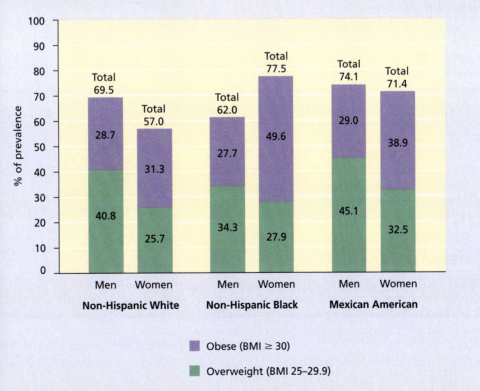

Prevalence of overweight and obesity by sex and racial group (ages 20–74). SOURCE: Centers for Disease Control and Prevention, *Health, United States,* 2005.

an epidemic level. The paradoxes of these facts reveal the complexity of America's weight issues.

Maintaining a reasonable body weight is a definite wellness issue. Your body is the vehicle by which you function in society. Being overweight can affect you physically, emotionally, socially, and occupationally. The purpose of wellness is to strive toward full potential, and so maintaining a reasonable body composition is one step toward achieving wellness. Knowledge gives you the tools to plan your lifetime weight-management scheme. It is important that you understand body composition facts, effective weight-loss principles, weight-management guidelines, and the influence of culture, heredity, environment, and behavior on weight control.

UNDERSTANDING BODY COMPOSITION

Your body is composed of body fat and fat-free mass. **Fat-free mass** includes muscle, bone, body fluids, and organs. Muscles, part of fat-free mass, are often specifically referred to as **lean-body mass** or **muscle mass.** **Body fat** is classified as either essential fat or storage fat. **Essential fat,** required for normal body functioning, is stored in major body organs and tissues such as the heart, muscles, intestines, bones, lungs, liver, spleen, and kidneys and throughout the central nervous system. Females have additional essential fat in the breasts and pelvic region for childbearing and other hormone-related functions. **Storage fat** is the extra fat that accumulates in adipose cells (or fat cells) around internal organs and beneath the skin surface to insulate, pad, and protect the body from trauma and extreme cold. As you learned in Chapter 3, there are different ways to assess body composition. Knowing your body composition (especially your percentage of body fat) can help you set realistic weight goals.

Overweight Versus Obesity

Too often, the terms *overweight* and *obesity* are used interchangeably. **Overweight** refers to a body weight in excess of a recommended range for good health. **Obesity** refers specifically to having an excessive accumulation of body fat.

Because these explanations are somewhat vague, the National Institutes of Health has adopted the **body mass index (BMI)** as a method of classifying overweight and obesity. BMI is a direct calculation based

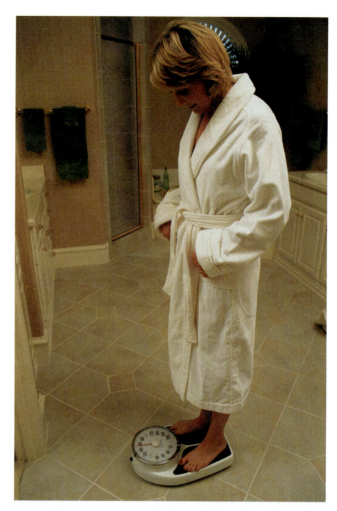

Although people seem concerned about their weight, obesity is on the rise.

on height and weight and has been universally adopted by health professionals to determine healthy weights and risky weights. BMI is computed from the following equations:

$$BMI = \frac{\text{weight in kilograms}}{(\text{height in meters})^2}$$

or

$$BMI = \frac{\text{weight in pounds}}{(\text{height in inches})^2} \times 703$$

Table 12-1 allows you to determine your BMI quickly. Note the classifications below the chart. These standards have been adopted worldwide. In this way, overweight and obesity are clearly defined. Notice that BMI is not gender specific. For example, a 5'6" woman who weighs 155 pounds is considered overweight. If she weighs 186 pounds, she is classified as obese. A 6'0" man weighing 184 pounds is overweight. At 221 pounds, he is considered obese.

One disadvantage of using the BMI is that it remains a measure of weight and height, not fatness (i.e., it doesn't

TABLE 12-1 ***Find Your Body Mass Index (BMI)***

Find your height, then look across that row. Your BMI is at the top of the column that contains your weight.

	BODY MASS INDEX (BMI)													
	19	**20**	**21**	**22**	**23**	**24**	**25**	**26**	**27**	**28**	**29**	**30**	**35**	**40**
Height	Weight (pounds)													
4'10"	91	96	100	105	110	115	119	124	129	134	138	143	167	191
4'11"	94	99	104	109	114	119	124	128	133	138	143	148	173	198
5'0"	97	102	107	112	118	123	128	133	138	143	148	153	179	204
5'1"	100	106	111	116	122	127	132	137	143	148	153	158	185	211
5'2"	104	109	115	120	126	131	136	142	147	153	158	164	191	218
5'3"	107	113	118	124	130	135	141	146	152	158	163	169	197	225
5'4"	110	116	122	128	134	140	145	151	157	163	169	174	204	232
5'5"	114	120	126	132	138	144	150	156	162	168	174	180	210	240
5'6"	118	124	130	136	142	148	155	161	167	173	179	186	216	247
5'7"	121	127	134	140	146	153	159	166	172	178	185	191	223	255
5'8"	125	131	138	144	151	158	164	171	177	184	190	197	230	262
5'9"	128	135	142	149	155	162	169	176	182	189	196	203	236	270
5'10"	132	139	146	153	160	167	174	181	188	195	202	207	243	278
5'11"	136	143	150	157	165	172	179	186	193	200	208	215	250	286
6'0"	140	147	154	162	169	177	184	191	199	206	213	221	258	294
6'1"	144	151	159	166	174	182	189	197	204	212	219	227	265	302
6'2"	148	155	163	171	179	186	194	202	210	218	225	233	272	311
6'3"	152	160	168	176	184	192	200	208	216	224	232	240	279	319
6'4"	156	164	172	180	189	197	205	213	221	230	238	246	287	328
	NORMAL						**OVERWEIGHT**					**OBESE**		

INTERPRETING YOUR BMI

- **≤18.9 Underweight**
- **19–24.9 Healthy weight (little health risk)**
- **25–29.9 Overweight (increased health risk)**
- **≥30 Obesity (greatest health risk)**

SOURCE: National Institutes of Health, National Heart, Lung, and Blood Institute.

distinguish between body fat and muscle mass). Nor does it take into account the *location* of fat. Therefore it may not be appropriate for an athlete or body builder with a lot of muscle mass. Also, for the elderly who have lost a lot of muscle mass, their BMI may reflect a "healthy weight," when in actuality they have reduced nutritional reserves. Therefore, an analysis of your body fat percentage using the skinfold calipers gives a more accurate body composition assessment (i.e., body fat versus lean body mass). A woman over 30 percent body fat and a man over 25 percent are considered obese. (See Chapter 3 for more on skinfold measuring and body composition.)

Risks Associated with Obesity

Obesity is rapidly becoming the most serious public health issue for both adults and children. The health implications of excess weight have become quite clear. Obesity is identified as a risk factor in 4 of the 10 leading causes of death. The major killers associated with obesity are heart disease, several types of cancer, stroke, type 2 diabetes, and atherosclerosis. Obesity contributes to cardiovascular disease by causing changes in the body that increase the risk factors:

- ✔ Raises levels of LDL ("bad") cholesterol
- ✔ Raises levels of triglycerides (fats in the blood)
- ✔ Reduces levels of HDL ("good") cholesterol
- ✔ Elevates blood pressure

Obesity can aggravate liver disorders and arthritis and is often found in conjunction with gallbladder disease. Recent statistics show a staggering increase in the number of cases of type 2 diabetes (33 percent in the past decade), paralleling the increasing obesity rates in the United States. Although it once was considered an adult disease, the number of overweight children now being diagnosed with type 2 diabetes is staggering. This diabetes and obesity combination can lead to blindness, nerve damage, kidney failure, and cardiovascular disease.

Obesity complicates surgery and pregnancy. Pulmonary problems, sleep apnea, heat intolerance, and reduced fertility are more prevalent in the obese. Among obese women there is an increased risk of cervical, uterine, colon, breast, and pancreatic cancers. Obese men

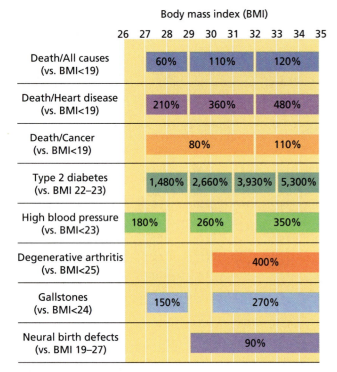

Body mass index (BMI)	26	27	28	29	30	31	32	33	34	35
Death/All causes (vs. BMI<19)			60%		110%			120%		
Death/Heart disease (vs. BMI<19)			210%		360%			480%		
Death/Cancer (vs. BMI<19)			80%					110%		
Type 2 diabetes (vs. BMI 22–23)			1,480%	2,660%	3,930%	5,300%				
High blood pressure (vs. BMI<23)	180%			260%			350%			
Degenerative arthritis (vs. BMI<25)						400%				
Gallstones (vs. BMI<24)		150%			270%					
Neural birth defects (vs. BMI 19–27)				90%						

FIGURE 12-2 Weighing the risks: Percent increase in risk by level of obesity. At BMIs of 27 and higher, one's risk for various disorders increases significantly. SOURCE: *New England Journal of Medicine, Annals of Internal Medicine, American Journal of Clinical Nutrition, Journal of the American Medical Association.*

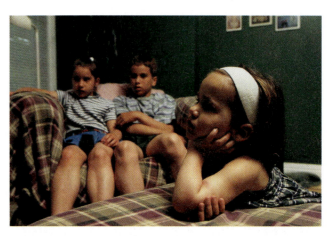

The percentage of obese children in the United States has almost tripled in the last 20 years. The 20-plus hours per week the average child spends watching TV and videos are a contributing factor.

face an increased chance of colon, stomach, rectal, and prostate cancers. In fact, according to the American Cancer Society, excess weight may account for as much as 20 percent of all cancer deaths in women and 14 percent in men. Obesity restricts mobility, increases fatigue, and decreases overall body efficiency. Figure 12-2 shows the percent increase in the risk of various conditions related to specific BMIs.

The high prevalence of obesity in the United States not only is linked to numerous chronic diseases but is responsible for a substantial portion of total health-care costs. According to the surgeon general's report, obesity health-care costs are $117 billion per year. This figure does not include the psychosocial costs of obesity—from lowered self-esteem to eating disorders to severe depression. The psychological and social consequences of obesity are often overlooked. Obese people also face a tremendous amount of prejudice and discrimination. Their educational and professional opportunities often suffer.

Until recently, modest weight gains throughout adulthood in initially lean individuals were overlooked and even culturally expected. Results from the ongoing Harvard Nurses' Health Study (a 25-year tracking of more than 100,000 nurses) have revealed that even *modest* weight gains (11 to 17 pounds) after 18 years of

age increase one's cardiovascular disease risk. The researchers concluded that there is a large fraction of the population falsely reassured that their weight is not a health concern because they are not "overweight." The study found that a person's weight at midlife (30 to 55 years) has the greatest influence on heart disease risk. Those with a BMI of 23 to 27 had a 31 percent increased risk; those with the lowest risk had a BMI below 21. Those with a BMI ≥ 30 have a 50 to 100 percent increased risk of death from *all* causes, compared with those with healthy BMIs (19 to 24.9).

Location of Fat

Studies suggest not only that body fat percentage and BMI are related to health but that the location of excess fat is a comparable risk factor as well. Fat distributed primarily in the abdominal area (called *apple-shape obesity*) is characteristic of many men (but also is present in some women). This so-called visceral fat is intermingled around the internal organs and is linked to increased risk for coronary heart disease, hypertension, high cholesterol, type 2 diabetes, and some forms of cancer. Fat distributed in the lower extremities, around the hips, buttocks, and thighs (called *pear-shape obesity*), does not present as great a risk. Pear-shape obesity is more common in women. The two types of fat have biochemical differences. Abdominal fat experiences much more enzyme and chemical activity, dumping more fatty acids into the bloodstream and increasing the prevalence of LDL cholesterol. Hip-thigh fat activity is more stagnant. Unfortunately, this hip-thigh fat is more difficult to lose than is abdominal fat. Some obesity experts now feel that one's waist-to-hip ratio is more important than the BMI in predicting potential weight-related health problems because abdominal fat is so heavily linked to diseases. A worldwide study revealed that abdominal

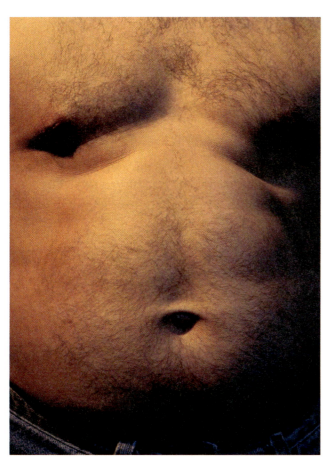

For a man or a woman, having a large amount of abdominal fat substantially increases the risk of heart disease, stroke, type 2 diabetes, and cancer.

TABLE 12-2	*Sample Waist-to-Hip Ratios*

$$\text{Waist-to-hip ratio} = \frac{\text{Waist circumference}}{\text{Hip circumference}}$$

(See Chapter 3 for specific measuring instructions.)

$\dfrac{\text{waist}}{\text{hip}} = \dfrac{28''}{38''} = 0.74$		$\dfrac{\text{waist}}{\text{hip}} = \dfrac{40''}{42''} = 0.95$
$\dfrac{\text{waist}}{\text{hip}} = \dfrac{32''}{40''} = 0.80$		$\dfrac{\text{waist}}{\text{hip}} = \dfrac{45''}{39''} = 1.15$
$\dfrac{\text{waist}}{\text{hip}} = \dfrac{38''}{42''} = 0.90$		$\dfrac{\text{waist}}{\text{hip}} = \dfrac{50''}{40''} = 1.25$

Higher risk is associated with a ratio > 0.8 for women and > 0.95 for men.

tack. Whereas the distribution of fat has a genetic link, a comprehensive program of a low-fat, reduced-calorie diet and regular exercise can help reduce body fat stores regardless of where they are located.

THE SURGEON GENERAL STEPS IN

One of the health goals in the government's publication *Healthy People 2010* was to reduce the number of obese people to 15 percent of the population by 2010. Unfortunately, current body weight trends are leading us away from this goal. Due to the alarming increase in weight in the United States, the government issued *The Surgeon General's Call to Action to Prevent and Decrease Overweight* in 2001. This document establishes five overarching principles to combat this critical public health issue. The five principles are:

1. Promote the recognition of overweight and obesity as major public health problems.
2. Assist Americans in balancing healthful eating with regular physical activity to achieve and maintain a healthy or healthier body weight.
3. Identify effective and culturally appropriate interventions to prevent and treat overweight and obesity.
4. Encourage environmental changes that help prevent overweight and obesity.
5. Develop and enhance public-private partnerships to help implement this vision.

This burden is not trivial. Strategies must be developed that involve schools, communities, restaurants,

obesity accounts for 90 percent of the risk for heart attack. A large amount of belly fat is a risk factor for cardiovascular disease even if the rest of the physique is skinny! This was true for men, women, all ages, and all ethnic groups. According to some scientists, if waist-to-hip ratios (rather than BMIs) were used currently to assess the risk of chronic disease, the number of people classified as obese worldwide would increase substantially. Waist-to-hip ratio can be calculated by dividing the number of inches around the waistline by the circumference of the hips. See Table 12-2 for examples of waist-to-hip ratios. For example, someone who has a 30-inch waist and 40-inch hips has a ratio of 0.75. A woman whose ratio is 0.80 or higher is at risk, as is a man whose ratio is 0.95 or above.

Many researchers feel that the waist circumference *alone* can be a predictor of risk. Men with a waist circumference over 40 inches and women with a waist circumference over 35 inches are classified as high risk no matter what their BMIs are. Men with a waist circumference over 40 inches are 12 times more likely to develop type 2 diabetes. An excess of abdominal fat in women has been linked to breast cancer and heart at-health professionals, and the media to attack this problem. A good start is to become educated about what causes obesity.

WHAT CAUSES OBESITY?

For years the simplistic explanation for obesity was that people became obese because they ate too much. Obesity was viewed as a condition resulting from a lack of self-control around food. In scientific terms, obesity occurs when a person's caloric intake exceeds the amount of energy that person burns. What causes this imbalance between consuming and burning calories is unclear. Evidence suggests that obesity is a complex combination of metabolic, genetic, psychological, behavioral, social, and environmental factors—not solely a result of a lack of individual willpower. It is clear that no single factor results in obesity. In an attempt to explain the causes of obesity, several factors have to be examined. They include energy balance, fat cells, set point, heredity, and metabolism.

The Energy Balance Equation

The energy balance equation states that energy input (calories consumed) must be equal to energy output (calories expended) for body weight to remain constant. Any imbalance in energy input or energy output will result in a change in body weight. If you eat more calories daily than your body expends in activity, you will store the excesses as fat. If you eat fewer calories than you burn, you will lose weight. It is unrealistic to assume that the equation must be exactly equal every day to maintain your weight. Some days you eat more, some days less. Some days you are more active than you are on other days. Several days of imbalance in one direction will produce a change in body weight.

This explanation assumes that a calorie is a calorie, whether it is from candy or from a vegetable. A **calorie** (actually a **kcal**) is a measure of energy. One pound of body fat equals 3,500 calories of stored energy. Therefore, consuming an extra 3,500 calories will cause you to gain 1 pound of fat. If you burn an extra 3,500 calories with activity, you will lose 1 pound. To cause a reduction in body weight, you (1) reduce calorie intake below the energy requirement, (2) increase the calorie output through additional physical activity above energy requirements, or (3) combine the two methods by reducing calorie intake and increasing calorie output. So how do you lose 10 pounds? By creating a calorie deficit of 500 calories daily (by increasing exercise or decreasing food intake) for 7 days, you will lose 1 pound (3,500 calories). By maintaining this deficit, you will be 10 pounds lighter in 10 weeks.

However, weight loss is not necessarily this simple. For some people, cutting calories causes feelings of fatigue, resulting in a decrease of energy expenditure. As body weight is reduced, the energy costs of movement go down proportionately, thus reducing caloric output. Also, individual differences in resting metabolic rates, cellular makeup, and lean tissue need to be considered. That is why knowledge about other factors is necessary to understand the complexities of weight loss fully.

Regardless of the problems that come with relying on the energy balance equation as the only way to understand weight loss and weight gain, this equation is the best way of explaining why, in this age of modernization and decreased physical demands, so many Americans are too fat. As Figure 12-3 shows, many factors contribute to our growing girth. Most are not active enough to use the calories consumed. Food in America is plentiful, available, and relatively inexpensive. It is also high in sugar, calories, and fat. More frequent eating is encouraged by numerous societal changes: The growth of the fast-food industry, 24-hour supermarkets, "pop-in" pantries, the increased incidence of snacking rather than sitting down to eat meals, the number of "all you can eat" buffets, and the growing tendency to socialize with food and drink have all added calories to our day. Although many people are consciously trying to eat lower-fat food items, *low fat* doesn't necessarily mean *low calorie*. Surveys indicate that our daily caloric intake is increasing, while our caloric expenditure is decreasing. Countless labor-saving devices at home and at work and our passive leisure-time activities (television, Internet, computer games, videos) have contributed to creeping obesity. Phoning, faxing, e-mailing, online shopping, and express mail don't burn many calories (unless you're the express mail delivery person!). Many neighborhoods lack sidewalks or bike lanes for safe walking and riding, and the automobile is used to travel even the shortest distances. There are fewer opportunities in daily life to burn calories. We live increasingly sedentary lives.

How many calories do you need to maintain a desirable body weight? Table 12-3 helps you estimate your daily caloric need based on your activity level. Remember, this is only an approximation and may vary between individuals. To lose or gain weight, the calorie intake must be adjusted upward or downward.

Fat-Cell Theory

The size and number of fat cells in the body determine degrees of fatness. **Fat cells** (also known as **adipose cells**) are storage sites for energy. The body increases fat storage in two ways: by increasing the *number* of fat cells and by increasing the *size* of fat cells. As might be expected, the body increases its number of fat cells during infancy and puberty growth spurts. Fat cells also expand and contract as energy is stored or burned. They can expand to two to three times their normal size, but they cannot enlarge endlessly. At some point, new fat cells can be created in response to the body's need to store more excess energy. This can occur in extremely obese individuals.

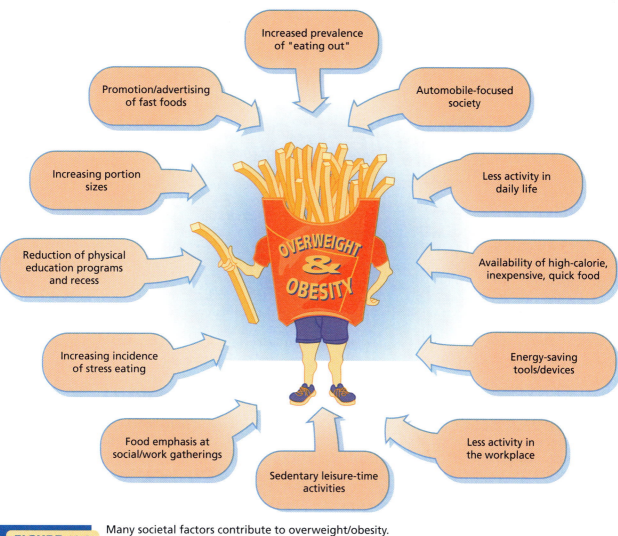

Increased prevalence of "eating out"

Promotion/advertising of fast foods

Automobile-focused society

Increasing portion sizes

Less activity in daily life

Reduction of physical education programs and recess

Availability of high-calorie, inexpensive, quick food

Increasing incidence of stress eating

Energy-saving tools/devices

Food emphasis at social/work gatherings

Less activity in the workplace

Sedentary leisure-time activities

OVERWEIGHT & OBESITY

FIGURE 12-3   Many societal factors contribute to overweight/obesity.

TABLE 12-3   *Determining Your Daily Caloric Needs*

The following is a method for estimating the caloric needs for healthy, nonpregnant adults. Older individuals (over age 50) should further reduce calories by 10 to 20 percent. These are only estimates. Individual activity factors and body frames vary from person to person.

Formula: Weight × Activity level = Calories needed daily

Activity Level	Calories Needed per Pound per Day	
	Female	Male
Inactive (little or no regular exercise; desk job; light work)	×12	×13
Moderately Active (20–30 minutes of exercise at least 3–4 times per week; or job dictates moderate activity)	×14	×16
Very Active (30–45 minutes of vigorous, sustained exercise 5–7 times per week; or job dictates considerable activity)	×16	×18

Example: female = 140 lbs (desired weight) × 14 (moderately active) = 1,960 calories per day

male = 180 lbs (desired weight) × 13 (inactive) = 2,340 calories per day

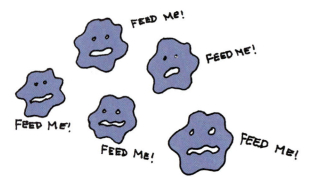

Fat cells are with you forever.

This capacity to increase cell numbers when a maximum cell size is reached depends on the age and sex of the person and the site of the fat tissue. Unfortunately, once a fat cell has been created, it exists for life. Fat cells do not seem to be destructible. An individual of normal weight has 30 to 50 billion fat cells, while an obese person can have as many as 60 to 100 billion fat cells.

Therefore, the fat-cell theory proposes that weight reduction in adults is a result of decreasing the size of the fat cells, shrinking them by using the energy stored in them or not filling them at all. This theory also explains why people who grow a large number of fat cells during childhood have a predisposition to obesity as adults. They can reduce the amount of fat stored in the cells, but the excess number of fat cells is still there, waiting to be filled again.

It is important to realize that fat tissue is not an inert storage depot. Fat is actually a dynamic organ that produces hormones, inflammatory proteins, and chemical messengers that contribute to a multitude of chronic diseases.

Set-Point Theory

The **set-point theory** maintains that every individual is programmed to be a certain weight and that the body regulates itself to maintain that "set" weight. Studies of people in alternating states of semistarvation and gorging have shown that once intervention ceases, they return to their former weights. What determines your set point? The hypothalamus in the brain may act as a body weight thermostat, lowering body metabolism and increasing hunger if fat levels fall below the set point. Here is where the set-point theory and fat-cell theory merge. The set-point mechanism is thought to respond to signals sent out by the fat cells as to the amount of fat in storage. The weight at which this occurs may depend on the number of fat cells. Consider two 180-pound women. Sara has a normal number of fat cells, which are enlarged. Mary has an excessive number of fat cells of normal size. Sara has a greater chance of weight loss, because she can reduce her cell size and still sustain adequate fat volume. Mary faces a harder battle because her body will work to maintain her cell size. This theory also helps explain why attempts at permanent weight loss by crash dieting are not successful. The body naturally fights against this starvation state.

The set-point theory is based on survival. How else could populations endure famine or our ancestors survive periods of food shortages? Heredity influences the set point, too. Some people have naturally higher set points, causing maintenance of higher levels of body fat, whereas other individuals have naturally low set points.

Can you change your set point? Some studies show that sustained consumption of a diet high in fats, refined carbohydrates, and perhaps even artificial sweeteners (the typical American diet?) raises the set

THE NUMBERS

$1,000	The additional annual medical costs for an obese person versus someone of normal weight.
335	The number of extra calories per day the average woman today consumes compared to a woman in 1971. (Men take in 168 more calories per day.)
50%	Portion of kids who walked to school in 1970. (Today only 15% walk to school.)
90,000	The number of yearly deaths from cancer that could be avoided if every U.S. adult could maintain a BMI under 25.0 throughout life.
$117 billion	The direct and indirect costs associated with obesity per year in the United States.
8	The average number of hours Americans age 13 years and older spend sitting each day.
2058	The year when everyone in the United States is predicted to be obese (if current obesity rates continue to rise as they have over the past 25 years).

point and that regular, vigorous exercise can lower the set point. Exercise stimulates changes in metabolism, causing the body to use fat rather than protect against its losses. Knowing this, it is easy to see how America's obesity problem is more connected to our sedentary lifestyles and dietary habits than to brain thermostat alterations. We've gone from lean to fat because we eat more and exert ourselves less.

Heredity

"I can't lose weight; it's in my genes!" Many would view this exclamation made by many obese persons as an excuse for their physical state. Research about genetic influences on obesity lends some (but not *total*) credibility to this exclamation. Children with obese parents do have a greater tendency to become obese adults. Is this an inherited tendency or a result of inappropriate behaviors learned and reinforced at home? Studies of families (especially twins) have provided insights into this question. A classic study conducted by Claude Bouchard showed that adult identical twins were similar in *total* fat gain and *distribution* of fat gain when consistently overfed for 100 days. There were huge differences between pairs of twins in body weight gains, body composition changes, and waist/hip circumference changes. Between twins, however, there were striking similarities. Similar research shows that adult twins tend to be similar in body weight and body mass index regardless of whether they were raised together in the same home or separated in early childhood and raised in different environments. Heredity seems to influence the number of fat cells in the body, how much fat is stored, where it is stored, and metabolic rates. However, scientists have concluded that genetics is responsible for only 25 percent of these factors.

Researchers are investigating how some of the body's hormones may be linked to obesity. One of those hormones, leptin, is secreted by fat cells and informs the brain about how large or small the body's fat stores are. As a result, the brain regulates appetite and metabolism accordingly. These studies give us more insight into the body's chemistry but do not fully explain the massive increases in weight across all age groups. Cases of obesity based solely on hormone abnormalities are rare. Centers for Disease Control and Prevention (CDC) former director Jeffrey Koplan, M.D., concurs by stating, "Genes related to obesity are clearly not responsible for the epidemic of obesity, because the gene pool in the U.S. did not change significantly after 1980."

Although these facts address the role heredity plays in obesity, heredity is only a *tendency* or predisposing factor that can be influenced by environmental components and behaviors. Those people predisposed to be overweight or obese will have more difficulty controlling their weight, but it is certainly not impossible for them to attain and maintain a healthy weight with healthy eating habits and regular exercise.

Metabolism

Every individual expends a certain amount of energy, even at rest, to sustain vital functions of the body such as brain activities, organ function, and temperature regulation. This energy requirement is called the **basal metabolic rate (BMR)** and accounts for approximately 60 to 75 percent of the calories burned in 1 day. A true measure of basal (resting) metabolism is taken when you have been lying quietly but awake and without food for 12 to 15 hours. Most men have a BMR requirement of 1,600 to 2,000 calories daily; most women need 1,200 to 1,500 calories daily. Lab Activity 12-3 provides an opportunity to determine your BMR. BMR is the largest component of your daily energy expenditure, and so it can significantly affect body weight over time.

Your BMR is a result of several interrelated factors, including age, gender, body size, nutritional status, musculature, activity level, and genetics. Pay particular attention to Table 12-4, which shows how BMR is affected by each of these factors.

Although some of your BMR is genetically inherited, you can affect it with exercise. An aerobic workout

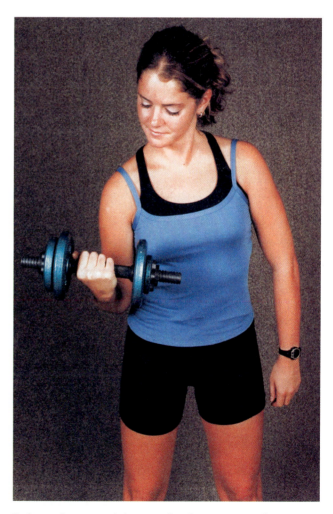

Doing resistance training exercises increases muscle mass, which in turn increases metabolism.

TABLE 12-4 *Factors That Affect Basal Metabolic Rate*

Gender	Women generally have lower BMRs than do men (about 5 to 10 percent lower) due to smaller size, more body fat, and less muscle mass.
Musculature	Increased muscle mass or tone increases BMR. Muscle tissue is more metabolically active than is fat. As muscles atrophy from inactivity, BMR declines.
Age	For both men and women, BMR declines by about 2 to 3 percent per decade after age 25. Loss of lean muscle mass typically occurs with aging as well. Maintaining a regular exercise program (including resistance training) can help prevent declines of lean muscle mass and BMR as you age.
Body size	Smaller body surface area results in lower BMR.
Nutritional status	Fasting, very low-calorie diets, and long-term undernutrition lower BMR.
Activity level	BMR increases during exercise and may remain elevated somewhat after exercising. The more vigorous the exercise, the longer your metabolism stays elevated.
Genetics	We inherit physiological tendencies, and as a result, BMR is inherently higher in some people and lower in others.

that includes resistance training (free weights, machines, or exercise bands) can increase muscle mass. The more muscle mass you have, the higher your BMR. Fat, being storage tissue, has a low metabolism, whereas muscle tissue is active and has a high metabolism. Women especially can counteract a slow metabolism by participating in exercise programs that include resistance training. In this way, they can increase their muscle mass. Middle-aged women often experience a dramatic slowdown of their metabolisms due to hormonal changes. They too can keep their "energy burners" fired up with regular exercise. The actual workout burns calories too! Your total daily caloric expenditure is influenced by:

1. Basal metabolism = 60 to 75 percent.
2. Digestion = 10 percent (e.g., if you consume 2,000 calories a day, you burn 200 of them by digesting the food).
3. Physical activity and exercise = anywhere from 15 to 40 percent (*you* control this!). Remember, *all* physical activity burns calories.

WHAT ABOUT "DIETING"?

Most people who want to lose weight think immediately of going on a diet. This notion is reinforced by the number of new fad diets advertised each year. In this connotation, the word *diet* implies a distinctive way of eating that involves special foods or food combinations; caloric or food restrictions; or special powders, pills, or shakes. In reality, the word *diet* should imply a way of eating for a lifetime. Popular weight-loss diets are viewed by the user as a temporary inconvenience that will be discontinued as soon as the weight goal has been reached. "Going on" a diet implies "going off" it. Dieters assume that weight will be lost quickly and immediately. Chances are, however, that the excess pounds have accumulated gradually over a period of years. These pounds are maintained by ingrained habits. Most fad diets rely on rigid food choices. Food becomes the enemy, and mealtime a battle to be fought. Continual deprivation can result in food cravings, binges, guilt, and self-deprecation. Many popular diets do not emphasize physical exercise. More than half the overweight adults trying to lose weight are doing so by restricting calories. Yet fewer than one-third are increasing physical activity. This is a reflection of our sedentary lifestyle and the emphasis on "going on a diet" as a means to control weight rather than increasing exercise. Diets have special appeal and sound easy. Many of them, however, are nutritionally inadequate, are too low in calories, are potentially dangerous, and most importantly, fail to teach lifelong eating habits. Even with programs that result in weight loss, the results are often short-term—and regaining weight is common if habits have not been permanently changed.

If you go on a very low-calorie diet, up to 70 percent of the weight loss during the first 3 days is water. This is predictable because your body needs carbohydrates for energy. Being starved of carbohydrates, it uses **glycogen** (stored carbohydrates) for energy. As you use this glycogen, you lose water, because each gram of carbohydrate is stored with 3 grams of water. Your body also uses protein for energy, resulting in a loss of muscle tissue. Crash dieting can cause headaches, ketosis, and loss of bone mineralization. If you go on a very low-

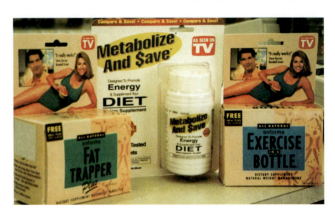

Be wary of diet aids that focus on a "quick fix."

calorie diet (less than 800 calories per day), your body slows its metabolism (BMR) significantly. After all, your body doesn't know that there is a grocery store a block away. It reacts as if you were suffering from starvation. Therefore, your body saves energy by burning fewer calories. This conservation of energy causes the diet to be even less effective. Depression, irritability, fatigue, and feelings of deprivation often follow. The survival urge to eat eventually wins out, and weight is regained.

There has been some debate in recent years (suggested primarily by proponents of low-carbohydrate diet plans) that the increasing obesity in the U.S. can be blamed on a shift to a low-fat, high-carbohydrate emphasis in the past few decades. In actuality, a recent long-range study shows that carbohydrates themselves do not cause weight gain. Excessive *calories* cause weight gain—whether they come from carbohydrates, protein, fats, jelly beans, or soda! Table 12-5 reviews some of the most

TABLE 12-5   *Diet Plans: Claims and Reality*

Diet Plan	Claims	Reality
Commercial weight-loss companies (Weight Watchers, L.A. Weight Loss, Jenny Craig, etc.)	Adheres to balanced and low-fat eating. Provides advice on portions, food choices, calorie intake. Moderate loss of 1–2 lbs. per week. Individual counseling and group support. (Note: Some commercial companies require purchase of their prepackaged foods, which can be expensive.)	Can be safe and effective if healthy lifelong eating habits and portion control are learned. The support system and personalized counseling are helpful.
Meal-replacement drinks/bars (Slim-Fast, etc.)	A liquid shake or bar replaces one or two meals a day. Contain sugar, protein, and vitamins and are low in calories.	May still be hungry; less satisfying. Calorie intake may be too low. Lacks fiber. Weight often regained when diet is stopped because proper food selection has not been learned.
"Fat-burning" diets (cabbage soup diet, grapefruit diet, etc.)	Certain foods can accelerate the body's ability to burn fat. Eating large quantities of these foods results in fast weight loss.	No food burns exclusively fat. Low in calories (which causes the weight loss). Boring and not nutritionally balanced. Weight is regained easily.
Low-carbohydrate/high-protein diets (Atkins, South Beach, Carbohydrate Addicts, etc.)	Restricts carbohydrates such as bread, cereals, starchy vegetables. Claims that carbs increase insulin, which promotes fat accumulation. Eat a lot of protein and fat. Transitions to phases that add complex carbohydrates and some fruits and vegetables.	Early phase is hard to stick with. Low calories. Loss of water and muscle causes weight loss. High fat and low calcium can contribute to future diseases. May cause bad breath, fatigue, dizziness, muscle weakness, headaches, and constipation in early phases. Weight is regained if eating returns to normal.
Low-fat diets (Ornish, Volumetrics, Pritikin)	Fat-free and low-fat foods and a lot of fruits, vegetables, whole grains, beans. Promotes foods high in fiber and water. Weight loss occurs despite eating ample amounts of low-calorie foods.	Healthy for heart and cancer prevention. Effective for weight loss but hard for some to adhere to due to lack of fats. May be low in calcium and iron if dieter is not careful. Exercise is emphasized.
Diet pills	Claim to burn fat, absorb extra fat, increase metabolism, and/or suppress appetite.	Promoted as a "quick fix." May contain amphetamine-like substances (ephedra, guarana, bitter orange), which may cause heart irregularities and jitters. Some herbs may help with appetite in some, but safety is an issue. Lifelong eating habits not learned.
Glycemic index ("The Glucose Revolution," "Good Carbs, Bad Carbs")	Carbohydrates that break down quickly (i.e., have a high glycemic index [GI]) cause a quick blood sugar and insulin rise, resulting in fat storage. Slow-release carbohydrates (low GI) fill you up, cause a slower release of glucose, decrease blood sugar fluctuations, and burn body fat.	Is a balanced approach of consuming adequate protein, low fat (under 30%), and 60% carbohydrate (of low GI: whole grains, legumes, vegetables, fruits) and reducing refined breads, cereals, rice, potatoes, and snacks). Is sensible and healthy but requires distinguishing high-GI from low-GI foods.
Insulin-resistance diets ("The Zone," etc.)	A low-carb, high-protein plan consisting of meals eaten with proper carb-to-protein-to-fat ratio (40:30:30) to combat the insulin production that may prompt fat storage.	No scientific evidence that a diet of precise ratios puts the body in a "zone" of enhanced or accelerated fat loss.

popular diet plans. It is important to know the facts before trying any specialized plan.

Weight Cycling

Weight cycling is the repeated loss and regaining of body weight. When weight cycling is the result of low-calorie or fad dieting, it is often called the **yo-yo syndrome.** There have been claims that weight cycling may make it more difficult to lose weight or keep it off, increase fat stores, slow metabolism, or even contribute to an increased risk of death from heart disease. Studies have not yet supported these claims conclusively. Most obesity experts believe that obese individuals should continue efforts to lose weight. Any weight loss is better than the potential risks of remaining obese or experiencing weight cycling.

Weight cycling should not affect the success of future weight-loss efforts. As with any attempt at changing behavior, you may experience cycles of success and lapses before finally succeeding. All people, whether they have dieted or not, experience a slowing of metabolism with aging. And a substantial weight loss results in a reduction in caloric needs. Therefore, it is important to monitor caloric intake and exercise habits to prevent weight cycling. This information accentuates even more dramatically the need to learn *skills* for maintaining weight loss and to *prevent* obesity from occurring altogether. Losing weight—and maintaining a healthy weight—is a lifelong commitment.

Reliable Weight-Loss Programs

Are there any reliable weight-loss programs? Yes. There are some good programs available, as long as the dieter understands the purpose and limitations of commercial plans. Enrolling in a weight-control program is an investment of time, energy, and money. Ask yourself if you are ready to lose the weight *and* do what it takes to keep it off. Losing the weight is only half the battle. Keeping it off demands lifestyle changes that are lifelong. It is especially important for the morbidly obese to seek professional help in losing weight. These persons would be wise to consult one of the hospital-based programs available in many communities or meet with a registered dietitian. New fad diets appear almost weekly and disappear almost as quickly, and so it is unrealistic to assess every particular diet for strengths and weaknesses. Instead, look at the Top 10 List "Guidelines for Evaluating a Weight-Loss Program." Many weight-management specialists view Weight Watchers as a reliable weight-loss program because it incorporates many of the principles that contribute to success: balanced eating, portion control, counseling and support, regular exercise, and teaching lifelong eating behaviors. It has been around since 1963 and was developed by registered dietitians and specialists in weight management.

TOP 10 LIST

Guidelines for Evaluating a Weight-Loss Program

1. It should use real, regular food available in supermarkets.
2. It should provide an energy deficit to allow slow, safe weight loss of 1 to 2 pounds per week.
3. It should encourage the reduction of fat in the diet.
4. It should encourage a safe, personalized exercise program.
5. It should not promise a quick fix or advertise claims that sound too good to be true.
6. It should teach lifelong changes that allow freedom and flexibility for individual lifestyles and not list "good" and "forbidden" foods. Allows for "favorite" foods in moderation.
7. It should make possible the enjoyment of social situations such as eating out, holidays, and special occasions.
8. It should allow for basic energy needs (never under 1,200 calories daily) and be nutritionally balanced.
9. It should not be too costly.
10. It should teach techniques and strategies for *maintaining* positive behavior change.

A final question to ask yourself when considering a diet plan should be, "Can I live with this program for the rest of my life?"

The goal of weight loss is fat loss, which takes time and long-term lifestyle change. Remember: It is not necessary for an overweight or obese person to reach an optimal body weight in order to begin experiencing health benefits. Even modest increments of weight loss are associated with improvements in blood pressure and other health parameters. Many diets are variations on the food restriction theme, are unpleasant, and fail to teach modification of eating behavior. Scarcity and deprivation often lead to bingeing and subsequent feelings of guilt and despair. Just about any type of food restriction will result in weight loss. The key is keeping the weight off by learning to live with food—forever!

LIFETIME WEIGHT MANAGEMENT: STAYING LEAN IN FATTENING TIMES

The factors that contribute to obesity are so numerous and complex that it is impossible to pinpoint one cause. Having knowledge of the theories of obesity should help you understand some of these complexities. Fat cells, metabolism, set points, genetics, and energy expenditure all play a role. Behaviors that have developed over time are also intricately involved. One unrefuted truth emerges in nearly all weight-control studies: *Permanent weight control involves a lifelong commitment to good eating habits and regular exercise.*

Dr. James O. Hill, director of the University of Colorado Center for Human Nutrition, states, "You need to use your intellect to *not* gain weight today. Social forces that promote overeating and our modern sedentary lifestyle are so persuasive that you always need to think about what you're buying, what you're eating, and how active you are." Weight management is a lifestyle. Maintaining a reasonable body composition is a result, not of isolated bouts of crash dieting or sporadic exercise, but of lifelong integration of three management components:

1. Food management
2. Emotional management
3. Exercise management

Food Management

We must eat to sustain life, and eating is one of life's pleasures. To lose or maintain weight, it is essential to have a good framework for making sensible, well-balanced food choices. Basic weight-management principles are not different from general good nutritional recommendations (low saturated fat, sugar, and salt and high complex carbohydrates, fruits and vegetables, and fiber). Cutting back on the fat in your diet reduces a tremendous number of calories. "I lost weight without eating less!" is often the exclamation of persons who substitute fiber-rich grains, fruits, and vegetables for fat in their diets. Fiber fills you up and slows the absorption of food, which regulates blood sugar and insulin levels.

This eating plan not only helps with weight; it helps prevent disease while ensuring adequate intake of all essential nutrients. The *2005 Dietary Guidelines for Americans* and MyPyramid (see Chapter 11) describe such an eating plan.

By consistently consuming more calories than are needed, creeping obesity occurs. This is what is happening in most industrialized countries in the world. Managing food intake in our modern world is a definite challenge. Understanding the following factors that contribute to this caloric imbalance may help you monitor your own food intake.

Recognizing Portion Distortion

Portion and serving sizes have increased tremendously in the past 25 years. As confirmed by a study published in the *Journal of the American Medical Association,* portion sizes since the 1980s have nearly doubled for most foods served in restaurants and at home, and portions are often "supersized" to be even larger for very little extra money! This makes larger portions seem like a bargain to the consumer. Restaurant plates are larger and are overfilled with pasta, nachos, and chicken wings. Parking lots at all-you-can-eat buffets are packed. And research shows: the more food that is put in front of us, the more we will eat. In 1957, a fast-food hamburger weighed 1 ounce and had 210 calories. Today's average burger is 6 ounces and has 618 calories. A typical restaurant serving of pasta exceeds the federal recommended serving size by 480 percent! And, with the introduction of fat-free foods, many people erroneously believe that they can eat the entire box of fat-free cookies, neglecting the fact that these foods have calories too. Overall calorie consumption cannot be ignored! Therefore, be aware of recommended serving sizes (see Chapter 11, Figure 11-1). It may be helpful to actually weigh and measure your food for several days to increase your awareness and help you monitor your intake.

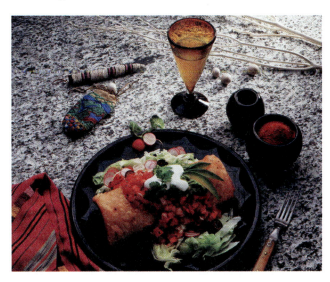

As restaurant portions become larger, Americans are "supersizing" their way to obesity.

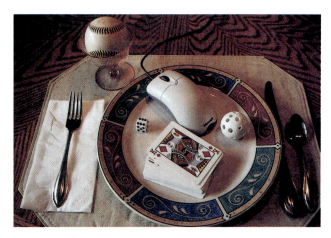

Be aware of recommended serving sizes. Using common everyday references (see Chapter 11, Figure 11-1 and Table 11-9) can help you manage your portion sizes.

Avoiding Mindless Eating

"I hardly eat anything! Why can't I lose weight?" This is a common complaint voiced by frustrated dieters. Because we have a culture of snacking and eating on the run, many people underestimate the calories they consume since they seldom sit down for a real meal. The doughnut in the break room, the mocha coffee from the coffee stand, the chocolate kisses from the candy dish, the taste-testing at the grocery store, and the sack of chips while watching television all count! The 2,000 calories consumed a day from a plate are reasonable, but another 1,000 calories nibbled, grazed on, or grabbed mindlessly throughout the day add up. Even though Americans are consciously consuming less fat as a percentage of total calories, today's average daily calorie intake is up about 300 calories as compared to 1970. Keeping an *honest* food journal for several days (see Lab Activity 12-1 for a sample journal) can help you see what and how much food/calories you are eating and drinking. By becoming conscious of everything you put into your mouth, you can begin to eat *mindfully* rather than *mindlessly*!

Understanding Our "Toxic" Environment

We live in an environment that provides food most everywhere and at any time of the day. It's conveniently packaged, inexpensive, good-tasting, and served in ample portions. Unfortunately much of it is poor quality in terms of nutrition. Dr. Kelly Brownell, director of the Yale Center for Eating and Weight Disorders, has termed our food environment "toxic." We are surrounded by temptations to eat wherever we go—on street corners, along highways, at gas stations, at the office, at the malls, and in school hallways. We are barraged by over 10,000 food advertisements each year on television—most of which are from fast-food chains or from soft drink and snack food companies. The commercials say, "Eat, eat, eat" but show an actress who is so thin that it appears she never eats! Food messages often drown out health messages. For example, more than $33 billion per year is spent on advertising sugary soft drinks, candy, and fatty snacks. In contrast, the National Cancer Institute's maximum annual advertising budget to promote the "5-to-9-a-Day" (fruit and vegetable) campaign is $1 million. So, what can you do? First of all, tune into your natural hunger signals and vow not to eat just because you are driving past the doughnut shop, walking past a vending machine, or talking with friends who are snacking. Pay attention to the social and environmental influences that confront you, and do not accept cultural reality as a license to splurge! And finally, become an advocate for environmental change. Education and public information are not enough to change the environment. Support new laws that regulate advertising, prohibit the sale of fast foods and soft drinks in schools, subsidize healthy foods, and require the posting of nutrition information in restaurants.

Whereas many people look to structured weight-loss diets for their "food management," such programs often feature a lot of "can have" and "cannot have" foods. Sensibility in food choices does not mean that you will never again eat chocolate cake. There should never be guilt or forbidden foods. Instead, lifetime food management means seeing how much or where chocolate cake fits into your total diet. Reduce, don't eliminate, certain foods. Balance your food choices over time. Gradual rather than drastic changes in dietary patterns lead to successful maintenance. Healthful eating does not happen by accident, and it is not always easy. In our "land of plenty" it is essential to learn about the nutritive value of foods, portion sizes, and why we are eating and devise strategies for making good choices over the course of each day.

Emotional Management

Why do you eat? "Because I am hungry!" you answer. If all people ate only when they were in the physiological state of hunger, few would have a weight problem. Not only are we surrounded with opportunities to eat more food than we need, eating behavior is strongly influenced by psychological, social, and emotional factors. We eat out of emotional needs. We eat when we're happy; we eat when we're sad. Food becomes a substitute for other things. We confuse physical hunger with emotional hunger. Whereas it is true that food affects the brain's production of certain "feel good" chemicals, habitually using food as a "drug" to cope with emotional feelings can be destructive.

Controlling eating habits begins with having an understanding of why you eat and what cues trigger eating. Do you eat when you are bored? Lonely? Angry? Stressed? Do you eat when you turn on the television? Read? Do you eat when something smells good? When others are eating? To avoid studying? Even positive feelings can trigger eating—earning an A on a paper, celebrating the end of final exams, looking forward to the weekend. For emotional eaters, food serves as a comfort. Their "fix" is food, a means of self-nurturing.

For emotional management, spend time observing your eating behavior. Keep a journal, recording the food you are eating and the feelings that accompany that moment. (Use the food journal in Lab Activity 12-1 at the end of this chapter.) Learn to recognize the cues and connections between your thoughts, feelings, and behaviors. Before you eat, ask yourself: "Why am I reaching for food at this time?" Learn to differentiate between hunger and appetite. *Hunger* is an actual physical need for food. *Appetite* is a desire for food that usually is triggered by anxiety, boredom, depression, stress, habit, or the mere availability of food. No diet plan works if it doesn't help you understand and resolve the reasons you turn to food when you aren't physically hungry. If

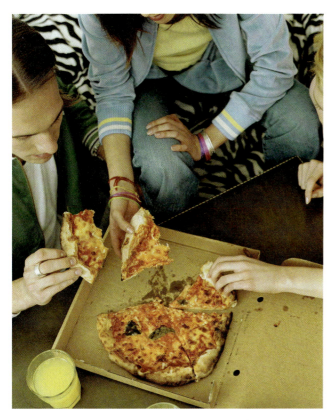

Many times we eat in social situations even when we're not really hungry.

TABLE 12-6 *Behavior Modification Techniques*

1. Keep a food journal to maximize awareness of eating.
2. Eat in one room only; sit at a table—don't stand.
3. Prepackage healthy snacks or meals and take them with you.
4. Keep a weight, fat gram, or calorie graph.
5. Never read or watch TV while eating.
6. Use smaller plates.
7. Always leave some food on your plate.
8. Drink a lot of water throughout the day and during meals.
9. Prepare, serve, and eat one portion at a time.
10. Do not place serving dishes on the table.
11. Grocery shop from a list and never on an empty stomach.
12. Leave the table after eating and clear dishes directly into the compost pile or garbage; brush your teeth immediately or chew gum.
13. Keep problem food out of sight or not in the house.
14. Keep healthy food accessible and visible.
15. Make eating a conscious experience (i.e., eat slowly, chew each bite thoroughly, put utensils down between bites, eat with your nondominant hand, cut food into smaller pieces).
16. Rehearse strategies in advance for eating out, special occasions, and high-risk situations.
17. Substitute alternative activities for eating (write a letter, go for a walk, jog, pay bills, sew, play tennis, etc.).
18. Don't do non-food-related activities in the kitchen; stay out of the kitchen as much as possible; close the kitchen down after a meal.
19. When eating out, plan to share large portions with a companion. Or take extras home for another meal.
20. Eat and snack from a plate, not the package, so you don't absentmindedly eat more than you realize.

you are one of those people who experience occasional food cravings, try using the 3 Ds+S.

- ✔ *Delay* at least 10 minutes before you eat so that your action is conscious, not impulsive.
- ✔ *Distract* yourself by engaging in an activity that requires concentration (e.g., play the guitar, surf the Internet, do a crossword puzzle, read a magazine)
- ✔ *Distance* yourself from the food.
- ✔ *Substitute* a small portion or healthier version of the craved food (e.g., a chocolate kiss instead of a whole candy bar, frozen yogurt rather than premium ice cream, veggie pizza instead of pepperoni).

Using behavior modification strategies can help emotional eaters. **Behavior modification** is the use of techniques to enhance awareness or consciousness of a behavior and subsequently alter that behavior. Behavior modification is based on the premise that all behaviors are learned responses to environmental cues or antecedents. In using these techniques, people make eating a more conscious act, and healthier behavior patterns are integrated into the day-to-day routine. These patterns include slowing the act of eating, altering susceptibility to the cues (separating eating from other activities, such as watching TV), and breaking behavior chains. Set

yourself up for success by managing your environment. For example, throw out the cookies stashed in your desk drawer, the chips in your cabinet, and the candy in your glove compartment. It is true that our "food frenzy" culture is a temptation-rich environment, but it is an environment over which *you* have control! Table 12-6 gives examples of some behavior modification techniques.

Changing eating behavior demands commitment and perseverance (unlike the magic potions or easy pitches delivered in many popular magazines). Too often, commercial weight-loss programs reward persons for the total number of pounds lost, creating undesirable behaviors such as going on crash diets, skipping meals, and using drugs and diuretics. According to some weight-management researchers, the use of rewards for weight loss is inappropriate because weight loss is not a behavior. It is the outcome of a complex interaction of emotions and behaviors over time. As discussed in Chapter 2, behavior change is a complex process that involves stages and coping techniques within each stage. You may want to go back to Chapter 2 and review the transtheoretical model of behavior change to see which techniques can be incorporated into managing

TABLE 12-7	*Tips for Behavior Change: Losing Weight*

STAGES OF CHANGE: IN WHAT STAGE ARE YOU?

1. Precontemplation: "As far as I'm concerned I'm not too heavy. I'm just big-boned."
2. Contemplation: "I think I should probably lose some weight. Maybe I'll try after the holidays."
3. Preparation: "I am currently planning my weight-loss program."
4. Action: "I have been making the lifestyle changes I need to make to lose weight (dietary change and exercise) for 3 months, and it is working."
5. Maintenance: "I have been successful at losing weight and maintaining that loss for over 6 months."

PROCESSES OF CHANGE

After identifying your current stage, try using some of the following selected processes and behavior strategies that are appropriate for your particular stage—to facilitate your transition into the next stage (refer to Figure 2-2):

- Consciousness-raising: Read about people who have lost weight.
- Social liberation: Check out low-fat and low-calorie options at your favorite lunch/dinner spots.
- Self-reevaluation: Assess and write down your feelings and disappointments due to your dependence on food.
- Reward: Treat yourself to a low-fat frozen yogurt or a small piece of chocolate every Saturday after a week of healthy food choices.
- Environment control: Throw out junk-food snacks stored in desk drawer/shelves.
- Helping relationships: Ask roommate to refrain from storing/eating snacks in your room; invite a friend to join you in making dietary/exercise changes.

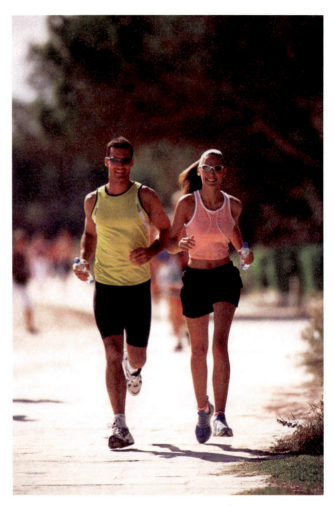

Participating in regular vigorous exercise is essential for lifelong weight management.

emotional eating. Table 12-7 may help you identify your stage of change in terms of weight loss. Some example techniques are listed with selected processes as well. To continue with or maintain weight loss, you must be able to identify your high-risk situations in which difficulties with feelings or social situations can lead to a relapse. Developing and practicing coping strategies for dealing with these situations is an essential part of emotional management. Remove yourself from former patterns of behavior and develop new rituals that will ensure your success. Food stops taking on the role of nurturer when people learn to nurture themselves. Long-lasting change can occur only through kindness to yourself, mindfulness about what you are doing and why, and a willingness to act on your own behalf.

Exercise Management

Exercise is crucial to losing weight and maintaining weight. Americans have become fatter because calorie output has declined drastically. Most of our work, daily activities, and even some of our leisure pursuits do not burn many calories. Television viewing, which substantially decreases activity levels and may influence diet, is a strong factor in obesity, especially among children and adolescents. In adults there is a direct relationship between the number of hours spent watching television and a person's level of obesity. The Internet, computers, video games, and DVDs and videos have decreased overall activity levels. American technology has been ingenious in discovering ways for us to save energy, thus throwing off our energy balance. Electric garage-door openers, riding lawn mowers, elevators, and drive-up banks are a few examples of activity-robbing conveniences.

The importance of physical activity in the prevention and treatment of obesity receives less attention than restrictive "dieting." There is certainly no scarcity of diet books, programs, and articles from which to choose. And studies have shown that physical activity *alone* (without a change in diet) produces only modest weight loss. However, for lifetime weight management to occur, exercise (accompanied by dietary management) is imperative. According to the National Weight Control Registry, a group of women and men who have lost at least 30 pounds and maintained that weight loss for at least one year, regular exercise is a common trait of successful "losers." This group reports that they average 1 hour or more of moderate- to vigorous-intensity physical activity every day. Although the immediate effects of exercise are sometimes limited, the long-term cumulative effects of small changes in activity level are key components in lifetime weight management. By reengineering some physical activity back into our daily routine (called "lifestyle physical activity") and by fitting in 30–60 minutes of moderate-intensity activity every day, lifetime weight goals can be reached. Plus, living a physically active lifestyle substantially reduces the risk for a variety of other chronic diseases! Look at how regular exercise contributes to fat loss.

✔ **It Burns Calories**   Table 12-8 shows how many calories you burn per minute in various activities. Note that the larger person burns more energy than does the lighter person engaged in the same activity. Also notice how aerobic activities burn considerably more calories per minute than do light, day-to-day tasks. Most people burn approximately 100 calories

per mile whether walking or jogging. If this does not seem like a lot, look at it this way: You burn only about 1 calorie per minute while sitting. Remember that weight gain does not occur overnight, nor does weight loss. A pound of fat is lost by burning 3,500 calories. No one ever said it must all be done at once and only by jogging. Liberating large amounts of energy from body reservoirs requires time—typically measured in months, if not years. Whereas the Centers for Disease Control and Prevention recommends 30 minutes of exercise per day for heart and overall health, recent research reveals that to lose weight and maintain weight loss, much more caloric expenditure from exercise is necessary. Studies indicate that burning approximately 2,800 calories a week with exercise (about 400 calories daily) should be the goal if weight is an issue. This would equate to about 1 hour of moderate-intensity activity per day or walking 4 miles. If more vigorous exercise is preferred (e.g., jogging, aerobic dance, lap swimming), about 40 minutes per day is recommended. As exercise intensity becomes more vigorous, an added benefit is that your metabolism

TABLE 12-8   *Caloric Expenditure per Minute for Selected Activities*

The figures in this table are only for the *time* you are engaged in the activity (not standing, waiting, resting). Variances may occur if you are running uphill, walking with hand weights, biking into a strong head wind, and so on. There may be small differences between males and females, but not enough to make a significant difference. You can approximate your expenditure if you are between the body weights listed. For information on calories burned in a more expansive list of activities, go to www.caloriesperhour.com or www.caloriecontrol.org.

Body Weight	120	150	180	210
Sitting and writing	1.5	1.9	2.3	2.7
Standing with light work, cleaning, etc.	3.3	4.1	4.9	5.7
Aerobic dance	7.3	9.1	10.9	12.7
Basketball (recreational)	6.0	7.5	9.0	10.5
Bicycling (10 mph; 6 min/mile)	5.1	6.4	7.6	8.9
Bicycling (15 mph; 4 min/mile)	8.7	10.9	13.1	15.3
Dancing (active, square, disco)	5.4	6.8	8.2	9.5
Deep water treading/running	12.0	15.0	18.0	21.0
Golf (foursome, carrying clubs)	3.3	4.1	4.9	5.7
Racquetball	7.8	9.8	11.7	13.7
Roller skating (9 mph)	5.1	6.4	7.6	8.9
Running (6 mph; 10 min/mile)	8.7	10.9	13.1	15.4
Running (7 mph; 8:35 min/mile)	10.2	12.8	15.4	17.9
Running (8 mph; 7:30 min/mile)	11.6	14.6	17.6	20.5
Skiing, downhill; cross country (4 mph; 15 min/mile)	7.8	9.9	11.9	13.8
Soccer	7.2	9.0	10.8	12.6
Stair step machine	5.7	7.0	8.7	10.2
Stationary cycling (vigorous)	7.8	9.7	11.7	13.6
Swimming (crawl, 35 yds/min)	5.9	7.3	8.8	10.2
Swimming (crawl, 45 yds/min)	6.9	8.7	10.4	12.2
Tennis (recreational singles)	6.0	7.5	9.0	10.6
Walking (3 mph; 20 min/mile)	3.3	4.1	4.9	5.7
Walking (4 mph; 15 min/mile)	5.1	6.4	7.6	8.9
Walking (5 mph; 12 min/mile)	6.5	8.2	9.8	11.5
Water aerobics	7.2	9.0	10.8	12.6
Weight training	6.2	7.8	9.4	11.2

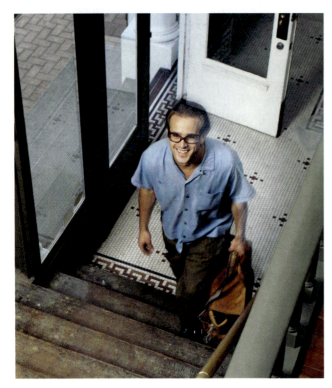

Regularly taking the stairs rather than the elevator is one way to add more activity to your day.

(rate of calorie burning) is increased for several hours after you have completed the exercise bout. However, regardless of intensity level, doing regular, sustained exercise on a consistent basis (on most days of the week) is the best strategy for maintaining weight. And don't forget that doing intermittent activity throughout the day also burns calories. Find ways to weave increased energy expenditure into day-to-day living: Walk to work or during breaks, take stairs instead of elevators, ride a bike on errands. Wear a pedometer and try to accumulate the recommended 10,000 steps per day.

✔ **It Prevents Loss of Lean Muscle Mass**   As you age, you lose about 2 percent of your muscle mass each year. By the time you are 55, you could be down 15 pounds of muscle and burning about 600 fewer calories per day. Exercise builds and helps maintain muscle tissue. And since muscle cells are metabolically active, they burn more calories in basal metabolism (at rest) than do fat cells. At rest, muscle tissue burns approximately 40 calories per day per pound. At rest, fat tissue burns approximately 2 calories per day per pound. As a result, someone with a lot of muscle mass burns more calories throughout the day *outside* the exercise session. This is a key factor especially for women of all ages (who typically have less muscle mass and more fat than men) and for *both* men and women during middle age, when metabolism can slow down due to loss of muscle tissue. Doing

resistance training exercises 2 to 3 days per week, using free weights, machines, or an exercise band, along with daily aerobic exercise can accelerate weight loss.

✔ **It Decreases Abdominal Fat**   Excessive fat in the abdominal area (apple-shape obesity) is linked to increased risk of heart disease, many cancers, and type 2 diabetes. Studies show that most of the positive effects of physical activity on heart disease risk factors (especially blood pressure and cholesterol) have to do with reductions in this intra-abdominal fat. This is true for both men and women. Since fat around the abdominal area is easier to mobilize than is fat in the hip-thigh area, regular physical activity attacks abdominal fat very effectively.

✔ **It Is a Natural Appetite Suppressor**   Moderate exercise has a tendency to decrease the appetite for a time after the workout because blood is diverted from digestive organs to skeletal muscles. You may feel thirsty but not usually hungry. This is why exercising during a lunch break helps you control weight. After exercising, you feel satisfied with a light lunch. Extremely intense exercise tends to lower blood sugar, which may stimulate appetite. To burn fat, keep your exercise at a moderate intensity and work to increase the duration. (Be sure not to view exercise as an excuse for eating more!)

✔ **It May Lower Your Set Point**   Set-point theorists believe that regular, vigorous exercise is the one sure way to lower your body's fat level. Maintaining an active lifestyle stabilizes the set point at this lower level.

✔ **It Helps Maintain Weight Loss**   Most health professionals agree that losing weight is easy; keeping it off is more difficult. To avoid the negative consequences of weight cycling, more attention is being given to *maintenance* of weight loss. Exercise has been shown to be one of the few factors correlated with long-term weight maintenance. A change in lifestyle that includes a consistent exercise regimen across the life span is the fundamental key to successful weight-loss maintenance.

✔ **It Improves Self-Esteem**   For overweight, sedentary individuals, exercise may not be a richly reinforcing experience at first. It may be difficult for them to get out and exercise in public. They may feel self-conscious about their bodies. They may have negative feelings about exercise because of past embarrassing experiences. As exercise becomes a satisfying habit, the individual begins to experience a new sense of well-being and power. Anxiety and depression are reduced. As weight comes off, self-image is enhanced. Self-esteem and self-confidence are improved. These psychological benefits received from regular participation in physical activity often supply the

Prescription for Action

Date *Do one or more today*

✔ Keep a food journal to see *what, how much,* and *why* you are eating.

✔ Count the calories you are eating (calories in) and compare it to your basal metabolic rate plus activity calories (calories out).

✔ Take a favorite recipe and investigate ways to make it less caloric and more nutritious.

✔ Resign from the "clean plate club." Even if it feels somewhat uncomfortable, leave a small amount of food on your plate.

✔ Do some form of exercise that burns a minimum of 300 calories.

Prescribed by _____*YOU*_____

---

additional impetus necessary for adhering to a weight-loss/maintenance program. This positive self-concept helps reinforce all other areas of weight management, including food selection, feelings of anxiety, and feelings of control.

As you incorporate food management, emotional management, and exercise management into your life, you'll forget the "dieting mentality" and incorporate a set of behaviors and attributes that are necessary for permanent weight control. This "non-diet mentality" incorporates looking at your body intelligently (i.e., developing a positive but realistic image of yourself), eating intelligently, and moving your body intelligently (i.e., finding ways to weave daily activity into your life). Check out the Top 10 List "Tips from Successful Losers and Maintainers." Like them, when you structure and program your environment and life for success, managing your weight becomes part of your lifestyle. Through deliberate actions and specific strategies, you can learn to quash the saboteurs and temptations that our environment presents.

GAINING WEIGHT: A HEALTHY PLAN FOR ADDING POUNDS

While many overweight people face the challenge of shedding extra pounds, those who are underweight face the challenge of trying to hold on to each pound and perhaps add more. The key to gaining weight is shifting the body weight equation so that you take in more calories than you burn. Add two to three substantial snacks

---

TOP **10** LIST

Tips from Successful Losers and Maintainers

People succeed at weight loss through conscious effort. These tips from successful losers and maintainers address *lifetime* weight management—how to lose weight *and* keep it off forever!

1. Focus on an overall *healthy* eating style, not a specialized "diet."
2. Choose low-fat over higher-fat foods when available (e.g., dairy, salad dressing, sauces, sour cream, cream cheese, cooking spray).
3. Control portions. Everything has calories, even fat-free foods. Take half of that huge restaurant portion home with you or split it with your dining partner.
4. Plan for up to an hour of exercise every day (include both aerobic and resistance training exercises). Look for ways to add additional activity to daily life.
5. Allow favorite foods—in moderation.
6. Fill up on fiber (fruits, vegetables, whole grains) and eat a little protein with each meal.
7. Don't skip meals (especially breakfast). "Grazing" or eating smaller but more frequent meals or snacks improves metabolism and blood sugar levels and reduces cravings and bingeing.
8. Set realistic goals. Working on losing 5 pounds at a time is easier than focusing on losing all 50 pounds.
9. Evaluate your relationship with food. Are you truly physiologically hungry, or are you eating because of stress, boredom, anxiety, or habit? Develop coping and problem-solving strategies.
10. Keep a written or mental record of what is eaten each day and the amount of exercise that is done each day.

Note: Finally, if you've eaten one too many chocolate chip cookies or haven't made it to the gym for a few days, don't give up. Take lapses in stride. Try to ascertain why the lapse occurred, learn from it, and move on. Weight management is a lifelong process, not an all-or-nothing contest. Remember, small changes can bring big results.

---

between three moderate-size meals. Rather than eating high-fat and sugary foods, choose "calorie-dense" foods packed with nutrients. Even skinny people need to be concerned about heart disease and cancer. Here are some dietary suggestions:

✔ Mix beans, nuts, cheese, peas, or lean meats into casseroles, side dishes, and pasta.

✔ Combine yogurt, fruit, wheat germ, peanut butter, and ice in a blender to make a shake or smoothie.

✔ Spread peanut butter on bananas, apples, toast, or bagels.

✔ Replace sodas with fruit juices or skim milk.

✔ Replace cookies and doughnuts with nuts, raisins, dried fruits, bran muffins, yogurt, puddings, and fruit.

✔ Replace hamburgers and fries with thick-crust vegetable-topped pizza.

✔ Prepare hot cereals with milk instead of water; add nuts, peanut butter, fruit, and wheat germ.

✔ Top cold cereal with bananas or raisins.

✔ Eat hearty soups.

✔ Add garbanzo beans, seeds, tuna, croutons, cottage cheese, and lean meat to salads.

In addition to dietary alterations, adding strength-training exercises two to three times a week will add muscle mass to your frame. (See Chapter 6 for suggestions.)

CULTURE AND WEIGHT

Why people diet and other weight-related issues are shaped by cultural environments. In earlier times, the female figures painted by Renoir and other artists were soft and fleshy. Rounded bellies and dimpled thighs were the feminine ideal. For both men and women, a surplus of fat was equated with wealth and success. The 20th century brought about a decline in fatness as a social asset. Insurance companies began observing the increased death rate among the overweight. The socially elite began diminishing the enormousness of banquet menus. Corsets gave way to exercise and raised hemlines. Hollywood stars became the ideals. Thinness became equated with glamour, success, and desirability. As weight reduction became a national pastime, mail-order companies began making large profits with their weight-loss gimmicks. The market eventually gave way to new low-calorie foods and drugs designed to fool the body's hunger sensations. At the same time, labor-saving machines reduced the energy output necessary in daily life. The message that emerged by the 1960s was "Thin is in." The desire for an unrealistic slimness, particularly among women, has caused many to be preoccupied with their bodies and with dieting. Diet books become instant best-sellers.

There She Is . . . Miss Unrealistic America

Open up any fashion magazine or clothing catalog. The models are thin. This thin standard is perpetuated in all channels of social influence: families, peers, and the media. The message is pounded home over and over: "You can never be thin enough." This notion has been documented in studies of *Playboy* centerfolds and Miss America Pageant contestants from 1959 to the present, indicating a shift toward a thinner ideal shape for women in our culture. At the same time, there has been a significant increase in diet articles in popular women's magazines. The cultural "ideal" for women's body size keeps getting thinner, though the average woman weighs 144 pounds and wears a size 12 to 14. This cultural index of the "ideal" woman's body is 13 to 19 percent below the expected weight for age and height. A body weight below 15 percent of expected weight is one of the criteria for diagnosing anorexia nervosa, so what does this say about our cultural ideals?

With extreme slimness as a cultural obsession, it becomes clear why fear of fat, fad dieting, surgical fat removal, and eating disorders abound. In our society that puts such a premium on thinness, overweight, obese, and even normal-weight individuals evaluate themselves in society's mirror, defining themselves as unattractive and as failures. Such harsh evaluations are a result of an acceptance of society's distorted concept of the ideal body. Every day we see pictures of models in magazines that are airbrushed and electronically altered—a "manufactured ideal." The readers, however, have "real-life" bodies! One study found that 3 minutes spent looking at models in a fashion magazine caused 70 percent of women to feel depressed, guilty, and shameful. Advertisements suggest that we invest money, time, and hope in trying to reach this ideal. Unfortunately, the results are often feelings of despair and inferiority. The first step toward a healthy weight is acceptance of your body type. Only about 5 percent of the population can look like the models and actresses we are exposed to daily. Twenty years ago fashion models weighed 8 percent less than the average woman; today they weigh 23 percent less. Our bodies are genetically programmed to be a certain build—tall, skinny, stout, short, muscular, big-boned, and so on. Everyone needs to accept his or her body type and then maximize it to be the best it can be rather than trying to achieve the impossible.

The media and the fashion industry need to take responsibility for using models who depict fitness and health rather than emaciation. Some already have. With the popularity of fitness and wellness programs in our country, we hope the image is changing. The "one size fits all" standard *must* change.

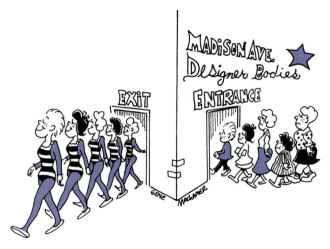
Many feel pressured to pursue a model-like body.

Men Are Joining In

Body image concerns are no longer confined to women. Millions of teenage boys and men are worried that their muscles aren't big enough or their bodies aren't lean enough. Bombarded with images of muscular half-naked men on the covers of men's magazines and in advertisements, men are facing the cultural pressures that women have felt for decades. Whereas both men and women experience a similar degree of body dissatisfaction, women universally want to lose weight while men tend to be evenly split between those wanting to lose weight and those desiring larger muscle mass. As a result, an increasing number of men are dieting, compulsively weight training, and abusing supplements and steroids as they strive for this ideal. This obsession for some goes beyond working out for health. It can affect schoolwork, jobs, personal relationships, and self-esteem and become a full-blown eating disorder.

EATING DISORDERS

Obsession with weight and the desire to be thin begin early in life. Even third-graders are dieting and fretting about their weight. Our culture especially socializes girls to be concerned about their physical appearance. For them, thinness equates with attractiveness and social approval. The message is, "Work hard in school, but be popular and pretty." In contrast, a male's self-concept is linked to physical dominance, power, and sports competence.

Few measure up to the fashion industry's ideal, and so dieting is commonplace. At the same time, obesity is dramatically rising. The dilemma of preventing obesity yet avoiding a fostering of "thin mania" presents a tremendous challenge.

The frequency of dieting among young women is alarming. It is estimated that two-thirds of adolescent girls in the United States have dysfunctional or abnormal eating behaviors. One survey of teenage girls revealed that most were more afraid of becoming fat than they were of cancer, nuclear war, or losing their parents! Fear of fat, obsessive dieting, and a distorted body image can lead to a psychological eating disorder. An **eating disorder** is defined as a disturbance in eating behavior that jeopardizes a person's physical or psychosocial health. Bear in mind that preoccupation with weight and dieting are not synonymous with an eating disorder. An eating disorder is an extremely serious psychopathological state. Most professionals agree, however, that dieting precedes the onset of an eating disorder. Eating disorders are viewed as multidimensional in cause and nature. Factors that increase vulnerability can be genetic, biological, psychological, personality, sociocultural, and familial. Thus, the treatment must include all components. Some of the general causes for eating disorders include:

1. Society's definition of the "perfect body" as unrealistically thin and lean.
2. Family characteristics such as overinvolvement and high expectations; overvaluing physical appearance; emotionally rigid and cold.
3. Personality traits like "perfectionism," the desire to achieve; feelings of inadequacy and loneliness.
4. A genetic propensity to being overweight.
5. Pressure from others to lose weight, including media images.
6. Appearance-obsessed friends (dance troupes, school cliques, sororities, cheerleaders).
7. Inherent low self-esteem.

It is estimated that 8 to 10 million Americans struggle with eating disorders. One million are men. All segments of society are affected—including minorities—and 86 percent report onset by age 20. However, eating disorders have been reported in children as young as age 6 and individuals as old as 76. Certain populations are especially at risk. They include gymnasts, dancers (especially ballet), cheerleaders, pom-pom performers, distance runners, and models. Although more women than men suffer from eating disorders, there is a higher

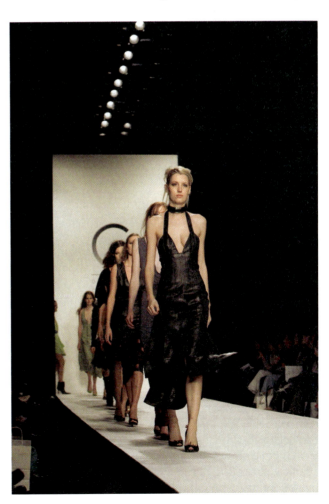

The fashion industry perpetuates the unrealistic ideal of extreme thinness, especially for women.

than normal incidence of eating disorders in certain subgroups of males where slenderness is encouraged: models, dancers, wrestlers, and distance runners.

High school and college-age students are also vulnerable due to academic and social stresses and peer pressure to conform. Most social events take place around eating and drinking: parties, dates, late-night snacks. Physical attractiveness is important, and the stresses of growing up and leaving home intensify these pressures. Rather than a strict addiction, eating disorders are a response to societal influences, dieting culture, fat discrimination, overachieving perfectionism, and media images. Two of the most common eating disorders are bulimia nervosa and anorexia nervosa. They may occur separately or together. A third eating disorder is called binge eating disorder.

Bulimia Nervosa

Bulimia is a Greek word meaning *ox* and *hunger.* The disorder was so named because the sufferer eats like a hungry ox. That is, **bulimia nervosa** is characterized by a compulsive need to eat large quantities of food (bingeing) to the point of gorging, followed by purging through vomiting, use of laxatives, or fasting. Often, the binge is a response to an intense emotional experience, such as stress, loneliness, or depression, rather than the result of a strong appetite. Nevertheless, most bulimics are not aware of what precipitates these uncontrollable binges and are not able to stop them. The diagnostic criteria for bulimia are as follows:

1. Recurrent episodes of binge eating (rapid consumption of a large amount of food in a discrete period).
2. A feeling of lack of control over eating behavior during the eating binges.
3. Self-induced vomiting, misuse of laxatives or diuretics, strict dieting or fasting, or excessive exercise to prevent a weight gain.
4. Two binge episodes a week for at least 3 months.
5. Self-evaluation unduly influenced by body shape and weight.
6. The bingeing and purging are not accompanied by anorexia nervosa.

Bulimia frequently starts as normal, voluntary dieting that later becomes compulsive, uncontrollable, and pathological. The bulimic's eating binge involves a rapid gulping of enormous quantities of food. Preferred foods are high in calories and sweet-tasting and can be eaten rapidly without preparation: ice cream, cookies, candy, bread, cheese, chips, doughnuts. The consumption of this food is not a pleasurable pastime but a compulsion. Up to 10,000 calories can be consumed in one sitting, followed by abdominal pain and discomfort. The binge generates guilt, depression, and anxiety. Purging follows, reducing the anxiety and fear. Then the cycle begins again.

The bulimic is aware of his or her abnormal behavior and has great fear of not being able to stop. He or she has feelings of guilt and shame about the behavior. Bulimia is a secret habit and can continue for many years undetected. The weight of most bulimics is normal or fluctuates within 10 pounds as a result of the binge-purge cycle.

The physical effects of bulimia include electrolyte imbalance (especially potassium), low blood sugar, esophageal lacerations, dehydration, and nerve and liver damage from low potassium. Tooth enamel is eroded by the stomach acid brought up with vomiting. Severe abdominal pain is common. In rare cases, actual rupture of the stomach has occurred. Bone density is lost if the disorder continues for many years.

People with bulimia need professional help and are often tearful and desperate when they finally seek help. Psychotherapy is necessary to understand the underlying cause of the disorder and to help restore the bulimic's feelings of self-worth and self-confidence. Bulimics tend to be extroverted perfectionists—high achievers—and are often academically or vocationally successful. Yet bulimics have troubled interpersonal relationships, low self-esteem, poor impulse control, and high levels of anxiety and depression and are self-critical and sensitive to rejection. It is not uncommon to see other impulsive behaviors among bulimics, including kleptomania, alcohol and drug use, and sexual promiscuity. The treatment goal is to get bulimics to cope with their stresses and body image insecurities through less destructive ways and to feel more comfortable with who they are. Bulimia is difficult to cure, and some struggle with this disorder for life.

Anorexia Nervosa

Far less common than bulimia, **anorexia nervosa** is a psychological disorder in which self-inflicted starvation leads to a drastic loss of weight. Although anorexia is less prevalent than bulimia, it is associated with more frequent physical problems and greater mortality. The mortality rate from anorexia—estimated at 10 to 20 percent—is the highest of any mental disorder. Whereas the bulimic has a general dissatisfaction with his or her body weight, the anorexic is obsessed with achieving thinness. Individuals with anorexia nervosa have an iron determination to become thin and an intense, irrational fear of becoming fat. They vehemently deny their impulse to eat, their appetite, and their enjoyment of food. The term *anorexia* is a misnomer, because loss of appetite is usually rare until late in the illness. While bulimics feel shame about their abnormal behavior, anorexics justify their weight-loss efforts.

Found primarily in early and middle adolescent females, anorexia may result in physical deterioration to the point of hospitalization or even death. Anorexia carries a 19:1 female-to-male ratio, with a prevalence estimated at

1 percent among adolescent girls. The diagnostic criteria for anorexia are as follows:

1. Refusal to maintain body weight at or above a minimal normal level for age and height (i.e., a body weight that is 15 percent below normal).
2. Intense fear of weight gain or becoming fat despite being significantly underweight.
3. A disturbed perception of body weight, size, or shape (i.e., feeling "fat" although emaciated).
4. In females, amenorrhea (lack of menstrual periods) for at least three consecutive cycles.

Anorexia often starts as innocent dieting that turns into irrational behavior characterized by severe caloric restriction, fasting, relentless exercising, diuretic and laxative use, and, in some cases, self-induced vomiting. The anorexic pursues and maintains thinness despite an emaciated appearance that is apparent to others.

Anorexics display an extraordinary amount of energy for exercise and schoolwork in spite of their starvation state. However, they avoid social relationships, have low self-esteem, and are fearful of change. Despite an aversion to eating, anorexics are preoccupied with food. They may prepare elaborate meals for others, collect recipes, carry or hide snacks, and memorize the caloric content of various foods. Bizarre eating habits are commonplace. Anorexics have been known to cut a raisin in two and chew each half for several minutes. In many situations, they may pretend to be eating while putting food into a napkin or feeding the dog under the table.

Family stress and social pressure contribute to this disorder. Most anorexics come from middle- to upper-class families that place a high premium on achievement, perfection, and physical appearance. Their families are often overcontrolling and overprotective. Anorexics exhibit extreme perfectionism accompanied by a profound sense of ineffectiveness. Only by restricting food intake do they feel a sense of control and feel capable of coping with life's stresses.

Anorexia causes the physiological complications that accompany any malnutritive state: chronic fatigue, dry and scaly skin, hair falling out, lack of menstruation, drops in blood pressure, and cardiac complications. Constipation is commonplace. Bone growth is retarded, increasing the risk of fractures and osteoporosis. Anorexics have an unusual sensitivity to cold due to their low body-fat percentage.

Treatment for anorexia nervosa involves medical, psychological, and nutritional help. The major obstacle to treatment is the patient's denial that any problem exists. The entire family must be involved, because the anorexic's behavior has deep psychological origins: low self-esteem, struggle for control and independence, and fear of physical sexual development.

Binge Eating Disorder

Classified separately from anorexia or bulimia, binge eating disorder (sometimes called *compulsive overeating*) has become a serious problem. It is now the most common eating disorder. **Binge eating disorder** (BED) is defined as recurrent episodes of eating characterized by eating, in a discrete period, an amount of food much larger than most people would eat in a similar period and accompanied by a sense of lack of control or a feeling that one cannot stop. The criteria for this disorder include:

1. Eating much more rapidly than normal.
2. Eating until uncomfortably full.
3. Eating large amounts of food when not hungry.
4. Eating alone because of embarrassment about how much is eaten.
5. Feeling disgusted with oneself, depressed, or guilty about eating.
6. The binge eating occurs, on average, at least 2 days a week for 6 months.

Most people overeat from time to time, and many feel that they eat more than they should. Compulsive overeaters, however, experience marked distress regarding their bingeing behavior and engage in binge eating on average at least 2 days a week for 6 months. They tend to overeat when home alone, while normal eaters tend to overeat in restaurants and social situations that are associated with positive feelings.

In some ways, people with binge eating disorder are similar to bulimics. Both engage in frequent binges, are preoccupied with food and body weight, experience intense feelings of body dissatisfaction, and set unrealistically high dieting standards. Both use food to fill an emotional void. However, some important differences distinguish bulimics from people with BED. People with BED do not regularly compensate for their behavior by dieting or purging. Whereas bulimics dwell on the importance of thinness, serious binge eaters would be happy to have an average body weight. Individuals with BED are usually very overweight, and most seek treatment for obesity. Compulsive overeaters make up approximately 30 percent of Americans who seek treatment for obesity and 5 to 8 percent of obese people in general. They eat even if they aren't hungry. Whereas bulimics engage in the extremes of severe dieting and eventual bingeing, people with BED rarely restrict food. Table 12-9 will help you assess whether you have a problem with compulsive overeating.

The goal in treating binge eaters is to normalize eating—to help them say no to overeating. They need help in adopting a plan of healthy eating and overall moderation *without* rigid rules. Binge eaters need help in learning to cope with the underlying emotions that perpetuate this eating problem—anxiety, loneliness, depression, shame, inferiority, and fear of criticism. Finally, binge eaters need to learn to accept that which cannot be changed about their bodies.

TABLE 12-9	*Are You a Compulsive Overeater?*

1. Do you eat when you're not hungry but don't know why?
2. Do you constantly think about food throughout the day?
3. Do you go on eating binges for no apparent reason and find yourself unable to stop?
4. Do you have feelings of guilt and remorse after overeating?
5. Do you look forward with pleasure and anticipation to the time when you can eat alone?
6. Do you eat sensibly in front of others and then binge when you're alone?
7. Is your weight affecting the way you live your life?
8. Do you eat to escape from worries or trouble?
9. Does your eating behavior make you or others unhappy?
10. Have you tried "dieting," only to fall short of your goal?

If you answered yes to over half these questions, you may want to think seriously about your relationship with food and consult a professional.

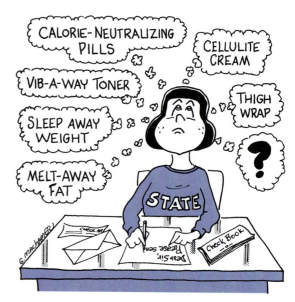

Weight-loss gimmicks reduce your wallet, not your waist.

Eating Disorders Not Otherwise Specified (EDNOS)

The fact that a person does not meet the exact diagnostic criteria for anorexia, bulimia, or binge eating disorder does not mean that the person does not have an eating problem. As a matter of fact, most people will not meet the full criteria. For example, a person with EDNOS may purge himself or herself after eating, but do so with less frequency or intensity than will someone diagnosed with bulimia. Or a person may exhibit occasional anorexic-type behaviors yet be near normal in weight. These varied types of behaviors are called **disordered eating.** The incidence of disordered eating is increasing and far exceeds that of the clinically diagnosed eating disorders. Exact statistics are unavailable because most of these behaviors are unreported, secretive, and difficult to define. Since about 80 percent of American women are dissatisfied with their weight, disordered eating behaviors have become a popular way of dealing with food issues. Those who exhibit disordered eating may diet, binge, purge, fast, exercise excessively, eat in secret, or gain and lose weight off and on. A considerable proportion of their lives is consumed by preoccupation with weight, body image, and food. If disordered eating becomes long-lasting and interferes with normal life, help should be sought.

What Can Be Done?

Eating disorders appear to be increasing in incidence, and so implementation of prevention programs is desperately needed. The most obvious and effective site for prevention is the schools. However, all segments of society need to absorb some of the responsibility, including parents, coaches, advertising executives, the media, and the entertainment business. Society needs to send the message of healthy acceptance of self and body. Not everyone is meant to be a size 6. You may want to do Lab Activity 12-5 at the end of the chapter to assess your risk for developing an eating disorder.

If you suspect a friend, roommate, or relative of having an eating disorder, you probably wonder what you can do to help. Eating disorders are not solely about food and eating but are manifestations of emotional distress. Therefore, just begging someone to start eating or put on some weight is futile. Ignoring the situation or waiting to see what happens also will not solve the problem.

The first step to recovery is indisputable: Locate professional help as soon as possible. Congress has mandated that every state establish a system of community mental health centers to assist people with a variety of psychological problems. These centers are a good source for providing treatment or helping you locate professionals who specialize in treating eating disorders. Even though psychotherapy has become more prevalent and accepted in the last 25 years, some still avoid it. For whatever reason, psychotherapy still carries a stigma with some people. Most college campuses have counseling services available as well.

Your anorexic or bulimic acquaintance may deny the condition or balk at your suggestion to seek help; therefore, it may be difficult to persuade her or him to seek help. However, both physical and psychological evaluation are crucial at the onset of treatment. You cannot force someone to get help. It is important, however, to be direct and honest while showing sincere concern and support. You may have to be tough, even make the appointment, and insist on accompanying the anorexic or bulimic to see a specialist.

Frequently Asked Questions

Q. Is it true that anything eaten after 8:00 P.M. will be stored as fat?

A. *What* and *how much* you eat affect weight control, not *when* you eat. If you balance total daily calories consumed with calories burned, it doesn't matter how late you eat. This myth probably stems from the tendency for people to snack "mindlessly" in the evening on high-fat, high-calorie foods such as chips, cookies, and ice cream, which add considerable additional calories to their day. Some people eat sparingly during the day and then consume several thousands of calories at night due to built-up hunger.

Q. I have cellulite on my thighs. Is there any special way to remove it?

A. There is no such thing as **cellulite.** It is a slang term used to describe the dimpled fat found primarily on the buttocks and thighs of women. Concentrated areas of fat tend to bulge in some women because, with age, their connective fibers become taut and their skin thin. This fat is like any other fat in that only a comprehensive program of exercise and calorie reduction will remove it. No miracle cream, sauna, diet, or device specifically breaks up cellulite. Buying a product that claims to do this reduces only your wallet.

Q. The only place I feel I have too much fat is on my abdomen. Is there any way to just lose fat there? How about trying one of those abdominal muscle stimulators?

A. The concept of *spot reduction* (that is, selectively burning off fat from a particular body area) is a myth. No one can dictate where body fat will accumulate or from where it will be removed. Genetics determine your body build and preferred fat storage sites. Exercising a specific body area does not burn fat in just that area. Fat stores from throughout the body are mobilized during exercise. Thus, your abdomen will lose fat only after a combined program of total-body aerobic exercise and calorie management, not solely by doing 100 crunches a day. It is possible to "spot tone," however. Those 100 crunches create stronger abdominals. As far as those abdominal stimulators go, don't waste your money!

Q. My friend had gastric bypass surgery and lost a considerable amount of weight. What about this and other surgical treatments of obesity?

A. Surgery for obesity should not be taken lightly and should be considered only as a last resort for the morbidly obese (those at least 100 pounds above ideal weight). Even the nonsurgical means of jaw wiring and inserting balloons in the stomach are drastic measures in tackling obesity. Also, their long-term effectiveness is questionable unless a drastic lifestyle change accompanies the procedure.

Liposuction (suctioning fat from under the skin) has become popular as a method of removing body fat from selected body parts. This surgical procedure is performed by physicians who specialize in cosmetic surgery. Interestingly, liposuction performed on abdominal fat does not eliminate the risks for heart disease, type 2 diabetes, or cancer. Since liposuction removes only the subcutaneous fat, the deeper, more dangerous intra-abdominal fat remains. Therefore, abdominal liposuction does not result in the metabolic benefits that fat loss through diet and exercise accomplishes. As with any major medical procedure, these surgeries have inherent risks and medical complications.

Q. What about body wraps, rubberized suits, and other special weight-reducing apparel? I've worn some of these, and they seem to work.

A. Waist belts and body wraps do nothing more than squeeze water out of one tissue area and into another. Think about the indentation that occurs on your wrist after wearing a rubber band there for several minutes. This circumference loss is only temporary until rehydration occurs. Rubberized or vinyl suits can be dangerous, especially if worn while exercising. These suits trap the heat and perspiration given off by the body, not allowing the natural process of evaporation—the body's normal cooling process. Water, not fat, is lost by the body, and the danger of life-threatening overheating is possible. Again, as soon as the body is rehydrated, weight is regained.

Q. I am heavily involved in competitive sports. As a result, I am very muscular. When I stop competing, how do I avoid having all that muscle turn into fat?

A. Your concern is fueled by a common misconception. Muscle can no more turn into fat than a cat can turn into a dog. Neither can fat become muscle. The cellular makeup of each is different. If you stop activity altogether, your muscles will atrophy and lose tone. Calories not needed to fuel your body will be stored as fat. To avoid this, continue doing some regular exercise and modify your calorie consumption, being sure your energy input and output are relatively equal.

Q. I have heard that I will burn more fat if I work out at the lower end of my target heart rate range rather than at a high intensity. Is this true?

A. This low-intensity fat-burning idea is a misunderstanding based on an oversimplification. It is true that at higher exercise intensities, the body prefers to use more glycogen rather than fat for fuel. Some have interpreted this to mean that to burn fat, low-intensity exercise is best. However, the type of fuel used during exercise does not make a huge difference. You burn calories *and* fat during both types of exercise. The most important exercise variable is *total* caloric expenditure. Higher-intensity exercise does burn more calories, but you may not be able to sustain that intensity for very long. Because you don't fatigue as quickly when exercising at a lower intensity, you may be able to work out for a longer period and feel more comfortable while doing it. The result is more total calories expended due to the longer workout time. Even though all types of exercise can help in weight management, most people find that a program of regular low- to moderate-intensity activity is easier to maintain over time. The key is doing it every day!

Q. I am concerned because my sister is very much overweight. She doesn't act like it bothers her, but I think it does. What can I do to motivate her to lose weight?

A. Often we have relatives or friends who have health-robbing habits (smoking, being overweight, not exercising). Because we care about them, it is natural to want to help. In the case of your sister, do not nag or criticize her. Instead, set a good example and talk about why you do the things you do (select certain foods, behavior modification tricks, etc.). Try to include her in your practices. Invite her to go on a walk, bike riding, or to an aerobics class. Grocery shop or eat out together. Share recipes and food preparation ideas. Show that you care. Make a pact with her (you will try to stop biting your fingernails, while she tries to lose weight). Be there for her. However, realize that she is ultimately responsible for herself. Nevertheless, be her friend, confidant, and number one cheerleader. A strong support system is essential in any weight-management program.

Q. I am 26 years old and weigh 40 pounds more than I should. Obesity runs in my family. Is it possible for me to achieve a normal weight or am I always going to fight being overweight because of my heredity?

A. Yes, you can achieve normal weight, but you will have to work much harder than some people because of your genetics. It may seem unfair, but you will have to exercise for 60 or more minutes a day and be vigilant in your calorie intake. Think positive, though; you have the opportunity to also lower your risk of heart disease, cancer, and type 2 diabetes. Genetic influences are real, but diet and exercise habits have far more impact on weight than heredity. Embrace your opportunity to take control of what you can—your lifestyle.

Summary

Obesity is acknowledged as this country's most important nutrition-related disease. It is a complex disorder that no longer is considered only a problem of overeating or lack of willpower. It is caused by multiple factors—some within your control and some beyond it. Environment, culture, and genetics combine to complicate the act of nourishing our bodies. It is important to understand body composition and be able to differentiate between overweight and obesity. Many health problems are associated with obesity, and so concern with weight control should begin sufficiently early in life to reduce the risk of developing obesity. Prevention is the treatment of choice. The factors affecting obesity give us insight into the complexities of losing excess body fat.

"Monday I start my diet" is far too often the battle cry for losing weight. This diet mentality has contributed to the obesity problem. Dieting and concerns about appearance have also contributed to the increasing incidence of eating disorders. Because successful weight management has been elusive for many people, the marketplace has provided many legitimate as well as unfounded claims about products and services. Therefore, consumer education is essential. Effective weight management involves food management, emotional management, and exercise management. Whereas dieting is temporary, restrictive, and negative, lifestyle weight management is a positive, flexible means of dealing with food for life. It is a lifestyle of calorie-controlled, nutritious eating and regular exercise amid established cultural patterns and social and economic forces. No gimmick or gadget can replace this lifestyle approach.

Regular exercise is the key ingredient in maintaining a healthy body composition. Technological advances have increased the quality of our lives in many ways but have eliminated much daily physical exertion. It is a challenge to find ways to fit activity into your life. However, lifelong weight management and total wellness depend on it. Only when we start considering food as fuel, regarding exercise as a daily necessity, and accepting a range of healthy body weights will weight concerns finally disappear.

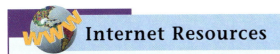

Internet Resources

American Obesity Association

www.obesity.org

A very comprehensive site that provides information, news, statistics, and the latest research on obesity and overweight.

Calorie Control Council

www.caloriecontrol.org

Loaded with articles on cutting calories and weight management. Has many interactive tools: calories burned during various exercises, BMI, caloric content of foods.

The Calorie King

www.calorieking.com

Has a huge database with nutritional and calorie information for thousands of generic and name-brand foods, including fast foods.

Calories Per Hour

www.caloriesperhour.com

Calculates calories burned for any activity as well as BMI and BMR. Also features a nutrition calculator for food items and a Q & A about diets and dieting.

The Diet Channel

www.thedietchannel.com

A terrific site loaded with information on fad diets, successful weight-loss tips, interactive tools for BMI, ideal weight, and links to over 600 reliable diet sources.

Food Nutrition Information Center/Obesity

www.nal.usda.gov/fnic/reports/obesity.html

A government site that features numerous reports and studies on obesity as well as current statistics.

Medline Plus/Weight Loss

www.nlm.nih.gov/medlineplus/weightlossdieting.html

From the U.S. National Library of Medicine, this site has the latest research and studies on all weight-management topics.

National Center for Chronic Disease Prevention and Health Promotion–Obesity

www.cdc.gov/nccdphp/dnpa/obesity

Covers definitions, BMI, trends, contributing factors, health consequences, and resources for overweight and obesity.

National Association of Anorexia Nervosa and Associated Disorders

www.anad.org

Provides comprehensive information and resources (including treatment referrals) on eating disorders.

National Eating Disorders Association

www.nationaleatingdisorders.org

A not-for-profit organization working to prevent eating disorders. Offers information on a variety of eating disorders, including body image issues, athletes, prevention, and treatment.

The National Weight Control Registry

www.nwcr.ws/

A registry of over 5,000 individuals who have lost significant amounts of weight and kept it off for long periods of time. Includes research findings and success stories.

Obesity in America

www.ObesityinAmerica.org

A very thorough site covering all aspects of overweight and obesity–facts, trends, causes, surgical options, myths, medications, etc.

Shape Up America

www.shapeup.org

Provides a wide range of information on exercise, healthy eating, lifestyle change, and weight management.

Something Fishy

www.something-fishy.org

Covers anorexia, bulimia, and compulsive overeating with news, research, dangers, treatment, options, and cultural issues.

Three Fat Chicks

www.3fatchicks.com

Three sisters have collaborated to offer a wide range of obesity/overweight articles, research, news, dieting information, recipes, and support. Has a lot of information on popular diet programs.

Weight-Control Information Network (WIN)

http://win.niddk.nih.gov/

As an information service of the National Institute of Diabetes and Digestive and Kidney Diseases, this site features a wide range of weight-loss and weight-control topics/articles, including dieting tips, suggestions for controlling food portions, and successful weight-loss programs.

The following restaurants have caloric information for their foods online:

www.arbys.com

www.blimpie.com

www.bostonmarket.com

www.carlsjr.com

www.chick-fil-a.com

www.churchs.com

www.dairyqueen.com

www.dominos.com

www.dunkindonuts.com

www.fazolis.com

www.hardees.com

www.jackinthebox.com

www.kfc.com

www.krispykreme.com

www.longjohnsilvers.com

www.mcdonalds.com

www.panerabread.com

www.papajohns.com

www.pizzahut.com

www.popeyes.com

www.schlotzskys.com

www.sonicdrivein.com

www.steaknshake.com

www.subway.com

www.tacobell.com

www.whitecastle.com

Bibliography

Abramson, E. *Body Intelligence.* New York: McGraw-Hill, 2005.

American Psychiatric Association. *Diagnostic and Statistical Manual of Mental Disorders,* 4th ed. Washington, D.C., 2000.

Blair, S. N., and E. A. Leermakers. "Exercise and Weight Management." In Wadden, T. A., and A. J. Stunkard, eds. *Handbook of Obesity Treatment.* New York: The Guilford Press, 2002.

Bouchard, C., et al. "The Response to Long-Term Overfeeding in Identical Twins." *New England Journal of Medicine* 322 (May 24, 1990): 1477–1482.

Bray, G. "Medical Consequences of Obesity." *The Journal of Clinical Endocrinology and Metabolism* 89 (June 2004): 2583–2589.

Calle, E. E., et al. "Overweight, Obesity, and Mortality from Cancer in a Prospectively Studied Cohort of U.S. Adults." *New England Journal of Medicine* 348 (April 24, 2003): 1625–1638.

Centers for Disease Control and Prevention. National Center for Chronic Disease Prevention and Health Promotion. *Behavioral Risk Factor Surveillance–United States, 2004.* www.cdc.gov/brfss

Centers for Disease Control and Prevention. National Center for Chronic Disease Prevention and Health Promotion. *Health, United States, 2005,* December 2005. www.cdc.gov/nchs

Centers for Disease Control and Prevention. National Center for Chronic Disease Prevention and Health Promotion. *National Health and Nutrition Examination Survey, 2003–2004.* Hyattsville, MD, 2005.

Centers for Disease Control and Prevention. National Center for Chronic Disease Prevention and Health Promotion. *Prevalence of Overweight and Obesity Among Adults: United States, 1999–2002.* Hyattsville, MD, October 2004.

Eckel, R. H. "Obesity." *Circulation* 111 (April 19, 2005): e257–e259.

Eckel, R. H., et al. "America's Children: A Critical Time for Prevention." *Circulation* 111 (April 19, 2005): 1866–1868.

Ewing, R., et al. "Relationship Between Urban Sprawl and Physcial Activity, Obesity, and Morbidity." *American Journal of Health Promotion* 18 (September/October 2003): 47–57.

Flegal, K. M., et al. "Excess Deaths Associated with Underweight, Overweight, and Obesity." *Journal of the American Medical Association* 293 (April 20, 2005): 1861–1867.

Flegal, K. M., et al. "Prevalence and Trends in Obesity Among U.S. Adults, 1999–2000." *Journal of the American Medical Association* 288 (October 9, 2002): 1723–1727.

Fletcher, A. M. *Thin for Life: 10 Keys to Success from People Who Have Lost Weight and Kept It Off.* New York: Houghton Mifflin Co., 2003.

Hedley, A. A., et al. "Prevalence of Overweight and Obesity Among U.S. Children, Adolescents, and Adults, 1999–2002." *Journal of the American Medical Association* 291 (June 16, 2004): 2847–2850.

Horgen, K. B., and K. D. Brownell. "Confronting the Toxic Environment: Environmental and Public Health Actions in a World Crisis." In Wadden, T. A., and A. J. Stunkard, eds. *Handbook of Obesity Treatment.* New York: The Guilford Press, 2002.

Howard, B. V., et al. "Low-Fat Dietary Pattern and Weight Change Over 7 Years: The Women's Health Initiative Dietary Modification Trial." *Journal of the American Medical Association* 295 (January 4, 2006): 39–49.

Jakicic, J. M., et al. "Effect of Exercise Duration and Intensity on Weight Loss in Overweight, Sedentary Women." *Journal of the American Medical Association* 290 (September 10, 2003): 1323–1330.

Kaminsky, L. A., ed. *ACSM's Resource Manual for Guidelines for Exercise Testing and Prescription.* Philadelphia: Lippincott Williams & Wilkins, 2006.

Klein, S., et al. "Absence of an Effect of Liposuction on Insulin Action and Risk Factors for Coronary Heart Disease." *New England Journal of Medicine* 350 (June 17, 2004): 2549–2557.

Kruskall, L. J., L. J. Johnson, and S. L. Meacham. "Eating Disorders and Disordered Eating–Are They the Same?" *ACSM's Health & Fitness Journal* 6 (May/June 2002): 6–12.

Lissau, I., et al. "Body Mass Index and Overweight in Adolescents in 13 European Countries, Israel, and the United States." *Archives of Pediatrics and Adolescent Medicine* 158 (January 2004): 27–33.

Mark, D. H. "Deaths Attributable to Obesity." *Journal of the American Medical Association* 293 (April 20, 2005): 1918–1919.

Melanson, K., and J. Dwyer. "Popular Diets for Treatment of Overweight and Obesity." In Wadden, T. A., and A. J. Stunkard, eds. *Handbook of Obesity Treatment.* New York: The Guilford Press, 2002.

Newman, C. "Why Are We So Fat?" *National Geographic* 206 (August 2004): 46–61.

Nielson, S. J., and B. M. Popkin. "Patterns and Trends in Food Portion Sizes, 1977–1998." *Journal of the American Medical Association* 289 (January 22/29, 2003): 450–453.

Pescatello, L. S., S. L. Volpe, and N. Clark. "Which Is More Effective for Maintaining a Healthy Body Weight: Diet or Exercise?" *ACSM's Health & Fitness Journal* 8 (September/October 2004): 9–14.

Preston, S. H. "Deadweight?–The Influence of Obesity on Longevity." *New England Journal of Medicine* 352 (March 17, 2005): 1135–1137.

Racette, S. B., S. S. Deusinger, and R. H. Deusinger. "Obesity: Overview of Prevalence, Etiology, and Treatment." *Physical Therapy* 83 (March 2003): 276–288.

Rolls, B. J., L. S. Roe, and J. S. Meengs. "Reduction in Portion Size and Energy Density of Foods Are Additive and Lead to Sustained Decreases in Energy Intake." *American Journal of Clinical Nutrition* 83 (January 2006): 11–17.

"The Skinny on Popular Diets." *Harvard Heart Letter* 16 (February 2005): 4–6.

Somer, E. *10 Habits That Mess Up a Woman's Diet.* New York: McGraw-Hill, 2006.

Stein, C. J., and G. A. Colditz. "The Epidemic of Obesity." *The Journal of Clinical Endocrinology and Metabolism* 89 (June 2004): 2522–2525.

Stunkard, A. J., et al. "The Body-Mass Index of Twins Who Have Been Reared Apart." *New England Journal of Medicine* 322 (May 24, 1990): 1483–1487.

U.S. Department of Health and Human Services. *The Surgeon General's Call to Action to Prevent and Decrease Overweight and Obesity.* Rockville, MD, December 13, 2001.

Wadden, T. A., and A. J. Stunkard, eds. *Handbook of Obesity Treatment.* New York: The Guilford Press, 2002.

"Waist-to-Hip Ratio Predicts Heart Risk Better Than BMI." *Tufts University Health & Nutrition Letter* 23 (January 2006): 1–2.

Wang, Y., et al. "Comparison of Abdominal Adiposity and Overall Obesity in Predicting Risk of Type 2 Diabetes Among Men." *American Journal of Clinical Nutrition* 81 (March 2005): 555–563.

Weinbrenner, T., et al. "Circulating Oxidized LDL Is Associated with Increased Waist Circumference Independent of Body Mass Index in Men and Women." *American Journal of Clinical Nutrition* 83 (January 2006): 30–35.

Williams, P. T., and P. D. Wood. "The Effects of Changing Exercise Levels on Weight and Age-Related Weight Gain." *International Journal of Obesity* 30 (March 2006): 543–551.

Yan, L., et al. "Midlife Body Mass Index and Hospitalization and Mortality in Older Age." *Journal of the American Medical Association* 295 (January 11, 2006): 190–198.

Young, L., and Nestle, M. "The Contribution of Expanding Portion Sizes to the U.S. Obesity Epidemic." *American Journal of Public Health* 92 (February 2002): 246–249.

Yusuf, S., et al. "Obesity and the Risk of Myocardial Infarction in 27,000 Participants from 52 Countries: A Case-Control Study." *Lancet* 366 (November 5, 2005): 1640–1649.

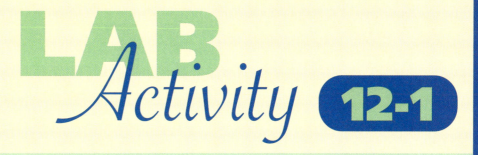

Why Do You Eat? (A Food Journal)

Use the following food journal to record your food intake for a day. This will allow you to see the number of calories you are eating and analyze the reasons you eat. Knowing the cues and factors that affect eating can help you manage your eating behavior. Don't forget to record "liquid" calories! (Make copies of this diary as needed to record multiple days.)

Date: _____

Time of Day	Location	Companion(s) (if any)	Food	Portion Size/ Quantity	Calories	Hunger Level (0–5) 0 = not hungry 5 = very hungry	Feelings/Mood (before eating)	Feelings/Mood (after eating)

Observations:

Strategies for change:

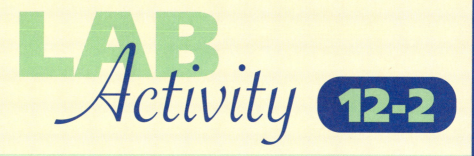

LAB Activity 12-2

How Active Are You?

Finding the time to exercise can be a challenge. However, there are several times during a day when you can weave activity into your life (walking rather than driving, riding a stationary bike while watching TV, taking the stairs rather than the elevator, getting up 45 minutes earlier in the morning to jog). Use the following log to keep track of your activity during the day. Use Table 12-8 or go to www.caloriesperhour.com or www.caloriecontrol.org (go to "Exercise Calculator") for the caloric expenditure for various activities. Then analyze *when* and *how* you could adapt your lifestyle to include more activity. (Make copies of this log as needed to record multiple days.)

Date: _____

Activity	Time of Day	Location	Duration	Calories Expended	Positive Outcomes	Negative Outcomes (if any)

Assess your activity level today (was it a typical day?):

Describe ways you could fit more activity into your day:

What obstacles do you face in trying to be active?

What are your strategies for combating these obstacles and adhering to a lifetime of activity/exercise?

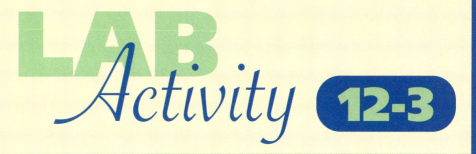

LAB Activity 12-3

Name _____ **Class/Activity Section** _____ **Date** _____

Estimating Your Basal Metabolic Rate (BMR)

Precise measurement of your BMR can be achieved only in a laboratory. However, you can compute an estimate of your BMR by using the following equation from the World Health Organization. Figured into the equation are factors that influence your BMR: age, gender, and weight.

STEP 1

Convert your body weight in pounds to kilograms (kg):
_____ lb ÷ 2.2 = _____ kg

STEP 2

Select the appropriate formula from the table below, using your age and gender:

Age Range	Male Formulas	Female Formulas
10–18	BMR = (17.5 × wt in kg) + 651	BMR = (12.2 × wt in kg) + 746
19–29	BMR = (15.3 × wt in kg) + 679	BMR = (14.7 × wt in kg) + 496
30–59	BMR = (11.6 × wt in kg) + 879	BMR = (8.7 × wt in kg) + 829
60 +	BMR = (13.5 × wt in kg) + 487	BMR = (10.5 × wt in kg) + 596

Example: For a 23-year-old male weighing 195 pounds:

195 lbs ÷ 2.2 = 88.6 kg
BMR = (15.3 × 88.6 kg) + 679 = 2,034.5 calories/day

Now figure your BMR:

BMR = (_____ × _____ kg) + _____ = [_____] calories/day

Remember, BMR does not include any calorie expenditure from activity or exercise that you do throughout the day. This is just your basal need (i.e., calories needed *at rest* just to sustain vital functions of the body).

If you want to approximate your TOTAL caloric expenditure in a day, use Table 12-8 and accompanying websites to calculate the calories you burn in daily activities and exercise. Then:

$$\frac{}{\text{BMR}} + \frac{}{\substack{\text{activity} \\ \text{calories}}} = \boxed{} \; \substack{\text{total daily} \\ \text{calories expended}}$$

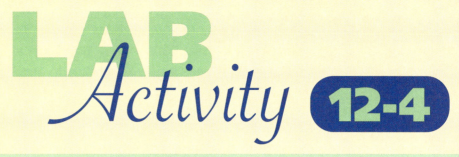

Weight Management Plan

Date: _____

Current weight: _____

  Goal weight: _____

Current body fat percentage: _____

  Goal body fat percentage: _____

Current body mass index (BMI): _____

  Goal body mass index (BMI): _____

Waist: _____ Hip: _____

  Current waist-to-hip ratio: _____ (waist ÷ hip)

  Goal waist-to-hip ratio: _____

  Goal waist measurement: _____

I. FOOD MANAGEMENT

- Calories per day: _____ (goal)

- Fat grams per day: _____ (goal)

- MyPyramid compliance and strategies for improvement:

- Snack strategy:

- Food preparation adjustments:

II. EMOTIONAL MANAGEMENT

Behavior modification and coping strategies:

1.   4.

2.   5.

3.   6.

III. EXERCISE MANAGEMENT

Physical activity strategies:

Sunday	Monday	Tuesday	Wednesday	Thursday	Friday	Saturday

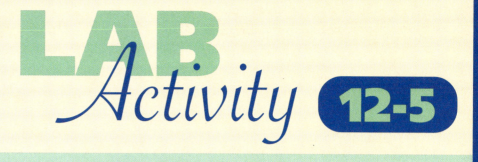

Name _____ **Class/Activity Section** _____ **Date** _____

Are You at Risk for an Eating Disorder?

Check the following statements that describe you.

_____ I feel fat even if people tell me I'm not.

_____ If I were thinner, I would like myself better.

_____ If I gain weight, I get anxious and depressed.

_____ I worry about what I will eat.

_____ I feel extremely guilty after eating.

_____ I am terrified of being overweight.

_____ I often wish I were someone else.

_____ I get anxious if I cannot exercise.

_____ I find myself preoccupied with food.

_____ I am preoccupied with a desire to be thinner.

_____ I binge eat sometimes.

_____ I have a secret stash of food.

_____ I don't like to be bothered or interrupted when I'm eating.

_____ I like to read recipes, cookbooks, calorie charts, and books about dieting.

_____ I would rather eat by myself than with family or friends.

_____ I am hardly ever satisfied with myself.

_____ I have dieted to lose weight.

_____ I want to be thinner than my friends.

_____ I vomit, use laxatives, or take diet pills to control my weight.

_____ When I eat, I worry that I may not be able to stop.

_____ I have perfectionist tendencies.

_____ I have a hard time saying no to others.

_____ I avoid eating even if I am hungry.

_____ Sometimes I feel worthless.

_____ I have a tendency to hide my feelings or have trouble expressing them.

This questionnaire is not meant to be a diagnostic tool, but if you checked many of the statements, that may be indicative of an eating disorder. The more items you checked, the more serious your problem may be. Don't be afraid to seek the advice of a counselor or physician who has experience in treating eating disorders. It takes courage to take this initial step, but it is essential to prevent severe medical and psychological problems.

Appendix 1

Outside Reading Assignment

Note: You may want to make extra copies of this form for future outside reading assignments.

Name _____ Class/Activity Section _____

Select a research article on fitness, health, or wellness. This article should be from a professional/scientific journal (not a popular newsstand magazine). A copy of the article or abstract should be attached to this form. Use a current journal, that is, dated 2003 to the present. Complete the following:

I. Bibliographic information:
   Example: Powers, D. L., G. C. Robbins, and S. Burgess. "Living the Wellness Way of Life." *Journal of Health and Behavior* 25 (June 2005): 25–31. (If the article is from the Internet, give the website address and date when retrieved.)

II. Summarize the research/study and its most important findings (in your words):

III. Explain how you can apply this information to your life:

Outside Reading Assignment

Note: You may want to make extra copies of this form for future outside reading assignments.

| Name _____ | Class/Activity Section _____ |

Select a research article on fitness, health, or wellness. This article should be from a professional/scientific journal (not a popular newsstand magazine). A copy of the article or abstract should be attached to this form. Use a current journal, that is, dated 2003 to the present. Complete the following:

 I. Bibliographic information:
     Example: Powers, D. L., G. C. Robbins, and S. Burgess. "Living the Wellness Way of Life." *Journal of Health and Behavior* 25 (June 2005): 25–31. (If the article is from the Internet, give the website address and date when retrieved.)

 II. Summarize the research/study and its most important findings (in your words):

III. Explain how you can apply this information to your life:

Appendix 2

Reaction Paper to Guest Speaker

Note: You may want to make extra copies of this form for future guest speakers.

Name _____ Class/Activity Section _____

Answer the following questions concerning the presentation by _____
(name of speaker)

titled _____ on _____.
(name of presentation)   (date)

  I. List and discuss three important points the speaker made.

     a.

     b.

     c.

 II. What was the *most* important information you heard at this presentation?

III. Was there anything that the speaker said that you disagreed with? Explain.

IV. How can you incorporate what you learned into your lifestyle?

Reaction Paper to Guest Speaker

Note: You may want to make extra copies of this form for future guest speakers.

Name _____ Class/Activity Section _____

Answer the following questions concerning the presentation by _____

                                                                                                                (name of speaker)

titled _____ on _____.

              (name of presentation)   (date)

   I. List and discuss three important points the speaker made.

     a.

     b.

     c.

  II. What was the *most* important information you heard at this presentation?

 III. Was there anything that the speaker said that you disagreed with? Explain.

 IV. How can you incorporate what you learned into your lifestyle?

Photo Credits

Glossary

a

action stage is the fourth stage in the transtheoretical model of behavior change. In this stage, individuals are overtly changing their behaviors; taking conscious action; and using strategies to resist temptations, remain motivated, and cope with everyday challenges.

active stretching is a stretch in which you use your own muscle forces to stretch yourself. For example, you can stretch calves by sitting and pulling the toes back.

acute stress is a form of stress in which the body responds or reacts to imminent danger.

aerobic literally means "with oxygen." Aerobic activities are activities that demand large amounts of oxygen, follow the FITT factors, and improve cardiorespiratory endurance.

aerobic capacity *see* maximal oxygen uptake.

agonist is a muscle primarily responsible for producing a movement. For example, in a biceps curl, the biceps muscle is the agonist.

amenorrhea is a menstrual abnormality that results in the absence of menses.

anaerobic means "without oxygen." This type of activity demands more oxygen than the body can supply while exercising, causing an oxygen debt. Start-and-stop activities, such as sprinting, are examples of anaerobic exercise.

angina pectoris is chest pain and is caused primarily by atherosclerosis.

anorexia nervosa is an eating disorder characterized by self-inflicted starvation and dramatic weight loss. An anorexic is obsessed with achieving thinness.

antagonist is a muscle opposing a movement. For example, in a biceps curl, the triceps muscle is the antagonist.

antioxidants are compounds that help protect the body's cells from the damaging effects of the normal oxygenation process. Vitamins A, C, E, and beta-carotene and selenium are antioxidants.

arteriosclerosis is thickening and hardening of the arteries.

atherosclerosis is a type of arteriosclerosis and is a progressive condition that results in a buildup of plaque in the blood vessels.

atrophy is the condition of diminished muscle size and strength due to lack of use.

autogenic training and imagery is a self-induced relaxation technique. This method uses mental concentration exercises to bring about sensations of warmth and heaviness in the limbs and torso and then uses relaxing images (e.g., clouds drifting by) to expand the relaxed state.

b

ballistic stretching involves jerking and bouncing movements and is not the recommended type of stretching.

basal metabolic rate (BMR) is the amount of energy (calories) expended by the body at rest to sustain vital functions.

behavior modification is the use of techniques to enhance awareness or consciousness about a behavior and then to alter the behavior. For example, a behavior modification technique for weight management would be refraining from grocery shopping while hungry.

binge eating disorder is recurrent episodes of eating characterized by eating, in a discrete period, an amount of food much larger than most people would eat in a similar period—and accompanied by a sense of lack of control or a feeling that one cannot stop.

biofeedback training is a technique in which machines measure certain physiological processes of the body. The machines convert this information to an understandable form and feed it back to the individual. This process gives a person access to biological information not usually available through consciousness alone.

blisters are inflamed burns caused by the friction of skin against a fabric or surface (such as a shoe).

body composition refers to the amount of body fat in proportion to fat-free weight.

body fat is tissue made up of billions of cells filled with varying amounts of triglyceride. If triglyceride is added to or removed from a fat cell, the cell will increase in size or shrink accordingly.

body mass index (BMI) is a ratio between weight and height. It is calculated as weight (in kg) divided by the square of height (in m). BMI is used by health professionals as a measure of overweight and obesity.

bulimia nervosa is an eating disorder characterized by alternating bouts of eating large quantities of food (bingeing) and purging through vomiting, use of laxatives, or fasting.

bursitis is inflammation of a bursa, a fluid-filled sac that lies between tissues and allows tendons, ligaments, muscles, and skin to glide smoothly over one another during activity.

C

calorie (kcal) is a measure of food energy. One pound of body fat equals 3,500 calories.

carbohydrates are the major source of energy for the body. Starches (such as potatoes, rice, and grains) and sugars are the main sources of carbohydrates in our diet.

cardiac output is the volume of blood pumped by the heart per minute.

cardiorespiratory endurance (CRE) is the ability to deliver essential nutrients, especially oxygen, to the working muscles of the body and remove waste products during prolonged physical exertion. It involves efficient functioning of the heart, blood vessels, and lungs.

cardiovascular disease refers to diseases of the heart and blood vessels.

cellulite is a slang term used to describe dimpled fat found primarily on the buttocks and thighs of women. It is no different from any other body fat.

cholesterol is a fatlike waxy substance found in animal tissue. Although it plays a vital role as a structural component of cell membranes, too much cholesterol has been linked to CVD.

chronic diseases are diseases that develop over many years and are strongly influenced by lifestyle.

Examples are heart disease, cancer, type 2 diabetes, and osteoporosis.

chronic stress is prolonged physical and emotional stress that is more than the individual can cope with. It may lead to a psychosomatic disease.

collagen is fibrous connective tissue found within muscles. Collagen is relatively inelastic.

collateral circulation is a process in which new blood vessels develop to nourish the areas of the heart muscle that are starved of oxygen and other nutrients.

complex carbohydrates are nutritionally dense foods (grains, rice, pasta, potatoes, fruits, and vegetables) that are a rich source of vitamins and minerals and provide a steady amount of energy for many hours. Complex carbohydrates are an important source of fiber.

concentric contraction occurs when a muscle shortens as it overcomes resistance. For example, the biceps muscle contracts concentrically during arm flexion in a biceps curl.

conditioning bout is the middle part of a three-segment workout. It contains vigorous aerobic exercise that stimulates the cardiorespiratory system and should follow the FITT formula.

constant resistance exercise is exercise in which a constant resistance (weight) is used throughout the range of motion, but the force needed to move the weight varies with leverage determined by the angle of the joint. Doing a biceps curl with free weights is an example.

contemplation stage is the second stage in the transtheoretical model of behavior change. In this stage, individuals have an awareness of their problem behavior and are thinking about changing it—but are not ready to do that.

contraindicated exercises are exercises indicated to be injurious to some people.

cool-down is the final segment of the three-segment workout. The purpose of the cool-down is to ease your body safely back to its resting state.

cramp is a sharp, painful, involuntary muscle contraction.

C-reactive protein (CRP) is a marker for inflammation of the blood vessels. It is recognized as increasing the risk for heart attack and stroke.

cross training involves participating in two or more types of exercise in one session or alternate sessions for balanced fitness. For example, lift weights, do 20 minutes of walking, and finish by stretching.

d

daily hassles are the events or interactions in daily life that are bothersome, annoying, or negative in some way. Examples are losing things, having too many things to do, filling out paperwork, chronic car trouble, and computer problems.

daily uplifts are the counterpart to daily hassles. These are positive events that make us feel good. Examples are payday; being visited, phoned, or sent a letter; being complimented; and having fun with a friend.

diabetes mellitus is a condition characterized by the body's inability to produce insulin or use the hormone properly.

diastolic blood pressure is the resting blood pressure and is the force of blood against the artery wall when the heart relaxes between beats. It is recorded as the lower number.

disordered eating is a classification of disturbed eating behaviors (bingeing, purging, fasting, excessively exercising, etc.) that are not as common or intense as in a diagnosed eating disorder.

distress refers to unpleasant or harmful stress under which health and performance begin to decline.

dynamic flexibility is the range of motion achieved by quickly moving a limb to its limits as in a bouncing hamstring stretch.

dynamic (isotonic) exercise is exercise in which the muscle contracts and shortens as movement occurs, such as push-ups or weight lifting.

dysmenorrhea is painful menstruation.

e

eating disorder is a disturbance in eating behavior that jeopardizes a person's physical or psychosocial health.

eccentric contraction occurs when a muscle lengthens and contracts at the same time, gradually allowing a force to overcome muscular resistance. For example, the biceps contracts eccentrically during the lowering phase of a biceps curl.

elastic elongation, the temporary lengthening of soft tissue, occurs when muscle is stretched and returns to its resting length.

elastin is elastic connective tissue found within a muscle.

electrolytes are chemicals, such as calcium, potassium, and sodium, dissolved in blood or cellular fluids that act as a vital messenger for many bodily processes. Electrolytes are essential, for example, in maintaining heart rhythm and kidney function; dehydration and certain drugs can disrupt electrolyte balance.

emotional dimension is the dimension of wellness that deals with the ability to control or cope with the vast array of human feelings/emotions. Adjusting to life's ongoing changes is one sign of emotional wellness.

endorphins are pain-relieving chemicals produced by the brain. Some individuals report experiencing their effects during aerobic exercise. They are also released during the fight-or-flight response when faced with a stressor.

environmental dimension is the dimension of wellness that deals with the preservation of natural resources and the protection of plant and animal wildlife as well as the defining of one's relationship with the environment. Practicing recycling is evidence of environmental wellness.

essential fat is the body fat required for normal functioning. This fat is stored in major body organs and tissues such as the heart, muscles, intestines, nervous system, and breasts.

estrogen is a female sex hormone.

eustress refers to happy or pleasant events under which health and performance improve even as stress increases.

exercise addiction is a chronic loss of perspective on the role of exercise in a full life.

exercise tolerance test is a test of aerobic capacity in which a person exercises while heart rate and oxygen consumption are measured. A maximal effort on a treadmill or bicycle ergometer is an example. This test gives an excellent measure of overall physiological functioning.

f

fast-twitch (FT) muscle fiber contracts quickly and strongly. It is recruited and developed mainly in short-burst anaerobic activities such as sprinting and weight training.

fat is the most concentrated form of food energy, providing 9 calories per gram—more than twice the energy provided by carbohydrates and proteins. Diets high in fat have been linked to coronary heart disease, some cancers, and obesity.

fat cells (adipose cells) are storage sites for energy. This type of cell shrinks and enlarges depending on the amount of excess calories (energy) in storage.

fat-free mass is all body tissue except fat (muscle, bones, etc.).

fat soluble vitamins are vitamins that are stored in the fatty tissues of the body. Vitamins A, D, E, and K are fat soluble.

faulty perception occurs when an individual assesses a situation (or stressor) as threatening regardless of its actual threat. It is seeing a situation as hopeless, harmful, or negative.

female athlete triad is a life-threatening syndrome marked by three disorders: disordered eating habits (inadequate food energy intake to meet metabolic demands), amenorrhea, and osteoporosis. This condition may be found in extremely physically active women.

fiber is the part of plant food that is not digested in the small intestine. It helps the movement of solid waste through the digestive tract.

fight-or-flight response (Alarm Reaction Stage) is the first stage in the Stress Response, in which the body prepares to cope with a stressor. Physiological and psychological responses appear. It is a basic survival mechanism.

FITT factors should be followed to develop cardiorespiratory endurance. The factors include recommendations about the frequency, intensity, time, and type of exercise.

flexibility refers to the movement of a joint through a full range of motion.

free radicals are singlet oxygen molecules that can produce tissue and cellular damage.

g

General Adaptation Syndrome (GAS) was described by Hans Selye and is today known as the Stress Response. It is the body's reaction or adaptation to stress and includes three stages: the fight-or-flight response, the stage of resistance, and the stage of exhaustion.

glycemic index (GI) is a scale that measures the extent to which a food affects blood sugar levels.

glycogen is the storage form of carbohydrates. It is found in the muscles and liver.

Golgi tendon organ (GTO) is a type of stretch receptor located within the muscle tendon that detects the amount of tension in a muscle. When excessive tension is placed on the muscle, the GTO triggers the inverse stretch reflex, causing the muscle to relax to prevent injury.

h

hardiness is an ability to resist the ill effects of stress.

Hatha yoga, or physical yoga, is the most familiar form of yoga. It is a discipline that involves the use of various exercises or postures (called *asanas*) in combination with proper breathing rhythm to remove tension and inflexibility in the body.

health is a state of complete physical, mental, and social well-being and not merely the absence of disease or infirmity.

health promotion involves the systematic efforts made by organizations to help people change their lifestyles to achieve a state of optimal well-being. Smoking cessation workshops, stress management classes, low-fat cooking demonstrations, and bulletin boards with cholesterol information are examples of health promotion efforts.

healthy life expectancy is the number of years a person is expected to live in *good* health.

heart rate reserve is the difference between your maximal and resting heart rates.

heel spur is a bony growth on the underside of the heel.

hemoglobin is the oxygen-carrying component of red blood cells.

high-density lipoprotein (HDL) is considered to be the good form of cholesterol because of its dense structure. It cleans out plaque and debris (i.e., atherosclerotic buildup) from the blood vessel walls.

homocysteine is an amino acid in the blood and a natural by-product of protein metabolism. Too much homocysteine in the blood is related to a higher risk of CVD. Homocysteine levels in the blood are strongly influenced by diet and genetic factors.

hot reactors are apparently healthy individuals who are prime candidates for stress-related heart attack or stroke because of the extreme reactions they demonstrate in response to daily stress.

hydrogenation is a manufacturing process in which hydrogen atoms are added to unsaturated fats, making them more saturated. Manufacturers use hydrogenated oils to extend the shelf life of products. Consumption of hydrogenated oils has been shown to increase blood cholesterol levels.

hypercholesterolemia is a term for high cholesterol levels in the blood.

hypertension is high blood pressure that is acknowledged to be equal to or greater than 140/90.

hyperthermia is a life-threatening condition in which the body temperature rises to a dangerously high level.

hypertrophy is an increase in muscle size due to enlargement of existing muscle fibers. Muscles exhibit hypertrophy when exercised.

hypokinetic diseases are lifestyle diseases resulting from inadequate physical fitness. Examples are heart disease, diabetes, osteoporosis, stroke, back pain, and cancer.

hyponatremia is water intoxication caused by drinking too much water. It can be life-threatening as it dilutes the sodium content of the blood too much. Although not common, it is seen in exercisers during extreme conditions (heat) and in people who exercise 3 hours or more.

hypothermia is a life-threatening condition in which the body temperature drops to a dangerously low level.

i

iliotibial band is a long tendon that begins in the buttocks, runs down the outside of the thigh, and attaches just below the knee. When inflamed, it causes tightness, burning, and pain on the side of the knee or hip.

insoluble fiber absorbs water as it passes through the digestive tract, increasing fecal bulk. By quickening the passage of food through the system, insoluble fiber is a good deterrent to digestive disorders, including cancer.

intellectual dimension is the dimension of wellness that involves ongoing curiosity and the pursuit of knowledge. Attending lectures, reading newspapers, discussing new ideas with people, and visiting museums are a few practices that reflect intellectual wellness.

intervertebral disc is a fluid-filled cushion that separates each bony vertebra in the back.

ischemia means "insufficient oxygen." It is used in reference to conditions in which cells are deprived of oxygen, resulting in pain or discomfort (heart angina, side stitch, etc.).

isokinetic exercise controls the speed of movement as force is applied through a range of motion. Cybex or Orthotron equipment employs isokinetic contraction to strengthen muscles.

k

Karvonen equation is used to determine the target heart rate (THR) for exercise. It takes into account the current fitness level of the exerciser by using his or her resting heart rate. (Karvonen was a Finnish researcher.) The formula is $THR = HR_{max} - RHR \times IF_2 + RHR$.

Kegel exercises strengthen the pelvic floor muscles and may prevent or cure stress incontinence. They are done by contracting the perineal muscles, which surround the bladder and vagina. The exercises are named after the physician who invented them.

ketone bodies are a toxic waste product that builds up in the body if fats are burned for energy in the absence of carbohydrates. This buildup, or *ketosis,* can result in fatigue, nausea, and nerve and brain damage.

l

lactovegetarian is the type of vegetarian who will consume plant foods and dairy products, but no meat or eggs.

LDL cholesterol receptors, primarily in the liver cells, bind and remove cholesterol from the blood.

lean-body mass (muscle mass) is specifically the *muscle* part of the fat-free body mass.

ligament is the fibrous connective tissue that binds bones together to form a joint.

liposuction is a surgical procedure in which fat is removed/suctioned from selected parts of the body.

locus of control is an individual's belief about how much power he or she has in regard to what happens to him or her.

low-density lipoprotein (LDL) is considered the bad form of cholesterol because it more easily attaches to the blood vessel wall, thereby increasing the atherosclerotic process.

m

macrominerals are minerals needed in large doses (more than 100 mg daily). Examples are calcium, magnesium, and potassium.

maintenance stage is the fifth and final stage in the transtheoretical model of behavior change. In this stage, individuals have been able to sustain their new behavior for over 6 months. Their habits are becoming automatic.

maximal heart rate (HR$_{max}$) is the highest possible heart rate. Maximal heart rate can be estimated by subtracting age from 220 bpm.

maximal oxygen uptake (V$_{O_2}$max) is the greatest amount of oxygen that can be used by the body during intense exercise.

meditation is a mental exercise that elicits the body's relaxation response. The purpose of meditation is to gain control over one's attention—to internally quiet down, allowing the individual to choose what to focus on and block out distracting thoughts.

menarche is the start of a young female's menstrual cycle. Menarche is usually experienced between 11 and 12 years of age.

metabolic syndrome (syndrome X) is a cluster of symptoms that increase the risk of heart disease, stroke, diabetes, and some cancers.

mindfulness meditation involves focusing on whatever a person happens to be experiencing at the time and learning to experience anything calmly, whether it is pleasant or unpleasant. This type of meditation was popularized by Dr. Jon Kabat-Zinn. Traditional meditation involves training the mind on a single point of focus, such as a word or phrase.

minerals are inorganic substances critical to many enzyme functions in the body.

moderate physical activity is activity that uses approximately 150 calories of energy per day, equivalent to walking 2 miles in 30 minutes. This produces significant health benefits but not physical fitness.

monounsaturated fats are fatty acids that have one double bond between carbon atoms, thus reducing the number of hydrogen atoms attached. Monounsaturated fats are better for the heart than are saturated fats. Olive oil and peanut oil are monounsaturated.

muscle spindles are stretch receptors within the muscle cells that sense the amount and speed of stretch. If a muscle is overstretched or stretched too fast, they activate the stretch reflex to prevent injury.

muscular endurance is the ability of a muscle to exert a submaximal force repeatedly against resistance or to sustain muscular contraction.

muscular power, a function of strength and speed, is the ability to apply force rapidly. Jumping requires muscular power.

muscular strength is the ability of a muscle to exert one maximal force against resistance.

myocardial infarction is a heart attack.

n

nutrient density is a description of foods that provide substantial nutrients with relatively few calories, fat, and sugar.

o

obesity is an excessive accumulation of body fat. A woman with over 30 percent body fat or a man with over 25 percent body fat is considered obese. Having a body mass index (BMI) of 30 or over is generally classified as obesity.

occupational dimension is the dimension of wellness that entails the ability to integrate skills, interests, and values that will heighten job satisfaction. Identifying a "well" work environment and balancing work time and personal leisure time are important skills in the occupational dimension.

oligomenorrhea is a menstrual abnormality that results in infrequent or irregular menses.

omega-3 is a polyunsaturated fat that is prevalent in fish. Omega-3 fatty acids inhibit atherosclerosis and can reduce blood cholesterol levels.

optimal stress is the point at which stress is intense enough to motivate and physically prepare us to perform optimally yet not intense enough to cause the body to overreact or sustain harmful effects.

orthotics are shoe inserts specially molded to the foot to correct foot, arch, or leg abnormalities.

osteopenia is low bone mass.

osteoporosis is an age-related condition in which the formation of bone fails to keep pace with lost bone tissue. The result is brittle, porous bone susceptible to fracture.

overpronation is a condition in which the foot rolls inward excessively on contact with the ground during walking, jogging, or running.

overuse is a condition of excessive overloading of fitness activities, resulting in nagging injuries. It often means doing too much, too soon—before the body is ready. The body and muscles must be given time to adapt gradually to new demands with *gradual* overloading.

overweight is a term that refers to an excess of body weight compared to a recommended range for good health. A body mass index (BMI) of 25 to 29.9 is considered overweight.

ovo-lactovegetarian is the type of vegetarian who will consume plant foods, dairy products, and eggs.

p

passive stretching is stretching in which someone or something else assists with a stretch. The assist could be gravity, body weight, a strap, or leverage; for example, using gravity or a slant board to assist with a calf stretch.

patellofemoral syndrome causes pain and stiffness around and under the kneecap.

physical dimension is the dimension of wellness that deals with the functional operation of the body. Committing to a regular exercise program, not smoking, and maintaining a normal weight are signs of physical wellness.

physical fitness is the capacity of the heart, lungs, blood vessels, and muscles to function at optimal efficiency.

phytoestrogens are plant estrogens that have a structure similar to that of the body's hormones. Found particularly in soy products, they may help reduce the risk for some cancers.

plantar fasciitis is an inflammation of the plantar fascia—the long thick band of connective tissue on the undersurface of the foot.

plaque is an accumulation of cholesterol on the inner walls of coronary arteries.

plastic elongation, a semi-permanent lengthening of tissues, can be produced by relatively long or intense stretching.

polyunsaturated fats are fatty acids that have two double bonds between carbon atoms, thus reducing the number of hydrogen atoms attached. Corn oil, soybean oil, and safflower oil are examples.

precontemplation stage is the first stage in the transtheoretical model of behavior change. In this stage, individuals deny any need to change or resist change.

prediabetes is a condition that is sometimes called insulin resistance. In this metabolic condition, the blood-glucose level is only slightly elevated but will develop into full-blown diabetes unless healthy lifestyle changes are implemented.

prehypertension is blood pressure equal to or greater than 120/80. It is considered unsafe and calls for lifestyle changes and monitoring.

preparation stage is the third stage in the transtheoretical model of behavior change. In this stage, individuals are intending to take action in the immediate future and are putting together a plan of action.

P.R.I.C.E., an acronym for Protect, Rest, Ice, Compress, and Elevate, is the recommended treatment for many injuries.

primary risk factors are linked directly to the development of CVD; they increase the possibility of having a heart attack more than do the secondary risk factors. All primary risk factors are controllable.

principle of individual differences People vary in their ability to develop fitness components.

principle of reversibility Changes occurring with exercise are reversible. If a person stops exercising, the body will decondition and adapt to the decreased activity level.

principle of specificity means that only the muscles or body systems being exercised will show beneficial change.

processes of change are the covert and overt activities and experiences that individuals engage in when they attempt to modify problem behaviors.

progressive overload is a gradual increase in physical activity to stress a muscle group or body system beyond accustomed levels. Gradual adaptation occurs, resulting in improved physiological functioning. Follow the rules on order of overload and 10 percent increase per week to overload correctly.

progressive relaxation is a series of exercises designed by the physician Edmund Jacobson for his tense patients. The method emphasizes the relaxation of the voluntary skeletal muscles by contracting a muscle group and then relaxing it, progressing from one muscle group to another until the total body is relaxed. Individuals eventually learn to recognize tenseness and consciously relax whenever that is needed.

pronation is the slight inward roll of the foot as it contacts the ground. It is natural for the foot to pronate slightly.

proprioceptive neuromuscular facilitation (PNF) is a type of flexibility exercise in which you perform a static stretch, contract the muscle to produce fatigue, and then relax while a partner stretches your limb.

protein builds and repairs tissue; maintains chemical balance; and regulates the formation of hormones, antibodies, and enzymes. Large amounts of protein are found in both animal sources (meat, dairy) and plant sources (beans, nuts, grains).

psychoneuroimmunology is the study of the effects of emotions, behavior, and mental attitudes on the immune system and the onset/course of illness.

psychosomatic disease is a physical ailment that is mentally induced. *Psycho* refers to the mind, and *somatic* refers to the body. This type of disease is frequently called a *stress disease.*

r

rate of perceived exertion (RPE) is a method of measuring exercise intensity developed by Gunnar Borg. Using this method, exercisers are able to sense (or perceive) their exercise intensity levels accurately.

reciprocal innervation Muscles work in pairs, and when one muscle contracts, through reciprocal innervation, its opposing muscle relaxes to permit movement. For example, during a biceps curl, the triceps relaxes to permit the biceps to shorten.

reframing is a way of looking at life in a positive manner. For example, seeing the glass as half full is a reframing of seeing it as half empty.

relaxation response is the body's built-in defense mechanism against the harmful effects of the inappropriate elicitation of the fight-or-flight response caused by everyday living. Dr. Herbert Benson of Harvard University discovered that with training, the healing mechanism can be summoned at will.

repetition (rep) is the performance of an exercise one time, such as lifting a weight once.

repetition maximum (1 RM) is the heaviest weight you can lift once with correct form.

risk factors are the conditions, situations, and behaviors that increase the likelihood that an undesirable outcome (injury, illness, or death) will occur.

s

sarcopenia means loss of muscle and decreased quality of muscle tissue. Strength training can restore or at least slow this loss as a person ages.

saturated fats are fatty acids that have hydrogen atoms attached to every carbon atom. Consumption of saturated fats has been shown to increase blood cholesterol levels. Coconut oil, butter, cheese, bacon, and meats are high in saturated fat.

secondary hypertension is high blood pressure caused by a specific condition, such as kidney disease, a tumor of the adrenal gland, or a defect of the aorta.

secondary prevention refers to early detection of cancer, such as by knowing cancer's warning signals and performing a monthly self-exam.

secondary risk factors contribute to the development of CVD but not as directly as do primary risk factors.

self-efficacy is a belief in the ability to successfully take action or perform a specific task.

semivegetarian is the type of vegetarian who excludes only red meat from his or her diet.

set is a group of several repetitions of an exercise. For example, lifting a weight eight times might be one set.

set point is a fat amount or weight level that the body physiologically works to maintain. It is thought that the brain regulates a "weight thermostat" for the body's metabolism. The set point can be altered, especially by engaging in regular exercise.

shin splint is a condition of pain along the front of the lower leg (shin). Involving the anterior tibialis muscle, the pain may range from mild discomfort to acute burning.

side stitch is pain that sometimes occurs on the side of the body just below the ribs during vigorous exercise. A variety of conditions may contribute to this spasm of the diaphragm—poor conditioning, shallow breathing, inadequate warm-up, and exercising too soon after eating.

simple carbohydrates are sugars that provide energy but lack much nutritional value. Honey, corn syrup, sucrose, fructose, dextrose, and brown sugar are examples.

skinfold calipers are devices that measure skinfold thickness to determine body fat percentage.

slow-twitch (ST) muscle fibers have good endurance but low power. They are recruited mainly in endurance-type activities.

social dimension is the dimension of wellness that deals with the ability to get along with other people regardless of their race, ethnic background, or beliefs. It involves appreciating the uniqueness of others as well as demonstrating sensitivity to the needs of others.

societal norms are the behaviors or practices expected in a culture and accepted and supported by its members. The practice of giving candy in heart-shaped boxes on Valentine's Day is an example of an American cultural norm.

soluble fiber travels through the digestive tract in a gel-like form, pacing the absorption of carbohydrates. This prevents dramatic shifts in blood sugar levels.

spiritual dimension is the dimension of wellness that involves looking within and exploring one's values and beliefs to discover a source of inner strength and serenity. It includes the ongoing search for personal meaning and purpose in life. Exhibiting honesty and having a clear sense of right and wrong are signs of spiritual wellness.

sprain is a partial or complete tear of a ligament. Both ankles and knees are vulnerable to sprains because of the sudden force or twisting motion that these joints often endure.

stage of exhaustion is the third stage of the General Adaptation Syndrome (GAS), now known as the Stress Response. During this stage, adaptation energy is exhausted and the organ system involved in the repeated stress response breaks down. Disease or malfunction of the organ system or death may occur.

stage of resistance is the second stage of the General Adaptation Syndrome (GAS), now known as the Stress Response. During this stage, the body actively resists and attempts to cope with the stressor.

static flexibility refers to the range of motion you can achieve through a slow controlled stretch, as in a sitting hamstring stretch that you hold for 15 to 30 seconds.

static (isometric) exercise is exercise in which the muscle contracts but does not change in length and little or no movement occurs. For example, if you push your palms together hard, your pectorals will contract but your arms will not move.

static stretching is the recommended method of stretching for flexibility. Each stretch is held for 15 to 30 seconds with no bouncing or jerking movements.

storage fat is the extra fat that accumulates in fat (adipose) cells around internal organs and beneath the skin surface to insulate, pad, and protect the body from trauma and extreme cold.

strain is a partial or complete tear of muscle fibers and/or a tendon. Sometimes referred to as a *pull*, a strain is often a result of a violent contraction of a muscle.

stress is the response of the body to any type of change and any new, threatening, or exciting situation. Dr. Hans Selye, one of the foremost authorities on stress, defined stress as the "nonspecific biological response of the human organism to any demand made upon it." *Nonspecific* means that the body reacts the same way regardless of the cause.

stress fracture is a microscopic break in a bone caused by overuse. Rather than being a result of a distinct traumatic event, a stress fracture results from cumulative overload on a bone (typically the lower leg and foot) that has not been able to adjust to the repeated force.

stress incontinence is an involuntary leakage of urine when laughing, coughing, sneezing, or exercising. It is a common problem, particularly in women over 30 who have given birth.

Stress Response, once known as the General Adaptation Syndrome (GAS), is the body's adaptation (reaction) to stress. Regardless of the cause, the reaction to stress is psychological and physiological.

stressors are factors causing stress. They may be pleasant or unpleasant, real or imagined, and physical, psychological, or emotional in nature.

stretch reflex is a reflex tightening of a muscle (to protect it from injury) when it is quickly stretched. For example, when you do a bouncy stretch, the muscle reflexively tightens as you reach the limit of your range of motion to prevent muscle strain.

strict vegetarian (vegan) is the type of vegetarian who consumes only plant foods.

stroke occurs when blood flow to the brain is blocked. It is primarily caused by atherosclerosis.

subcutaneous fat is fat that underlies the skin.

systolic blood pressure is the pumping pressure of the heart as it pushes the blood out of the heart. It is recorded as the upper number.

t

talk test is used to adjust exercise intensity. You should be able to talk with a friend while exercising. If you are too breathless to talk, you are exercising too hard.

target heart rate (THR) is the recommended heart rate range (or intensity level) for exercise. It is the range of intensity that assures adequate stimulation of the cardiorespiratory system yet is not so strenuous that symptoms of overtraining develop.

task specific activity is an exercise (or activity) using the same muscles that will be used in the conditioning bout. Warm-up and cool-down should be task specific. For example, if you jog during the conditioning bout, a period of jogging at a lower intensity should precede (warm-up) and follow (cool-down).

tendinitis is the inflammation of a tendon from repeated stress.

tendons are fibrous cords that connect muscle to bone. The most familiar tendon in the body is the Achilles tendon, which connects the calf muscle to the heel.

three-segment workout is the recommended pattern for exercise workouts. It should include a warm-up, a conditioning bout, and a cool-down.

trace minerals are minerals needed in small amounts. Examples are iron, zinc, copper, iodine, and fluoride.

training effect is the total beneficial change or physiological adaptation that results from regular aerobic exercise.

transcendental meditation (TM) is a form of meditation that originated in the cultures of India and Tibet. It was exported to the West by the Maharishi Mahesh Yogi. It involves training the mind on a single point of focus, such as a word or phrase.

trans-fatty acids (trans fats) are a type of fat found in many processed foods. During the manufacturing process of hydrogenation, some fatty acid molecules become rearranged into trans fats. Foods typically high in trans fats include margarine, crackers, cookies, doughnuts, french fries, chips, and candy.

transtheoretical model of behavior change is a five-stage progression that one passes through on the way to making a permanent lifestyle change. The five stages are precontemplation, contemplation, preparation, action, and maintenance.

triglycerides are known as *free fatty acids* and contribute to the atherosclerotic process. They are manufactured in the body and stored as excess fat.

Type A personality (and/or Type A emotional behavior) is described as competitive, ambitious, driven, impatient, workaholic, and always rushed. Type As put big demands on themselves to accomplish more and more in less and less time. They have little time for or interest in hobbies or leisure pursuits and have few intimate friends. The key problem with Type A behavior is stress. Type As put themselves under constant pressure, and their bodies react by producing extra amounts of stress hormones, which can be harmful.

Type B personality (and/or Type B behavior) is the opposite of Type A personality. Type Bs are relaxed, casual, unaggressive, and patient. They tend to deal more effectively with stressful situations.

Type C personality (and/or Type C behavior) is a Type A personality who has stress-resistant, "hardiness" traits and thus is not prone to the deleterious effects of stress, even though he or she lives a highly stressed life. Type Cs have five common traits called the *Five Cs* (control, commitment, challenge, choices in lifestyle, and connectedness).

Type D personality (for "distressed") is a person who possesses two negative emotional states: negative affectivity (worry, irritability, gloom) and social inhibition (discomfort in social interactions, reticence, and a lack of social poise). Type Ds are at increased risk of cardiovascular disease.

u–z

underpronation is insufficient outward roll of the foot on contact with the ground.

Valsalva maneuver involves holding your breath while you strain against a closed epiglottis, as in holding your breath while lifting a weight. You should avoid doing this because it can cause a dangerous elevation of blood pressure. When you lift weights, exhale on the exertion.

variable resistance exercise is exercise in which the force needed to move a weight is changed to provide a maximum load throughout the range of motion. Using Nautilus machines is an example.

vigorous physical activity is exercise that follows the FITT formula and not only provides health benefits but also increases cardiorespiratory fitness.

vitamins are organic catalysts necessary to initiate the body's complex metabolic functions.

warm-up is the first part of the three-segment workout. It prepares the exerciser physically and mentally for the conditioning bout.

water soluble vitamins are vitamins that remain in the body tissues for a short time. Excesses are excreted. Vitamin C and the B complexes are water soluble.

weight cycling (yo-yo syndrome) is the repetitive cycle of weight loss and weight gain. Off-and-on fad dieters typically experience weight cycling.

wellness is an integrated and dynamic level of functioning oriented toward maximizing potential, dependent on self-responsibility. It is a mind-set of self-empowerment and lifelong growth in the emotional, spiritual, physical, occupational, intellectual, environmental, and social dimensions.

Index

Note: Page numbers followed by *f* indicate figures; those followed by *t* indicate tables; and those followed by *a* indicate Lab Activities.

abdominal breathing, 334*t*
abdominal curl crunch, 195
abdominal curls, 72, 189
    evaluating, 97*a*
    fitness norms of, 74*t*
    oblique, 196
abdominal fat, 426
abdominal stimulators, 433
abdominal strengthening exercises, 194–196
abdominal/core strengthening workout,
    217*a*–218*a*
abuse, 32
aches, 160
Achilles tendonitis, 255
ACSM. *See* American College of Sports
    Medicine
action, 34–35
    back plan for, 275*a*–276*a*
    for eating disorders, 432
    prescription for, 42
    transtheoretical model of behavior change,
      34–35
active stretching, 162
activities. *See also* physical activity
    cardiorespiratory endurance, 60
    high impact, 245
    moderate physical, 61
    for relaxation, 351–352*a*
    task-specific, 65
    for wellness, 21*a*–30*a*
activity pyramid
    illustration of, 63*f*
    for physical activity, 62
activity step equivalents, 119*t*
acute stress, 317
addiction, 232
adipose cells, 414
aerobic capacity, 108
aerobic dance, 118–122
    advantages/disadvantages of, 118–119
    beginning/progress for, 120–121
    indoor cycling classes, 121–122
    step aerobics in, 121
    techniques/safety tips for, 120
    variety of, 121
    what to wear for, 119–120
aerobic exercise
    benefits of, 108
    body composition/physical appearance
      benefits with, 109
    cancer, 110
    cardiovascular disease and, 110
    chronic diseases reduced by, 110
    high blood pressure, 110
    immune system function, 110
    improved body composition, 110
    improved cognitive function, 110
    improved mental health with, 109

osteoarthritis, 110
osteoporosis and, 110–111
psychological/mental/emotional
    benefits, 109
weight management, 110
age, 162, 297
age-related flexibility declines, 160
aging, 239–242, 388–389
agonists, 181
alarm reaction, 317–319
alcohol, 337
alcohol consumption, 289
alternate arm/leg lift, 196
amenorrhea, 227
American College of Sports Medicine
    (ACSM), 60
anaerobic exercise, 115
anger, 296
angina pectoris, 281–282
angioplasty, 300
angry behavior modification, 328–329
ankle sprain, 258
anorexia nervosa, 430–431
antagonists, 181
anticipated high-risk situations, 50*a*
anticipated obstacles, 50*a*
antioxidants, 378
appearance, 178
appetite suppressor, 426
apples, 378
aqua aerobics, 142–144
    advantages/disadvantages of, 142
    beginning/process, 143
    common discomforts with, 144
    technique/safety tips for, 142–143
    variety, 143–144
    what to wear, 142
arousal, 38, 52*a*
arthritis, 110, 242
asanas, 334
aspirin, 258
assessment, 12
asthma, 242–243
atherosclerosis, 280–281
    causes of, 281
    progression of, 281
athletic performance, 160, 179
atrophy, 182
autogenic training/imagery, 333–334
awareness, 12

back. *See also* lower back
    action plan for, 275*a*–276*a*
    extension, 189, 191, 196
    health, 268
    strengthening, 246
    tips, 268–269
balance, 179–180
ballistic stretching, 65
basal metabolic rate (BMR), 417
    estimating, 443*a*
    factors that affect, 418*t*

    formula for, 443*a*
basic fitness, 164–165
basic resistance training programs, 186*t*
beans, 397*a*
BED. *See* binge eating disorder
behavior
    hostile, modification, 328–329
    learned, 32
    log, 53*a*–54*a*
    new, 32
    for stress, 361*a*–362*a*
    tips for, 384*t*
    transtheoretical model of, 33–39,
      51*a*–52*a*
behavior change
    contract, 40*f*, 51*a*–52*a*
    excuses for, 34
    journal, 53*a*–54*a*
    keys for success with, 41
behavior modification, 328–329, 423
    angry, 328–329
    changes, 423
    hostile, 328–329
    techniques, 423*t*
bench press, 187, 189
    fitness norms of, 74*t*
    strength test, 72, 75, 100*a*, 189
bent-knee sit-up, 72
bent-over rowing, 189
BIA. *See* bioelectrical impedance analysis
biceps curl, 181*f*, 189, 191
bicycle exercise, 195
bicycling, 122–125
    advantages/disadvantages of, 122
    beginning/progress, 124–125
    braking, 124
    bumps, 124
    common discomforts with, 125
    maintenance for, 123
    pedaling, 124
    shifting, 123–124
    technique/safety tips for, 123–124
    variety of, 125
    what to wear for, 123
bicycling test, 3-mile, 70, 73*t*
binge eating disorder (BED), 430, 431
    emotions of, 431
    symptoms of, 432*t*
bioelectrical impedance analysis (BIA), 78
biofeedback training, 335
blisters, 259–260
blocked coronary arteries
    angioplasty, 300
    drug therapy for, 300
    treatment for, 299–300
blood flow, 108
blood pressure. *See also* high blood pressure;
    hypertension
    DASH, 382–383
    diastolic pressure, 285
    nondrug approaches to, 287
    stress and, 322

systolic pressure, 285
blueberries, 378
BMI. *See* body mass index
BMR. *See* basal metabolic rate
body composition, 64
    body girth measures, 79
    evaluating, 103a–104a
    tests, 77–78
    understanding, 410–411
    using skinfold calipers, 78–79
body fat, 410
body fat percentage
    evaluating, 104a
    norm, 80t
body girth measures, 79–80
body mass index (BMI), 410
    evaluating, 104a
    lean, 77
bone strength, 179, 376
brain attack, 282
braking, 124
breast support, 231
breathing, 185
    abdominal, 334t
    thoracic, 334
broccoli, 378
Brussels sprouts, 378
bulimia nervosa, 430
    dynamic of, 430
    physical effects of, 430
bulk, 368
bumps, 124
bursitis, 260

cabbage, 378
calcium, 374–376, 376t
calf flexibility, 76f, 255
calf raise, 189
calorie, 414
    burning, 424–425
    determining needs, 415t
    expenditure, 425t
cancer
    aerobic exercise and, 110
    stress and, 322
canola oil, 371
carbohydrate-electrolyte replacement solutions
    (CES), 237
carbohydrates, 367
    complex, 367
    simple, 367
cardiac output, 108
cardiopulmonary resuscitation, 120
cardiorespiratory benefits, 103
cardiorespiratory endowment, 108
cardiorespiratory endurance (CRE)
    importance of, 64
    maximum oxygen uptake and, 108–111
    tests, 68–69
cardiorespiratory endurance activity, 60
cardiorespiratory exercise log, 157a
cardiorespiratory fitness, 68
    aerobic dance, 118–122
    bicycling, 122–125
    CRE and, 108–111
    evaluating, 91a–95a
    fitness swimming, 125–127
    fitness walking, 127–132
    FITT prescription for, 111–115
    frequently asked questions for, 145–146

indoor exercise equipment, 133–137
in-line skating, 137–140
Internet resources for, 147
jogging, 140–142
lifetime exercise activities, 115–116
maximizing, 107–148
summary of, 146–147
10,000 steps for, 116–118
water exercise, 142–144
cardiovascular disease (CVD), 4
    aerobic exercise and, 110
    deaths from, 279t
    frequently asked questions for, 302–303
    impact of, 278–279
    lifestyle changes for, 300–301
cardiovascular health, 180
cardiovascular system, 322
carrots, 378
CDC. *See* Centers for Disease Control and
    Prevention
cells, 414
cellulite, 433
Centers for Disease Control and Prevention
    (CDC), 283–284
cerebral hemorrhage, 282
CES. *See* carbohydrate-electrolyte replacement
    solutions
CGMP. *See* Current Good Manufacturing
    Practices
chafing, 260
change, 32, 33. *See also* behavior change;
        transtheoretical model of behavior
        change
    algorithm for stage of, 36f
    identifying current state, 47a–50a
    plan for, 39–42
    process of, 35–39
    strategies for, 29a–30a
CHD. *See* coronary heart disease
cholesterol, 286–291, 373
    guidelines, 289t
    HDL, 287–289
    high, 289
    hypercholesterolemia, 287
    LDL, 287
    triglycerides, 290–291
chronic compartment syndrome, 270
chronic diseases, 3, 110
chronic fatigue, 252
chronic stress, 317
cigarette(s), 337
    secondhand smoke, 291
    smoking, 291–292
circuit training, 144
circulation, 282
cognitive function, 110
collapse, 44
collateral circulation, 282
common injuries, 258–264
    ankle sprain, 258
    blisters, 259–260
    bursitis, 260
    chafing, 260
    frequently asked questions for, 270–271
    heel spur, 260
    iliotibial band syndrome, 260
    Internet resources for, 271
    medical help for, 264–265
    muscle cramp, 260
    muscle strain, 261

patellofemoral syndrome, 261
plantar fasciitis, 261
preventing, 251–271
recovering from, 265
side stitch, 263
stress fracture, 263
summary of, 271
symptoms/treatment, 259t
tendonitis, 255, 263–264
complex carbohydrates, 367–368
composition. *See* body composition
compress, 258
concentric contraction, 182
conditioning bout, 66
confusion, 115
consciousness, 36t
constant resistance exercise, 183
Consumer Product Safety Commission
    (CPSC), 140
contemplation, 34
contraction, 182
contract-relax-agonist contract, 166
contraindicated exercises, 167–171
    diagrams for, 168–170f
    donkey kicks, 169
    flexibility, 167–171
    full squat, 167
    head roll, 167
    hurdler stretch, 167
    knee tuck to chest, 167
    leg stretches, 167
    swan arch, 169
    yoga plow, 167
control, 320–321
control locus, 13
cool-down, 66
coping skills
    measuring, 353–354a
    scoring, 354–355a
coronary arteries. *See* blocked coronary arteries
coronary bypass surgery, 300
coronary heart disease (CHD), 58, 280
countering, 37t, 44, 52a
CPSC. *See* Consumer Product Safety
    Commission
cramp, 260
cravings, 43
CRE. *See* cardiorespiratory endurance
C-reactive protein (CRP), 299
cross training, 67
CRP. *See* C-reactive protein
culture, 428–429
curls
    abdominal, 72, 74t, 97a, 195
    hamstring, 187
    oblique abdominal, 196
Current Good Manufacturing Practices
    (CGMP), 379
CVD. *See* cardiovascular disease

daily hassles, 325–326
daily planning, 360a
daily time study log, 358a
daily uplifts, 325–326
DASH. *See* Dietary Approaches to Stop
    Hypertension
decision making, 33
deep tissue massage, 335
dehydration, 253
desirable weight, 104a

DEXA. *See* dual energy X-ray absorptiometry
diabetes, 58
  complications of, 295*t*
  exercising with, 110, 243
  mellitus, 243–244, 293–295
  obesity and, 293
  pre, 294
  risk for, 313*a*–314*a*
  type 2, 110
diastolic pressure, 285
diet
  analyzing, 397*a*–398*a*
  pills, 419
  plans, 419*t*
  well-balanced, 379–386
Dietary Approaches to Stop Hypertension
    (DASH), 382–383
dietary guidelines, 366*t*
dieting, 418–420
differences, 67, 164
dips, 197–198
disease(s). *See also* cardiovascular disease
  chronic, 3, 110
  coronary heart, 58, 280
  hypokinetic, 58
  psychosomatic, 321
  resistance, 233
distress, 317
distribution, 417
donkey kicks, 169
drugs, 287, 300, 337, 379
dual energy X-ray absorptiometry
    (DEXA), 77
dynamic flexibility, 162
dynamic isotonic exercise, 182–183
dynamic stretching, 162
dysmenorrhea, 227

eating. *See also* food
  binge, 430, 431, 432*t*
  changing times for, 364–367
  ethnic food choices, 388
  fast foods, 386, 405*a*–406*a*
  frequently asked questions, 389–390
  Internet resources for, 390
  mindless, 422
  out, 386–387
  summary of, 390
  for wellness, 363–393
eating disorders, 429–432
  actions for, 432
  anorexia nervosa, 430–431
  binge eating, 430, 431, 432*t*
  bulimia nervosa, 430
  risks for, 447*a*–448*a*
eating disorders not otherwise specified
    (EDNOS), 432
EDNOS. *See* eating disorders not otherwise
    specified
eggs, 302
elastic band exercises, 222*a*
elastic band workout, 221*a*–222*a*
elastic elongation, 164
elastic resistance, 201
elastic resistance exercises, 201–204
electrolytes, 236
  loss, 430
  replacement, 236–237
elevation, 258
elliptical trainers, 133

advantages/disadvantages of, 136
beginning/progress, 136–137
selecting, 136
technique/safety tips for, 136
elongation, 164
emotional arousal, 38, 52*a*
emotional dimension, 10
emotional management, 422–424
endorphins, 227
energy, 77, 179
energy balance equation, 414
enhanced athletic performance, 160
environmental conditions, 4
  exercise and, 233–238
  toxic, 422
environmental control, 37*t*, 52*a*
environmental dimension, 11
erector spinae muscle group, 269
essential fat, 410
estrogen, 227
ethnic food choices, 388
ethnic groups, 409
eustress, 317
exercise(s). *See also* aerobic exercise; fitness;
    physical activity; wellness
  abdominal strengthening, 194–196
  activity log for, 441*a*–442*a*
  addiction, 232
  alternate arm/leg lift, 196
  anaerobic, 115
  aqua aerobics, 142–144
  arthritis and, 242
  asthma and, 242–243
  bench press, 72, 74*t*, 75, 100*a*, 187, 189
  benefits for older adults, 241*t*
  bent-knee sit-up, 72
  bent-over rowing, 189
  biceps curl, 181*f*, 189, 191
  bicycling, 122–125, 195
  for bone strength, 376
  calf raise, 189
  chronic health conditions and, 242–246
  in cold, 233–235
  constant resistance, 183
  diabetes and, 110, 243
  disease resistance and, 233
  dynamic isotonic, 182–183
  elastic band, 222*a*
  elastic band workout, 221*a*–222*a*
  environmental conditions and, 233–238
  females and, 226–231
  fitness swimming, 125–127
  fitness walking, 127–132
  flexibility, 165*f*
  free weight, 189, 190–191*f*, 215*a*
  hamstring curl, 187
  in heat, 235
  hip/thigh, 196–197
  hot weather, 236
  hypertension and, 244
  importance of, 58–59
  indoor exercise equipment, 133–137
  in-line skating, 137–140
  isokinetic, 183
  isometric, 182
  jogging, 140–142
  Kegel, 230–231
  lat pull, 189
  leg press, 74*t*, 187
  life span increase from, 241–242

lifetime, 115, 116, 128
for lower back, 266*f*
males and, 231–232
military press, 189
osteoporosis and, 244–245
overload, 253*f*
partner resistance, 204–206, 224*a*
performance, 226
Pilates, 145, 201
postpartum and, 231
pregnancy and, 229–230
results with, 115
reverse crunch, 195
rowing machines, 133–136
run test, 1.5-mile, 69–70
self-esteem and, 426–427
shoulder shrugs, 198
side plank, 195
ski machines, 133, 135
special considerations, 225–248
squats, 167, 189
stability ball, 198–200, 220*a*
static, 182
stationary bikes, 133–134
sticking with, 117
stress management and, 332
sun salutations, 176*a*
sweating during, 235–236
toe press, 187
toe squat, 167
tolerant tests, 68–69
traveling tips for, 62
triceps press, 189, 191
upper body, 197–198
variable resistance, 183
vertical leg crunch, 195
walking, 127–132
water, 142–144
weight training, 187, 188*f*, 189, 214–215
exercise management, 424–428
  abdominal fat decreased by, 426
  as appetite suppressor, 426
  calorie burning and, 424–425
  lean muscle mass loss prevented by, 426
  self-esteem improved by, 426
  set-point lowering, 426
  for weight loss management, 426
exhaustion, 318, 320

fashion magazines, 428
fast foods, 386
  eating healthy, 405*a*–406*a*
  fast tips for, 386
fast-twitch (FT), 181
fat, 370–372
  abdominal, 426
  body, 80*t*, 104*t*, 410
  body location of, 412
  comparison of, 371*t*
  consumption of, 399*a*–400*a*
  essential, 410
  gram allowance, 373
  monounsaturated, 371
  polyunsaturated, 371
  saturated, 371
  storage, 410
  subcutaneous, 78
  total, gain, 417
  trans, 372
fat-cell theory, 414–415

fat-free mass, 410
fat-free tissue, 77
fatigue, 252
faulty perception, 320
FDA. *See* Food and Drug Administration
females
    athlete triad, 228–229
    exercise and, 226–231
fiber, 181, 368
    reasons, 368
    in selected foods, 369*t*
    soluble, 368, 388
fight-or-flight response, 317–319
    examples of, 319
    physical reaction of, 318*f*
fish oils, 372–373
fit ride, 121–122
fitness. *See also* cardiorespiratory fitness;
        muscular fitness
    basic, 164–165
    goals, 105*a*
    health, 187
    health-related components of, 64
    muscle gains and, 181
    personal profile of, 89*a*
    profile, 89*a*
    test norms, 73–74*t*
fitness development
    cross training, 67
    individual differences, 67
    principles of, 66–67
    progressive overload, 66
    reversibility principle, 66
    specificity principle, 66
fitness norms
    of abdominal curls, 74*t*
    of bench press, 74*t*
    of bicycling test, 3-mile, 73*t*
    of push-ups, 74*t*
    of run test, 1.5-mile, 73*t*
    of swim test, 500-yard, 73*t*
    tests for, 73–74*t*
    of walk test, 1-mile, 73*t*
    of water run test, 500-yard, 73*t*
fitness swimming, 125–127
    advantages/disadvantages of, 125–126
    beginning/progress, 126
    discomforts with, 127
    technique/safety tips for, 126
    variety with, 126
    what to wear, 126
fitness walking, 127–132
    advantages/disadvantages of, 127
    beginning/progressing, 130–131
    common discomforts with, 132
    correct walking form for, 129*f*
    pace increasing, 129–130
    technique/safety tips for, 128–129
    variety of, 131–132
    weight additions for, 130–131
    what to wear, 128
FITT. *See* frequency intensity time and type
flexibility, 64, 179
    age and, 162
    balance and, 164
    for basic fitness, 164–165
    benefits of, 160–161
    calf, 76*f*, 255
    cautions with, 161
    contraindicated exercises, 167–171

developing, 159–172
development, 163
dynamic, 162
evaluating, 101*a*–102*a*
exercises, 165*f*
factors affecting, 161
frequently asked questions for, 171
gender and, 162
genetics and, 162
individual differences, 164
injury/scar tissue, 162
Internet resources for, 172
joint structure with, 161
obesity and, 162
principles of, 164
programs for enhancing, 166–167
reversibility principle, 164
sample program for, 173*a*–174*a*
soft tissues, 161
specificity, 164
static, 162
summary of, 172
temperature for, 161–162
tips for developing, 163
types of, 162–163
flexibility quick checks
    equipment needed for, 102*a*
    evaluating, 102*a*
    procedure, 102*a*
flexibility tests
    hamstring, 76*f*
    hip flexor, 76*f*
    lower back, 76*f*
    quick checks for, 75
    sit and reach, 75–76
    sit and reach wall, 77
flours, 369
fluid pyramid, 238*f*
fluid replacement, 237
folacin, 299
food. *See also* antioxidants; fiber; nutrition
        basics
    apples, 378
    beans, 397*a*
    blueberries, 378
    broccoli, 378
    Brussels sprouts, 378
    calcium-fortified, 376
    fruits, 381, 397*a*
    grains, 397
    grapes, 378
    hamburgers, 386
    journal, 439*a*–440*a*
    kale, 378
    log, 395–396*a*
    management, 421
    meat, 397*a*
    Mexican, 386
    milk, 397*a*
    nutrition basics for, 367–377
    onions, 378
    oranges, 378
    peppers, 378
    pizza, 386, 390
    raisins, 378
    raspberries, 378
    refined flours, 369
    spinach, 378
    strawberries, 378
    sweet potatoes, 378

tomatoes, 378
    wellness associations of, 364*t*
Food and Drug Administration (FDA), 379
footwear, 254
form, 184
forward bending, 245
free radicals, 378
free weight exercises, 189, 190–191*f*, 215*a*
frequency, 111
frequency intensity time and type (FITT)
    exercise prescription for, 111–115
    frequency, 111
    intensity, 111–112
fruits, 381, 397*a*
FT. *See* fast-twitch
full body scan, 302
full squat, 167

GAS. *See* General Adaptation Syndrome
gastric bypass surgery, 433
gel packs, 258
gender. *See also* females
    differences, 182
    flexibility and, 162
    males, 297
General Adaptation Syndrome (GAS), 317
genetics, 162
GI. *See* glycemic index
glucose, 293
glute squeeze, 196
gluteal stretch, 166
glycemic index (GI), 369, 419
glycogen, 367, 418
goals
    fitness, 105*a*
    of *Healthy People, 2010*, 60
    of leg press strength test, 72
    road maps for, 39
    S.M.A.R.T., 41
    weekly, 359*a*
    yearly, 357*a*
golgi tendon organ (GTO), 162
grains, 397
grapes, 378
GTO. *See* golgi tendon organ

hamburgers, 386
hamstring curl, 187
hamstring flexibility test, 76*f*
hamstring stretch, 164, 166
hardiness, 330, 349*a*–350*a*
hassles, 325–326
Hatha yoga, 175*a*–176*a*, 334–335
HDL. *See* high-density lipoprotein
head roll, 167
health. *See also* wellness
    assessment, 87*a*
    cardiovascular, 180
    clubs, 146
    determinants of, 4
    disparity, 7
    environmental conditions for, 4
    fitness, 187
    lifestyle behaviors for, 5
    lower back, 269
    medical care and, 5
    mental, 109
    physical activity and, 59–63
    prevention, 5
    promotion, 5

social circumstances for, 4
health life expectancy, 3
healthy lifestyle assessment, 21a–23a
Healthy People 2010
    goals of, 60
    health objectives for, 6t
healthy weight
    achieving, 407–437
    body composition, 410–411
    culture/weight, 428–429
    eating disorders and, 429–432
    emotional management and, 422–424
    exercise management and, 424–428
    frequently asked questions for, 433–434
    Internet resources for, 435
    obesity and, 414–420
    summary of, 434
    surgeon general on, 413–414
heart
    attack, 282, 299–300
    maximal, rate, 114
    RHR, 112
heart disease, 2t, 307a–308a, 309a–310a. *See
    also* cardiovascular disease; coronary
    heart disease
heart health
    cardiovascular disease and, 278–279, 300–303
    frequently asked questions for, 302–303
    Internet resources for, 303
    lifestyle and, 300–301
    maximizing, 277–305
    mending, 311a–312a
    risk factors, 283–299
    summary of, 303
heart rate reserve (HRR), 112
heat
    exercise in, 235
    illnesses, 235t
    relievers, 258
    safety illness, 236f
    tolerance, 226
heavy lifting, 245
heavy sweating, 235–236
heel spur, 260
helping relationships, 37t, 52a
hemoglobin, 226
hemorrhage, 282
heredity, 4, 417
high blood lipid level, 286–291
high blood pressure, 110, 285–286. *See also*
    hypertension
high cholesterol, 289
high-impact activities, 245
high-level wellness, 7–8
high-density lipoprotein (HDL), 287–289
high-risk situations, 50a
hip flexor flexibility test, 76f
hip flexor stretch, 164
hip/thigh exercises, 196–197
homocysteine, 298–299
hostile behavior modification, 328–329
hostility, 296
hot reactors, 296, 327–328
hot stone massage, 335
hot weather exercise, 236
HRR. *See* heart rate reserve
hurdler stretch, 167
hydrogenation, 372
hypercholesterolemia, 287
hypertension, 244, 285–286

DASH, 382–383
    exercise and, 244
    secondary, 286
hyperthermia, 235
hypertrophy, 182
hypokinetic diseases, 58
hyponatremia, 238
hypothermia, 234

ibuprofen, 258
ice, 257
iliotibial band syndrome, 260
immune system, 321
immune system function, 110
improved body composition, 110
improved cognitive function, 110
improved mental health, 109
improved sleep, 110
individual differences, 67, 164
indoor cycling classes, 121–122
indoor exercise equipment, 133–137
    advantages/disadvantages of, 133
    considerations for, 133–134
    equipment for, 133
    what to wear for, 133
inflexibility, 254–255
injuries, 160, 162, 258–264. *See also* common
    injuries
    flexibility, 162
    lower back, 269
    specialists, 264
injury prevention, 179, 252–256
    case study for, 273–274a
    footwear, 254
    frequently asked questions for, 270–271
    heat/pain relievers, 258
    mechanics of, 255–256
    top 10 ways for, 256
    weakness/inflexibility, 254–255
in-line skating, 137–140
    advantages/disadvantages of, 137–138
    bearing replacement, 139
    beginning process of, 139
    brake replacement, 139
    common discomforts with, 139–140
    necessary gear, 138
    safety guidelines for, 138t
    techniques/safety tips for, 138–139
    tools for, 139
    variety, 139
    what to wear for, 138
    wheel rotation, 139
inner thigh stretch, 166
innervation, 162
insoluble fiber, 368
Institute of Medicine (IOM), 284
intensity, 111–112
intervertebral disc, 269
inverse stretch reflex, 162
IOM. *See* Institute of Medicine
iron, 377
ischemia, 263, 282
isometric exercise, 182

Jacobson's progressive relaxation, 334
Jenny Craig, 419
jogging, 140–142
    advantages/disadvantages of, 140
    beginning/progress, 141
    common discomforts with, 142

technique/safety tips for, 140–141
    variety, 141–142
    water, 144
    what to wear for, 140

kale, 378
Karvonen equation, 112–113
Kegel exercises, 230–231
ketone bodies, 371
knee tuck to chest, 167
knowledge, 12

label reading assignment, 401a–402a
lactose intolerance, 376
lactovegetarian, 387
lapse, 44
lat pull, 189
LDL. *See* low-density lipoprotein
LDL cholesterol receptors, 290
lean body mass, 77, 411
lean muscle mass, 426
learned behaviors, 32
learned optimism, 42
leg extension, 187
leg press, 74t, 187
leg press strength test, 72, 75
    evaluating, 99a
    goal/directions for, 72
leg stretches, 167
lifestyle abuse, 32
lifetime exercise
    achievements, 115–116
    reasons for, 128
lifetime goals, 357a
lift(s)
    alternate arm/leg, 196
    daily, 325–326
    rear leg, 196
    up, 325–326
lifting
    heavy, 245
    techniques, 267
ligament, 258
lipids
    total amount of, 287
    transportation of, 287–288
liposuction, 433
live event stress test, 324t, 345
log(s)
    activity, 441a–442a
    behavior, 53a–54a
    cardiorespiratory exercise, 157a
    daily time study, 358a
    food, 395–396a
    sheet, 348a
    training, 211a
long arm crunch, 195
longevity
    determinants of, 4
    factors affecting, 4f
low-density lipoprotein (LDL), 287
lower back
    caring for, 251–271, 265–269
    core in, 269
    exercises for, 266f
    frequently asked questions for, 270–271
    health, 269
    injuries, 269
    Internet resources for, 271
    pain, 265–266

stretch, 164, 166
summary of, 271
lower back flexibility test, 76f
lunge, 189

macrominerals, 373
maintenance, 35
males
    exercise and, 231–232
    gender, 297
management
    emotional, 422–424
    exercise, 424–428
    food, 421
    lifetime weight, 420–428
    self, skills, 13
    stress, 331–332, 335–339
    time, 336–337, 357a–360a
    weight, 445a–446a
massage
    deep tissue, 335
    hot stone, 335
    sports, 335
    Swedish, 335
maximal heart rate, 114
maximum oxygen uptake, 108–111
meat, 397a
medical care, 5
meditation, 332–333
    log sheet, 348a
    mindfulness, 331
    relaxation response and, 347–348a
    TM, 332–333
memory bank, 339
menarche, 227
menstruation, 226–228
mental health, 109
metabolic syndrome, 298
metabolism, 417–418
Mexican food, 386
MI. *See* myocardial infarction
military press, 189
milk, 397a
mind/body connection, 301
mindfulness meditation, 331
mindless eating, 422
minerals, 373
moderate physical activity, 61
monosodium glutamate (MSG), 377
monounsaturated fats, 371
motivation, 13
movement speed, 185
MSG. *See* monosodium glutamate
muscle
    atrophy, 182
    balance, 184–185
    cramp, 260
    fiber recruitment, 181
    fibers, 181
    fitness gains, 181
    function, 181
    imbalances, 255t
    major, 185f
    ass, 41
    ess, 160–161, 260–261
    162

push-ups test, 98a
muscular fitness, 177–209
    determinants of, 181–183
    frequently asked questions for, 206–207
    guidelines for developing, 183–185
    Internet resources for, 208
    programs for, 185–193
    resistance training for, 178–181
    shaping/toning without weights for, 193–204
    summary of, 207
muscular power, 184
muscular strength, 64, 99a–100a
muscular strength/endurance tests, 72–75
    abdominal curls, 72
    bench press strength test, 75
    leg press strength test, 72, 75
music, 335
myocardial infarction (MI), 282
MyPyramid, 380f

negative pull-ups, 198
nervous system, 322
new behavior, 32
nutrient density, 383
nutrition
    behavior change using theoretical model
        for, 403a–404a
    frequently asked questions for, 389–390
    labeling, 384–386
    summary of, 391
    supplements, 378–379
nutrition basics, 367–377
    calcium, 374
    carbohydrates, 367
    cholesterol, 373
    fish oils, 372–373
    iron, 377
    nutritional supplements, 378–379
    protein, 370
    sodium, 377
    vitamins, 373
    water, 377
nutritional wellness, 383t

obesity, 58
    causes of, 414–420
    diabetes and, 293
    energy balance equation, 414
    fat-cell theory, 414–415
    flexibility and, 162
    healthy weight and, 414–420
    heredity, 417
    metabolism, 417–418
    percentage risk increased with, 412t
    as primary risk factors, 292–293
    risks associated with, 411–412
    set-point theory, 416–417
oblique abdominal curls, 196
obstacles, 50a
oil
    canola, 371
    fish, 372–373
Old Order Amish community, 284
oligomenorrhea, 227
omega-3 fatty acids, 373
onions, 378
optimal calcium requirements, 376t
optimal stress, 317
optimism, 42
oranges, 378

orthotics, 255
osteoarthritis, 110
osteopenia, 374
osteoporosis, 58, 374
    aerobic exercise and, 110–111
    exercise and, 244–245
    progression of, 375
    risk for, 228–229
overpronation, 255
overtraining, 252, 254t
overuse, 252, 254t
overweight, 410–411
ovolactovegetarian, 387
oxygen uptake, 108–111

pain, 160
    lower back, 265–266
    relievers, 258
partner resistance exercises, 204–206, 224a
partner resistance workout, 223a–224a
passive stretching, 163
patellofemoral syndrome, 261
pectoral stretch, 166
pedaling, 124
pedometer, 117, 151a–153a
peppers, 378
perception, 320–321
performance, 239–240
performance aids, 193, 193t
peroneal area, 231
personal decision making, 33
personal fitness profile, 89a
personalities
    Type A, 326
    Type B, 326
    Type C, 330
    Type D, 327
physical activity
    activity pyramid for, 62
    in adolescence, 58–59
    aging and, 238–239
    benefits of, 59–60
    frequently asked questions for, 82
    health and, 59–63
    Healthy People 2010 goals for, 60–61
    Internet resources for, 83
    moderate, 59f, 61
    skill-related, 63
    summary of, 82
    three-part workout for, 65–66
    time for, 61
physical fitness
    assessing, 67–68
    benefits of, 65t
    definition of, 63
    developing/assessing, 57–85
    tests, 68
    wellness and, 64
physician-approved exercise clearance form, 88a
phytochemicals, 378–379
phytoestrogens, 378
Pilates, 145, 201
pizza, 386, 390
plan, 39–42
plank, 195
planning, 360a
plantar fasciitis, 261
plaque, 280–281
plastic elongation, 164
plyometrics, 144

PNF. *See* proprioceptive neuromuscular facilitation
polyunsaturated fats, 371
portion distortion, 421
postpartum
    ACOG guidelines for exercise during, 230*t*
    exercises during, 231
precontemplation, 33–34, 45
prediabetes, 294
pregnancy, 387–388
    ACOG guidelines for exercise during, 230*t*
    exercise and, 229–230
prehypertension, 285
preparation, 34
pressure. *See also* blood pressure
    diastolic, 285
    systolic, 285
pretest instructions, 69
P.R.I.C.E. (protect, rest, ice, compress, elevate), 256–258
primary risk factors, 283–295
    cholesterol, 286–291
    cigarette smoking, 291–292
    diabetes mellitus, 293–295
    hypertension, 285–286
    inactivity, 283–285
    obesity, 292–293
principles
    of fitness development, 66–67
    of flexibility, 164
process of change, 35–39
progression, 33
progressive overload, 66, 164, 183
progressive relaxation
    Jacobson's, 334
    routine, 334*t*
pronation, 255
proprioceptive neuromuscular facilitation (PNF), 155*f*, 165
protect, rest, ice, compress, elevate. *See* P.R.I.C.E.
protein, 370
    CRP, 299
    HDL, 287–289
    LDL, 287
    nutrition basics and, 370
psychological benefits, 180
psychoneuroimmunology, 321
psychosomatic disease, 321
pull-ups, 198
push-ups, 197
    evaluating, 98*a*
    fitness norms of, 74*t*

quadriceps flexibility test, 76*f*
quadriceps stretch, 165

race, 297–298
raisins, 378
raspberries, 378
rate of perceived exertion (RPE), 113, 114*t*
rear leg lift, 196
reciprocal innervation, 162
recovery, 183
reduced peroneal area, 231
refined flours, 369
reflex, 162
reframing, 339
relapse
    factors contributing to, 43
    preventing, 42–45

tips for getting back on track, 44*t*
relationships
    helping, 37*t*, 52*a*
    stress management and, 338
relaxation
    activities for, 351–352*a*
    Jacobson's progressive, 334
    meditation response and, 347–348*a*
    progressive, 334
    training, 331
relaxation response, 331
    experience on, 347–348*a*
    meditation, 332–333
relaxation techniques, 332–335. *See also* meditation
    biofeedback training, 335
    massage, 335
repetitions, 183
resistance
    basic, training programs, 186*t*
    constant, exercise, 183
    diseases, 233
    elastic, 201
    elastic, exercises, 201–204
    partner, exercises, 204–206, 224*a*
    partner, workout, 223*a*–224*a*
    stages of, 318–320
    stress, 349*a*–350*a*
    training log, 211*a*
    variable, exercise, 183
resistance training
    benefits/cautions for, 178–181
    common discomforts/training errors with, 193
    disadvantages of/cautions for, 180–181
    equipment, 186
    frequently asked questions for, 206–207
    mistakes to avoid, 187
    performance aids, 193
    principles of, 183
    program, 182, 185
    progressing with, 191
    psychological benefits of, 180
    safety guidelines for, 184*t*
    social benefits, 180
    variety, 192
rest, 257
rest between sets, 184
resting heart rate (RHR), 112
resuscitation, 120
reverse crunch, 195
reversibility principle, 66, 164
reward, 37*t*, 52*a*
rhomboid rolls, 198
RHR. *See* resting heart rate
risk factors, 283–299
    cigarette smoking, 291–292
    diabetes mellitus, 293–295
    obesity, 292–293
    primary, 283–295
    secondary, 295–298
risks, 50*a*
    for diabetes, 313*a*–314*a*
    for eating disorders, 447*a*–448*a*
    for heart health, 283–299
    obesity and, 411–412, 412*t*
    for osteoporosis, 228–229
roughage, 368
rowing, 189
rowing machines, 133–136

advantages/disadvantages of, 135
selecting, 135
technique/safety tips for, 135–136
RPE. *See* rate of perceived exertion
run test, 1.5-mile, 69–70
    evaluating, 91*a*
    fitness norms of, 73*t*

saturated fats, 371
scar tissue, 162
secondary hypertension, 286
secondary risk factors, 295–298
    emotional behavior, 296–297
    male gender, 297
    race, 297–298
    stress, 295–296
secondhand smoke, 291
self-efficacy, 32, 44
self-esteem, 426–427
self-evaluation strategies, 38
self-liberation, 37, 52*a*
self-management skills, 13
self-reevaluation, 37*t*, 52*a*
self-responsibility, 13
self-talk, 42
semivegetarian, 387
serving sizes, 385*f*
setbacks, 55*a*–56*a*
set-point theory, 416–417, 426
shiatsu, 335
shifting, 123–124
shin splints, 262–263
shoulder shrugs, 198
side plank, 195
side stitch, 263
simple carbohydrates, 367
sit and reach, 74*t*
sit and reach test
    directions for, 75–76
    evaluating, 101*a*
sit and reach wall test, 77
ski machines, 133
    advantages/disadvantages of, 135
    selecting, 135
    technique/safety tips for, 135
skinfold calipers, 78
sleep
    developing, 338*t*
    improved, 110
    stress and, 337–338
sleeping position, 267
Slimfast, 419
slow-twitch (ST), 181
S.M.A.R.T, 41
    goal, 45
    identifying specific, 49*a*
smoking, 291–292
social circumstances, 4
social dimension, 10
social liberation, 51*a*
    description of, 36*t*
    strategies, 38
social situations, 43
societal norms, 14–15, 14*t*
    unwritten codes of, 29–30
    wellness and, 15–16
sodium, 377
soft tissues, 161
soluble fiber, 368, 388
soreness, 160–161, 260–261

special exercise considerations, 225–248
  aging, 239–242
  environmental, 233–238
  exercise addiction, 232
  exercise/chronic health conditions, 242–246
  exercise/disease resistance, 233
  exploring, 249a–250a
  females and, 226–231
  frequently asked questions for, 246–247
  Internet resources for, 247
  males and, 231–232
  summary of, 247
special nutritional concerns, 387–389
  pregnancy, 387–388
  sports/fitness, 389
specificity, 183
specificity principle, 66
spinach, 378
spinal twist, 164
spinning, 121–122
spirituality
  components of, 10
  dimension, 10–11
sports, 335, 389
spot reduction, 433
sprain, 258
squats, 167, 189
squeeze, 196
ST. *See* slow-twitch
stability ball
  exercises, 198–200, 220a
  workout, 219a–220a
stages of exhaustion, 318, 320
stages of resistance, 318, 319–320
standing toe squat, 167
static exercise, 182
static flexibility, 162
static stretching, 65, 162
stationary bikes, 133
  advantages/disadvantages of, 134
  selecting, 134
  technique/safety tips for, 134
step aerobics, 121
step test, 3-minute, 71, 95a
steppers, 133
  advantages/disadvantages of, 134
  selecting, 134
  technique/safety tips for, 134
steps
  activity, equivalents, 119t
  aerobics, 121
  reaching 10,000, 119t
  recommended daily number of, 116–118
stimulators, 433
storage fat, 410
strain, 261
strategies for change, 29a–30a
strawberries, 378
strength, 226
  bone, 179, 376
  muscular, 64, 99a
  ...ining, 246
  ... 295–296
  ...17
  ...r, 361a–362a
  ... and, 322

daily hassles/uplifts, 325–326
definition of, 317
distress, 317
eustress, 317
fracture, 263
frequently asked questions for, 340–341
harmful effects of, 321–322
hot reactors, 327–328
incontinence, 230
Internet resources for, 341
live event test for, 324t, 345
managing, 332t
measuring, 322–325, 353–355a
optimal, 317
reduction tips, 329
resistance, 349a–350a
resistant hardy person, 329–331
response, 317–320, 347
secondary risk factors, 295–296
sleep and, 337–338
summary of, 341
stress management, 331–332
  exercise and, 332
  laughter/humor, 339
  lifestyle change, 335–336
  memory bank, 339
  reframing, 339
  relationships and, 338
  sleep and, 337–338
  time management, 336–337
stressors, 317, 318f
stretch(es)
  gluteal, 166
  hamstring, 164, 166
  hip flexor, 164
  hurdler, 167
  inner thigh, 166
  inverse, reflex, 162
  leg, 167
  lower back, 164, 166
  pectoral, 166
  quadriceps, 165
stretching
  active, 162
  ballistic, 65
  dynamic, 162
  passive, 163
  static, 65, 162
strict vegetarian, 387
stroke, 282
student precourse health assessment, 87a
subcutaneous fat, 78
sun salutations, 176a
support, 13
surgery
  coronary bypass, 300
  gastric bypass, 433
swan arch, 169
sweating, 235–236
Swedish massage, 335
sweet potatoes, 378
swim test, 500-yard, 70
  evaluating, 94a
  fitness norms of, 73t
swimming, 125–127
  advantages/disadvantages of, 125–126
  beginning/progress, 126
  discomforts with, 127
  technique/safety tips for, 126
  variety with, 126

what to wear for, 126
syndrome(s)
  chronic compartment, 270
  GAS, 317
  iliotibial band, 260
  metabolic, 298
  patellofemoral, 261
  X, 298
  yo-yo, 420
systolic pressure, 285

Tai Chi, 145, 166
talk test, 113
target heart rate (THR), 66
  calculating, 149a
  equation for, 112–113
  estimated, 113f
task-specific activity, 65
temporary muscular failure, 181
tendonitis, 255, 263–264
tendons, 263–264
tennis elbow, 263
test(s)
  bicycling, 3-mile, 70, 73t
  body composition, 77–78
  cardiorespiratory endurance (CRE), 68–69
  exercise tolerant, 68–69
  fitness, norms, 73–74t
  flexibility, 75–77
  hamstring flexibility, 76f
  hip flexor flexibility, 76f
  leg press strength, 72, 75, 99a
  live event stress, 324t, 345
  lower back flexibility, 76f
  muscular strength/endurance, 72–75
  physical fitness, 68
  quadriceps flexibility, 76f
  run, 1.5-mile, 69–70, 73t, 91a
  sit and reach, 75–76, 101a
  sit and reach wall, 77
  step, 3-minute, 71, 95a
  swim, 500-yard, 70, 73t, 94a
  talk, 113
  walk, 1-mile, 70
  water run, 500-yard, 70–71, 73t, 93a
thoracic breathing, 334
THR. *See* target heart rate
three-part workout, 65–66
  conditioning bout, 66
  cool-down, 66
  warm-up, 65
time, 114
  economy, 178
  evaluating, 357a–360a
  management, 336–337
tissue(s)
  fat-free, 77
  scar, 162
  soft, 161
TM. *See* transcendental meditation
toe press, 187
toe squat, 167
tomatoes, 378
total cholesterol/HDL ratio, 290
total fat gain, 417
toxic environment, 422
trace minerals, 373
training. *See also* resistance training; weight
    training

autogenic, 333–334
basic resistance, 186*t*
biofeedback, 335
circuit, 144
cross, 67
effect, 108
over, 252, 254*t*
relaxation, 331
strength, 246
trans fat, 372
transcendental meditation (TM), 332–333
transfatty acid, 372
transtheoretical model of behavior change
action, 34–35
behavior-change contract of, 51*a*–52*a*
contemplation, 34
frequently asked questions for, 44–45
Internet resources for, 45
maintenance, 35
precontemplation, 33–34
preparation, 34
process of change, 35–39
processes of, 51*a*–52*a*
summary of, 44–45
traveling, 62
treadmill, 133
advantages/disadvantages of, 134–135
selecting, 135
technique/safety tips for, 135
treadmill workouts, 155*a*–156*a*
triceps press, 189, 191
triglycerides, 290–291
twisting, 245
type personalities, 326–328

underpronation, 255
unhealthy norm, 29*a*–30*a*
United States
health-care costs in, 3
health disparity in, 7
leading causes of death in, 2
United States Pharmacopoeia (USP), 379
unwritten codes, 29*a*–30*a*
uplifts, 325–326
upper body exercises, 197–198
U.S. Department of Agriculture (USDA), 381
USDA. *See* U.S. Department of Agriculture
USP. *See* United States Pharmacopoeia

Valsalva maneuver, 185
variable resistance exercise, 183
vegan, 387
vegetables
eating, 381
intake, 6, 397*a*
vegetarianism
lacto, 387
ovolacto, 387
semi, 387
strict, 387
vegan, 387
vertical leg crunch, 195
vitamins, 299, 373, 374–375*t*

waist circumference, 413
waist girth
evaluating, 103*a*
measurements for, 80*t*, 81
waist-to-hip ratio
evaluating, 103*a*
measurements for, 80*t*, 81
walk test, 1-mile, 70
evaluating, 92*a*
fitness norms of, 73*t*
walking
advantages/disadvantages of, 127
beginning/progressing, 130–131
common discomforts with, 132
correct walking form for, 129*f*
equipment, 131*t*
pace, 130
pace increasing, 129–130
technique/safety tips for, 128–129
variety of, 131–132
weight additions for, 130–131
what to wear for, 128
W.A.L.K.S. program, 132
water, 237–238, 377
water run test, 500-yard, 70–71
evaluating, 93*a*
fitness norms of, 73*t*
water exercise, 142–144
advantages/disadvantages of, 142
beginning/process, 143
common discomforts with, 144
technique/safety tips for, 142–143
variety, 143–144
what to wear, 142
water jogging, 144
weakness, 254–255
weekly goals, 359*a*
weight. *See also* healthy weight
control, 178, 408
culture and, 428–429
desirable, 104*a*
differences, 409
overweight, 410–411
weight cycling, 420
weight gain, 178, 427–428
weight loss
programs, 420
tips for, 424*t*
tips from successful losers/
maintainers, 427
weight management, 110
aerobic exercise and, 110
emotional management, 422–424
exercise management, 424–428
food management, 421
lifetime, 420–428
mindless eating, 422
plan, 445*a*–446*a*
portion distortion, 421
weight room etiquette, 186–187
weight training, 185
exercise, 187, 188*f*, 189, 214*a*–215*a*
experience, 213*a*–215*a*

frequently asked questions for, 206–207
Internet resources for, 208
summary of, 207–208
Weight Watchers, 419
weight-bearing, 245
well-balanced diet, 379–386
wellness
assessing, 12, 25–28*a*, 25*a*–28*a*
awareness, 12
continuum, 9*f*
definition of, 11
dimensions of, 9
eating for, 363–393
emotional dimension of, 10
environmental dimension of, 11
factors affecting, 12*f*
frequently asked questions for, 16–17
growth in, 11–12
high level, 7–8
intellectual dimension, 9
Internet resources for, 17–18
knowledge, 12
lab activities for, 21*a*–30*a*
lifestyle practices of, 5
motivation of, 13
nutritional, 383*t*
occupational dimension of, 11
physical dimension of, 9
physical fitness and, 64
self-management skills of, 13
self-responsibility, 13
social dimension of, 10
societal norms and, 15–16
spiritual dimension of, 10–11
summary of, 17
support/opportunity, 13
WHO. *See* World Health Organization
whole grains, 369
willpower, 32
windchill temperatures, 234*f*
witness, 52*a*
women. *See also* females
average size of, 428
fashion magazines and, 428
workload, 191–192
workout(s)
abdominal curl crunch, 195
abdominal/core strengthening, 217*a*–218*a*
elastic band, 221*a*–222*a*
partner resistance, 223*a*–224*a*
stability ball, 219*a*–220*a*
three part, 65 66
treadmill, 155*a*–156*a*
World Health Organization (WHO), 3

yearly goals, 357*a*
yoga, 145
hatha, 175*a*–176*a*, 176, 334–335
plow, 167
yo-yo syndrome, 420

Flexibility Exercises

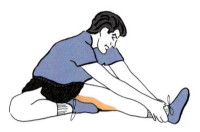

(a) Hamstring stretch

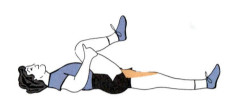

(b) Lower back/hip flexor stretch

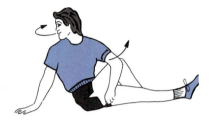

(c) Spinal twist

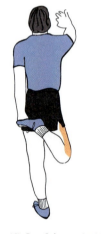

(d) Quadriceps stretch

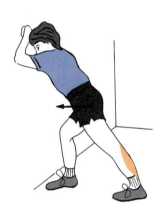

(e) Calf/Achilles stretch

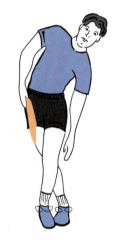

(f) Iliotibial band stretch

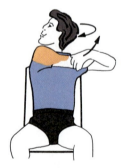

(g) Deltoid stretch

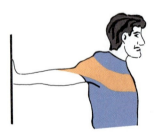

(h) Pectoral stretch

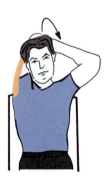

(i) Triceps stretch

Exercises for the Lower Back

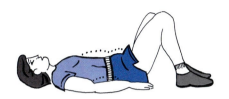

(a) Pelvic tilt
Lie on back, knees bent. Press small of back firmly down to floor by tightening the abdominal muscles. Hold for a count of five.

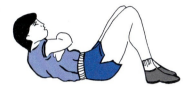

(b) Abdominal curl
Do a pelvic tilt and, while holding this position, curl head and shoulders up until shoulder blades have been lifted from the floor. Hold briefly. Lower slowly.

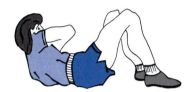

(c) Oblique abdominal curl
Do a pelvic tilt and, while holding this position, curl head and shoulders up, twisting right shoulder toward left knee. Hold briefly. Lower slowly. Repeat other side.

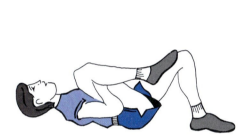

(d) Low back stretch
(a) Lie on back. Pull one knee toward chest. Hold for a count of five. Repeat other leg.
(b) Double knee pull. Pull both knees to chest; hold for a count of five.

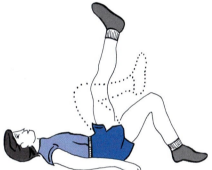

(e) Lying hamstring stretch
Lie on back. Bring knee toward chest and extend leg toward ceiling. Flex foot. (You may grasp the back of your thigh with your hands.) Hold 20 seconds. Repeat with other leg.

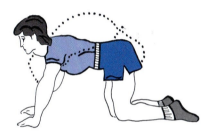

(f) Cat stretch
Start on all fours. Round the back upward like a cat. Tighten abdominals. Hold for 5 seconds. Relax and return to starting position. Do not let back sag.

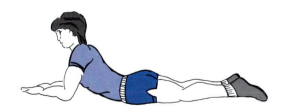

(g) Upper back lift
Lie on your stomach with forearms flat on the ground. Tighten abdominals. Lift upper body using back muscles. Do not press with arms. Hold for a count of five.

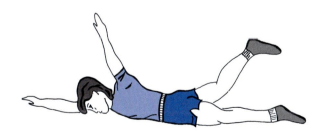

(h) Alternate arm/leg lift
Lie on your stomach with arms extended in front. Raise one arm overhead toward ceiling while simultaneously lifting the opposite leg. Hold for a count of five. Repeat with the other arm and leg.

Free Weight Exercises

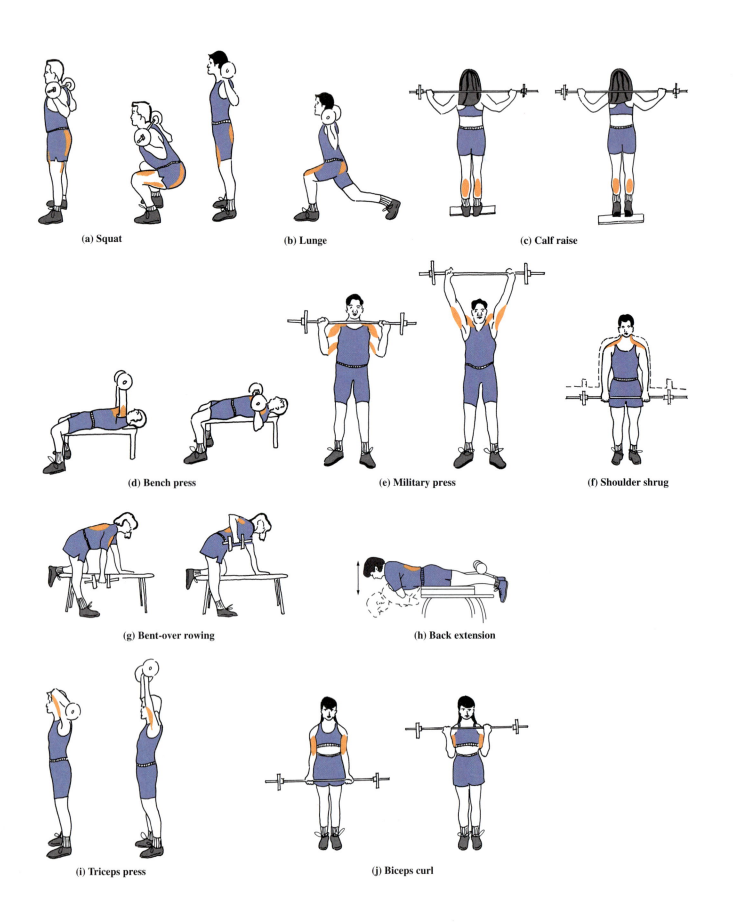

(a) Squat

(b) Lunge

(c) Calf raise

(d) Bench press

(e) Military press

(f) Shoulder shrug

(g) Bent-over rowing

(h) Back extension

(i) Triceps press

(j) Biceps curl

Abdominal/Core Strengthening Exercises

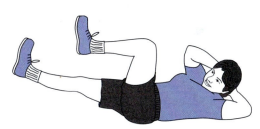

(1) Bicycle exercise

Lie on your back with hands beside your head. Raise knees to a 45-degree angle and slowly do a bicycle pedaling motion as shown. Touch right elbow to left knee and left elbow to right knee.

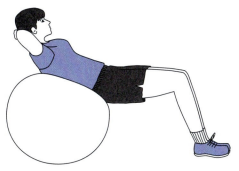

(2) Abdominal crunch on stability ball

Lie on stability ball with feet flat on floor, thighs and trunk parallel to floor. Cross arms behind shoulders or across chest; contract abdominals by raising trunk about 45 degrees. Spread feet apart for better balance. To work obliques more, bring feet closer together.

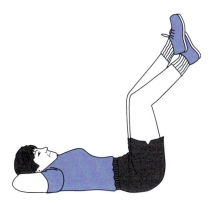

(3) Vertical leg crunch

Lie on your back with legs raised in the air, knees slightly bent and crossed at the ankles. Cross hands behind the shoulders to support the head. Keep chin lifted to prevent jerking the head. Lift the trunk and slowly lower.

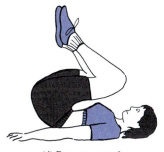

(4) Reverse crunch

Lie on the back with ankles crossed, feet off the ground, and knees at about a 90-degree angle. Place arms on the floor beside your trunk. Press lower back to the ground, contract the abdominals, and rotate hips 1 to 2 inches. Your feet will lift slightly toward the ceiling with each contraction.

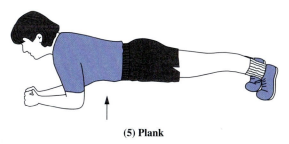

(5) Plank

Lie face down, propped with elbows under chest, palms down. Lift up on toes and tighten back and abdominals, keeping body straight and head and spine neutral. Hold 10 to 60 seconds, rest, repeat. If a straight-back position is too difficult, begin with hips hiked up or hold the contraction a shorter amount of time. Do not let the hips sag.

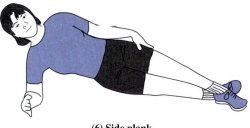

(6) Side plank

Lie on side with weight balanced between forearm, palm, and feet. Contract back and abdominals to hold body straight. Do not push hips out behind the body. Hold 10 to 30 seconds, rest, repeat on the other side. If a full-body position is too difficult, begin with the half-plank, balancing weight between knees and forearm. For an advanced version, try lifting the top foot in the air for 5 to 10 seconds.

Abdominal/Core Strengthening Exercises

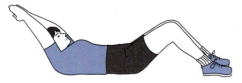

(7) Long arm crunch

Lie on your back with knees bent, heels next to buttocks. Extend arms alongside your ears, chin raised, eyes focused on ceiling. Contract abdominals, keeping lower back to floor, lift shoulders as for a basic crunch, lower slowly.

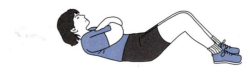

(8) Abdominal curl "crunch"

Lie on your back with knees bent. Place hands across chest or behind shoulders. Keep eyes focused on ceiling, chin up and about a fist's distance from your chest. Contract your abdominals; do not jerk your head forward as you curl. Keeping lower back on the ground, curl shoulders up to 3 inches and slowly lower.

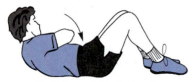

(9) Oblique abdominal curl

Lie on the back as for the basic crunch but add a twist, bringing right elbow toward left knee, then left elbow toward right knee. Elbow does not have to touch knee.

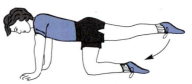

(10) Rear leg lift

On hands and knees, hollow abdomen and round back to protect it. Extend right leg to the rear. Tense gluteus. Raise and lower leg slowly six to eight counts. Repeat left.

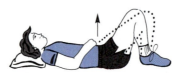

(11) Glute squeeze

Lying on back with knees bent, squeeze gluteus hard, raising hips no more than 3 inches from floor. Do not arch back. Hold for a count of five, relax, repeat.

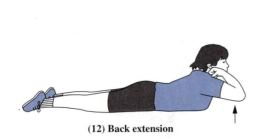

(12) Back extension

Lie on your stomach with feet on the floor, head neutral, hands touching shoulders. Slowly lift head, shoulders, and chest. Hold 5 to 10 seconds, then slowly lower. Variation: Squeeze shoulder blades in toward spine while holding trunk lift.

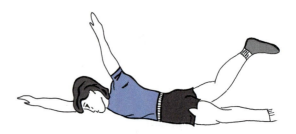

(13) Alternate arm/leg lift

Lie on your stomach with arms extended in front. Raise right arm while lifting left leg. Hold 5 to 10 seconds. Repeat on other side. Keep head neutral.